MW00562081

Musculoskeletal Disease Test and Syllabus

William A. Murphy, Jr., M.D.
Section Chairman

Lawrence W. Bassett, M.D.
Terry M. Hudson, M.D.
Phoebe A. Kaplan, M.D.
Sheila G. Moore, M.D.

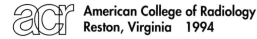 **American College of Radiology**
Reston, Virginia 1994

Sets Published

Chest Disease
Bone Disease
Genitourinary Tract Disease
Gastrointestinal Disease
Head and Neck Disorders
Pediatric Disease
Nuclear Radiology
Radiation Pathology and
    Radiation Biology
Chest Disease II
Bone Disease II
Genitourinary Tract Disease II
Gastrointestinal Disease II
Head and Neck Disorders II
Nuclear Radiology II
Cardiovascular Disease
Emergency Radiology
Bone Disease III
Gastrointestinal Disease III
Chest Disease III
Pediatric Disease II
Nuclear Radiology III
Head and Neck Disorders III
Genitourinary Tract Disease III

Diagnostic Ultrasound
Breast Disease
Bone Disease IV
Pediatric Disease III
Chest Disease IV
Neuroradiology
Gastrointestinal Disease IV
Nuclear Radiology IV
Magnetic Resonance
Radiation Bioeffects and
    Management
Genitourinary Tract Disease IV
Head and Neck Disorders IV
Pediatric Disease IV
Breast Disease II
Musculoskeletal Disease

Sets in Preparation

Diagnostic Ultrasonography II
Chest Disease V
Neuroradiology II
Gastrointestinal Disease V
Emergency Radiology II
Genitourinary Tract Disease V
Nuclear Radiology V

Note: While the American College of Radiology and the editors of this publication have attempted to include the most current and accurate information possible, errors may inadvertently appear. Diagnostic and interventional decisions should be based on the individual circumstances of each case.

SET 37:
Musculoskeletal Disease Test and Syllabus

Editor in Chief
BARRY A. SIEGEL, M.D., Professor of Radiology and Medicine and Director, Division of Nuclear Medicine, Mallinckrodt Institute of Radiology, Washington University School of Medicine, St. Louis, Missouri

Associate Editor
DAVID H. STEPHENS, M.D., Professor of Radiology, Mayo Medical School; Department of Diagnostic Radiology, Mayo Clinic, Rochester, Minnesota

Section Chairman
WILLIAM A. MURPHY, M.D., Professor of Radiology and John S. Dunn, Sr. Chair; Head, Division of Diagnostic Imaging; and Chairman, Department of Diagnostic Radiology, University of Texas, M.D. Anderson Cancer Center, Houston, Texas

Coauthors
LAWRENCE W. BASSETT, M.D., Professor of Radiological Sciences, UCLA School of Medicine, Los Angeles, California
TERRY M. HUDSON, M.D., Professor of Radiology, Emory University School of Medicine; Section of Radiology, The Emory Clinic, Atlanta, Georgia
PHOEBE A. KAPLAN, M.D., Professor of Radiology and Orthopedics, Division of Musculoskeletal Radiology, University of Virginia Health Sciences Center, Charlottesville, Virginia
SHEILA G. MOORE, M.D., Director, Pediatric Radiology, Cedars-Sinai Medical Center, Los Angeles, and Assistant Clinical Professor of Radiology, Stanford University, Stanford, California

AMERICAN COLLEGE OF RADIOLOGY
PROFESSIONAL SELF-EVALUATION AND CONTINUING EDUCATION PROGRAM

Publishing Coordinators:	*G. Rebecca Haines and Thomas M. Rogers*
Administrative Assistant:	*Marcy Olney*
Production Editor:	*Sean M. McKenna*
Copy Editors:	*Yvonne Strong and John N. Bell*
Text Processing:	*Fusako T. Nowak*
Composition:	*Karen Finkle*
Index:	*EEI, Inc., Alexandria, Va.*
Lithography:	*Lanman Progressive, Washington, D.C.*
Typesetting:	*Publication Technology Corp., Fairfax, Va.*
Printing:	*John D. Lucas Printing, Baltimore, Md.*

Library of Congress Cataloging-in-Publication Data

Musculoskeletal disease test and syllabus / William A. Murphy, Jr., section chairman ; Lawrence W. Bassett ... [et al.].

    p. cm. — (Professional self-evaluation and continuing education program; set 37)

    "Committee on Professional Self-Evaluation and Continuing Education, Commission on Education, American College of Radiology"—Cover.

    Includes bibliographical references and index.

    ISBN 1-55903-036-4 : $200.00. — ISBN 1-55903-000-3 (series)

    1. Musculoskeletal system—Radiography—Examinations, questions, etc. 2. Musculoskeletal system—Radiography—Outlines, syllabi, etc. I. Murphy, William A. II. Bassett, Lawrence W. (Lawrence Wayne), 1942– . III. American College of Radiology. Commission on Education. Committee on Professional Self-Evaluation and Continuing Education. IV. Series.

    [DNLM: 1. Musculoskeletal diseases—radiography—examination questions. 2. Musculoskeletal diseases—radiography—atlases. W1 PR606 set 37 1994 / WE 18 M985 1994]

    RC925.7.M869 1994

    616.7'07572'076—dc20

    DNLM/DLC   94-796

for Library of Congress   CIP

v

Additional Contributors

CATHERINE BRANDON, M.D., Assistant Professor of Radiology and Radiological Sciences, Vanderbilt University School of Medicine, Nashville, Tennessee

WALTER A. CARPENTER, Ph.D., M.D., Assistant Professor of Radiology, Emory University School of Medicine; Section of Radiology, The Emory Clinic, Atlanta, Georgia

VIJAY P. CHANDNANI, M.D., Chief of Skeletal Radiology, Tripler Army Medical Center, Honolulu, Hawaii

JULIA R. CRIM, M.D., Clinical Assistant Professor of Radiology, Bowman Gray School of Medicine, Wake Forest University, Winston-Salem, North Carolina

ROBERT G. DUSSAULT, M.D., Professor of Radiology and Orthopedics, and Co-Director, Division of Musculoskeletal Radiology, University of Virginia Health Sciences Center, Charlottesville, Virginia

WILLIAM A. FAJMAN, M.D., Associate Professor of Radiology, Emory University School of Medicine, and Chief, Diagnostic Radiology, Grady Memorial Hospital, Atlanta, Georgia

RICHARD H. GOLD, M.D., Professor of Radiological Sciences, UCLA School of Medicine, Los Angeles, California

THOMAS L. POPE, Jr., M.D., Professor of Radiology and Orthopedics, Bowman Gray School of Medicine, Wake Forest University, Winston-Salem, North Carolina

MAHVASH RAFII, M.D., Clinical Associate Professor, New York University Medical Center, New York, New York

LEANNE L. SEEGER, M.D., Associate Professor, Chief of Musculoskeletal Radiology, UCLA School of Medicine, Los Angeles, California

NEAL R. STEWART, M.B., Ch.B., Radiologist, Auckland Hospital, Auckland, New Zealand

RICHARD G. STILES, M.D., Assistant Professor of Radiology, Emory University School of Medicine; Section of Radiology, The Emory Clinic, Atlanta, Georgia

CRAIG W. WALKER, M.D., Assistant Professor of Radiology, University of Nebraska Medical Center, Omaha, Nebraska

O. CLARK WEST, M.D., Instructor of Radiology, Mallinckrodt Institute of Radiology, Washington University School of Medicine, St. Louis, Missouri

ANTHONY J. WILSON, M.B., Ch.B., Associate Professor of Radiology, Mallinckrodt Institute of Radiology, Washington University School of Medicine, St. Louis, Missouri

Section Chairman's Preface

This syllabus is the fifth in the Bone Disease sequence of the American College of Radiology's Professional Self-Evaluation and Continuing Education series. The bone disease syllabi have become progressively more detailed and sophisticated as our knowledge and technologies have also grown, expanded, and matured. We currently pay as much attention to the soft tissues as we do to bone. It is now proper to refer to the subspecialty as musculoskeletal radiology and to this syllabus as *Musculoskeletal Disease* in recognition of our changed perspective, practice, and contribution to patient care. We no longer image "just bone."

As the primary contributors gathered to consider the content for this syllabus, several goals were specified. First, we made a conscious attempt not to duplicate questions or content already adequately covered in the four prior bone disease syllabi. We chose topics that would interest a broad spectrum of radiologists, topics that are timely or that are not adequately discussed in other usually referenced resources. Some of the test cases are quite challenging, but all can be diagnosed. Several should provoke very careful study.

Second, we tried to reach a balance of factors. The cases and questions surveyed are representative of the major themes in musculoskeletal radiology. We included a broad sampling of experience with musculoskeletal disease and tried to avoid too great a concentration in any one area. Although much of the current syllabus is devoted to sectional imaging, a substantial portion of the book was reserved for conventional imaging, as this is still the foundation upon which all other imaging knowledge is built. Conceptual themes were enriched by detailed discussions. Standard radiologic observations were interwoven with anatomic features, pathophysiologic explanations, and practical clinical information, including physical and laboratory findings, management options, and anticipated outcomes.

Third, much attention and care were directed toward selection of the most representative images. In some areas, the syllabus is fairly comprehensive in its illustrations because we felt it might well be the single best source of such information.

Syllabus development is a long process from conceptualization to final publication. Inadvertent delays occur due to the usual exigencies of people's lives and the complex production schedules. Each person gave a great measure to the final product. It is a good feeling to reach fruition. This musculoskeletal syllabus is timely, and we trust it will be as well received and studied as were the four prior bone disease syllabi.

Sincere and great thanks go to my coauthors, Drs. Lawrence W. Bassett, Terry M. Hudson, Phoebe A. Kaplan, and Sheila G. Moore. Each contributed a great deal of time and expertise. Harold G. Jacobson, M.D., provided guidance as the syllabus content was shaped. Barry A. Siegel, M.D., deserves special thanks. He has been a friend, colleague, and teacher for over 20 years. I never fail to marvel at Barry's dedication, industry, efficiency, and mastery of medicine and English. A better editor does not exist. David H. Stephens, M.D., critiqued every question and sentence in the syllabus and became a friend in the process. Ms. Rebecca Haines, Director of Publications, and Mr. Thomas M. Rogers, Associate Director of Publications, were unequivocally committed to this project. Becky made sure every step occurred as it should, and Tom guided each case through the rigorous editing process with great skill and unending humor.

This syllabus is a pinnacle of satisfaction for us all as it brought us together, stimulated our creativity, caused us to critically examine our beliefs, made us learn, and provided a product of which we will always be proud.

William A. Murphy, Jr., M.D.
Section Chairman

Editor's Preface

On behalf of the Editors of the American College of Radiology Professional Self-Evaluation and Continuing Education Program, I am pleased to introduce the *Musculoskeletal Disease Test and Syllabus* to our readers. This volume is the 37th in the College's series of diagnostic radiology syllabi. Its publication also marks the initiation of the fifth cycle of the self-evaluation program, now in its 23rd year. This syllabus covers many of the key developments in musculoskeletal radiology that have occurred since publication of the *Bone Disease (Fourth Series) Test and Syllabus* in 1989. As is noted by Dr. Murphy in his preface, one such important development is reflected in the title of the current volume; the tools now available in this radiologic arena allow for assessment of not only bones but the entire musculoskeletal system. Hence, this book includes discussions of alterations in bone marrow, muscles, tendons, and ligaments as the imaging signs of many different musculoskeletal disorders. Additionally, this syllabus devotes considerable attention to the radiologic evaluation of several different orthopedic interventions, emphasizing the need for effective communication between radiologists and our colleagues in orthopedic surgery.

The underlying principles of the self-evaluation program that formed the ground rules for development of this test and syllabus have remained essentially unchanged over the last several years. The lead questions in each case are carefully designed to reproduce the types of clinical problems that diagnostic radiologists must solve daily in their own practices. Accordingly, the lead questions are generally constructed so that the participant must first critically analyze one or more images from an individual patient, then integrate the radiologic data with pertinent clinical information, and finally select the most likely diagnosis from a list of clinical differential diagnoses. The lead question in each case is generally followed by one or more satellite questions; these are designed to challenge the participant's fund of cognitive knowledge, chiefly in relation either to the diseases comprising the case's differential diagnosis or to the specific imaging modality under discussion. The authors and editors strive for a syllabus that will represent more than just a compilation of answers to the test questions. Rather, the discussions are intended to guide the reader through the logical steps to the correct diagnosis used by the experts. Syllabus discussions of satellite questions represent concise reviews of each question's topic so as to help participants keep abreast of advances in radiologic knowledge.

The process for developing a self-evaluation test and its accompanying syllabus is an arduous one designed to ensure a final product of high quality. This process begins with a series of intensive, but intellectually stimulating and spirited, meetings of the authors and editors for selection of cases and scrutiny of questions for appropriate content and style. The subsequently generated syllabus discussions, although reflecting the individual labor of one or two principal authors, are subjected to critical review by the section chairman and the series editors, leading to one or more revision cycles. An important feature of the College's self-evaluation program is the ability authors and editors have to make changes in their material essentially until the moment the press run begins. By allowing for this, we hope that the currency of the material in these volumes will be virtually up to the minute.

As our reader's work their way through this volume, they will surely recognize that extraordinary thanks are due to Dr. William A. Murphy, Jr., for his consummate efforts in developing this self-evaluation package. The College was fortunate indeed to have such a master clinician take on the role of Section Chairman for this volume. He approached this task with a clear vision of purpose and brought it to fruition with great leadership skills and with exceptional editorial acumen. Our readers also must greatly appreciate the long hours of voluntary effort contributed by Dr. Murphy's principal coauthors—Drs. Lawrence W. Bassett, Terry M. Hudson, Phoebe A. Kaplan, and Sheila G. Moore. Working with this group of high-caliber musculoskeletal radiologists, who thoroughly devoted themselves to this project, was a distinct pleasure and made my job, and that of my Associate Editor for this volume, Dr. David H. Stephens, quite easy indeed.

As always, special thanks are due to the dedicated staff responsible for the publications of the American College of Radiology. This group of skilled professionals, working under the highly competent leadership of G. Rebecca Haines, hone the manuscripts delivered by the authors and editors into the highly polished final product that each syllabus volume represents. In particular, I personally thank Thomas M. Rogers, who is charged with principal editorial responsibility for each syllabus, for his infinite patience, attention to detail, and unflagging pursuit of excellence. Thanks also are due to Dr. Anthony V. Proto, who, as chairman of the Professional Self-Evaluation and Continuing Education Committee, kept this project and the entire program on track. The continuing support and encouragement of Dr. Joseph Ferrucci, and of the College's Commission on Education, are also gratefully acknowledged.

Finally, and most importantly, thanks are due to the thousands of radiologists who have enthusiastically supported the self-evaluation program for more than two decades. This support is demonstrated by the nearly 192,000 subscriptions since publication of the first syllabus in 1972. Knowing that we, as authors and editors, have contributed to the continuing education and professional development of so many radiologists is more than enough justification for our efforts.

Barry A. Siegel, M.D.
Editor in Chief

Musculoskeletal Disease Test

For you to derive the maximum benefit from this program, you should complete the following test, and send your answer sheet to the ACR for scoring, before you proceed to the syllabus.

If for any reason you refer to the syllabus material, or any other references, in answering the questions, please be sure to so indicate when answering Question 126, the first demographic question. Your score will then not be used in developing the norm tables.

NOTE: You must return your answer sheet for scoring, whether or not you use reference materials, in order to claim the 25 hours of Category 1 credit.

Category 1 credit is valid for this publication from April 1994 through April 1997. Category 1 credit review will be conducted in April 1997 and every three years thereafter.

CASE 1: Questions 1 through 7

For each numbered MR scan (Figures 1-1 through 1-4), select the *one* lettered description (A, B, C, D, or E) that is MOST closely associated with it. Each lettered description may be used once, more than once, or not at all.

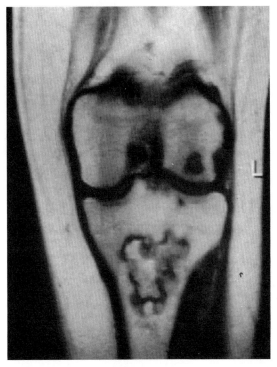

SE 500/20

Figure 1-1

1. Figure 1-1
2. Figure 1-2
3. Figure 1-3
4. Figure 1-4

(A) Chronic medullary infarct
(B) Sickle-cell anemia with infarct
(C) Focal lymphoma
(D) Late radiation effect on marrow
(E) Aplastic anemia

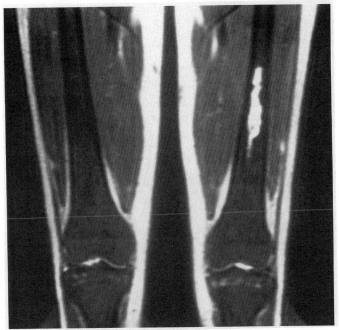

SE 2,500/60

Figure 1-2

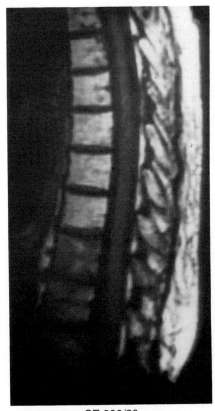

SE 300/20

Figure 1-3

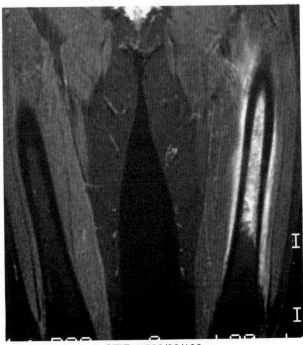

STIR 1,500/30/100

Figure 1-4

CASE 1 (Cont'd)

QUESTIONS 5 THROUGH 7: MARK YOUR ANSWER SHEET TRUE (T) OR FALSE (F) FOR EACH OF THE RESPONSE CHOICES.

5. Concerning marrow distribution patterns on T1-weighted spin-echo MR images,

   (A) in children, ossified epiphyses almost always contain fatty marrow
   (B) at 10 years of age, intermediate-intensity metaphyseal red marrow in the femur is typical
   (C) at 20 years of age, homogeneous low-intensity marrow in the clivus is normal
   (D) at 40 years of age, red marrow in the proximal humeral metaphyses is probably abnormal
   (E) in adults, the signal intensity of vertebral marrow should be lower than that of the adjacent disk

6. Concerning the MR evaluation of leukemic marrow,

   (A) leukemia is reliably distinguished from diffuse metastatic disease
   (B) the calculated vertebral T1 relaxation time is prolonged
   (C) the signal intensity is increased on chemical-shift fat-fraction images
   (D) volume-selected proton spectroscopy shows an increase in the water peak
   (E) post-treatment aplastic anemia usually results in diffuse low signal intensity

7. Concerning MRI of marrow,

   (A) the susceptibility effect of trabecular bone is negligible on gradient-recalled-echo images
   (B) focal metastatic lesions are usually bright on short-tau inversion-recovery (STIR) images
   (C) fatty marrow has low signal intensity on fast-acquisition spin-echo images obtained with a TR of 2,500 msec
   (D) fat-suppression techniques exploit the inherent resonant frequency differences of fat and water protons

This 35-year-old man injured his right shoulder. You are shown an anteroposterior radiograph of the shoulder (Figure 2-1).

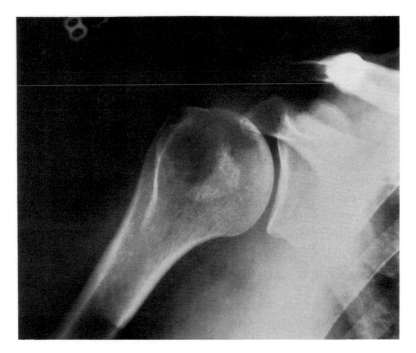

Figure 2-1

8. Which *one* of the following is the MOST likely diagnosis?

   (A) Tuberosity avulsion fracture
   (B) Giant cell tumor
   (C) Chondroblastoma
   (D) Humeral pseudocyst
   (E) Hill-Sachs deformity

CASE 2 (Cont'd)

QUESTIONS 9 AND 10: MARK YOUR ANSWER SHEET TRUE
(T) OR FALSE (F) FOR EACH OF THE RESPONSE CHOICES.

9. Concerning fractures of the proximal humerus,

   (A) in the Neer classification, a comminuted nondisplaced
       fracture is a two-part fracture
   (B) most are nondisplaced
   (C) isolated tuberosity avulsions are usually pathologic
       fractures
   (D) a four-part fracture is associated with a greater than
       50% chance of avascular necrosis

10. Pseudocysts are often seen in the:

   (A) proximal humerus
   (B) calcaneus
   (C) proximal femur
   (D) radius
   (E) ulna

This 2-year-old child has a heart murmur. You are shown a posteroanterior radiograph of the hands (Figure 3-1).

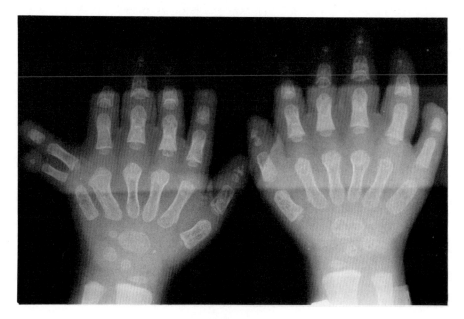

Figure 3-1

11. Which *one* of the following cardiac abnormalities is the MOST likely diagnosis?

    (A) Tetralogy of Fallot
    (B) Peripheral pulmonic stenosis
    (C) Septal defect
    (D) Patent ductus arteriosus
    (E) Coarctation of the aorta

CASE 3 (Cont'd)

QUESTIONS 12 THROUGH 14: MARK YOUR ANSWER SHEET TRUE (T) OR FALSE (F) FOR EACH OF THE RESPONSE CHOICES.

12. Concerning syndromes with combined skeletal and cardiac abnormalities,

    (A) lower-extremity skeletal abnormalities are more common than cardiac abnormalities in patients with the cardiomelic (Holt-Oram) syndrome
    (B) cardiac abnormalities are more common than skeletal abnormalities in patients with Turner's syndrome (monosomy X)
    (C) short stature is more common than septal defects in patients with Down's syndrome (trisomy 21)
    (D) skeletal abnormalities produce more important long-term sequelae than do cardiac anomalies in patients with congenital rubella syndrome
    (E) aortic root disorders are common in patients with Marfan's syndrome

13. Congenital heart disease is associated with:

    (A) clubbing
    (B) articular erosions
    (C) osteosclerosis
    (D) premature fusion of sternal ossification centers
    (E) accelerated bone age
    (F) scoliosis
    (G) rib notching

14. Concerning upper-extremity musculoskeletal anomalies,

(A) duplication of the little finger is an example of preaxial polydactyly

(B) failure of separation of the long and ring fingers is the most common form of syndactyly

(C) lunotriquetral carpal coalition is usually syndrome related

(D) the carpal angle is increased in patients with Madelung deformity

(E) the frequency of associated anomalies in patients with congenital radial defects is less than 10%

This 55-year-old man has severe pain in his left shoulder. You are shown proton-density (A) and T2-weighted (B) coronal oblique MR images of the left shoulder (Figure 4-1).

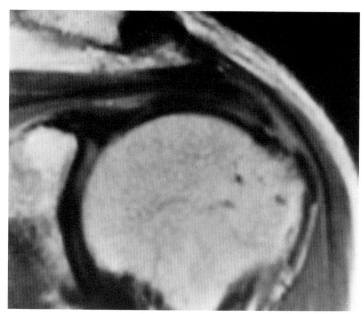

SE 1,800/20

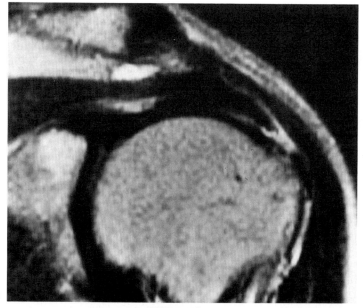

SE 1,800/80

Figure 4-1

CASE 4 (Cont'd)

QUESTIONS 15 THROUGH 17: MARK YOUR ANSWER SHEET TRUE (T) OR FALSE (F) FOR EACH OF THE RESPONSE CHOICES.

15. The test images demonstrate abnormalities of the:

    (A) supraspinatus tendon
    (B) infraspinatus tendon
    (C) subscapularis tendon
    (D) subacromial bursa
    (E) long head of biceps tendon

16. Concerning impingement syndrome of the shoulder,

    (A) it is the underlying cause of most rotator cuff tears
    (B) a low-lying acromion predisposes to this condition
    (C) early surgical intervention is required in most cases
    (D) radiographic changes occur early
    (E) arthrography is an effective method for early detection

17. Concerning glenohumeral joint stability,

    (A) the glenoid labrum is the major soft tissue support for the glenohumeral joint
    (B) CT arthrography is an effective method of evaluating the anatomic structures of the glenohumeral joint
    (C) tears of the anterior labrum are more common than tears of the posterior labrum
    (D) the presence of a labral tear implies a previous dislocation
    (E) the term "Bankart lesion" is limited to osseous fractures of the glenoid rim

CASE 5: Questions 18 through 23

This 10-month-old chronically ill infant was anemic. You are shown anteroposterior radiographs of the left forearm (A) and both femora (B) taken at diagnosis (Figure 5-1), as well as similarly positioned radiographs obtained 6 months later (Figure 5-2).

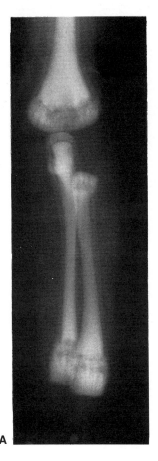
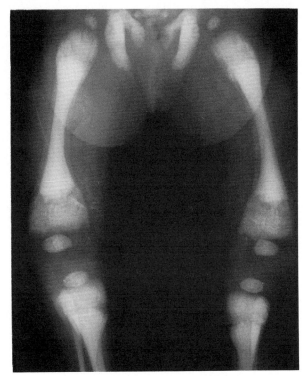

A   B

Figure 5-1

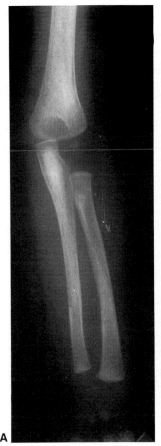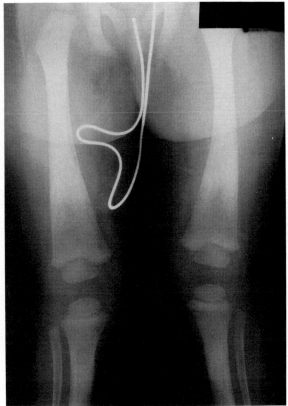

A   B

Figure 5-2

18. Which *one* of the following is the MOST likely cause of the change in skeletal pattern?

   (A) Tissue transplantation
   (B) Radiation therapy
   (C) Steroid therapy
   (D) Antibiotic therapy
   (E) Withdrawal of noxious agent

CASE 5 (Cont'd)

QUESTION 19: MARK YOUR ANSWER SHEET TRUE (T) OR
FALSE (F) FOR EACH OF THE RESPONSE CHOICES.

19. Effects of radiotherapy on the skeleton include:

   (A) arrest of epiphyseal chondrogenesis
   (B) periosteal reaction
   (C) asymptomatic fractures
   (D) formation of exostoses
   (E) induction of chondrosarcoma more frequently than os-
         teosarcoma

For each numbered medication listed below (Questions 20 through
23), select the *one* lettered musculoskeletal manifestation (A, B, C,
D, or E) that is MOST closely associated with it. Each lettered
musculoskeletal manifestation may be used once, more than once,
or not at all.

   20. Isotretinoin
   21. Phenytoin
   22. Sodium fluoride
   23. Prostaglandin E_1

      (A)   Growth arrest lines
      (B)   Osteomalacia
      (C)   Periostitis
      (D)   Intra-articular calcification
      (E)   Hyperostosis

This 54-year-old woman complained of pain in the right sterno-clavicular region. You are shown a posteroanterior chest radio-graph (A) and a CT scan (B) through the region of the sternoclav-icular joint (Figure 6-1).

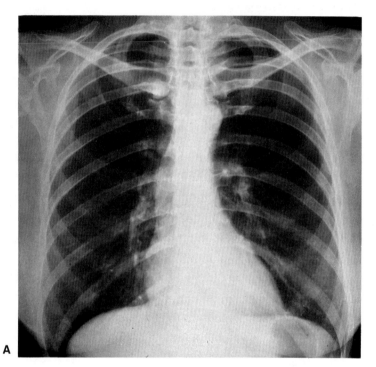

Figure 6-1

24. Which *one* of the following is the MOST likely diagnosis?

   (A) Sternocostoclavicular hyperostosis
   (B) Osteitis condensans
   (C) Osteomyelitis
   (D) Paget's disease
   (E) Osteosarcoma

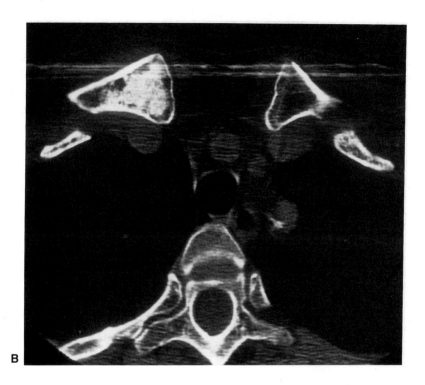

B

QUESTIONS 25 THROUGH 27: MARK YOUR ANSWER SHEET TRUE (T) OR FALSE (F) FOR EACH OF THE RESPONSE CHOICES.

25. Concerning sternocostoclavicular hyperostosis,

    (A) it is more common in women than in men
    (B) it is associated with pustular lesions of the palms and soles
    (C) an associated spondyloarthropathy is common
    (D) histocompatibility antigen HLA B27 is usually present
    (E) histologically it is identical to osteitis condensans

26. Concerning osteitis condensans of the clavicle,

    (A) it is a response to mechanical stress
    (B) histologically the lesion consists of thickened trabecu-
        lae
    (C) the width of the sternoclavicular joint is normal
    (D) bone scintigraphy is usually normal
    (E) treatment with anti-inflammatory medications usually
        relieves symptoms

27. Concerning the sternoclavicular joint,

    (A) it is a synovial joint
    (B) posterior dislocations are more common than anterior
        ones
    (C) it is involved in about 5% of patients with rheumatoid
        arthritis
    (D) it is a common site of septic arthritis in drug abusers

CASE 7: Questions 28 through 32

You are shown an oblique radiograph of the right knee in a 16-year-old athlete with right knee pain (Figure 7-1).

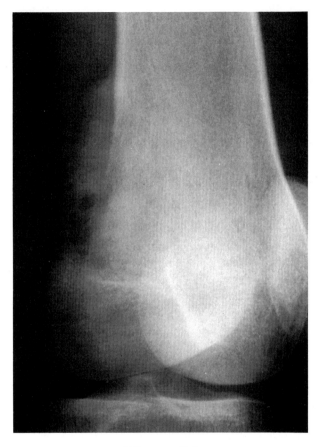

Figure 7-1

28. Which *one* of the following is the MOST likely diagnosis?

   (A) Well-differentiated osteosarcoma
   (B) Osteoblastoma
   (C) Aneurysmal bone cyst
   (D) Nonossifying fibroma
   (E) Chondrosarcoma

QUESTIONS 29 THROUGH 32: MARK YOUR ANSWER SHEET TRUE (T) OR FALSE (F) FOR EACH OF THE RESPONSE CHOICES.

29. Concerning well-differentiated osteosarcoma,

   (A) the distal femur is the most common site
   (B) it is most commonly a lytic lesion
   (C) it is often expansile
   (D) it is histologically similar to parosteal osteosarcoma
   (E) it is commonly misdiagnosed as a benign lesion

30. Concerning osteoblastoma,

   (A) there is a male predominance
   (B) recurrence is common following surgical resection
   (C) about 30% occur in the vertebrae
   (D) epidural extension occurs with vertebral lesions
   (E) appendicular lesions are usually lytic

31. Concerning nonossifying fibromas,

   (A) they most often occur in the metadiaphyseal region
   (B) they are most common about the knee
   (C) the inner boundary is usually poorly defined
   (D) there is associated marrow edema on MR images
   (E) most lesions show homogeneous high signal intensity on T2-weighted MR images

32. Concerning benign neoplasms of bone,

   (A) periosteal reaction distal to the lesion is often seen with chondroblastoma
   (B) intra-articular osteoid osteoma of the elbow is usually predominantly osteolytic
   (C) marrow edema is seen on T2-weighted MR images of osteoid osteoma
   (D) the perichondrium has low signal intensity on both T1- and T2-weighted MR images of osteochondroma
   (E) aneurysmal bone cysts rarely occur in a subperiosteal location

CASE 8: Question 33

This 3-year-old girl presented with a tumor of the right femur. You are shown a transaxial T2-weighted MR image of the right femur (Figure 8-1).

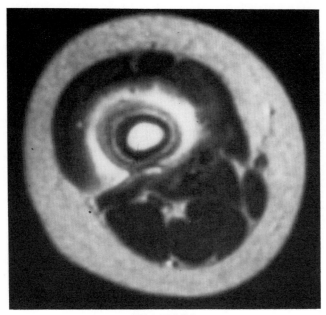

SE 2,500/80

Figure 8-1

QUESTION 33: MARK YOUR ANSWER SHEET TRUE (T) OR FALSE (F) FOR EACH OF THE RESPONSE CHOICES.

33. The test image demonstrates:

   (A) "onion skin" periosteal reaction
   (B) tumor within the medullary cavity of the femur
   (C) edema of the vastus intermedius muscle
   (D) cortical penetration by tumor
   (E) sparing of the femoral neurovascular bundle

CASE 9: Question 34

This 58-year-old man has adenocarcinoma of the lung. Bone scintigrams and radiographs of the lumbar spine were normal. You
are shown sagittal T1-weighted (A) and T2-weighted (B) MR images of the lumbar spine (Figure 9-1).

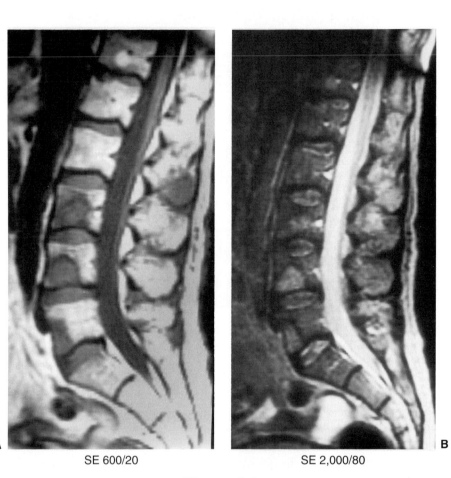

A   B

SE 600/20   SE 2,000/80

Figure 9-1

CASE 9 (Cont'd)

34. Which *one* of the following statements concerning bone biopsy of this patient is correct?

 (A) It is not indicated because the negative results of bone scintigraphy make metastatic disease highly unlikely.
 (B) Percutaneous biopsy is feasible even though the lesions cannot be seen on radiographs.
 (C) It is not indicated because the diagnosis is obvious on the MR images.
 (D) Biopsy of the L3 body is inappropriate because of the high risk of vertebral collapse.
 (E) Open biopsy would be safer than percutaneous biopsy.

You are shown radiographs obtained at 7 (A) and 18 (B) months of age. The patient received no treatment between these studies (Figure 10-1).

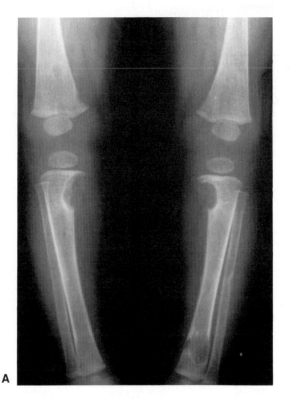

Figure 10-1

35. Which *one* of the following is the MOST likely diagnosis?

    (A) Fibrous dysplasia
    (B) Congenital multiple fibromatosis
    (C) Neurofibromatosis type 1
    (D) Cystic angiomatosis
    (E) Multiple hemangioma of bone

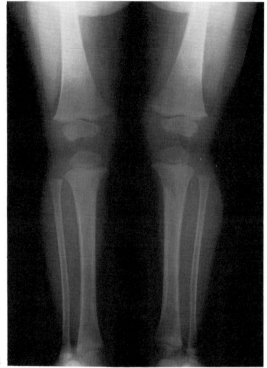

B

For each of the following clinical features (Questions 36 through 40), indicate whether it is more closely associated with the monostotic or polyostotic forms of fibrous dysplasia, equally associated with both, or associated with neither (A, B, C, or D). Each option may be used once, more than once, or not at all.

36. Soft tissue myxoma
37. Frequent resolution of the lesion
38. High signal intensity on T2-weighted images
39. Involvement of the spine
40. Malignant transformation

   (A)   Monostotic
   (B)   Polyostotic
   (C)   Both
   (D)   Neither

CASE 10 (Cont'd)

QUESTIONS 41 AND 42: MARK YOUR ANSWER SHEET TRUE
(T) OR FALSE (F) FOR EACH OF THE RESPONSE CHOICES.

41. Concerning congenital multiple fibromatosis,

(A) lesions occur primarily in the soft tissues
(B) osseous lesions are typically metaphyseal in location
(C) lesions are usually similar in size
(D) there is an association with pathologic fractures
(E) the lesions resolve spontaneously in nearly all patients

42. Concerning juvenile fibromatosis,

(A) it causes pressure erosions of the bone
(B) nearly all lesions have low signal intensity on T2-
weighted MR images
(C) recurrence after surgical resection is uncommon
(D) aponeurotic lesions tend to calcify
(E) the foot is a common site of occurrence

This 17-year-old jogger was hit in the knee by a moving car. You are shown T1-weighted sagittal (Figure 11-1), gradient-echo sagittal (Figure 11-2), and T1-weighted coronal (Figure 11-3) MR images of the knee.

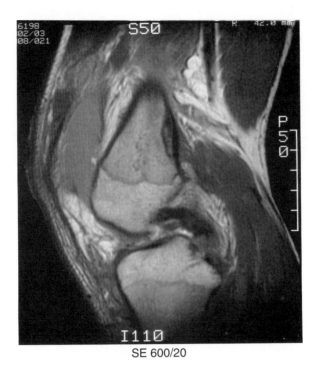

SE 600/20

Figure 11-1

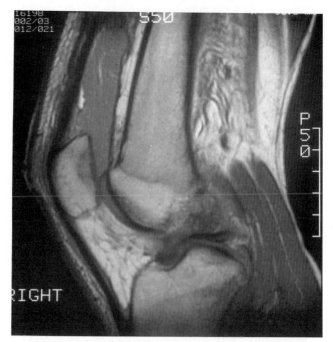

SE 600/20

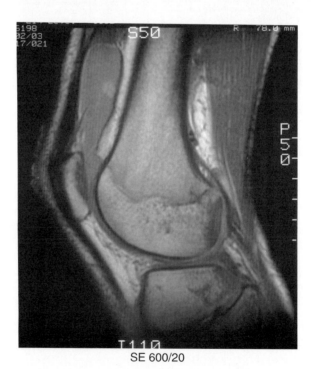

SE 600/20

Figure 11-1 *(Continued)*

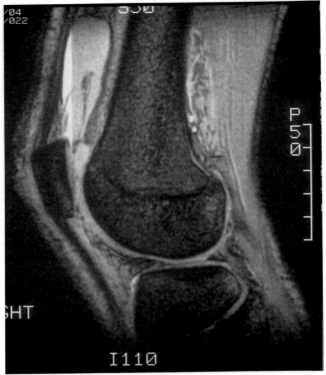

GRE 480/20/30°

Figure 11-2

QUESTIONS 43 THROUGH 46: MARK YOUR ANSWER SHEET TRUE (T) OR FALSE (F) FOR EACH OF THE RESPONSE CHOICES.

43. Abnormalities demonstrated in the test images include:

    (A) anterior cruciate ligament tear
    (B) posterior cruciate ligament tear
    (C) medial collateral ligament tear
    (D) lateral collateral ligament tear
    (E) quadriceps tendon tear
    (F) patellar tendon tear
    (G) medial meniscus tear
    (H) lateral meniscus tear
    (I) bone marrow contusion
    (J) lipohemarthrosis

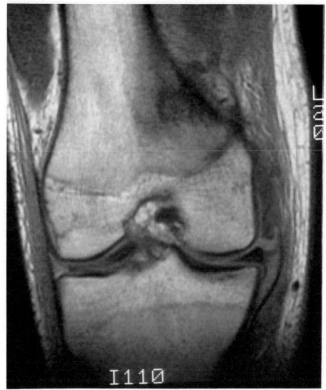

SE 600/20

Figure 11-3

44. Concerning MRI of meniscal injuries of the knee,

   (A) a "double cruciate" sign indicates a horizontal cleavage tear
   (B) meniscal tears are simulated by the ligament of Humphry
   (C) tears in the periphery of the meniscus are treated differently from those on the free edge
   (D) following conservative management of meniscal tear, persistent high signal intensity indicates failure to heal
   (E) a tear is present when the anterior horn of the medial meniscus is smaller than the posterior horn

45. Concerning tendons and ligaments of the knee,

  (A) patellar tendon ruptures generally occur in the mid-substance of the tendon rather than at either end
  (B) quadriceps tendon ruptures occur in an older population than do patellar tendon ruptures
  (C) lateral collateral ligament tears are more common than medial collateral ligament tears
  (D) the most common MR sign of a complete anterior cruciate ligament tear is inability to identify the ligament
  (E) on MRI, alternating bands of high and low signal intensity are normally seen in the anterior cruciate ligament

46. Concerning bone marrow contusions,

  (A) they have no prognostic significance
  (B) medial contusions of the femur and tibia are commonly associated with anterior cruciate ligament tears
  (C) bone scintigraphy is usually normal in areas of bone contusion seen by MRI
  (D) follow-up MR examinations show resolution of abnormal signal intensity by about 3 months after the injury
  (E) the abnormal signal intensity is postulated to be the result of endosteal callus formation

This 57-year-old woman has chronic musculoskeletal pain and increasingly frequent fractures. You are shown anteroposterior radiographs of her left knee (A) and hip (B) (Figure 12-1).

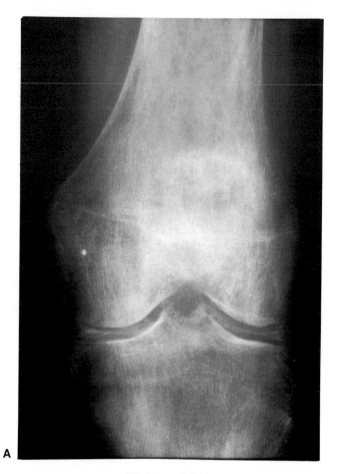

Figure 12-1

47. Which *one* of the following is the MOST likely diagnosis?

    (A) Postmenopausal osteoporosis
    (B) Osteogenesis imperfecta tarda
    (C) Mastocytosis
    (D) X-linked hypophosphatemia
    (E) Hypophosphatasia

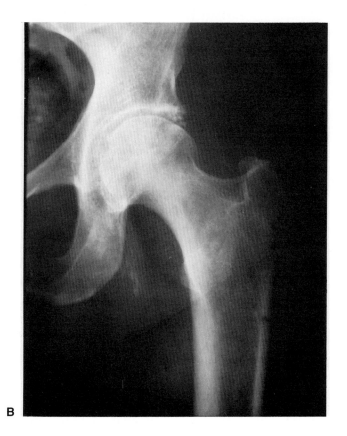

B

QUESTIONS 48 THROUGH 51: MARK YOUR ANSWER SHEET TRUE (T) OR FALSE (F) FOR EACH OF THE RESPONSE CHOICES.

48. Concerning mastocytosis,

(A) approximately 90% of patients have cutaneous manifestations

(B) systemic symptoms are caused by release of chemical mediators

(C) only 25% of patients with multiorgan involvement have skeletal lesions

(D) its manifestations include both osteopenia and osteosclerosis

(E) bone lesions are symptomatic in about 75% of patients

49. Concerning X-linked hypophosphatemia,

   (A) proximal renal tubules fail to reabsorb filtered phosphate
   (B) it is typically diagnosed before 12 months of age
   (C) affected men have more severe deformities than do affected women
   (D) most affected adults have measurably diminished bone mass
   (E) enthesopathy is a characteristic feature
   (F) the principal cause of morbidity in affected adults is lower extremity degenerative joint disease

50. Concerning hypophosphatasia,

   (A) the plasma concentration of inorganic phosphate is decreased
   (B) half of patients with the infantile form die in infancy
   (C) the childhood form is characterized by the combination of rachitic deformities and premature loss of deciduous teeth
   (D) nearly 100% of patients with the adult form have a history of symptoms during infancy or childhood
   (E) in patients with the adult form, some pseudofractures progress to complete fractures
   (F) soft tissue calcification is common

51. Concerning osteomalacia,

   (A) it is characterized by defective mineralization of osteoid matrix
   (B) it is usually caused by excessive hydroxylation of vitamin D in the kidneys
   (C) it is occasionally caused by a mesenchymal tumor
   (D) deficient quantities of osteoid result in a coarsened and unsharp trabecular pattern
   (E) the presence of Looser's zones differentiates it from Paget's disease
   (F) bone pain is infrequent

This 39-year-old woman has pain radiating down the lateral aspect of the left leg. You are shown coronal T1-weighted (A) and transaxial T2-weighted (B) MR images of the knee (Figure 13-1).

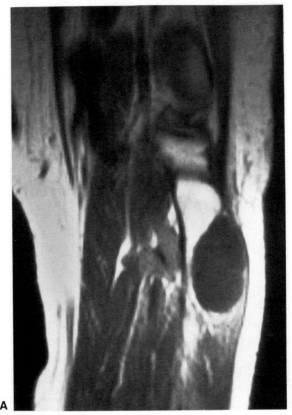

SE 480/30

Figure 13-1

52. Which *one* of the following is the MOST likely diagnosis?

   (A) Cavernous hemangioma
   (B) Ganglion cyst
   (C) Meniscal cyst
   (D) Baker's cyst
   (E) Lipoma

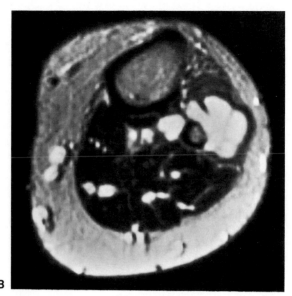

B

SE 2,000/85

For each of the descriptions listed below (Questions 53 through 58), indicate whether it is MORE closely associated with meniscal cyst (A) or synovial cyst (B), equally associated with both types of cyst (C), or associated with neither cyst (D). Each lettered option may be used once, more than once, or not at all.

53. Easily diagnosed by arthrography
54. Common on the lateral aspect of the knee
55. Recurs after surgical resection
56. Rupture resembles thrombophlebitis clinically
57. Congenital in origin
58. Gelatinous contents

(A)   Meniscal cyst
(B)   Synovial cyst
(C)   Both
(D)   Neither

QUESTION 59: MARK YOUR ANSWER SHEET TRUE (T) OR
FALSE (F) FOR EACH OF THE RESPONSE CHOICES.

59.   Concerning angiovenous dysplasias of the extremities,

   (A)   hemangiomas are the most common type
   (B)   they are associated with leg length discrepancies
   (C)   calcification is uncommon
   (D)   periosteal new bone formation is a typical feature
   (E)   they are best categorized by the caliber of their vessels
   (F)   hemangiomas and venous malformations have a simi-
         lar appearance on angiography
   (G)   MRI commonly shows fat between the vascular chan-
         nels
   (H)   synovial hemangiomas occur most frequently in the hip

CASE 14: Questions 60 through 62

This 21-year-old man has pain and swelling of his left knee. You are shown anteroposterior (A) and lateral (B) radiographs of the left knee (Figure 14-1).

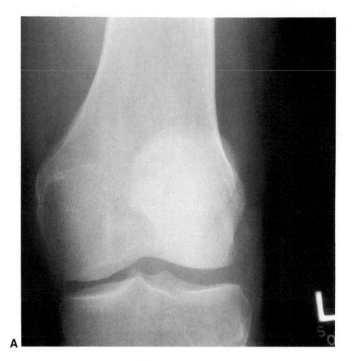

Figure 14-1

60. Which *one* of the following is the MOST likely diagnosis?

   (A) Bipartite patella
   (B) Osteochondritis dissecans
   (C) Chondromalacia patellae
   (D) Dorsal defect
   (E) Osteoid osteoma

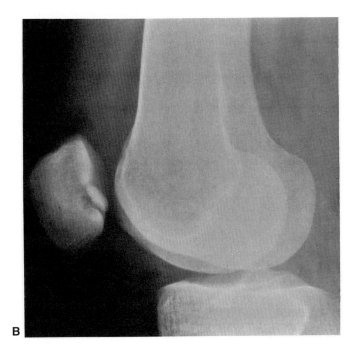

B

QUESTIONS 61 AND 62: MARK YOUR ANSWER SHEET TRUE (T) OR FALSE (F) FOR EACH OF THE RESPONSE CHOICES.

61. Concerning osteochondritis dissecans,

(A) remote or subacute infection is considered the cause
(B) it usually affects patients under 10 years of age
(C) the most common site is the medial femoral condyle
(D) the stability of the osteochondral fragment determines management
(E) premature osteoarthritis is a sequela

62. Concerning lesions of the patella,

    (A) chondromalacia patellae is the most common cause of pain

    (B) chondromalacia patellae is best evaluated on T2-weighted spin-echo MR images

    (C) medial patellar plicae are more likely than other plicae to be symptomatic

    (D) acute dislocations are associated with fractures of the lateral patellar facet

    (E) enchondroma is the most common primary tumor

This patient sustained trauma to the left knee. You are shown an-teroposterior (A) and lateral (B) radiographs of the knee (Figure 15-1).

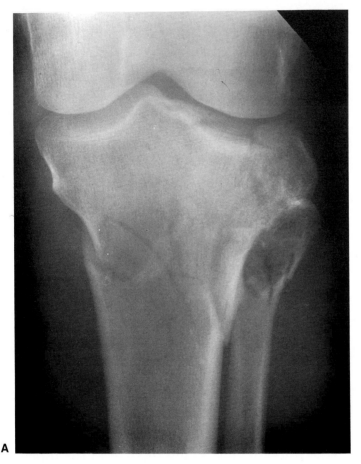

Figure 15-1

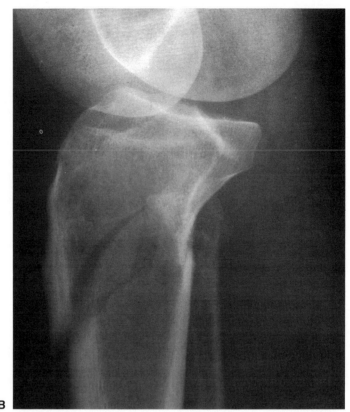

B

QUESTIONS 63 THROUGH 65: MARK YOUR ANSWER SHEET TRUE (T) OR FALSE (F) FOR EACH OF THE RESPONSE CHOICES.

63.   Concerning the injury to the test patient,

    (A)   the fracture affects only the lateral tibial plateau and fibula

    (B)   the lateral collateral ligament is likely to be ruptured

    (C)   closed treatment by traction and early motion should not be used

    (D)   an associated distal fibular fracture is likely

    (E)   knee instability is a likely long-term complication of inadequate treatment

CASE 15 (Cont'd)

64. Concerning complications of tibial plateau fractures,

    (A) popliteal artery damage is likely
    (B) peroneal nerve palsy occurs in about 5% of cases
    (C) the medial collateral ligament is the most commonly torn ligament
    (D) tears of the menisci are unlikely
    (E) there is a high frequency of nonunion

65. Concerning the treatment of tibial plateau fractures,

    (A) nonoperative treatment of uncomplicated fractures with less than 4 mm of displacement yields good results
    (B) residual varus deformity correlates with a poor functional result
    (C) collateral ligament tears usually heal well with nonoperative treatment by immobilization
    (D) cast immobilization of the knee joint for 8 to 12 weeks is required to ensure solid bony union
    (E) open reduction is required in less than 25% of patients

This 36-year-old man injured his right foot while under the influence of alcohol. You are shown direct coronal CT scans displayed with bone and soft tissue windows of the ankle (A and B) and hind foot (C and D) (Figure 16-1).

QUESTIONS 66 THROUGH 68: MARK YOUR ANSWER SHEET TRUE (T) OR FALSE (F) FOR EACH OF THE RESPONSE CHOICES.

66. Concerning the injury to the test patient,

   (A) the fracture involves both the posterior and middle cal-
        caneal articular facets
   (B) peroneal tendinitis is likely to develop
   (C) subtalar osteoarthritis is a likely complication
   (D) forced dorsiflexion was the mechanism of injury
   (E) assessment for possible vertebral fracture is appropri-
        ate

67. Concerning the subtalar joint,

   (A) the sinus tarsi separates the anterior and middle calca-
        neal facets
   (B) the anterior and middle calcaneal facets are in the
        same joint space
   (C) the facets are best shown by CT images parallel to the
        long axis of the calcaneus
   (D) Boehler's angle is estimated by drawing lines parallel
        to the middle and posterior facets

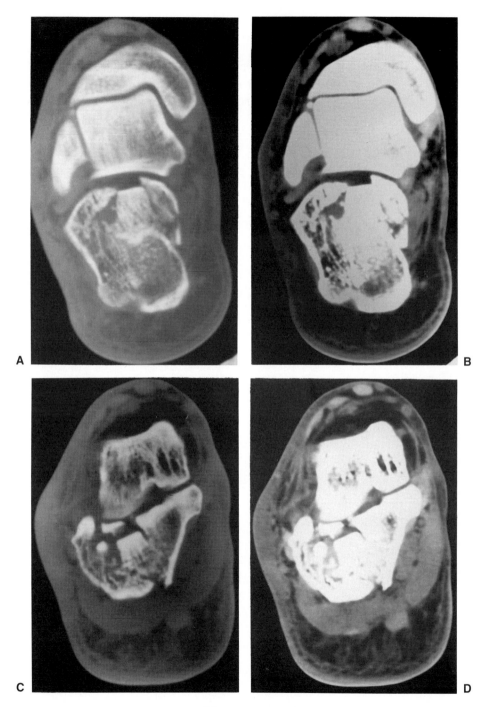

Figure 16-1

68. Concerning calcaneal fractures,

   (A) forces at the angle of Gissane result in either joint depression- or tongue-type fractures
   (B) approximately 75% are extra-articular
   (C) extra-articular fractures have an excellent overall clinical outcome
   (D) restoration of Boehler's angle is predictive of an excellent surgical result
   (E) an abnormal Boehler's angle indicates a requirement for open reduction and internal fixation

This is a 19-year-old man. Additional history is withheld. You are shown T1- and T2-weighted MR images of the right thigh (Figure 17-1).

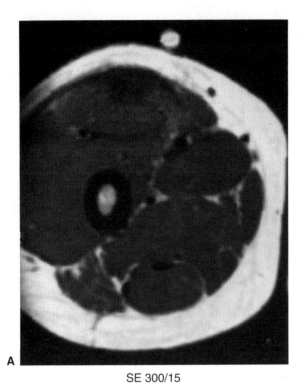

SE 300/15

Figure 17-1

69. Which *one* of the following is the MOST likely diagnosis?

(A) Rhabdomyosarcoma
(B) Muscular dystrophy
(C) Muscle tear
(D) Plexiform neurofibroma
(E) Hemangioma

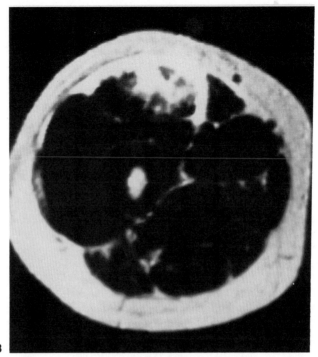

B

SE 2,500/80

QUESTIONS 70 AND 71: MARK YOUR ANSWER SHEET TRUE (T) OR FALSE (F) FOR EACH OF THE RESPONSE CHOICES.

70. Concerning rhabdomyosarcoma,

   (A) the median age at presentation is 5 years
   (B) most arise within the striated muscle of the extremities
   (C) at clinical presentation, skeletal metastases occur in over 50% of patients
   (D) direct cortical bone invasion by the primary tumor is common

71. Concerning the MR evaluation of muscle,

(A) increased signal intensity on both T1- and T2-weighted images likely represents subacute hemorrhage or fat

(B) on T2-weighted images, acute muscle tears are accompanied by increased signal intensity

(C) neuromuscular disorders are characterized by focal muscle atrophy and fatty replacement

(D) in acute myonecrosis, muscle signal is frequently normal on T1-weighted images

(E) exercise increases muscle signal intensity on short-tau inversion-recovery (STIR) images

This patient presented with progressive low back and leg pain 3 years after back surgery. You are shown radiographs of the lumbar spine obtained 1 month apart (Figures 18-1 and 18-2).

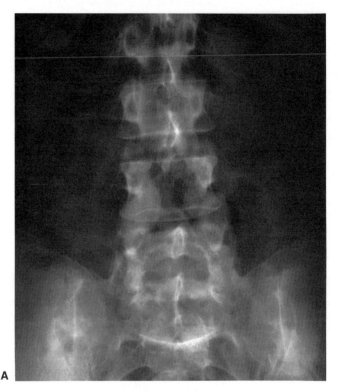

A

Figure 18-1

72. Which *one* of the following was the MOST likely clinical diagnosis leading to the surgical procedure shown in Figure 18-2?

   (A) Degenerative disk disease
   (B) Failed back syndrome
   (C) Postoperative infection
   (D) Segmental spine instability
   (E) Diskogenic pain

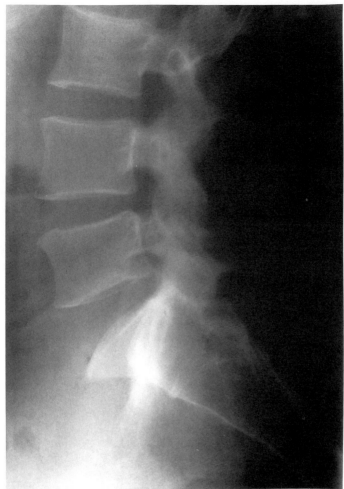

B

73. The fixation system shown in Figure 18-2 (page T-50) is:

   (A) Harrington
   (B) Cotrel-Dubousset
   (C) Transpedicular screw
   (D) Anterior interbody
   (E) Luque

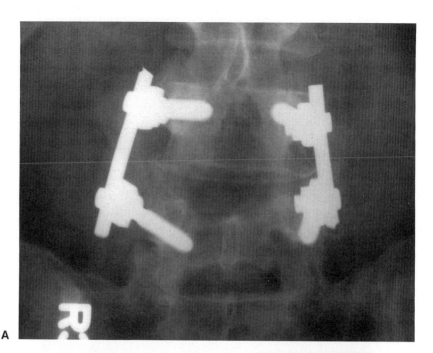

A

B

Figure 18-2

CASE 18 (Cont'd)

QUESTION 74: MARK YOUR ANSWER SHEET TRUE (T) OR FALSE (F) FOR EACH OF THE RESPONSE CHOICES.

74. Concerning the Harrington system of spinal fusion,

    (A) it has been used to treat both vertebral fractures and scoliosis

    (B) postoperative braces are required

    (C) stabilization is inadequate

    (D) short-segment fixation cannot be achieved

    (E) postoperative mobility is facilitated

75. Which *one* of the following is a characteristic of BOTH transpedicular screw and anterior interbody fixation systems?

    (A) Simple surgical procedure

    (B) Low complication rate

    (C) Usefulness in treating scoliosis

    (D) Stable short-segment fixation

    (E) Few vascular complications

QUESTIONS 76 THROUGH 78: MARK YOUR ANSWER SHEET TRUE (T) OR FALSE (F) FOR EACH OF THE RESPONSE CHOICES.

76. Advantages of the Cotrel-Dubousset spine fixation system include:

    (A) derotation of the scoliotic curve

    (B) correction of the rib-hump deformity

    (C) no postoperative brace

    (D) use in a variety of spinal problems

    (E) short operative time

77. Fracture of a posterior fixation rod is frequently associated with:

    (A) pseudarthrosis
    (B) postoperative infection
    (C) neurologic injury
    (D) severe preoperative deformity

78. Manifestations of pseudarthrosis developing after spinal fusion for scoliosis include:

    (A) loss of correction of the scoliotic curve
    (B) pain
    (C) fracture of fixation hardware
    (D) loss of lumbar lordosis
    (E) no symptoms

This 40-year-old man underwent a leg-lengthening procedure to correct a deformity due to a malunited fracture. You are shown an anteroposterior radiograph of the leg within the lengthening device (Figure 19-1).

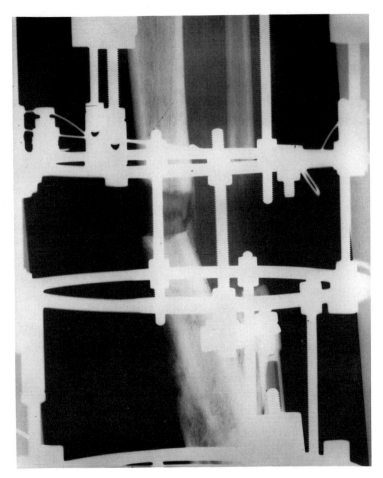

Figure 19-1

79. Which *one* of the following BEST describes this method of bone lengthening?

    (A) Chondrodiatasis
    (B) Callotasis
    (C) Tension-stress
    (D) Epiphysiolysis
    (E) Hemichondrodiatasis

CASE 19 (Cont'd)

80. The regenerate bone in the test image is BEST designated as:

(A) normal
(B) atrophic
(C) hypertrophic
(D) fractured
(E) infected

QUESTIONS 81 THROUGH 83: MARK YOUR ANSWER SHEET TRUE (T) OR FALSE (F) FOR EACH OF THE RESPONSE CHOICES.

81. Concerning bone lengthening by the Ilizarov procedure,

(A) distraction begins immediately after surgery
(B) osteotomies and corticotomies are equally effective in the production of regenerate bone
(C) the average distraction rate is 0.25 mm every 6 hours
(D) distraction is limited to a total of 10 mm per surgical site
(E) purulent pin tract drainage indicates osteomyelitis

82. Concerning regenerate bone formed by the Ilizarov procedure,

(A) it is primarily the result of membranous repair
(B) bone marrow is the largest source of interfragment callus
(C) radiographically it appears as longitudinally oriented trabeculae
(D) its formation is compromised by smoking

83. Complications of the Ilizarov procedure include:

(A) nerve damage
(B) muscle contracture
(C) joint subluxation
(D) vascular damage
(E) premature consolidation of bone across the surgical site
(F) refracture

CASE 20: Questions 84 through 87

This ballet dancer presented with ankle pain. You are shown transaxial T1-weighted (A) and gradient-echo (B) MR images of the ankle (Figure 20-1).

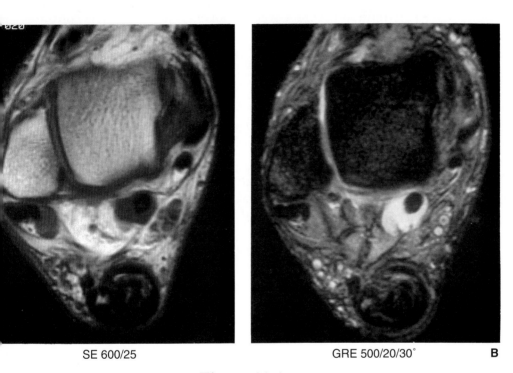

SE 600/25   GRE 500/20/30°   **B**

Figure 20-1

QUESTIONS 84 THROUGH 87: MARK YOUR ANSWER SHEET TRUE (T) OR FALSE (F) FOR EACH OF THE RESPONSE CHOICES.

84.   Concerning the test images,

(A)   there is diffuse soft tissue edema
(B)   there is a partial tear or tendinitis of the flexor hallucis longus tendon
(C)   the posterior tibial tendon is normal
(D)   there is a partial tear or tendinitis of the Achilles tendon
(E)   there is an ankle joint effusion

CASE 20 (Cont'd)

85. Concerning MR findings of tendon abnormalities,

    (A) ankle joint effusion is a cause of fluid in the sheath of the flexor hallucis longus tendon
    (B) the presence of fluid surrounding the peroneus longus tendon is considered abnormal only if there is concomitant abnormal signal intensity within the tendon
    (C) tendon enlargement is required to diagnose a partial tear
    (D) high signal intensity within the tendon is required to diagnose a partial tear
    (E) fluid in the Achilles tendon sheath is a sign of partial tear

86. Concerning the anatomy of the foot and ankle,

    (A) the Achilles tendon uses the anterior tuberosity of the calcaneus as a pulley
    (B) the flexor hallucis longus tendon uses the sustentaculum tali as a pulley
    (C) the peroneus longus tendon attaches to the base of the first metatarsal
    (D) the flexor digitorum longus tendon uses the lateral malleolus as a pulley
    (E) the tibialis posterior tendon uses the medial malleolus as a pulley

87. Concerning tendons of the foot and ankle,

    (A) posterior tibial tendon abnormalities are most common in ballet dancers
    (B) the flexor hallucis longus tendon is the principal everter of the foot
    (C) peroneal tendon abnormalities are a common cause of pain in patients with a history of calcaneal fractures
    (D) an abnormal flexor digitorum longus tendon is a common cause of a painful flat foot in patients with rheumatoid arthritis
    (E) downhill hiking is a common cause of Achilles tendon injuries

This 32-year-old man presented with swelling of the left ankle. You are shown lateral radiographs of the ankle obtained at presentation (A) and 1 month later (B) (Figure 21-1).

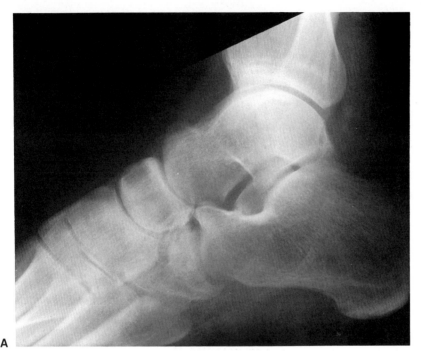

A

Figure 21-1

88. Which *one* of the following is the MOST likely diagnosis?

   (A) Septic arthropathy
   (B) Calcium pyrophosphate arthropathy
   (C) Neuropathic arthropathy
   (D) Reiter's arthropathy
   (E) Hemophilic arthropathy

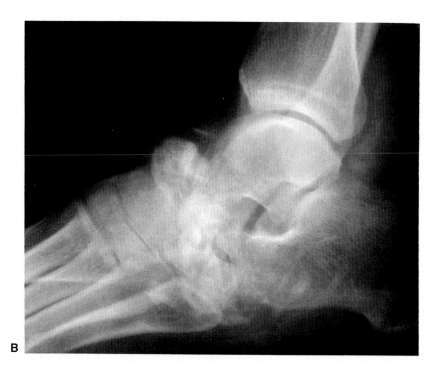

B

QUESTIONS 89 THROUGH 91: MARK YOUR ANSWER SHEET TRUE (T) OR FALSE (F) FOR EACH OF THE RESPONSE CHOICES.

89. Concerning calcium pyrophosphate dihydrate crystal deposition,

(A) pseudogout and pyrophosphate arthropathy are synonyms
(B) it is associated with diabetes mellitus
(C) it is associated with scapholunate collapse
(D) it is associated with scalloped erosion of the anterior cortex of the distal femur
(E) tophaceous deposits are a rare manifestation

CASE 21 (Cont'd)

90. Concerning Reiter's syndrome,

    (A) it is a reactive arthritis
    (B) it typically subsides within 6 months
    (C) upper extremity involvement is more common in men than in women
    (D) periarticular osteopenia accompanies the acute phase
    (E) unilateral sacroiliitis is more common than bilateral sacroiliitis

91. Concerning fractures of the midfoot,

    (A) they are typically isolated to one tarsal bone
    (B) lateral stress injury typically results in cuboid dislocation
    (C) dorsal cortical avulsion fractures of the navicular are most frequent
    (D) medial tuberosity fractures of the navicular are typically displaced
    (E) about 80% of navicular stress fractures occur in the lateral third

This 45-year-old woman complained of foot pain. You are shown an anteroposterior weight-bearing radiograph of the forefoot (Figure 22-1).

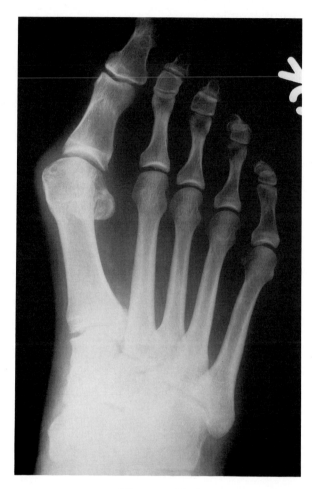

Figure 22-1

92. Which *one* of the following is the MOST likely diagnosis?

    (A) Hammertoes
    (B) Hallux valgus deformity
    (C) Hallux rigidus deformity
    (D) Systemic lupus erythematosus
    (E) Traumatic dislocation

CASE 22 (Cont'd)

QUESTIONS 93 THROUGH 95: MARK YOUR ANSWER SHEET TRUE (T) OR FALSE (F) FOR EACH OF THE RESPONSE CHOICES.

93. Components of surgical correction of hallux valgus deformity include:

   (A) soft tissue release of lateral contracture
   (B) plication of medial capsular structures
   (C) removal of the medial eminence
   (D) osteotomy to correct metatarsus primus varus
   (E) removal of the sesamoid complex

94. Concerning the sesamoid bones of the great toe,

   (A) during walking they absorb most of the weight-bearing stresses on the medial forefoot
   (B) in patients with hallux rigidus deformity, the joints between the sesamoids and the metatarsal head are usually involved by degenerative arthritis
   (C) in patients with hallux valgus deformity, they are tethered to the second metatarsal head by the transverse metatarsal ligament
   (D) bipartite sesamoids and fractured sesamoids can usually be differentiated on standard radiographs
   (E) the anteroposterior radiograph provides adequate evaluation of most sesamoid disorders

95. Concerning deformities of the second through fifth toes,

   (A) a hammertoe results from a fixed flexion contracture at the proximal interphalangeal joint
   (B) a claw toe results from a fixed extension contracture at the distal interphalangeal joint
   (C) a second-digit crossover toe is the result of a hallux valgus deformity
   (D) a bunionette is characterized by a prominence of the lateral condyle of the fifth metatarsal head
   (E) constricting footwear is a major contributor to their formation and progression

This 22-year-old woman underwent a routine pre-orthodontic evaluation. You are shown a panoramic radiograph (Figure 23-1).

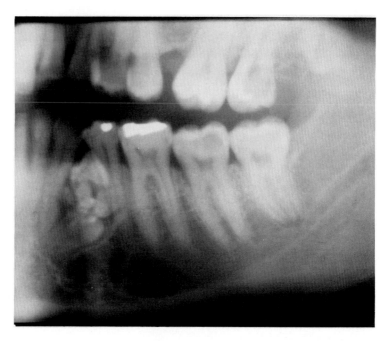

Figure 23-1

96. Which *one* of the following is the MOST likely diagnosis?

   (A) Cemental dysplasia
   (B) Compound odontoma
   (C) Condensing osteitis
   (D) Ossifying fibroma
   (E) Osteosarcoma

For each of the lesions of the osseous portion of the jaw listed below (Questions 97 through 101), select the *one* clinical feature (A, B, C, D, or E) that is MOST closely associated with it. Each clinical feature may be used once, more than once, or not at all.

97. Giant cell reparative granuloma
98. Fibrous dysplasia
99. Osteoma
100. Osteosarcoma
101. Langerhans cell histiocytosis

    (A)   It is limited to the jaws, hands, and feet.
    (B)   Its enlargement parallels skeletal growth.
    (C)   It readily responds to small doses of radiation therapy.
    (D)   A widened periodontal ligament space is an early finding.
    (E)   It is associated with intestinal polyposis.

QUESTIONS 102 THROUGH 105: MARK YOUR ANSWER SHEET TRUE (T) OR FALSE (F) FOR EACH OF THE RESPONSE CHOICES.

102. Concerning osteosclerotic odontogenic lesions of the jaw,

    (A) condensing osteitis occurs in response to dental infection
    (B) about 10% of odontomas have an amorphous appearance
    (C) cemental dysplasia progresses from osteosclerotic to osteolytic
    (D) hypercementosis is excessive formation of cementum on the surface of the tooth root
    (E) ossifying fibroma causes tooth migration

103. Concerning osteolytic odontogenic lesions of the jaw,

    (A) at least 60% of jaw cysts occur at the apex of a tooth root
    (B) radicular cysts arise most often in association with the roots of vital teeth
    (C) dentigerous cysts develop in association with unerupted teeth
    (D) odontogenic keratocysts should be surgically excised rather than curetted
    (E) ameloblastomas metastasize in about 20% of cases

104. Concerning mandibular trauma,

    (A) a panoramic radiograph is an adequate examination
    (B) a widened periodontal ligament space indicates a loosened tooth
    (C) single mandibular fractures are twice as common as multiple fractures
    (D) malocclusion resulting from fracture requires fracture reduction and stabilization
    (E) clinical and radiologic evidence of fracture healing occur simultaneously

105. Concerning periodontal disease,

    (A) it is the principal cause of tooth loss prior to age 30
    (B) it is typically painful
    (C) it is caused by loosening of the teeth
    (D) dentists rely on oral radiographs for early diagnosis
    (E) resorption of the alveolar crest is a typical radiologic feature
    (F) control of bacterial plaque is the most important preventive measure

CASE 24: Questions 106 through 109

This 33-year-old man has had pain and swelling of the knee for approximately 1 year. You are shown an anteroposterior radiograph obtained at initial evaluation (Figure 24-1) and a T2-weighted gradient-echo MR image obtained 9 months later (Figure 24-2).

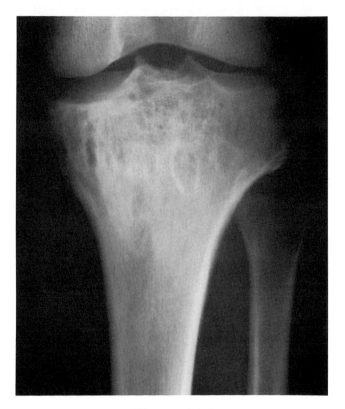

Figure 24-1

106. Which *one* of the following is the MOST likely diagnosis?

    (A) Fungal infection
    (B) Bone infarction
    (C) Langerhans cell histiocytosis
    (D) Pigmented villonodular synovitis
    (E) Subchondral cysts

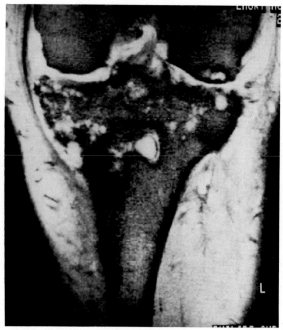

GRE 509/20/40°

Figure 24-2

QUESTIONS 107 THROUGH 109: MARK YOUR ANSWER SHEET TRUE (T) OR FALSE (F) FOR EACH OF THE RESPONSE CHOICES.

107. Concerning fungal osteomyelitis,

    (A) sporotrichosis of bone occurs primarily in immunocompromised patients

    (B) the incidence in the United States is decreasing

    (C) mycetoma most commonly affects the jaws

    (D) most opportunistic fungal infections are acquired from the hospital environment

    (E) coccidioidal osteomyelitis usually follows a primary pulmonary infection

108. Concerning diametaphyseal bone marrow infarction,

    (A) its radiologic appearance is easily confused with that of fibrous dysplasia
    (B) a lytic area nearly always represents cyst formation
    (C) pathologic fracture is a frequent complication
    (D) most patients also develop subarticular epiphyseal infarcts
    (E) it is usually associated with systemic corticosteroid therapy

109. Concerning Langerhans cell histiocytosis of bone,

    (A) a solitary bone lesion requires treatment by curettage or intralesional steroid injection
    (B) disseminated bone disease is usually treated with systemic chemotherapy
    (C) the spine is the most common site of bone involvement
    (D) the development of marginal sclerosis on serial radiographs suggests healing of a lesion
    (E) the lesions exhibit low signal intensity on T2-weighted MR images

This 17-year-old baseball player presented with wrist pain. You are shown a conventional posteroanterior radiograph (A) and coronal T1-weighted (B) and gradient-echo (C) MR images of the wrist (Figure 25-1).

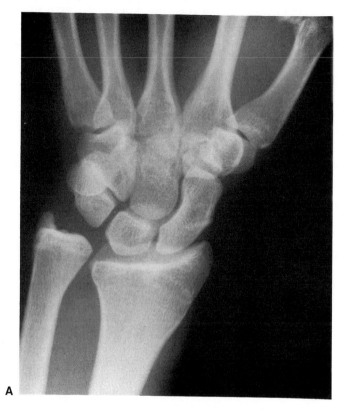

Figure 25-1

110. Which *one* of the following is the MOST likely diagnosis?

    (A) Kienböck's disease
    (B) Ulnar-minus variance
    (C) Ulnolunate impaction syndrome
    (D) Subluxation of the distal radioulnar joint
    (E) Scapholunate ligament tear

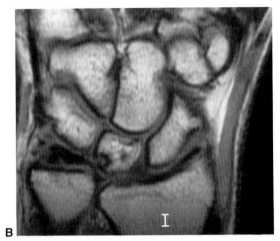

B

SE 600/20

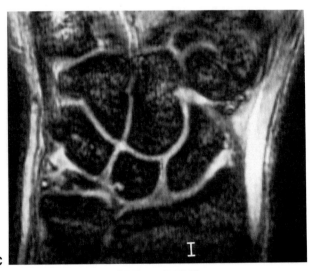

C

GRE 350/20/30°

QUESTIONS 111 AND 112: MARK YOUR ANSWER SHEET TRUE (T) OR FALSE (F) FOR EACH OF THE RESPONSE CHOICES.

111. MRI of the wrist is a sensitive method for detecting:

  (A) Kienböck's disease
  (B) radiographically occult fractures
  (C) triangular fibrocartilage tears
  (D) deQuérvain's tenosynovitis
  (E) chondrocalcinosis

112. Concerning ulnar variance,

  (A) positive variance is associated with triangular fibrocartilage tears
  (B) negative variance is associated with Kienböck's disease
  (C) its assessment is not influenced by wrist positioning during radiography
  (D) both proximal and distal radial fractures are associated with positive variance
  (E) with a normal relationship between the distal ulna and radius, 50% of the axial-loading forces pass through the radial side of the wrist

This 24-year-old man with human immunodeficiency virus infection has elbow pain. You are shown anteroposterior and lateral radiographs (Figure 26-1).

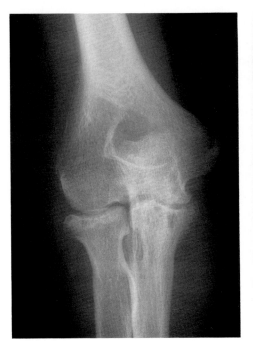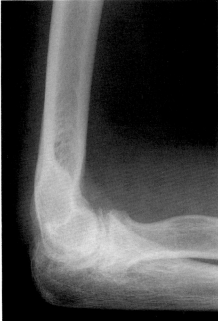

Figure 26-1

113. Which *one* of the following is the MOST likely diagnosis?

   (A) Rheumatoid arthritis
   (B) Gout
   (C) Pigmented villonodular synovitis
   (D) Hemophilia
   (E) HIV arthropathy

QUESTIONS 114 THROUGH 116: MARK YOUR ANSWER SHEET TRUE (T) OR FALSE (F) FOR EACH OF THE RESPONSE CHOICES.

114. Concerning pigmented villonodular synovitis,

    (A) the affected synovium has low signal intensity on MR images
    (B) the combination of bone erosions and intact joint space is a characteristic radiographic appearance
    (C) polyarticular involvement is the rule
    (D) bone erosions are found in about 50% of affected elbow joints
    (E) the elbow is the most commonly involved joint

115. Concerning the elbow,

    (A) hemophilia affects the elbow more commonly than does juvenile chronic arthritis
    (B) degenerative joint disease of the elbow is usually idiopathic
    (C) degenerative arthritic abnormalities of the elbow joint in a young man suggest the possibility of AIDS
    (D) golfer's elbow, tennis elbow, and Little Leaguer's elbow are all the same entity
    (E) the distal tendon of the brachialis muscle is the most commonly ruptured tendon about the elbow

116. Populations of patients with human immunodeficiency virus infection show an increased prevalence of:

    (A) ankylosing spondylitis
    (B) Reiter's syndrome
    (C) psoriasis
    (D) rheumatoid arthritis
    (E) septic arthritis

This 35-year-old woman complained of right hip pain. You are shown an anteroposterior radiograph of the pelvis (A) and a close-up view of the right hip (B) (Figure 27-1).

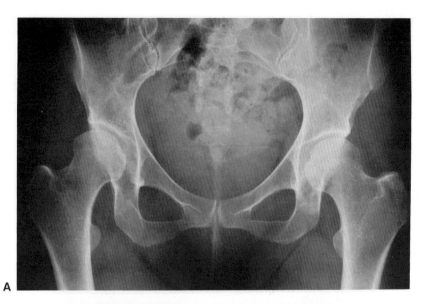

A

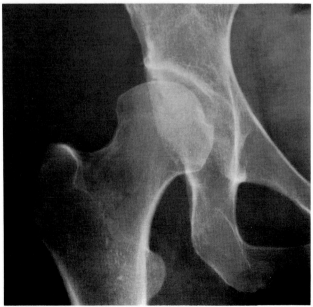

B

Figure 27-1

CASE 27 (Cont'd)

117. Which *one* of the following is the MOST likely diagnosis?

    (A) Synovial chondromatosis
    (B) Healed Legg-Calvé-Perthes disease
    (C) Transient osteoporosis
    (D) Infection
    (E) Developmental dysplasia of the hip

QUESTIONS 118 THROUGH 121: MARK YOUR ANSWER SHEET TRUE (T) OR FALSE (F) FOR EACH OF THE RESPONSE CHOICES.

118. Concerning synovial chondromatosis,

    (A) it is almost invariably a monoarticular disorder
    (B) the synovium is hypoplastic
    (C) conventional radiographs are frequently diagnostic
    (D) ossified intra-articular loose bodies are common
    (E) malignant transformation is rare

119. Concerning transient osteoporosis of the hip,

    (A) it is most common in young women
    (B) conventional radiographs are usually normal
    (C) it predisposes to fracture of the femoral neck
    (D) MRI shows marrow edema

120. Concerning developmental dysplastic hip disease in adults,

    (A) it usually develops during late adolescence
    (B) osteoarthritis is a common sequela
    (C) there is diminished weight-bearing area in the acetabulum
    (D) conservative management will diminish symptoms
    (E) the center-edge angle of Wiberg is increased

121. Concerning developmental dysplasia of the hip in the neonate,

    (A) the cartilaginous femoral head should normally be completely covered by the bony acetabular roof on coronal sonographic images
    (B) dynamic ultrasonography is best performed by the application of posterior force to assess posterior-to-anterior movement of the femoral head
    (C) MR diagnosis of "hourglass capsule" is made by identification of the iliopsoas muscle anterior to the femoral head
    (D) loss of the characteristic "rose thorn" appearance of the labrum on hip arthrography is seen in inverted limbus
    (E) ischemic necrosis occasionally occurs in the contralateral normal hip when both hips are immobilized

CASE 28: Questions 122 through 125

This 57-year-old woman with plasma cell (multiple) myeloma complained of bilateral hip pain. You are shown an anteroposterior radiograph of the pelvis (A) and a detail image of the left hip (B) (Figure 28-1).

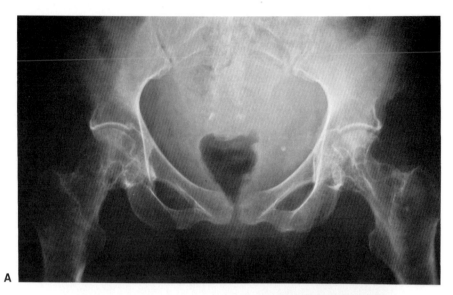

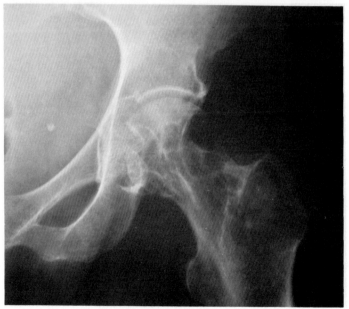

Figure 28-1

122. Which *one* of the following is the MOST likely explanation for the radiographic changes in the hips?

    (A) Tuberculosis
    (B) Amyloidosis
    (C) Plasma cell myeloma
    (D) Hemochromatosis
    (E) Gout

QUESTIONS 123 THROUGH 125: MARK YOUR ANSWER SHEET TRUE (T) OR FALSE (F) FOR EACH OF THE RESPONSE CHOICES.

123. Concerning joint tuberculosis,

    (A) radiographically apparent pulmonary tuberculosis is also present in most patients
    (B) it is associated with severe periarticular osteopenia
    (C) destruction of articular cartilage precedes marginal erosion
    (D) the hip is the most commonly affected appendicular joint
    (E) it is common in patients with AIDS

124. Concerning musculoskeletal amyloidosis,

    (A) it occurs in about 15% of patients with plasma cell myeloma
    (B) intra-articular amyloidosis is characterized by preservation of the joint space
    (C) joint involvement is associated with periarticular soft tissue masses
    (D) it is associated with carpal tunnel syndrome
    (E) joint involvement is usually monoarticular

CASE 28 (Cont'd)

125. Concerning plasma cell myeloma,

    (A) the mandible is involved in about 30% of patients

    (B) skull lesions are more uniform in size than are metastases

    (C) destruction of pedicles is a characteristic feature

    (D) diffuse osteosclerosis is a rare manifestation

DEMOGRAPHIC DATA QUESTIONS

Please answer all of the questions below. The data you provide will be used to supply information that will allow you to compare your performance on the examination with that of others at similar levels of training and with similar backgrounds, and for purposes of planning continuing education projects. Please answer each question as accurately and as objectively as possible. Please mark the *one* BEST response for each question. Recall, of course, that we do *not* want individual names. Our analyses will reflect only categories and groups; everything will remain completely anonymous, and no attempt will be made to identify any specific individual.

126. The ACR will be evaluating the questions in this examination to determine their degree of difficulty and to determine the success of the examination as an instrument of self-evaluation and continuing education. To assist the ACR, please indicate in which of the following ways you took this examination.

    (A) Used reference materials or read the syllabus portion of this book to assist in answering some portion of the examination
    (B) Did not use reference materials and did not read the syllabus portion of this book while taking the examination

127. How much residency and fellowship training in Diagnostic Radiology have you completed?

    (A) None
    (B) Less than 1 year
    (C) 1 year
    (D) 2 years
    (E) 3 years
    (F) 4 or more years

DEMOGRAPHIC DATA QUESTIONS (Cont'd)

128. When did you finish your residency training in Radiology?

    (A) More than 10 years ago
    (B) 5 to 10 years ago
    (C) 1 to 5 years ago
    (D) Less than 1 year ago
    (E) Not yet completed
    (F) Radiology is not my specialty

129. Have you been certified by the American Board of Radiology in Diagnostic Radiology?

    (A) Yes
    (B) No

130. Have you completed fellowship training in Musculoskeletal Radiology?

    (A) Yes
    (B) No

131. Which one of the categories listed below BEST describes the setting of your practice in the immediate past 3 years? (For residents and fellows, in which one did you or will you spend the major portion of your residency or fellowship?)

    (A) Community or general hospital—less than 200 beds
    (B) Community or general hospital—200 to 499 beds
    (C) Community or general hospital—500 or more beds
    (D) University-affiliated hospital
    (E) Office practice

DEMOGRAPHIC DATA QUESTIONS (Cont'd)

132. In which *one* of the following general areas of Radiology do you consider yourself MOST expert?

    (A) Musculoskeletal radiology
    (B) Chest radiology
    (C) Gastrointestinal radiology
    (D) Genitourinary radiology
    (E) Head and neck radiology
    (F) Neuroradiology
    (G) Breast Imaging
    (H) Pediatric radiology
    (I) Cardiovascular radiology
    (J) Other

133. In which *one* of the following radiologic modalities do you consider yourself MOST expert?

    (A) General angiography
    (B) Interventional radiology
    (C) Magnetic resonance imaging
    (D) Nuclear radiology
    (E) Ultrasonography
    (F) Computed tomography
    (G) Radiation therapy
    (H) Other

Musculoskeletal Disease

Table of Contents

The Table of Contents is placed in this unusual location so that the reader will not be distracted by the answers before completeing the test. A detailed index of the areas considered in this syllabus is provided (beginning on p. 787) for further reference.

Musculoskeletal Disease Syllabus

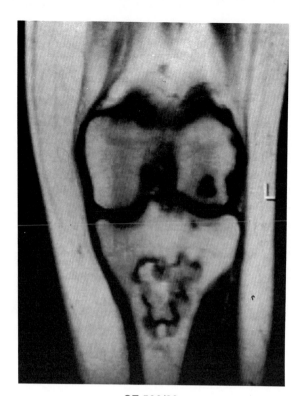

SE 500/20

Figure 1-1

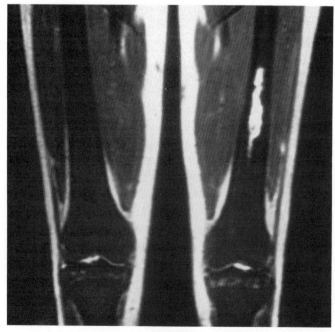

SE 2,500/60

Figure 1-2

Case 1: Bone Marrow

Questions 1 through 4

For each numbered MR scan (Figures 1-1 through 1-4), select the *one* lettered description (A, B, C, D, or E) that is MOST closely associated with it. Each lettered description may be used once, more than once, or not at all.

1. Figure 1-1
2. Figure 1-2
3. Figure 1-3
4. Figure 1-4

    (A) Chronic medullary infarct
    (B) Sickle-cell anemia with infarct
    (C) Focal lymphoma
    (D) Late radiation effect on marrow
    (E) Aplastic anemia

Figure 1-1, a coronal T1-weighted image of the left knee, reveals a well-defined lesion of the metaphyseal bone marrow characterized by a low-intensity border. The central portion of the lesion is isointense to surrounding normal marrow (Figure 1-5). There is no evidence of soft tissue or bone marrow edema. This constellation of findings is most consistent with a chronic medullary bone infarct **(Option (A) is the correct answer to Question 1)**. There is no evidence of bone marrow replacement by cellular tissue; therefore, this pattern does not represent sickle-cell anemia (Option (B)). Similarly, lymphoma (Option (C)) is most frequently encountered as focal or regional marrow replacement of low or intermediate intensity on T1-weighted images. Both late radiation effect on marrow (Option (D)) and aplastic anemia (Option (E)) are regional or diffuse phenomena and do not present as focal lesions.

Medullary bone marrow infarction occurs as a result of marrow ischemia. The time elapsed since the initial insult, the degree of ischemia, and the host response all influence the MR appearance. As documented by histologic studies, initial ischemic insult results in cell death followed by a host inflammatory response. Hematopoietic cells, the most sensitive

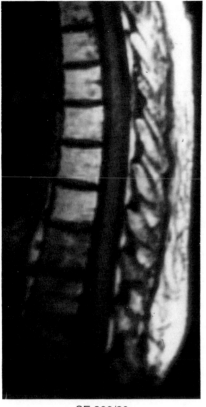

SE 300/20

Figure 1-3

STIR 1,500/30/100

Figure 1-4

to marrow ischemia, die in the first 6 to 12 hours. Osteoblasts, osteo-clasts, and osteocytes show evidence of cell death by 48 hours, and fat cells show evidence of cell death 2 to 5 days following the ischemic event. Granulation tissue, increased vascularity, and fibroblastic response can be seen at the interface between viable and necrotic tissue.

Acute medullary bone infarcts are frequently characterized as ill-defined regions of intermediate intensity within otherwise normal mar-row on T1-weighted images (Figure 1-6A). These regions show increased intensity on T2-weighted images (Figure 1-6B). As an infarct matures, its borders become better defined (Figure 1-7). At this stage, the infarct can be surrounded by a border with intermediate intensity on T1-weighted images and increased intensity on T2-weighted images. This border represents the reactive interface between normal and infarcted tissue and consists primarily of inflammatory cells. With further healing, the infarcted marrow is replaced by fatty marrow and the affected area

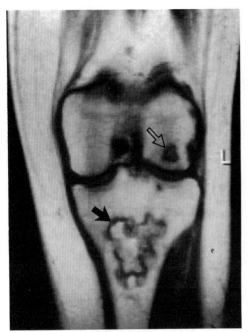

SE 500/20

Figure 1-5 (Same as Figure 1-1). Chronic medullary infarct on a T1-weighted coronal image through the left knee in a patient with knee pain following systemic treatment for lymphoma. A well-defined lesion in the proximal tibial metaphysis has a low-intensity border (solid arrow) with isointense central marrow compared with surrounding normal marrow. These findings are characteristic of a healing or healed infarct. A second rounded infarct is seen in the left lateral femoral epiphysis (open arrow).

thus becomes isointense with surrounding fatty marrow, as demonstrated in Figure 1-1. The border, now representing reactive bone, either resorbs or remains visible on both T1- and T2-weighted images as a low-intensity rim.

Figure 1-2, a T2-weighted coronal MR image of the femora and proximal tibiae, shows diffuse replacement of fatty marrow including the epiphyses, metaphyses, and diaphyses. The marrow has very low intensity rather than the normally higher intensity of fat such as is evident in the subcutaneous adipose tissue. Such diffuse marrow replacement can be caused by either neoplastic or hyperplastic cells. Excess iron deposition in bone marrow can further lower the signal intensity of marrow on both T1- and T2-weighted images as a result of a paramagnetic T2-shortening effect of the iron. A well-circumscribed, somewhat geographic area of increased signal intensity is identified in the left femoral shaft (Figure 1-8). This abnormality represents medullary bone infarct, probably acute or subacute in duration. Patients with sickle-cell anemia frequently have extensive marrow replacement as a result of hyperplastic cells and lower than usual marrow signal intensity from excess iron deposition due to local hemolysis. Medullary bone infarction is a frequent complication of this conditon **(Option (B) is the correct answer to Question 2).** A long-standing or chronic medullary infarct (Option (A)) usually has fatty-

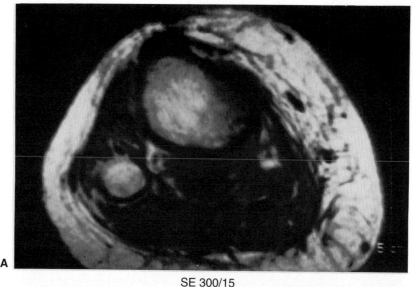

SE 300/15

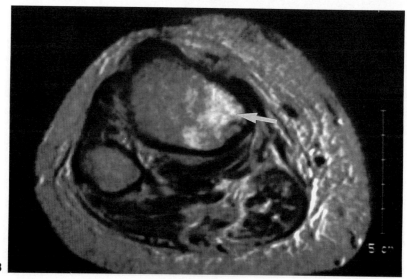

SE 2,500/80

Figure 1-6. Acute medullary infarct. T1-weighted (A) and T2-weighted (B) transaxial MR images through the right leg in a patient with acute marrow ischemia secondary to radiation therapy. Note the focus of low-intensity marrow on the T1-weighted image; this is ill defined and has increased signal intensity on the T2-weighted image (arrow in panel B). Extensive soft tissue edema is seen as high-intensity linear streaks on the T2-weighted image.

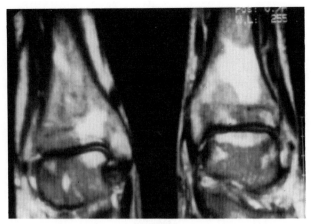

SE 2,000/80

Figure 1-7. Subacute medullary infarcts on a T2-weighted coronal MR image through the ankles in a patient with chronic myelogenous leukemia. Multiple subacute medullary infarcts are identified as well-defined geographic regions of increased signal intensity. The underlying bone marrow, which should have higher signal intensity, shows abnormally low intensity secondary to the patient's leukemia. (Reprinted with permission from Moore [4].)

marrow signal intensity and would not show increased intensity on T2-weighted images. Focal lymphoma (Option (C)) could present as a focal area of increased intensity, but this diagnosis would not explain the diffuse very-low-intensity marrow replacement seen in Figure 1-2. Both radiation therapy (Option (D)) and aplastic anemia (Option (E)) can cause fatty replacement of marrow (seen as a high-intensity area) but do not cause cellular infiltration of marrow (seen as a low-intensity area).

Chronic hemolysis in patients with sickle-cell anemia results in recruitment of what would otherwise be yellow marrow for the purpose of hematopoiesis. An intermediate-intensity area corresponding to "hematopoietic" or "hyperplastic" marrow is therefore seen in regions of marrow that, for the patient's age, would normally contain yellow marrow. The degree and distribution of marrow changes seem generally proportionate to the severity of disease. In more extreme examples, hematopoietic marrow can cause widening of the diploic space in the calvarium and will replace yellow marrow in the normally fatty epiphyses.

Medullary infarction is a common complication of sickle-cell disease. The metabolically active, hyperplastic hematopoietic marrow requires an increased blood supply to maintain its viability, and the subnormal oxygen delivery by sickled cells results in both periarticular and medullary

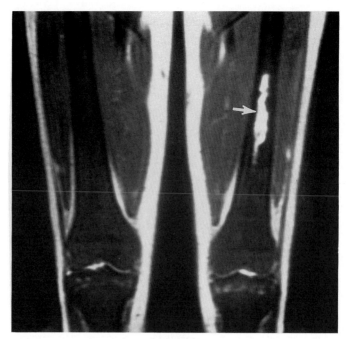

SE 2,500/60

Figure 1-8 (Same as Figure 1-2). Sickle-cell anemia with medullary infarction. A T2-weighted coronal MR image shows diffuse low-intensity hematopoietic marrow replacing all medullary spaces, including the epiphyses. The high-intensity lesion in the left femoral shaft (arrow) is geographic in appearance and is sharply demarcated from surrounding marrow. This is most consistent with an acute or subacute medullary infarction. (Courtesy of Vijay M. Rao, M.D., and Robert M. Steiner, M.D., Thomas Jefferson University, Philadelphia.)

infarctions. Focal regions of decreased signal intensity on short-TR/TE images with increased intensity on long-TR/TE images are thought to represent acute or subacute marrow infarction when seen in patients with sickle-cell anemia.

Figure 1-3, a T1-weighted sagittal MR image of an adult thoracolumbar spine, shows normal low-intensity hematopoietic marrow in the upper lumbar vertebral bodies. There is a sharp demarcation between this pattern and the homogeneous, high-intensity marrow seen in the lower thoracic vertebral bodies. The juxtaposition of these two patterns and the sharp transition between them (Figure 1-9) is most consistent with a sequela of radiation therapy that has resulted in diffuse fatty replacement of the marrow **(Option (D) is the correct answer to Question 3).** Aplastic anemia (Option (E)) can also result in fatty

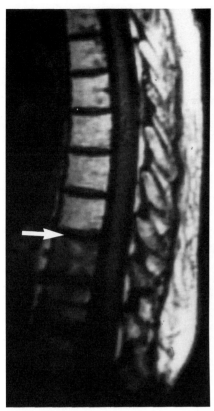

Figure 1-9 (Same as Figure 1-3). Effect of radiation therapy. A T1-weighted sagittal MR image of the thoracolumbar spine in a patient following radiation therapy for Hodgkin's disease shows a geographic distribution of homogeneous high-intensity fatty marrow where cellular marrow would otherwise be expected. This is characteristic of hematopoietic marrow extinction secondary to radiation therapy. Note the sharp transition (arrow) between the fatty marrow above and the hematopoietic marrow below.

SE 300/20

replacement of the marrow, but this is typically a diffuse process involving all, not just some, of the vertebral bodies. Aplastic anemia (Figure 1-10) often causes a more heterogeneous marrow appearance than is seen in Figure 1-3, since foci of marrow fibrosis are frequently present. Chronic medullary infarct (Option (A)) and focal lymphoma (Option (C)) would not involve multiple contiguous vertebral bodies. Sickle-cell anemia (Option (B)), with or without marrow infarction, would not spare large segments of marrow space in the spine.

Pathologic changes in the spine following fractionated radiation therapy of 2,000 to 4,000 rads (20 to 40 Gy) include initial edema, destruction of sinusoids, and suppression of hematopoiesis. Decreased hematopoietic cellularity and an increased amount of fat predominate at 1 month following therapy. Absence of hematopoietic cells and replacement of marrow by fibrosis and fat are complete at 3 months. The result is fatty marrow (of high signal intensity) in all bones included in the radiation port. This is a common MR pattern following radiation therapy in older

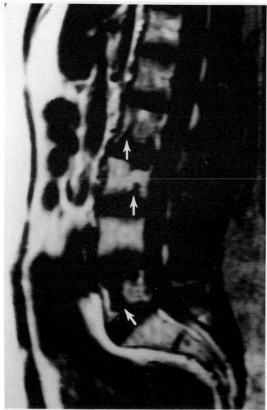

SE 300/30

Figure 1-10. Aplastic anemia with fibrosis. A T1-weighted sagittal MR image through the spine shows that the vertebral bodies are composed primarily of high-intensity fat and contain few hematopoietic cells. Regions of low signal intensity (arrows) within the vertebral marrow represent focal fibrosis, a common feature of aplastic anemia.

patients; however, a second postradiotherapy bone-marrow pattern can also be seen. This consists of a central region of high-intensity fatty marrow (surrounding the basivertebral vein) with intermediate-intensity marrow adjacent to the endosteal surface of the vertebral body (Figure 1-11). The intermediate-intensity subendosteal marrow may represent repopulation of this region of vertebral marrow with hematopoietic cells. It has been observed that 55% of patients have full hematopoietic marrow recovery and 85% of patients have at least partial marrow recovery within 2 years following radiation therapy. Marrow recovery is more likely to occur in younger patients.

Figure 1-4, a short-tau inversion-recovery (STIR) coronal MR image of the femora, reveals a region of increased intensity in the left proximal femoral diaphysis. The lesion is sharply demarcated from adjacent normal marrow. The normal marrow exhibits low intensity since yellow marrow (fat) signal is suppressed on STIR images. Increased intensity in

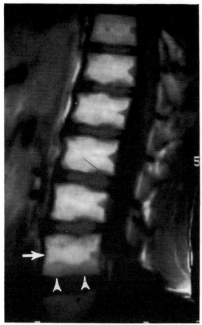

SE 300/15

Figure 1-11. Marrow recovery following radiation therapy. A T1-weighted sagittal MR image through the lumbar spine of a 20-year-old man 6 months after radiation therapy for seminoma shows a "band" pattern of central increased-intensity fatty marrow (arrow) and endosteal intermediate-intensity recovery marrow (arrowheads).

the soft tissues adjacent to the affected bone (Figure 1-12) reflects soft tissue edema. Chronic medullary infarcts (Option (A)) are seen as focal, well-defined lesions that are isointense with fat, not increased in signal intensity compared with surrounding marrow. Acute or subacute bone marrow infarcts can be seen as areas of increased signal intensity on STIR images, but they do not normally involve such a long segment of marrow cavity. In addition, the low-intensity marrow in Figure 1-4 reflects suppressed fatty marrow, not the hyperplastic marrow seen in patients with sickle-cell anemia (Option (B)), which would have higher intensity on this pulse sequence. Both radiation therapy (Option (D)) and aplastic anemia (Option (E)) result in diffuse replacement of marrow by fat, which would have low signal intensity on STIR images but would not result in a focal area of increased intensity.

Infiltration of marrow by neoplastic cells typically results in increased signal intensity on STIR images. Involvement of part but not all of the marrow cavity is typical in patients with lymphoma because of the focal or multifocal nature of the condition. When the spine is affected by lymphoma, vertebral body involvement tends to be isolated, unlike the diffuse vertebral marrow involvement typical of leukemia (Figure 1-13). Soft tissue edema is often seen in both neoplastic and inflammatory processes. Therefore, the constellation of focal increased-intensity marrow,

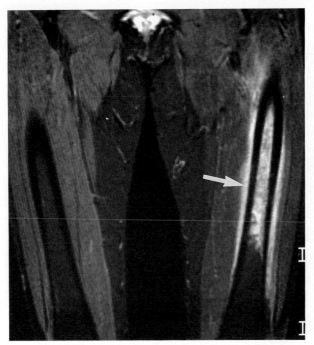

Figure 1-12 (left) (Same as Figure 1-4). Focal lymphoma. A STIR coronal MR image of the femora in a 38-year-old patient with lymphocytic lymphoma shows a region of increased signal intensity in the left proximal femoral diaphysis, representing marrow involvement by lymphoma. The normal fatty marrow is suppressed and is nearly black on this STIR image. Increased-intensity soft tissue edema surrounds the involved bone (arrow).

STIR 1,500/30/100

Figure 1-13 (right). Acute leukemia. A T1-weighted sagittal MR image through the lumbar vertebral marrow in a patient with acute lymphocytic leukemia shows that the signal intensity of the vertebral marrow is lower than that of adjacent intervertebral disks, which is evidence of diffuse replacement of the marrow space by a population of cells.

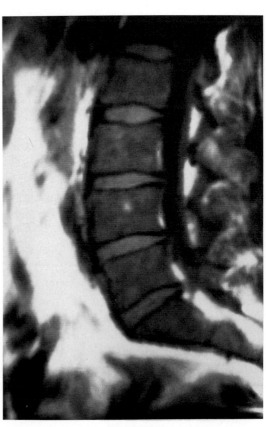

SE 300/30

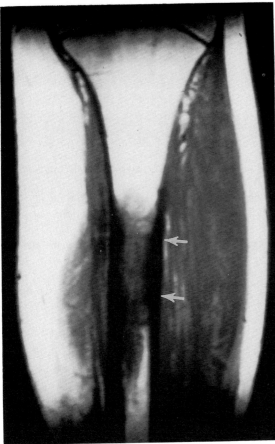

Figure 1-14. Lymphoma. A T1-weighted coronal MR image through the tibia in a 15-year-old with marrow involvement by non-Hodgkin's lymphoma shows abnormal low-intensity marrow in the diaphyseal region of the tibia. This appearance is typical of lymphoma, which often involves focal regions of marrow. Low-intensity cortical thickening is seen surrounding the involved marrow (arrows).

SE 300/15

adjacent soft tissue edema, and otherwise normal marrow in Figure 1-4 is most consistent with lymphoma **(Option (C) is the correct answer to Question 4).**

Lymphomatous infiltration of marrow most frequently occurs in regions of hematopoietic marrow. Diffuse infiltration is more common in patients with lymphocytic lymphoma than in those with Hodgkin's disease and results in decreased signal intensity on T1-weighted images and intermediate to increased intensity on T2-weighted, fat-saturation, and STIR images, as a result of the hypercellularity. Marrow involvement by non-Hodgkin's lymphoma is more common than involvement by Hodgkin's disease and is frequently more diffuse. Regions of diffuse marrow infiltration by non-Hodgkin's lymphoma can be punctuated by focal marrow sparing, so that substantial portions of a long bone may be spared and macroscopic areas of normal fatty marrow will separate regions of involved marrow (Figure 1-14). In the spine, several vertebral bodies can appear normal while the remainder appear affected. Bone lesions in patients with Hodgkin's disease are less frequent, usually focal, and most frequent in the spine and pelvis followed by the ribs, femora, and sternum.

Question 5

Concerning marrow distribution patterns on T1-weighted spin-echo MR images,

(A) in children, ossified epiphyses almost always contain fatty marrow
(B) at 10 years of age, intermediate-intensity metaphyseal red marrow in the femur is typical
(C) at 20 years of age, homogeneous low-intensity marrow in the clivus is normal
(D) at 40 years of age, red marrow in the proximal humeral metaphyses is probably abnormal
(E) in adults, the signal intensity of vertebral marrow should be lower than that of the adjacent disk

At birth, bone marrow consists entirely of hematopoietic cells (Figure 1-15). With growth and development, there is progressive conversion of this hematopoietic marrow to fatty marrow, so that by adulthood the normal sites of red marrow distribution are in the calvarium, flat bones, spine, and proximal humeral and femoral metaphyses (Figure 1-16). The remainder of the marrow, including the long bones and all epiphyses and apophyses, is composed primarily of yellow marrow, which is displayed as increased signal intensity on T1-weighted images.

Initially, epiphyses are cartilaginous and are seen as areas of intermediate signal intensity on T1-weighted MR images and intermediate to high intensity on T2-weighted and fat-suppression images. With progressive ossification, the epiphyseal ossification center usually appears to contain increased-intensity areas corresponding to yellow marrow **(Option (A) is true)** (Figure 1-17). This epiphyseal ossification center will remain high in intensity and will increase in size as the child grows, eventually replacing the intermediate-intensity cartilaginous epiphysis.

Histologic evaluation of ossifying epiphyses shows that they often contain some red marrow, especially at birth. Occasionally, intermediate-intensity red marrow is seen within the ossifying proximal humeral, proximal femoral, distal femoral, and proximal tibial epiphyses in T1-weighted images of newborns or very young infants (Figure 1-18). This finding can persist for as long as 2 to 3 months after the initiation of ossification and should not be considered abnormal. However, once the ossifying epiphysis has been present for more than 2 or 3 months, persistent

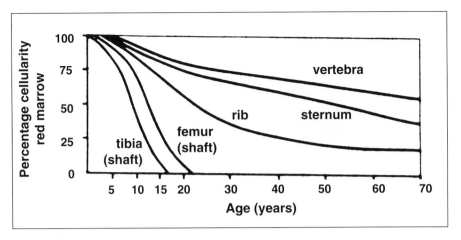

Figure 1-15. Normal conversion of hematopoietic marrow into fatty marrow. Diagram shows the relative amounts of macroscopic hematopoietic marrow in different anatomic sites. The percentage of hematopoietic marrow decreases with age. (Adapted with permission from Kricun [28].)

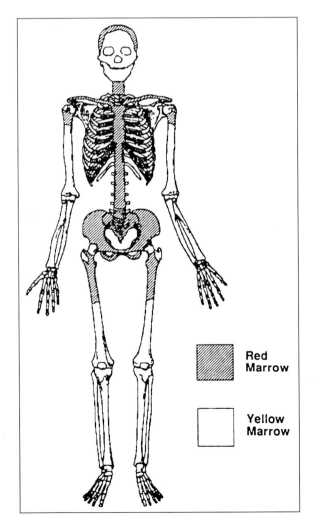

Red Marrow

Yellow Marrow

Figure 1-16. Macroscopic red and yellow marrow distribution. Diagram shows shaded macroscopic red marrow in the vertebral bodies, flat bones, and proximal metaphyses of the femora and humeri.

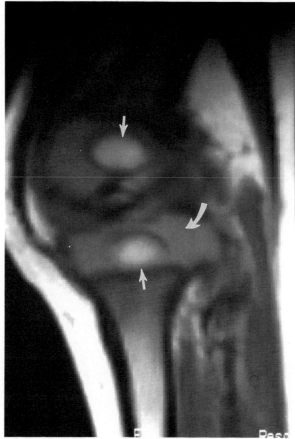

SE 600/15

Figure 1-17. Ossifying epiphyses with fatty marrow. A T1-weighted sagittal MR image through the knee in an infant with ossifying distal femoral and proximal tibial epiphyses shows high-intensity fatty marrow within the ossifying epiphyses (straight arrows). The cartilaginous portion of the tibial epiphysis has intermediate signal intensity (curved arrow).

intermediate-intensity "hematopoietic" marrow within the epiphysis is distinctly abnormal. Epiphyseal or apophyseal marrow that is not high-intensity fatty marrow in any patient other than a newborn or very young infant should be considered abnormal and indicates edema, infiltration of the marrow by tumor, or hyperplastic marrow resulting from abnormal conversion of yellow to red marrow. Ischemia and sclerosis can also result in abnormal intermediate- or low-intensity epiphyseal marrow. A densely sclerotic proximal femoral epiphysis that exhibits low intensity on both T1- and T2-weighted images can be seen in children with congenital dislocation of the hip and should not be misdiagnosed as a focus of abnormal marrow.

The long bones exhibit a normal pattern of marrow conversion (hematopoietic to fatty), which follows a "distal to proximal" trend for both anatomic site and marrow region. In general, conversion of extremity

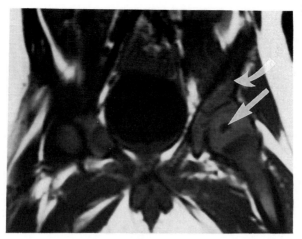

SE 600/15

Figure 1-18. Ossifying epiphysis with hematopoietic marrow. A T1-weighted coronal MR image through the proximal femora in an infant shows a low-intensity ossifying proximal left femoral epiphysis (straight arrow) within the slightly increased-intensity cartilaginous epiphysis. Note the intermediate-intensity marrow (similar to that of muscle) in the left pelvis (curved arrow) and the proximal left femoral metaphysis. (Courtesy Diego Jaramillo, M.D., Massachusetts General Hospital, Boston.)

bone marrow occurs first in the hands and feet and then progresses from the distal to the proximal long bones. Within a bone itself, marrow conversion occurs first in the diaphysis, then in the distal metaphysis, and finally in the proximal metaphysis.

Four general patterns of bone marrow distribution and signal characteristics have been described and can be used as a template for understanding marrow conversion in all of the long bones. These four patterns are: (1) the infant pattern, (2) the childhood pattern, (3) the adolescent pattern, and (4) the adult pattern. The infant pattern occurs during the first year of life and is visible on MR images as homogeneous intermediate-intensity hematopoietic marrow in all portions of the long bones (Figure 1-18). The childhood pattern consists of high-intensity diaphyseal marrow with intermediate-intensity proximal and distal metaphyseal marrow (Figures 1-19 and 1-20). The ossifying epiphyses always contain yellow marrow. This pattern can first become apparent as early as 1 year of age. Between the ages of 6 and 10 years, the conversion of diaphyseal red marrow to yellow marrow appears "complete," and the childhood pattern of diaphyseal yellow and metaphyseal red marrow should be seen by 10 years of age **(Option (B) is true).** Between the ages of 11 and 15

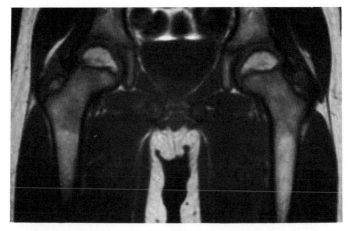

SE 800/15

Figure 1-19. Childhood pattern of proximal femur and pelvis. A T1-weighted coronal MR image through the hips and proximal femora in a 6-year-old girl shows intermediate-intensity red marrow in the ischia and proximal femoral metaphyses and higher-intensity yellow marrow in the epiphyses and diaphyses.

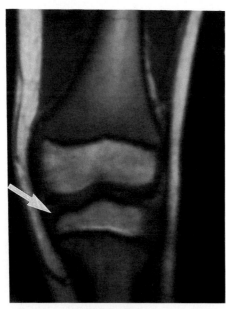

SE 800/20

Figure 1-20. Childhood pattern of normal knee. A T1-weighted coronal MR image through the knee in a 9-year-old girl shows increased signal intensity in the femoral diaphysis and epiphysis; intermediate-intensity hematopoietic marrow is seen in the distal femoral and proximal tibial metaphyses. Note the intermediate-intensity cartilaginous epiphysis (arrow) surrounding the increased-intensity ossified epiphysis in the proximal tibia.

years, the fat fraction in metaphyseal marrow increases with concomitant increases in signal intensity. The signal of metaphyseal marrow

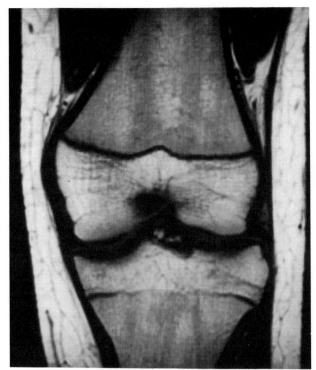

Figure 1-21. Adolescent pattern of normal knee. A T1-weighted coronal MR image through the knee in a 16-year-old girl shows focal areas of intermediate and slightly increased signal intensity in the distal femoral metaphysis. Heterogeneous distal femoral marrow is typical of the adolescent. The epiphyses contain high-intensity fatty marrow.

SE 800/20

tends to appear heterogeneous when compared with that seen before the age of 10. Between the ages of 16 and 20, patchy distal metaphyseal red and yellow marrow is expected and the adolescent pattern is fully expressed (Figure 1-21). The adult pattern of yellow epiphyseal, diaphyseal, and distal metaphyseal marrow is typically reached by 21 years of age (Figure 1-22). The proximal femoral metaphysis frequently appears as intermediate-intensity hematopoietic marrow, although after the age of 60 increasing intensity may reflect less active hematopoietic marrow in this region as well. However, residual hematopoietic marrow is "normal" in the proximal femoral metaphysis at any age.

Hematopoietic marrow within the skull accounts for approximately one-fourth of the marrow activity at birth and decreases to 12% of hematopoietic activity by age 10. The hematopoietic bone marrow in the clivus is homogeneous and of low to intermediate intensity on T1-weighted images in infants less than 1 year of age (Figure 1-23). Between the ages of 1 and 7 years the converting bone marrow in the clivus appears patchy with areas of low and high signal intensity (Figure 1-24). As a general rule, by age 15 there is homogeneous high-intensity fatty marrow in both the clivus and the calvarium (Figure 1-25) **(Option (C) is false).**

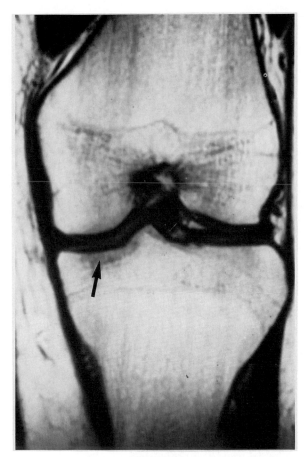

Figure 1-22 (left).
Adult pattern of normal knee. A T1-weighted coronal MR image of the knee in an adult shows increased-intensity yellow marrow in the metaphysis and epiphysis. Low-intensity sclerosis is seen in the medial tibial condyle (arrow).

SE 600/20

Figure 1-23 (right).
Hematopoietic clival marrow. A T1-weighted MR image through the clivus of a 17-month-old girl shows intermediate-intensity hematopoietic marrow (arrow). Increased-intensity fatty marrow is identified in the sphenoid sinus (arrowhead).

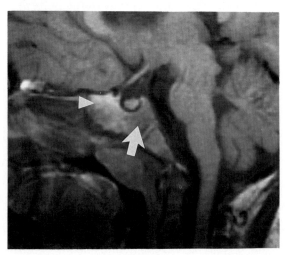

SE 800/20

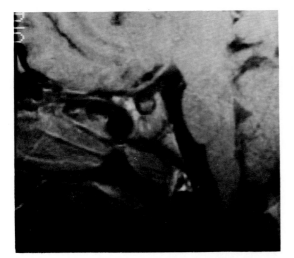

Figure 1-24 (left). Converting clival marrow. A T1-weighted sagittal MR image shows heterogeneous red and yellow marrow in the clivus of a 6-year-old child. Sphenoid aeration is noted.

SE 800/20

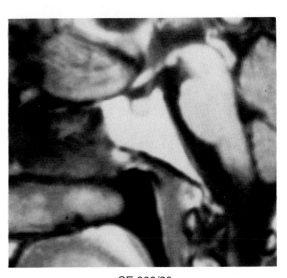

Figure 1-25 (right). Fatty clival marrow. A T1-weighted sagittal MR image shows homogeneous high-intensity yellow marrow in a normal adult.

SE 800/20

The adult pattern of red and yellow marrow distribution (Figure 1-16) consists of predominantly red marrow in the flat bones, spine, and proximal humeral and femoral metaphyses. Fatty marrow is seen in the remainder of the skeleton. Hematopoietic marrow contains variable percentages of both red and yellow marrow, so the hematopoietic marrow signal intensity on MR images will range from low to intermediate to relatively high depending on the amount of fat present. It is not unusual for the proximal humeral metaphyses to have the appearance of yellow marrow, especially in persons over the age of 60, but symmetric bilateral

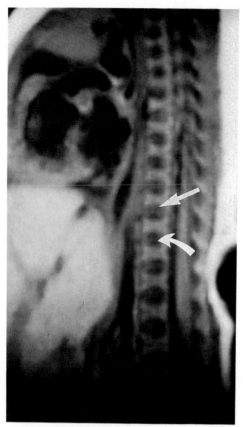

Figure 1-26. Hematopoietic vertebral marrow in the newborn. A T1-weighted sagittal MR image through the spine shows low-intensity hematopoietic vertebral marrow (straight arrow) surrounded by intermediate-intensity cartilaginous end plates. The high-intensity basivertebral vein is sometimes seen within the hematopoietic marrow (curved arrow).

SE 600/20

intermediate-intensity red marrow in the proximal humeral metaphyses is within the normal range for a 40-year-old individual **(Option (D) is false).** This proximal humeral metaphyseal marrow can be heterogeneous in appearance with patchy regions of mixed red and yellow marrow. This should not be interpreted as an abnormal marrow pattern in this region.

At birth, whatever marrow is in vertebral bodies is completely hematopoietic, and the signal intensity of the vertebral bodies in MR images is low (often lower than that of adjacent muscle) (Figure 1-26). With growth and development there is progressive conversion of red to yellow marrow, so that the signal intensity of vertebral marrow on T1-weighted images increases. As the primary hematopoietic reservoir, however, the vertebral bodies still contain considerable hematopoietic marrow. Vertebral marrow has a variable percentage of red and yellow marrow. Therefore, the spine exhibits a wide range of normal signal intensities on T1- and T2-weighted MR images. Marked heterogeneity of signal, focal fibrosis, sclerosis, and focal fatty marrow are all normal findings in the spine. Abnormal vertebral marrow signal intensity can range from the increased intensity of fatty marrow (as in patients with aplastic anemia) to the diffuse low intensity of neoplastic marrow, such as might be seen in patients with leukemia. Therefore, as a general guideline, the vertebral marrow in adults should be brighter than that of a normal adjacent disk on T1-weighted images **(Option (E) is false).** If this is not the case, either hyperplasia of marrow or infiltration of marrow by neoplastic cells should be considered.

Question 6

Concerning the MR evaluation of leukemic marrow,

    (A) leukemia is reliably distinguished from diffuse metastatic disease
    (B) the calculated vertebral T1 relaxation time is prolonged
    (C) the signal intensity is increased on chemical-shift fat-fraction images
    (D) volume-selected proton spectroscopy shows an increase in the water peak
    (E) post-treatment aplastic anemia usually results in diffuse low signal intensity

MR evaluation of leukemic marrow has been an active area of research since MR images of bone marrow were first obtained. Radiographically, periostitis, permeative bone changes, focal lytic lesions, and metaphyseal lucency can reflect underlying leukemic marrow (Figure 1-27); however, the radiographic appearance of involved bone is often normal. Leukemic cells are native to bone marrow tissue, and so MRI can readily display marrow changes in leukemic patients. Leukemic infiltrates are found predominantly in regions with normally high concentrations of hematopoietic cells, such as the spine, iliac crest, and proximal femur. These are the areas typically studied by MRI.

Leukemic infiltration of the marrow is seen most frequently as homogeneous marrow of intermediate to low intensity on MR images. This can be recognized in the spine because the signal intensity of the abnormal marrow is lower than that of the adjacent disk on T1-weighted images (Figure 1-13), or it can be recognized in the long bones as focal or diffuse decreased-intensity marrow in regions where fatty marrow is expected. The signal intensity of leukemic marrow may appear increased on T2-weighted, STIR, and fat-saturation images. The pattern of marrow replacement is usually diffuse, but leukemic marrow infiltration can also be focal or regional. This focal or regional marrow infiltration can be seen with any leukemic cell type but is more common in patients with acute

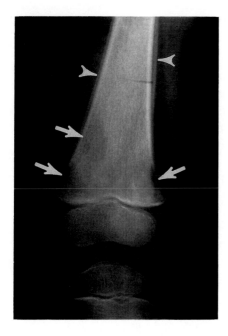

Figure 1-27. Leukemia. An antero-posterior radiograph of the distal femur in a child with acute lymphocytic leukemia shows lytic lesions (arrows) and periosteal reaction (arrowheads).

myelogenous leukemia (AML), in whom chloromas frequently develop in the marrow cavities of the long bones and skull.

MR images of the marrow in patients with leukemia are frequently abnormal, but the pattern of marrow replacement and the appearance of the marrow on both T1- and T2-weighted images can be identical to that seen in patients with any neoplastic marrow replacement. Specifically, patients with focal or diffuse metastatic disease can have marrow of homogeneous intermediate to low signal intensity on T1-weighted images and increased intensity on T2-weighted, STIR, or fat-saturation images **(Option (A) is false).** Cortical infiltration and development of adjacent soft tissue edema are common ancillary findings in patients with leukemia and metastases.

Marrow signal intensity alone cannot be reliably used to diagnose and determine the stage of leukemic disease (relapse versus remission). To further characterize leukemic infiltration of marrow on MR images, there have been attempts to increase the specificity of MRI and to quantify the degree of involvement of marrow. Approaches have included studies of calculated vertebral marrow T1 relaxation times, chemical-shift characteristics, and volume-selected proton spectroscopy.

Calculated T1 relaxation times can be used to identify and stage leukemic marrow disease. The T1 relaxation time of normal vertebral marrow is generally reported to range between 350 and 650 msec, depending

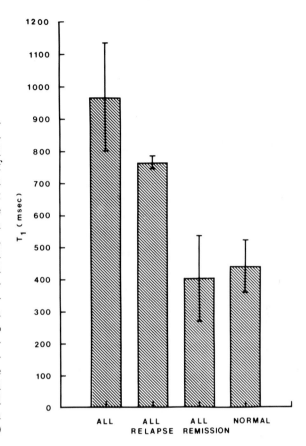

Figure 1-28. Histogram of the T1 relaxation time (mean and standard deviation) of vertebral marrow in each of four groups: newly diagnosed acute lymphocytic leukemia (ALL), ALL in relapse, ALL in remission, and normal age-matched controls. The T1 relaxation time is significantly prolonged in children with ALL compared with children having no evidence of active disease and with age-matched controls. (Reprinted with permission from Moore et al. [42].)

on the field strength of the magnet used. The T1 relaxation time of lumbar vertebral marrow is prolonged in patients with newly diagnosed and relapsed acute lymphocytic leukemia **(Option (B) is true),** whereas the T1 relaxation time of marrow in patients in remission is similar to that in age-matched normal controls (Figure 1-28). The etiology of this prolongation is uncertain. Both decreased marrow fat content and increased marrow cellularity have been suggested as contributors, since the T1 relaxation time of fat is shorter than that of cells. *In vitro,* leukemic blast cells show a longer T1 relaxation time than do normal marrow cells, suggesting that the T1 relaxation time of isolated leukemic cells is inherently prolonged. T1 relaxation time prolongation is not specific for leukemic cells; infiltration of the marrow by other types of neoplastic cells (e.g., rhabdomyosarcoma and neuroblastoma), as well as hyperplasia of myeloid cells, will also result in a prolongation of calculated marrow T1 relaxation time. No statistically significant differences between leukemic and normal marrow T2 relaxation times have been demonstrated.

Chemical-shift techniques allow acquisition of marrow images that reflect either the water (cellular marrow) or fat (fatty marrow) component of marrow. These images are referred to as "water-fraction" and "fat-fraction" images, respectively, and have been used to distinguish leukemic from normal marrow. When the percentage of hematopoietic or neoplastic cells in marrow is high, increased signal intensity is seen on the water-fraction image. The fat-fraction image shows a corresponding decreased signal intensity since there is little fatty marrow. On the other hand, when the percentage of fat cells in marrow is high, increased signal intensity is seen on the fat-fraction image, whereas a corresponding water-fraction image shows intermediate or low intensity. The relative signal intensities of the water- and fat-fraction images will reflect the relative percentages of cellular and fatty marrow. Therefore, marrow signal intensity in cell-rich leukemic marrow is generally decreased on fat-fraction images **(Option (C) is false)** and increased on water-fraction images. It may be more difficult to distinguish between normal and leukemic marrow in younger children, since the higher percentage of normal vertebral hematopoietic marrow in young children would necessarily increase the marrow signal intensity on water-fraction images whether or not leukemic infiltrate were present.

In addition to qualitative analysis of leukemic marrow on chemical-shift images, quantitative analysis of chemical-shift images in leukemic patients has been successful in further distinguishing normal from leukemic marrow. Calculation of the adult vertebral marrow T1 relaxation time for both the water and fat fractions shows a prolonged water-fraction T1 relaxation time in patients with acute leukemia and leukemia in relapse. Patients with leukemia in remission have a water-fraction T1 relaxation time similar to that of normal patients.

In vivo proton MR spectroscopy of tibial marrow and posterior iliac crest marrow in adult patients with leukemia shows a relative increase in the marrow water peak when compared with normal controls **(Option (D) is true)**. This increase reflects the predominant cellularity of leukemic marrow. With treatment, a decrease in the water peak reflects a decrease in the number of leukemic cells. This decrease in the water peak is accompanied by an increase in the fat peak (Figure 1-29).

Treatment for leukemia consists primarily of systemic chemotherapy and radiation therapy to the central nervous system. Following induction chemotherapy, the patient is treated with multiple cycles of chemotherapeutic agents and steroids; this is referred to as consolidation therapy. One of the major toxicities of the chemotherapeutic agents used in the treatment of leukemia is myeloid suppression. Therefore, aplastic anemia is a known complication of leukemia treatment. The aplastic anemia is often secondary to replacement of cellular marrow by fat. Less

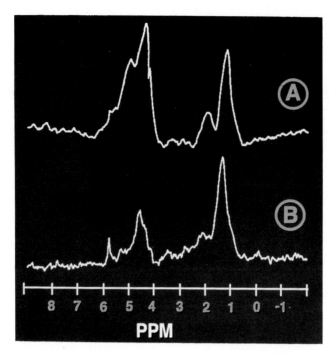

Figure 1-29. *In vivo* high-resolution, volume-selected hydrogen MR spectroscopy of human tibial marrow. (A) Large water peak representing cellular marrow (first peak) in a patient with leukemia. (B) MR spectrum following therapy for leukemia. There has been a decrease in the water (cellular) peak and a relative increase in the fat peak (second peak). This correlates with tumor response to therapy. (Reprinted with permission from Irving et al. [37].)

frequently, the marrow cavity is replaced by a combination of fat and fibrous tissue. On MR images, aplastic marrow usually has high signal intensity, reflecting the lack of hematopoietic cells. Occasionally, associated myelofibrosis results in patchy areas of high and low intensity on both T1- and T2-weighted images. Treated leukemia with resulting aplastic anemia does not manifest as low-intensity marrow **(Option (E) is false).** If diffuse low-intensity marrow is seen after therapy, relapsed leukemia or hemosiderosis should be considered.

Question 7

Concerning MRI of marrow,

(A) the susceptibility effect of trabecular bone is negligible on gradient-recalled-echo images
(B) focal metastatic lesions are usually bright on short-tau inversion-recovery (STIR) images
(C) fatty marrow has low signal intensity on fast-acquisition spin-echo images obtained with a TR of 2,500 msec
(D) fat-suppression techniques exploit the inherent resonant frequency differences of fat and water protons

Most MR images of marrow obtained in the clinical setting involve the use of a spin-echo technique; therefore, an understanding of marrow signal intensity on spin-echo images is necessary. When describing the signal intensity of marrow on spin-echo images, comparison is commonly made with the intensity of adjacent muscle. Marrow signal intensity that is lower than that of adjacent muscle is referred to as "low" signal intensity; marrow signal intensity that is equal to or slightly greater than that of adjacent muscle is referred to as "intermediate" signal intensity; and marrow signal intensity that approaches that of subcutaneous fat is referred to as "increased" or "high" signal intensity.

Yellow (fatty) marrow has a relatively short T1 relaxation time (ca. 400 to 600 msec) since most of the fat protons are in the form of hydrophobic CH_2 groups and therefore have an efficient spin-lattice relaxation. Spin-spin relaxation of fat is less efficient, and consequently the T2 relaxation time of fat is relatively longer than the T2 relaxation time of water. On T1-weighted MR images, fatty marrow has a signal intensity similar to that of subcutaneous fat; the intensity decreases slightly on T2-weighted images.

The signal intensity of hematopoietic marrow is complex compared with that of fatty marrow. Hematopoietic marrow contains cells, protein, and water. These components interact to give a relatively long T1 and a long T2 relaxation time. Therefore, the primarily hematopoietic marrow seen in the newborn has low signal intensity on T1-weighted images and has increased intensity on T2-weighted images. Hematopoietic marrow also contains a variable proportion of fat. The long T1 and T2 relaxation times of protein and water in the cellular component of hematopoietic marrow will be averaged with the short T1 and relatively long T2 relaxation times of this fat. Hematopoietic marrow will therefore range in signal intensity from low to increased depending on the relative percentages of hematopoietic and fatty marrow. Marrow that is completely hematopoietic, such as that seen in the newborn spine, usually has low signal intensity (Figure 1-26). As the percentage of fatty marrow

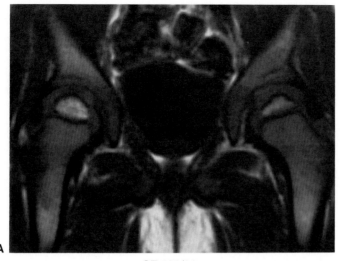

A

SE 600/20

Figure 1-30. Relative signal intensities of red and yellow marrow. (A) A T1-weighted coronal MR image through the pelvis in a 2-year-old girl shows intermediate-intensity red marrow in the proximal femoral metaphyses with increased-intensity yellow marrow in the epiphyses and proximal diaphyses. (B) The corresponding T2-weighted image shows that the signal intensity of the yellow marrow decreases, while that of the red marrow increases. There is greater contrast between the red and yellow marrow elements on the T1-weighted image than on the T2-weighted image.

increases, the signal intensity of the marrow on both T1- and T2-weighted images increases. On T2-weighted spin-echo images, the signal intensity of hematopoietic marrow remains unchanged to slightly increased compared with that on equivalent T1-weighted images (Figure 1-30). The contrast difference between yellow and red marrow diminishes and may nearly disappear on T2-weighted spin-echo images.

Gradient-recalled-echo (GRE) imaging exploits the use of a partial-flip-angle excitation pulse, which is typically less than 90°. This is followed by a gradient reversal to refocus the echo and generate the signal. Free induction decay is used for data acquisition so that the signal can be maximized. As a result, the marrow signal intensity will be dependent on the effective transverse relaxation time (T2*) and not on T2 as seen in spin-echo sequences. Two primary mechanisms affect the T2 and T2* tissue relaxation times: diffusion of spins and dephasing of the transverse magnetization. Diffusion of spins in the magnetic field gradients generated by susceptibility differences will cause an irreversible dephasing of

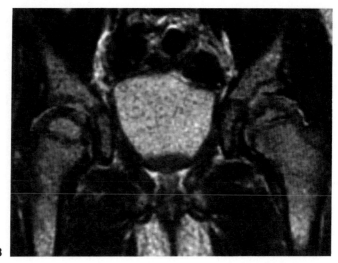

B

SE 2,000/70

T2*. This results in a shortening of T2* and a loss of signal on GRE images. The trabecular bone that forms the support matrix for marrow produces local field gradients resulting in inhomogeneous susceptibilities and T2* dephasing where the mineralized matrix interfaces with marrow. This shortened T2* time causes a loss of marrow signal in regions of marrow with the highest content of trabecular bone. Therefore, the susceptibility effect of trabecular bone on marrow can be a major factor in the determination of marrow signal intensity on GRE images (**Option (A) is false**).

The epiphyses, vertebral bodies, and other cancellous bones have the highest content of trabecular bone, whereas the metaphyses of long bones have a lower content and the diaphyses contain little or none. As a result, there is significant dephasing of protons in the epiphysis and vertebral body, intermediate dephasing of protons in the metaphysis, and little or no dephasing of protons in the diaphysis. This results in decreased-intensity marrow in the epiphyses and metaphyses on GRE images regardless of the character of the underlying marrow (whether fatty or hematopoietic), whereas the marrow in the diaphyseal region more accurately reflects the cellular composition of marrow (Figure 1-31).

GRE images of hematopoietic marrow reflect the magnetic susceptibility effect of iron as well as the susceptibility effect of trabecular bone. Iron present in hematopoietic marrow will cause local field gradients and T2* dephasing. This results in a greater decrease in marrow signal

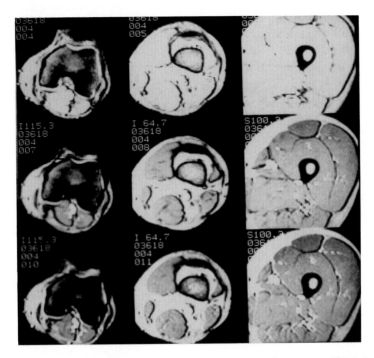

Figure 1-31. Susceptibility effect of trabecular bone on GRE images. Transaxial GRE (TR 60/30°) images through the femoral epiphysis (first column), femoral metaphysis (second column), and femoral diaphysis (third column) in a normal 28-year-old man. Images were acquired at a TE of 12 msec (first row), 16 msec (second row), and 20 msec (third row). With increasing TE, there is an increasing magnetic susceptibility effect on the marrow in the trabecular-rich epiphysis, whereas no magnetic susceptibilty effect is seen in the trabecular-poor diaphysis. An intermediate susceptibility effect is seen in the femoral metaphysis, which has a mild to moderate amount of trabecular bone. The trabecular susceptibility effect is manifested as progressive loss of marrow signal intensity. (Reproduced with permission from Sebag and Moore [49].)

intensity than would be expected from trabecular bone alone (Figure 1-32).

The susceptibility effect of trabecular bone on marrow can affect the appearance of marrow lesions on GRE images. Blastic lesions that occur in highly trabeculated regions of bone may not be readily identified, since dense trabecular bone and blastic bone both produce a susceptibility effect. This is most obvious in the epiphyses, where the density of trabecular bone is greatest. On the other hand, lytic lesions in regions of bone with high trabecular bone content may be seen as focal areas of increased signal intensity (Figure 1-33).

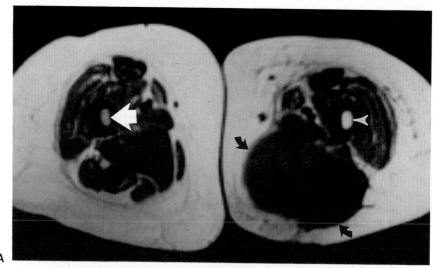

SE 300/15

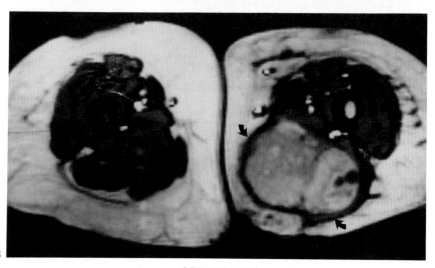

GRE 60/12/30°

Figure 1-32. Susceptibility effect of iron on GRE images. T1-weighted
(A) and GRE (B) transaxial MR images through the femora in a patient
following chemotherapy and radiation therapy for a left thigh liposarcoma. On the T1-weighted image, the signal intensity of marrow (white
arrow) in the right femoral diaphysis is increased but is less so than that
of subcutaneous fat, indicating some component of hematopoietic marrow. In the left diaphysis, the marrow shows even higher intensity (white
arrowhead). This feature is probably secondary to the radiation therapy
that the patient received for her liposarcoma (black arrows). On the GRE
image, a marked decrease in marrow signal intensity is seen in the right
mid-femur; since the diaphysis contains no trabecular bone, this susceptibility effect is probably secondary to iron within hematopoietic marrow.
The signal intensity of the marrow in the left femur remains high,
reflecting the absence of both trabecular bone and hematopoietic marrow
and therefore the lack of either susceptibility effect. (Reprinted with permission from Moore [3].)

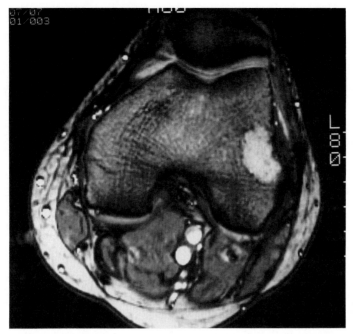

GRE 80/12/30°

Figure 1-33. Susceptibility effect and lesion recognition. A GRE trans-axial image through the distal femur in a 40-year-old man with intra-osseous lipoma shows that the susceptibility effect of the epiphyseal trabecular bone on the epiphyseal marrow results in a diminished signal intensity of otherwise yellow marrow. The intraosseous lipoma has high signal intensity, reflecting the lack of trabecular bone within the lesion. (Reprinted with permission from Moore [3].)

Short-tau inversion-recovery (STIR) images result from acquisition of signal following an initial 180° pulse, a 90° pulse, and a second 180° pulse to rephase the protons. The 90° pulse is given at a time when fat protons are at the "null point," so that fat protons and protons with a T1 relaxation time similar to that of fat (approximately 350 msec) do not emit a signal that can be received by the coil. The "null point" (phase re-construction) or the "bounce point" (magnitude reconstruction) is the in-version time (TI, or the time between the initial 180° pulse and the 90° pulse) which will result in suppression of signal from a species with a particular T1 relaxation time. The TI chosen will depend on the T1 relaxation time of the tissue for which suppression is desired and on the field strength of the magnet. Since signal intensity on the STIR image is dependent on T1, T2, and proton density, it can be described by the simplified formula $SI = N(H) [1 - 2e^{-TI/T1}] e^{-TE/T2}$, where SI = signal intensity and N(H) = proton density. The "null point" can therefore be approximated when $1 - 2e^{-TI/T1} = 0$ (i.e., when $1 = 2e^{-TI/T1}$ or when $e^{-TI/T1} = 0.5$). The TI can then be approximated as 0.69T1. For STIR images, TI is chosen so that fat signal is suppressed; it is approximately 150 msec at 1.5 T and 100 msec at 0.5 T.

The T1 and T2 contrast is additive in STIR images, and this, combined with the lack of signal from fatty marrow, results in increased marrow lesion conspicuity **(Option (B) is true).** On STIR images, the signal from fat and any tissue with a T1 relaxation time similar to that of fat is suppressed, resulting in very low signal intensity (black). Air, fibrosis, calcification, and paramagnetic substances (e.g., gadolinium and hemorrhage) all have low intensity on STIR images. Muscle has intermediate signal intensity on STIR images, and fluid, edema, lymph nodes, and neoplastic tissue all appear bright.

The spectrum of marrow signal intensity on STIR images depends on the relative percentages of hematopoietic and fatty marrow. Predominantly fatty marrow has very low intensity, and predominantly hematopoietic marrow exhibits intermediate to increased intensity (Figure 1-34). When trying to distinguish normal red marrow from a marrow lesion or abnormal infiltrated marrow, one can use the relative signal intensities of marrow and muscle. In general, the signal intensity of hematopoietic marrow is similar to that of adjacent muscle on STIR images, while the intensity of marrow lesions or abnormal marrow is brighter than that of adjacent muscle (Figures 1-4 and 1-34). Focal lesions that have high signal intensity, have adjacent marrow or soft tissue edema, and are not in regions of expected hematopoietic marrow are easy to recognize as abnormal. Not all focal lesions seen on STIR images are neoplastic; lesions such as aneurysmal bone cysts, Paget's disease, and fibrous dysplasia can also be seen as high-intensity foci on STIR images.

Fast-acquisition spin-echo (FSE) imaging produces high-resolution images with long TRs (in the range of 4,000 to 5,000 msec) in reasonable scan times. FSE images are acquired with use of altered k-space filling. k-space is defined as the amount of space that must be filled with information that can be mathematically manipulated (by Fourier transformation) to form an image. It can also be defined as image raw data or as the intersection of one frequency-encoded axis and one phase-encoded axis. The manner in which k-space is filled will affect the appearance of the final image, and FSE imaging uses altered k-space filling, or traversal, to provide conventional spin-echo type image contrast at rates up to 16 times higher than for conventional spin-echo sequences. In conventional spin-echo imaging, the phase-encoded gradient is applied only once regardless of the number of echoes being generated. Therefore, each echo possesses the same phase encoding, and only one line of k-space is filled

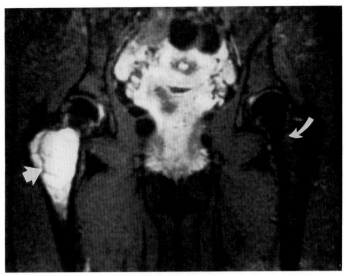

STIR 1,500/30/100

Figure 1-34. Relative signal intensity on a STIR coronal image through the pelvis in a child with a right proximal femoral aneurysmal bone cyst. The aneurysmal bone cyst has very high signal intensity (straight arrow) and is easily distinguished from the surrounding suppressed fatty marrow and mineralized bone. In the left proximal femur, intermediate-intensity hematopoietic marrow can be identified (curved arrow). The signal intensity of the hematopoietic marrow in this region and in the pelvic bones is similar to that of adjacent muscle.

for each repetition (TR interval). In the FSE pulse sequence, an initial 90° pulse is followed by the acquisition of 2 to 16 echoes, each acquired with a different value of the phase-encoding gradient. Multiple lines of k-space can therefore be filled for each TR interval repeated.

The number of lines of k-space filled per TR interval will depend on the number of echo acquisitions that follow each 90° pulse. This number is referred to as the "echo-train (ET) length," and the time between each echo is referred to as the "echo space." The greater the ET, the less time is required to obtain an image. The middle lines of k-space are associated with the greatest signal and therefore have the highest impact on image contrast. Peripheral lines of k-space, which are at high spatial frequency, are in fact acquired at a TE that is slightly different from the TE chosen by the operator for image acquisition. The TE actually used to obtain the FSE image is thus a complex averaging of multiple TEs, with most of the image signal and contrast acquired in the middle lines of k-space, at or near the TE defined by the operator. We therefore refer to the TE used in

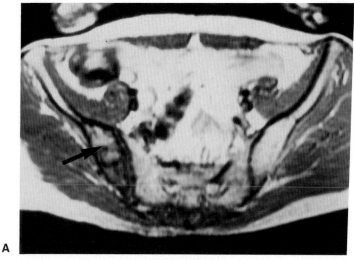

A

FSE 2,500/20

Figure 1-35. Relative signal intensity on FSE transaxial images through the pelvis in a patient with right iliac lymphoma. (A) A proton-density-weighted image shows heterogeneous intermediate signal intensity in the posterior right iliac crest (arrow), corresponding to the location of the lymphoma. (B) The signal intensity of the lesion increases on the T2-weighted image (arrow). Note the high signal intensity of fatty marrow on these FSE images.

acquisition of FSE images as the "effective TE." An image that has been acquired with an effective TE of 80 msec will have some signal contribution from the high-frequency lines acquired in the first 60 msec after excitation.

On FSE images, marrow signal intensity is similar to that on conventional spin-echo images, with increased-intensity fatty marrow and intermediate- to slightly increased-intensity hematopoietic marrow. At relatively long TRs (2,500 to 5,000 msec) the signal intensity of fatty marrow appears higher than that seen on conventional spin-echo MR images, without the expected drop-off in fat signal intensity **(Option (C) is false).** The reason for this is unclear, although the bright fatty signal may be the result of imaging with an averaged or effective TE as opposed to a single TE. When an effective TE of, say, 80 msec is selected for image acquisition, the contribution of fat signal acquired in the first 60 msec, which is fairly bright, may be enough to affect the overall appearance of fat on the effective-TE image of 80 msec or greater (Figure 1-35). Altered J-coupling of protons may also contribute to the high signal intensity of fatty marrow in FSE images. It can therefore be difficult to distinguish

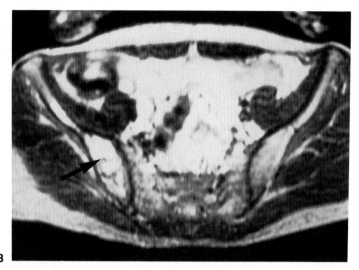

B

FSE 2,500/70

increased-intensity hematopoietic or abnormal marrow from fatty marrow on FSE images. To mitigate the effect of high-intensity fatty marrow on FSE images and to increase lesion conspicuity, FSE images are frequently obtained by fat-suppression techniques, which will suppress the signal from fatty marrow and therefore increase the conspicuity of hematopoietic marrow, infiltrated marrow, and marrow lesions containing higher water fractions.

Techniques that allow the acquisition of predominantly fat or predominantly water images exploit the chemical shift between fat and water protons. Fat and water protons have different chemical environments and therefore resonate at slightly different frequencies, providing the basis for the fat-suppression techniques used for conventional and fast spin-echo imaging **(Option (D) is true).** In clinical imaging, frequency-selective saturation of fat protons involves a typically long (several hundred milliseconds) low-intensity rectangular radiofrequency (RF) pulse. Fat and water protons dephase relative to each other following excitation, so the frequency of this pulse can be centered on the fat resonance. Fat magnetization is rotated multiple times in the direction of the applied RF field, which, when occurring simultaneously with T1 relaxation, will null the Z component of fat magnetization and block fat signal. This effect cannot be reversed until the fat protons return to equilibrium. The unexcited water component is then imaged with conventional spin-echo or fast spin-echo pulse sequences. Fatty marrow has low signal intensity, whereas hematopoietic marrow, marrow lesions, and

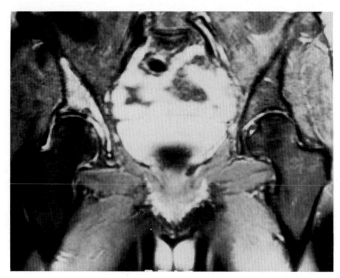

FSE 4,200/20 with fat saturation

Figure 1-36. Same patient as in Figure 1-35. FSE with fat saturation. A T2-weighted FSE coronal saturation image of the pelvis shows lymphoma as an area of bright signal intensity in the inferior right ilium; the fatty marrow is suppressed and has low to intermediate signal intensity.

abnormal marrow have high intensity (Figure 1-36). The major drawback of this technique is the need for a homogeneous magnetic field, so that currently images obtained with a field of view greater than 24 cm may show image inhomogeneity.

Discussion

In fetal life, most hematopoiesis occurs in the endodermal epithelium of the yolk sac. Beginning at the end of the fourth week, hematopoiesis is initiated in the liver, and until *in utero* bone ossification begins, the liver remains the primary organ of fetal hematopoiesis.

At birth, marrow found within the medullary cavity of ossified bone is hematopoietic and contains pluripotential stem cells that are capable of differentiating into discrete stem cell lines. These include erythroblasts, myeloblasts, and stem cells committed to the megakaryocyte line. In addition to these cellular elements, hematopoietic marrow contains some percentage of marrow fat cells and reticulum cells. Reticulum cells are a group of cells that characteristically form a reticulum or cytoplasmic network, a three-dimensional meshwork holding the vascular sinuses and hematopoietic elements in place. Some of these reticulum cells are phagocytic and contain multiple vesicles, liposomes, and a Golgi complex. These phagocytic reticulum cells are primarily responsible for the decreased MR signal intensity of marrow seen with iron loading, since ferritin aggregates are taken up by these cells and deposited primarily around the Golgi zone.

Yellow or fatty marrow is composed primarily of fat cells and reticulum and has a relatively short T1 relaxation time (approximate range 400 to 600 msec). T2 relaxation is relatively long, at least compared with that of water. The signal intensity of fatty marrow on conventional spin-echo images is similar to that of subcutaneous fat, being increased on T1-weighted images and slightly decreased on T2-weighted images. The complex structure of hematopoietic marrow accounts in large part for the variable signal intensity of hematopoietic marrow on spin-echo images.

The primary components of red or hematopoietic marrow are cellular elements, protein, and water. The interaction of these elements is complex and not completely understood; however, it has been observed that purely hematopoietic marrow has relatively long T1 and T2 relaxation times. These relatively long T1 and T2 relaxation times will be averaged with the short T1 and relatively long T2 relaxation times of any fat in hematopoietic marrow, so that the signal intensity of hematopoietic marrow on spin-echo MR images will range from low to increased. The exact contribution of fat cells to the overall signal intensity of hematopoietic marrow is unknown; however, observations of marrow signal intensity in the femur reveal that a relatively small percentage of fat cells within hematopoietic marrow will result in a marrow signal intensity that is higher than that of adjacent muscle. In general, hematopoietic marrow signal intensity is unchanged or slightly increased on T2-weighted images compared with T1-weighted images.

Following birth, there is progressive conversion of hematopoietic marrow to fatty marrow. It is thought that bone marrow fat is a primarily passive tissue that accommodates hematopoietic activity and maintains the constancy of marrow volume by decreasing in size and number of cells with active hematopoiesis and increasing in size and number of cells with decreased hematopoiesis. Conversion from red to yellow marrow occurs first in the distal long bones, then in the proximal long bones, and finally in the axial skeletal compartment. In addition to the "distal-to-proximal" trend for marrow conversion by anatomic site, marrow conversion occurs first in the diaphysis, then in the distal metaphysis, and finally in the proximal metaphysis. Epiphyseal marrow converts rapidly, so the epiphysis should be seen as increased-intensity yellow marrow at any age. The only exception to this would be in the newborn and young infant, when intermediate-intensity hematopoietic marrow is occasionally seen in ossifying epiphyses. The "adult pattern" of hematopoietic marrow includes residual red marrow in the vertebral bodies, flat bones, and skull, as well as in the proximal shafts of the femoral and humeral epiphyses.

In addition to the age-related MR patterns for marrow conversion in the long bones (Question 5), age-related patterns for conversion of pelvic marrow have been established. Conversion of red to yellow marrow in the pelvis occurs first in the anterior iliac crest and acetabulum, followed by the pubic symphysis, posterior iliac crest, and sacral alae. The symphysis, posterior iliac crest, and sacrum all maintain varying percentages of hematopoietic marrow with increasing patient age, so that the MR pattern of posterior pelvic marrow of intermediate to slightly increased intensity and anterior pelvic yellow marrow can persist in adults and should not be considered abnormal. During adolescence, significant pelvic marrow heterogeneity develops secondary to macroscopic foci of both hematopoietic and fatty marrow. This heterogeneity frequently persists in adult life and should be considered normal. To distinguish normal pelvic marrow heterogeneity from diffuse metastatic disease, T1- and T2-weighted spin-echo images should be compared. Normal marrow is usually more heterogeneous on T1-weighted images, in which signal intensity differences between normal red and yellow marrow are more pronounced, and more homogeneous on T2-weighted images. STIR or fat-saturation images can also be helpful in distinguishing normal pelvic heterogeneity from metastatic disease, since areas of metastatic disease can have significantly increased signal intensity on these sequences, whereas normal hematopoietic marrow may show only slightly increased intensity.

Hematopoietic disorders are often reflected in the MR signal intensity of the calvarial, sphenoid, and facial marrow, as well as the clival marrow. Initially, all bones of the face and skull contain red marrow. In healthy adolescents and adults, the calvarium and all facial bones except the maxilla, zygoma, and ethmoid contain contain primarily fatty marrow with some degree of hematopoietic marrow. The maxilla, zygoma, and ethmoid contain only fatty marrow. Calvarial marrow has uniformly low to intermediate signal intensity on T1-weighted images in most infants less than 1 year of age. There is progressive conversion of yellow to red calvarial marrow with age, so that by age 15 most patients have homogeneous high-intensity fatty marrow in the calvarium. The signal intensity of marrow in the occipital, parietal, and frontal regions in male subjects tends to be somewhat higher than that in female subjects in the second decade. Two normal subjects in one study had low- to intermediate-intensity calvarial marrow into the second decade of life, indicating that the normal range for MR signal intensity of calvarial marrow occasionally lies outside these guidelines. Fatty marrow is seen in the frontal region of the skull in about 5% of patients less than 1 year of age.

Vertebral marrow contains the greatest percentage of hematopoietic marrow and is among the first regions of marrow to respond to the need for increased hematopoiesis; therefore, specific MR patterns of marrow conversion with age have not been established. There are age-related trends of marrow signal intensity, beginning at birth, when low-intensity hematopoietic vertebral marrow is seen uniformly. There is a progressive increase in hematopoietic marrow signal intensity with increasing percentages of fat, so that the intensity of vetebral marrow on T1-weighted images begins to approximate that of muscle in early childhood. On T1-weighted images (at 0.5 T), the signal intensity of vertebral marrow is similar to or lower than that of the adjacent cartilaginous disk in about 90% of children less than 1 year of age, whereas the signal intensity of vertebral marrow is greater than that of the adjacent disk in about 90% of children between the ages of 5 and 15 years. In adults, the signal intensity of vertebral marrow should be greater than that of the adjacent disk; lower intensity probably indicates an abnormality. When suspicious low-intensity vertebral marrow is identified, abnormal low marrow signal intensity in the long bones or increased vertebral marrow signal intensity on T2-weighted or STIR images increases the level of confidence in diagnosing abnormal vertebral marrow.

The signal intensity of the vascular, largely hematopoietic vertebral bodies seen in the newborn can increase with gadolinium administration during the first year of life. This enhancement of normal hematopoietic marrow should not be confused with an abnormal marrow process, such as infiltration by malignant cells. Enhancement of the signal intensity of vertebral marrow in adults and older children should be considered abnormal. Marrow heterogeneity, focal fibrosis, sclerosis, and fatty deposition are all normal findings in the vertebral bodies. There may be one of several patterns of fatty marrow deposition along vertebral end plates, which may be the result of aging or the effect of local marrow ischemia adjacent to a degenerative lumbar disk.

Focal fatty vertebral marrow can be seen in children as young as 10 months, and these changes can be either isolated or multifocal, peripheral (located adjacent to the end plates) or central. About 15% of children under the age of 10 years have focal fatty vertebral marrow, whereas more than 90% of adult patients over the age of 50 exhibit this phenomenon. Focal fatty infiltration of vertebral marrow is more frequent in the lumbar spine. "Polka dot" spine (central focal areas of fat within vertebral marrow) is another normal finding on MR images of the vertebral bodies.

In the vertebral body, blood is supplied via a nutrient artery that enters the posterior aspect of the vertebral body and courses anteriorly with the basivertebral vein. Branches of the nutrient artery decussate at the vertebral end plates, forming endosteal sinusoids. Most hematopoietic cells are found in these endosteal sinusoids, and the central region of marrow, surrounding the basivertebral vein, is normally populated by fatty marrow. This is reflected on MR images of the spine, where focal regions of fat surround the basivertebral vein on sagittal or coronal T1-weighted images. Malignant cells, when present, may not respect the normal boundaries within the vertebral body, and therefore obliteration of the fatty marrow surrounding the basivertebral vein is not uncommon in patients with malignant infiltration of vertebral marrow. Preservation of central fat seems more characteristic of hyperplastic than malignant marrow.

Focal regions of intermediate-intensity "red" marrow can be seen in the distal femoral and proximal tibial metaphyses during MR examination of the knee in adult patients. Attempts have been made to correlate the appearance and amount of this hematopoietic marrow with underlying hematopoietic disease. The hematocrit and peripheral smear in many anemic patients are normal, and there has been no correlation between the amount of distal femoral metaphyseal "hematopoietic" marrow and the degree of anemia. This MR appearance of the knees is therefore a frequent normal finding, and although determination of the hematocrit and examination of the peripheral smear are not unreasonable, the frequency of hematopoietic abnormality does not appear sufficient to warrant further investigation such as bone marrow biopsy.

Adult marrow is predominantly yellow, but it forms a large reserve potentially available for the formation of blood cells. Marrow "reconversion" is a term used to describe the activation of quiescent hematopoietic precursors, resulting in repopulation of fatty marrow by active hematopoietic cells. Stress, anemia, or infiltration of red marrow by neoplastic cells can initiate this reconversion process. Reconversion tends to occur in a pattern converse to that of red-to-yellow marrow conversion (Figure 1-37). Reconversion occurs first in the spine and flat bones, followed by the long bones and finally the hands and feet.

Homogeneous low-intensity marrow is probably abnormal in an adult, except when it is confined to focal areas of expected hematopoiesis. In pathologic states when there has been either extensive reconversion of yellow to red marrow or replacement of normal marrow by neoplastic cells, the marrow signal intensity may be equal to or lower than that of muscle on T1-weighted images. The older the patient and the lower the

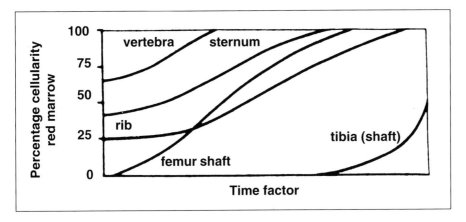

Figure 1-37. Reconversion of fatty marrow to hematopoietic marrow. Diagram shows relative amounts of macroscopic hematopoietic marrow in different anatomic sites. The percentage of hematopoietic marrow increases in proportion to the stimulus and progresses from proximal to distal. Bones that already have a significant hematopoietic fraction are recruited earlier and faster than those that do not.

marrow signal intensity compared with that of muscle, the more likely it is that an abnormality exists. Distal long bones, hands and feet, and epiphyses and apophyses show late recruitment of yellow to red marrow. The more severe the marrow abnormality, the more likely it is that peripheral regions of marrow will show abnormal marrow signal intensity.

   Disorders that affect bone marrow production and increase the need for reconversion and hematopoiesis can be divided into four major categories: stem cell failure, uncontrolled marrow hyperplasia, stem cell dysplasia, and malignant transformation. Causes of marrow stem cell failure include granulomatous and viral infection, chemical agents such as organic solvents, medications including chemotherapeutic agents, chloramphenicol, and ionizing radiation. These myelotoxic agents decrease the number of erythroid, myeloid, and platelet precursors and result in pancytopenia. Aplastic anemia may be irreversible but can respond to the administration of androgens, immunosuppressive therapy, high-dose steroids, or antithymocyte globulin. Hypocellular or aplastic bone marrow is characterized on MR images by increased signal intensity on T1- and T2-weighted images as a result of generalized replacement of hematopoietic marrow by fatty marrow. In children this may be appreciated in all regions, whereas in adults it is most noticeable in the spine, flat bones, and proximal femora. In addition to replacement of hematopoietic marrow by fatty marrow, regions of focal fibrosis frequently accompany marrow extinction. This is seen as patchy areas of low intensity on both T1- and T2-weighted images.

Uncontrolled proliferation of one or more of the normal bone marrow cell lines results in marrow hyperplasia and an increase in the number of circulating cells. This proliferation may be controlled, such as that seen in response to infection, or uncontrolled, such as that seen in patients with myelodysplastic syndromes. Acute and chronic myelogenous leukemia, polycythemia vera, and myelofibrosis all result from uncontrolled stem cell proliferation. On MR examination, the marrow most frequently has low signal intensity on T1-weighted images with slightly increased intensity on T2-weighted images or, in patients with myelofibrosis, low intensity on both T1- and T2-weighted images. Low-intensity marrow is present in regions that would normally show increased-intensity fatty marrow. Calculation of the T1 relaxation time of vertebral marrow in patients with polycythemia vera shows a prolongation of T1 relaxation similar to that seen in leukemic patients, with a range of relaxation times from 690 to 970 msec.

Bone marrow changes in patients with stem cell dysplasias such as sickle-cell anemia, thalassemia, and spherocytosis tend to be diffuse and indicative of disease severity. On T1-weighted images, the hyperplastic marrow has intermediate to low signal intensity, whereas on T2-weighted images the marrow signal typically increases in intensity. Hyperplastic marrow is frequently seen in the epiphyses and distal metaphyses. Medullary infarction is a common complication of these disorders, particularly sickle-cell anemia. Marrow infarction in patients without sickle-cell anemia generally occurs in regions of fatty marrow because of its decreased vascularity, but bone marrow infarction in patients with sickling disorder is unique in that it occurs primarily in regions of hematopoietic marrow. Acute infarction typically results in intermediate signal intensity on T1-weighted images and increased intensity on T2-weighted images. Hemosiderosis secondary to repeated transfusions in patients with stem cell dysplasias can result in very low marrow signal intensity on T2-weighted images, an MR characteristic of hemosiderosis (Figure 1-38).

Finally, the signal intensity of marrow in patients with malignant bone marrow infiltration and replacement is seen primarily as diffuse or focal low signal intensity on T1-weighted images and isointense or increased intensity on T2-weighted images. Either as a result of the inherent population of these cells in regions of hematopoietic marrow (e.g., in patients with leukemia or lymphoma) or as a result of the rich vascularity of hematopoietic marrow when compared with that of fatty marrow (for metastatic disease), malignant infiltration of marrow is expected first in the spine, flat bones, calvarium, and proximal humeral

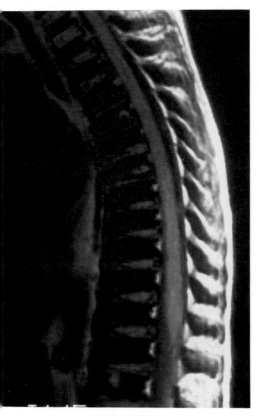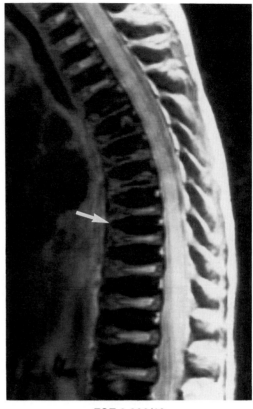

SE 800/20   FSE 3,000/18

Figure 1-38. Thalassemia. T1-weighted (A) and T2-weighted FSE (B) sagittal MR images show diffuse low-intensity vertebral bodies, which are flattened and exhibit anterior beaking (arrow in panel B). The diffusely decreased signal intensity of the marrow on both images is consistent with iron overload; the anterior beaking of the vertebral body is characteristic of thalassemia.

and femoral metaphyses. Late infiltration occurs in the remainder of the peripheral skeleton. Marrow changes in patients with leukemia are primarily diffuse, whereas those in patients with lymphoma are more regional or focal. Metastatic marrow infiltration such as that seen in patients with neuroblastoma can be diffuse or focal. When focal metastatic lesions are identified in marrow, they may be accompanied by marrow edema. In the final analysis, a biopsy is commonly necessary to arrive at a specific tissue diagnosis.

Sheila G. Moore, M.D.

SUGGESTED READINGS

MEDULLARY INFARCTION

1. Kirby CL, Meyer SJF, Dalinka MK. Magnetic resonance imaging evaluation of avascular necrosis of the hip. In: Bloem JL, Sartoris DJ (eds), MRI and CT of the musculoskeletal system: a text-atlas. Baltimore: Williams & Wilkins; 1992:324–336
2. Mitchell DG, Kressel HY. MR imaging of early avascular necrosis. Radiology 1988; 169:281–282
3. Moore SG. Pediatric musculoskeletal imaging. In: Stark DD, Bradley WG Jr (eds), Magnetic resonance imaging, 2nd ed. St. Louis: Mosby-Year Book; 1992:2223–2330
4. Moore SG, Sebag GH. Primary disorders of bone marrow. In: Cohen MD, Edwards MK (eds), Magnetic resonance imaging of children. Philadelphia: BC Decker; 1990:765–824
5. Totty WG, Murphy WA, Ganz WI, Kumar B, Daum WJ, Siegel BA. Magnetic resonance imaging of the normal and ischemic femoral head. AJR 1984; 143:1273–1280

SICKLE-CELL ANEMIA

6. Kirsch DL, Colletti PM, Zee CS, Destian S, Raval JK. MRI of the skull. Magn Reson Imaging 1990; 8:217–222
7. Rao VM, Fishman M, Mitchell DG, et al. Painful sickle cell crisis: bone marrow patterns observed with MR imaging. Radiology 1986; 161:211–215
8. Rao VM, Mitchell DG, Rifkin MD, et al. Marrow infarction in sickle cell anemia: correlation with marrow type and distribution by MRI. Magn Reson Imaging 1989; 7:39–44
9. Sebes JI. Diagnostic imaging of bone and joint abnormalities associated with sickle cell hemoglobinopathies. AJR 1989; 152:1153–1159
10. Steiner RM, Mitchell DG, Rao VM, Rifkin MD. Magnetic resonance imaging of bone marrow disorders. In: Bloem JL, Sartoris DJ (eds), MRI and CT of the musculoskeletal system: a text-atlas. Baltimore: Williams & Wilkins; 1992:108–129
11. Van Zanten TE, Statius van Eps LW, Golding RP, Valk J. Imaging the bone marrow with magnetic resonance during a crisis and in chronic forms of sickle cell disease. Clin Radiol 1989; 40:486–489

LYMPHOMA

12. Beatty PT, Bjorkengren AG, Moore SG, Gelb AB, Gamble JG. Case report 764: Primary lymphoma of bone, large cell, B-phenotype with articular involvement. Skeletal Radiol 1992; 21:559–561
13. Castellino RA, Parker BR. Non-Hodgkin's lymphoma. In: Parker BR, Castellino RA (eds), Pediatric oncologic radiology. St. Louis: CV Mosby; 1977:183–208

14. Linden A, Zankovich R, Theissen P, Diehl V, Schicha H. Malignant lymphoma: bone marrow imaging versus biopsy. Radiology 1989; 173:335–339

15. Olson DO, Shields AF, Scheurich CJ, Porter BA, Moss AA. Magnetic resonance imaging of the bone marrow in patients with leukemia, aplastic anemia, and lymphoma. Invest Radiol 1986; 21:540–546

16. Shields AF, Porter BA, Churchley S, Olson DO, Appelbaum FR, Thomas ED. The detection of bone marrow involvement by lymphoma using magnetic resonance imaging. J Clin Oncol 1987; 5:225–230

MARROW RADIATION EFFECT

17. Ramsey RG, Zacharias CE. MR imaging of the spine after radiation therapy: easily recognizable effects. AJR 1985; 144:1131–1135

18. Remedios PA, Colletti PM, Raval JK, et al. Magnetic resonance imaging of bone after radiation. Magn Reson Imaging 1988; 6:301–304

19. Stevens SK, Moore SG, Kaplan ID. Early and late bone marrow changes after irradiation: MR evaluation. AJR 1990; 154:745–750

20. Sykes MP, Chu FCH, Wilkerson WG. Local bone-marrow changes secondary to therapeutic irradiation. Radiology 1960; 75:919–924

APLASTIC ANEMIA

21. Cohen MD, Klatte EC, Baehner R, et al. Magnetic resonance imaging of bone marrow disease in children. Radiology 1984; 151:715–718

22. Kaplan PA, Asleson RJ, Klassen LW, Duggan MJ. Bone marrow patterns in aplastic anemia: observations with 1.5-T MR imaging. Radiology 1987; 164:441–444

MARROW DISTRIBUTION AND SPIN ECHO APPEARANCE

23. Algra PR, Bloem JL. Magnetic resonance imaging of metastatic disease and multiple myeloma. In: Bloem JL, Sartoris DJ (eds), MRI and CT of the musculoskeletal system: a text-atlas. Baltimore: Williams & Wilkins; 1992:218–235

24. Aoki S, Dillon WP, Barkovich AJ, Norman D. Marrow conversion before pneumatization of the sphenoid sinus: assessment with MR imaging. Radiology 1989; 172:373–375

25. Cristy M. Active bone marrow distribution as a function of age in humans. Phys Med Biol 1981; 26:389–400

26. Dawson KL, Moore SG, Rowland JM. Age-related marrow changes in the pelvis: MR and anatomic findings. Radiology 1992; 183:47–51

27. Dooms GC, Fisher MR, Hricak H, Richardson M, Crooks LE, Genant HK. Bone marrow imaging: magnetic resonance studies related to age and sex. Radiology 1985; 155:429–432

28. Kricun ME. Red-yellow marrow conversion: its effect on the location of some solitary bone lesions. Skeletal Radiol 1985; 14:10–19

29. Modic MT, Steinberg PM, Ross JS, Masaryk TJ, Carter JR. Degenerative disk disease: assessment of changes in vertebral body marrow with MR imaging. Radiology 1988; 166:193–199

30. Moore SG, Dawson KL. Red and yellow marrow in the femur: age-related changes in appearance at MR imaging. Radiology 1990; 175:219–223

31. Okada Y, Aoki S, Barkovich AJ, et al. Cranial bone marrow in children: assessment of normal development with MR imaging. Radiology 1989; 171:161–164

32. Ricci C, Cova M, Kang YS, et al. Normal age-related patterns of cellular and fatty bone marrow distribution in the axial skeleton: MR imaging study. Radiology 1990; 177:83–88

33. Steiner RM, Mitchell DG, Rao VM, et al. Magnetic resonance imaging of bone marrow: diagnostic value in diffuse hematologic disorders. Magn Reson Q 1990; 6:17–34

34. Sze G, Bravo S, Baierl P, Shimkin PM. Developing spinal column: gadolinium-enhanced MR imaging. Radiology 1991; 180:497–502

35. Trubowitz S, Davis S. The bone marrow matrix. In: Trubowitz S, Davis S (eds), The human bone marrow: anatomy, physiology, and pathophysiology. Boca Raton, FL: CRC Press; 1982:43–75

36. Vogler JB III, Murphy WA. Bone marrow imaging. Radiology 1988; 168: 679–693

LEUKEMIA

37. Irving MG, Brooks WM, Brereton IM, et al. Use of high resolution *in vivo* volume selected [1]H-magnetic resonance spectroscopy to investigate leukemia in humans. Cancer Res 1987; 47:3901–3906

38. Jenkins JP, Stehling M, Sivewright G, Hickey DS, Hillier VF, Isherwood I. Quantitative magnetic resonance imaging of vertebral bodies: a T1 and T2 study. Magn Reson Imaging 1989; 7:17–23

39. Jensen KE, Thomsen C, Henriksen O, Hertz H, Johansen HK, Yssing M. Changes in T1 relaxation processes in the bone marrow following treatment in children with acute lymphoblastic leukemia. A magnetic resonance imaging study. Pediatr Radiology 1990; 20:464–468

40. Kusnierz-Glaz C, Reiser M, Hagemeister B, Büchner T, Hiddemann W, van de Loo J. Magnetic resonance imaging follow-up in patients with acute leukemia during induction chemotherapy. Hamatol Bluttransfus 1990; 33:351–356

41. McKinstry CS, Steiner RE, Young AT, Jones L, Swirsky D, Aber V. Bone marrow in leukemia and aplastic anemia: MR imaging before, during, and after treatment. Radiology 1987; 162:701–707

42. Moore SG, Gooding CA, Brasch RC, et al. Bone marrow in children with acute lymphocytic leukemia: MR relaxation times. Radiology 1986; 160: 237–240

43. Nyman R, Rehn S, Glimelius B, et al. Magnetic resonance imaging in diffuse malignant bone marrow diseases. Acta Radiol 1987; 28:199–205

44. Rosen BR, Fleming DM, Kushner DC, et al. Hematologic bone marrow disorders: quantitative chemical shift MR imaging. Radiology 1988; 169: 799–804

45. Thomsen C, Sörensen PG, Karle H, Christoffersen P, Henriksen O. Prolonged bone marrow T1-relaxation in acute leukaemia. *In vivo* tissue characterization by magnetic resonance imaging. Magn Reson Imaging 1987; 5:251–257

46. Graif M, Pennock JM, Pringle J, et al. Magnetic resonance imaging: comparison of four pulse sequences in assessing primary bone tumours. Skeletal Radiol 1989; 18:439–444
47. Majumdar S, Thomasson D, Shimakawa A, Genant HK. Quantitation of the susceptibility difference between trabecular bone and bone marrow: experimental studies. Magn Reson Med 1991; 22(1):111–127
48. Rosenthal H, Thulborn KR, Rosenthal DI, Kim SH, Rosen BR. Magnetic susceptibility effects of trabecular bone on magnetic resonance bone marrow imaging. Invest Radiol 1990; 25:173–178
49. Sebag GH, Moore SG. Effect of trabecular bone on the appearance of marrow in gradient-echo imaging of the appendicular skeleton. Radiology 1990; 174:855–859
50. Szumowski J, Simon JH. Proton chemical shift imaging. In: Stark DD, Bradley WG Jr (eds), Magnetic resonance imaging. St. Louis: Mosby-Year Book; 1992:479–521

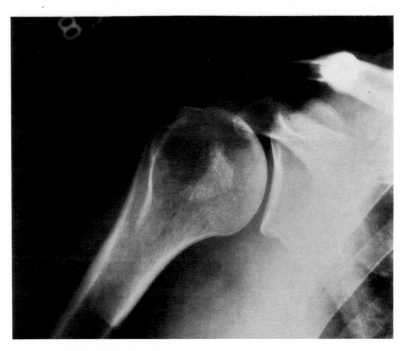

Figure 2-1. This 35-year-old man injured his right shoulder. You are shown an anteroposterior radiograph of the shoulder.

Case 2: Tuberosity Fracture

Question 8

Which *one* of the following is the MOST likely diagnosis?

(A) Tuberosity avulsion fracture
(B) Giant cell tumor
(C) Chondroblastoma
(D) Humeral pseudocyst
(E) Hill-Sachs deformity

The history of shoulder trauma suggests a diagnosis of fracture in the test case. However, nontraumatic shoulder lesions are often incidentally found in patients who are referred for radiography because of an injury, and other diagnoses must be considered as well. The anteroposterior radiograph, obtained in the posterior oblique position with external rotation of the humerus (Figure 2-1), shows a well-defined lucency at the lateral aspect of the humeral head, in the region of the greater and lesser tuberosities (Figure 2-2). The key to the correct diagnosis is the triangular area of increased density superimposed on the humeral head, just medial to the radiolucency. The radiolucency is due to a bony defect at the site of an avulsion fracture, and the triangular density represents the avulsed and displaced bone fragment superimposed on the humeral head. This combination of radiographic findings and the history of trauma is most consistent with the diagnosis of a tuberosity fracture **(Option (A) is correct).** On the basis of the anteroposterior radiograph alone, it cannot be determined whether the site of the avulsion is the greater or lesser tuberosity. However, an axillary view (Figure 2-3) revealed that the fragment was situated anteriorly, consistent with a fracture of the lesser tuberosity.

Giant cell tumor (Option (B)) and chondroblastoma (Option (C)) are lytic tumors that tend to involve bone epiphyses. Both of these tumors may involve the accessory epiphyses (also termed apophyses or tuberosities) of the proximal humerus. However, neither a giant cell tumor nor a chondroblastoma would have the triangular radiodensity seen in the test

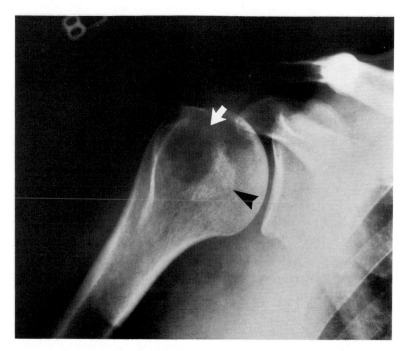

Figure 2-2 (Same as Figure 2-1). Avulsion fracture of the lesser tuberosity. An anteroposterior radiograph in the posterior oblique position with external rotation of the humerus shows a well-defined lucency (arrow) at the lateral aspect of the humeral head. Adjacent to the lucency is a triangular radiodensity (arrowhead), consistent with a fracture fragment superimposed on the humeral head.

image, and therefore these diagnoses are unlikely. Furthermore, chondroblastoma is rarely seen in patients over the age of 25 years.

A humeral pseudocyst (Option (D)) is a rarefaction of trabeculae often seen at the lateral aspect of the humeral head. This normal variant may mimic a lytic lesion in the humerus. Unlike the radiographic appearance of an avulsion fracture, a chondroblastoma, or a giant cell tumor, all of which are expected to show sharp margination from the surrounding normal bone, the radiolucency of a pseudocyst would be expected to merge gradually with the surrounding normal trabeculae. Furthermore, a pseudocyst would not explain the area of increased density seen in the test case, and it is therefore an unlikely diagnosis.

A Hill-Sachs deformity (Option (E)) is a wedge-shaped impaction fracture in the posterosuperior aspect of the humeral head; it is caused by anterior dislocation of the humerus. It usually appears as a triangular defect of the surface of the humeral head on neutral or internal rotation views. On radiographs taken with the arm in external rotation, an area

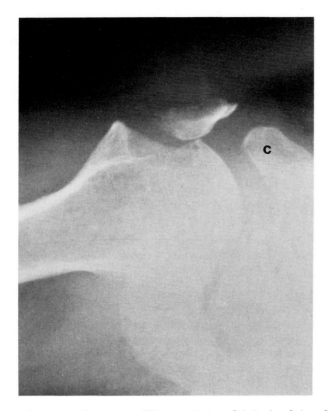

Figure 2-3. Same patient as in Figures 2-1 and 2-2. Avulsion fracture of the lesser tuberosity. Axillary radiograph reveals that the fracture fragment is avulsed anteriorly and rotated 180°. c = coracoid process.

of radiolucency due to the bone defect may be seen. However, the radiolucency resulting from a Hill-Sachs deformity would be located more superiorly than the radiolucency seen in the test image. A Hill-Sachs deformity is therefore not the most likely diagnosis.

Question 9

Concerning fractures of the proximal humerus,

    (A) in the Neer classification, a comminuted nondisplaced fracture is a two-part fracture
    (B) most are nondisplaced
    (C) isolated tuberosity avulsions are usually pathologic fractures
    (D) a four-part fracture is associated with a greater than 50% chance of avascular necrosis

The Neer classification is the most widely used system for classifying proximal humeral fractures. Its value lies in its clinical usefulness in predicting fracture prognosis and guiding treatment. In evaluating these fractures, the orthopedic surgeon is less concerned with the number of fracture fragments (comminution) than with the degree of displacement or angulation of major fragments. Nondisplaced fractures, even those with many fragments, do not require surgical intervention. However, surgery may be performed when there is significant separation or rotation of fragments that could lead to compromise of function or to chronic pain.

The Neer classification defines four potential major fracture fragments in the proximal humerus: the articular segment, the greater tuberosity, the lesser tuberosity, and the humeral shaft. Fractures of the proximal humerus can involve these four parts in a variety of combinations. By considering each of the four possible fragments independently, a fracture may be classified as a two-part, three-part, or four-part fracture depending on whether each fragment is displaced. Only a displaced fragment is considered to be a separate "part," and the four categories of the Neer classification are based on the number of fracture fragments that are either displaced by more than 1 cm from their usual location or rotated more than 45°. Therefore, nondisplaced fractures of the proximal humerus, regardless of how many fracture lines are seen in the radiograph, are considered one-part fractures **(Option (A) is false).**

More than 80% of fractures of the proximal humerus are nondisplaced, one-part fractures **(Option (B) is true).** This type is more commonly referred to as a nondisplaced fracture rather than as a one-part fracture. These fractures are treated conservatively, and the prognosis for complete recovery is good. In any proximal humeral fracture, the articular portion of the head can be dislocated out of the glenoid fossa, resulting in a fracture dislocation.

The isolated avulsion fracture of the lesser tuberosity in the test patient is a two-part fracture because of the displacement and angulation of the avulsed fragment. Most isolated avulsion fractures of the greater or lesser tuberosity are due to trauma, often sports related, and are not a result of an underlying pathologic condition **(Option (C) is false).** Isolated avulsion fractures of the greater tuberosity are common, but isolated fractures of the lesser tuberosity are rare.

Fractures of the lesser tuberosity are most often associated with posterior dislocations of the shoulder. The lesser tuberosity is protected from direct trauma by its small size and its location on the medial side of the humerus, and so the rare isolated fracture of the lesser tuberosity is usually due to avulsion by the attached tendon of the subscapularis muscle. The subscapularis muscle has its origin on the anterior surface of the scapula, and it is the only muscle to insert on the lesser tuberosity. This muscle causes internal rotation and adduction of the humerus. Avulsion of the lesser tuberosity occurs when the tendon is maximally stretched, with the arm externally rotated and abducted approximately 60°. The avulsed fragment is displaced anteriorly and medially by the attached subscapularis muscle, as in the test case.

The lesser tuberosity is depicted *en face* in anteroposterior radiographs performed in external rotation, and so small avulsions may not be recognized in this projection. A radiograph taken with the arm in internal rotation may bring the avulsed fragment into view. As demonstrated by the test patient, an axillary projection is important because it documents the anterior displacement of the avulsed fragment (Figure 2-3).

Individuals who suffer isolated avulsion of the lesser tuberosity are often involved in strenuous sports activities, and the actual event that resulted in the fracture may not be remembered. Typically, patients with this injury have point tenderness over the anterior aspect of the proximal humerus, limited rotation of the humerus, and pain during rotatory motion. In adults, this clinical presentation may lead to an incorrect diagnosis of calcific peritendinitis of the rotator cuff, a condition that often has similar symptoms. In children, isolated fractures of the lesser tuberosity probably occur through the relatively weak apophyseal plate of the tuberosity.

The prognosis is better for one- and two-part fractures than for three- and four-part fractures. In determining the classification of a fracture of the proximal humerus, CT scanning may be required to determine the exact relationship of fragments; CT scans are often useful in difficult cases where surgical intervention is contemplated (Figure 2-4).

Minimally displaced (one-part) fractures usually heal with conservative treatment with the arm in a sling. Two- and three-part fractures are usually treated by closed reduction in the operating room with percutaneous pinning if necessary. However, open reduction and internal fixation are indicated if reduction of these fractures cannot be obtained by closed means. In patients with three-part fracture-dislocations or four-

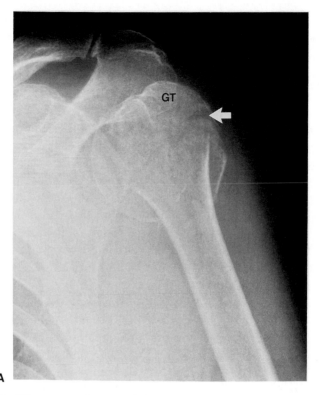

A

Figure 2-4. Three-part humeral fracture. A 50-year-old man injured his shoulder during a fall. (A) An anteroposterior radiograph demonstrates a comminuted proximal humeral fracture with greater than 45° angulation of the humeral head with respect to the proximal humeral shaft, indicating at least a two-part fracture. There is also a fracture (arrow) of the greater tuberosity (GT), but the degree of displacement of this fracture could not be fully determined from the radiograph. (B) A CT scan reveals a comminuted fracture of the greater tuberosity (GT) with displacement of the major fragment (arrow) by more than 1 cm. The radiologic classification was amended to a three-part proximal humerus fracture. Closed reduction was successfully accomplished in the operating room. C = coracoid process.

part fractures (which have displacement or rotation of all four major fragments), blood supply to the humeral head is severely compromised, and more than 50% of these patients develop osteonecrosis of the humeral head **(Option (D) is true).** Malunion is also common in patients with three-part fracture-dislocations or four-part fractures, even after internal fixation. Therefore, a humeral head replacement is usually considered for these patients.

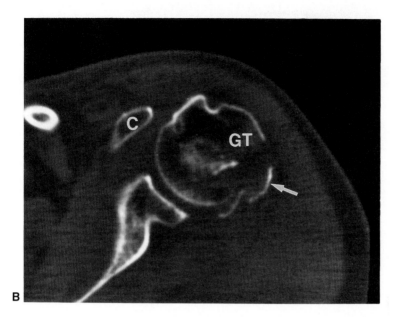

B

Question 10

Pseudocysts are often seen in the:

(A) proximal humerus
(B) calcaneus
(C) proximal femur
(D) radius
(E) ulna

Primary trabeculae develop along lines of stress. In areas with low stress, there may be such a paucity of trabeculae visible in radiographs that a lytic lesion is suspected. Such areas of trabecular rarefaction are called pseudocysts or pseudotumors. They are frequently observed in the proximal humerus, in the region of the greater tuberosity, and in the midportion of the calcaneus **(Options (A) and (B) are true).**

Humeral pseudocysts may be quite prominent in young individuals. Unlike a lytic bone lesion, the borders of a pseudocyst gradually merge with the surrounding normal trabeculae (Figure 2-5). A pseudocyst of the proximal humerus must be distinguished from chondroblastoma (Figure 2-6) and giant cell tumor (Figure 2-7), both of which are frequently located in the humeral head. These tumors are usually more sharply

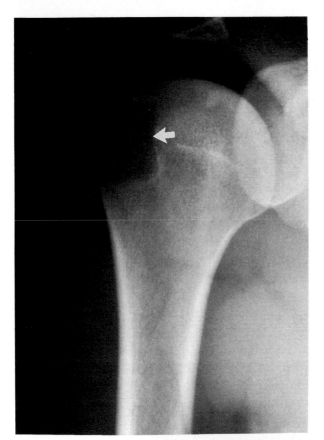

Figure 2-5 (left).
Pseudocyst. An antero-
posterior radiograph
of the proximal hu-
merus shows osseous
rarefaction (arrow),
characterized by mar-
gins that gradually
merge with surround-
ing trabeculae.

Figure 2-6 (right).
Chondroblastoma.
The patient had
pain in the shoul-
der. Radiographi-
cally, this tumor
was difficult to dif-
ferentiate from a
pseudocyst, but the
clinical history
and the moderately
thick sclerotic mar-
gin (arrow), a fea-
ture not expected
in a pseudocyst,
were clues to the
correct diagnosis.

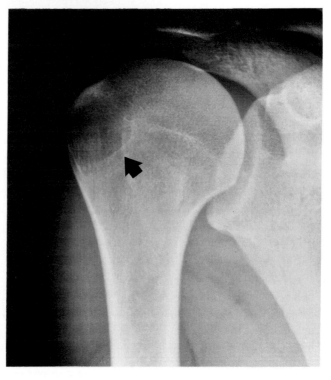

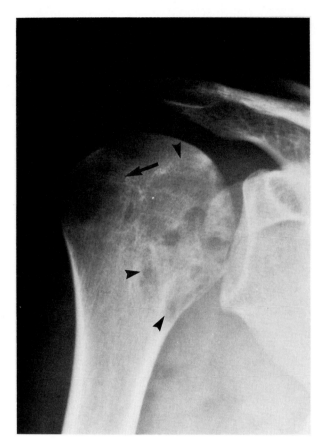

Figure 2-7. Giant cell tumor (arrowheads) and pseudocyst (arrow). The giant cell tumor, located medially, has an inhomogeneous "bubbly" appearance and a more defined margin than the pseudocyst of the greater tuberosity.

marginated and more radiolucent than a pseudocyst. The bilaterality of humeral pseudocysts may be helpful in differentiating them from osteolytic lesions. Therefore, if there is doubt whether a radiolucency of the proximal humerus is a pseudocyst, a comparison view of the contralateral humerus should be obtained.

As with the humeral pseudocyst, a normal area of rarefaction in the base of the neck of the calcaneus is due to a paucity of the trabeculae in the area (Figure 2-8). The major entity to be differentiated from a calcaneal pseudocyst is a simple (solitary) cyst, which occurs in the same location but features a more defined boundary or even a thin sclerotic rim (Figure 2-9). Simple cysts are asymptomatic, unless a pathologic fracture occurs.

Chondroblastoma, giant cell tumor, chondromyxoid fibroma, enchondroma, intraosseous lipoma, fibrous dysplasia, and eosinophilic granuloma may cause a geographic area of radiolucency in the calcaneus.

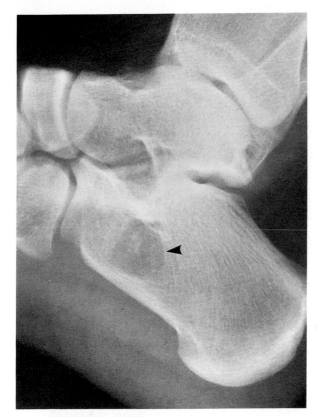

Figure 2-8. Pseudo-cyst of the calcaneus (arrowhead).

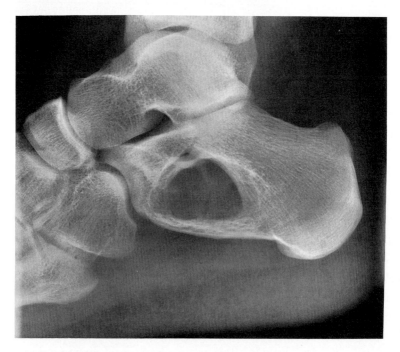

Figure 2-9. Solitary cyst of the calcaneus. The cyst has a well-defined, partially sclerotic margin. The patient had recurrent pain secondary to microfractures.

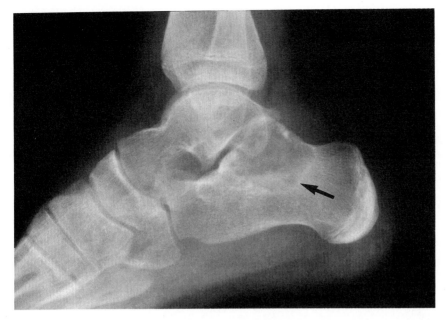

Figure 2-10. Chondroblastoma of the calcaneus. This lesion (arrow), located in the posterior subtalar region, has a thin, fuzzy, but slightly sclerotic margin.

Unlike pseudocysts and simple cysts of the neck of the calcaneus, these tumors tend to be symptomatic and can be found in other locations in the calcaneus. For example, chondroblastoma is often located in the subtalar region (Figure 2-10). Occasionally, CT or MRI is required to differentiate a pseudocyst, which should have normal trabeculae and bone marrow, from a tumor of the humerus or calcaneus, which does not.

The femoral neck often shows one or more well-circumscribed radiolucencies known as herniation pits (Figure 2-11). Herniation pits are usually ovoid and less than 1 cm in diameter. They are erosions on the surface of the bone that are caused by invagination of synovium into the anterior femoral neck, possibly secondary to repeated hyperextension of the hip. Histologically, the area is composed of collagenous tissue, neocartilage, and reactive new bone. Herniation pits of the femoral neck can be observed in radiographs of most adult patients. Unlike a pseudocyst, a herniation pit is a true defect located on the surface of the bone. The proximal femur is not a typical location for pseudocysts **(Option (C) is false).**

When seen *en face*, the tuberosity of the proximal radius presents as a pseudotumor or pseudocyst in radiographs (Figure 2-12) **(Option (D) is true).** The pseudocyst of the proximal radius can be easily identified

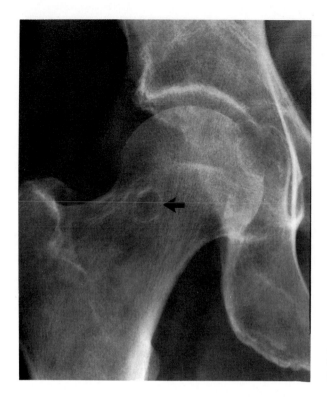

Figure 2-11. Herniation pit (arrow) of the femoral neck.

because it occurs exactly at the location of the tuberosity and is not reproducible in other radiographic projections.

Pseudocysts do not occur in the ulna **(Option (E) is false).**

Julia R. Crim, M.D.
Lawrence W. Bassett, M.D.

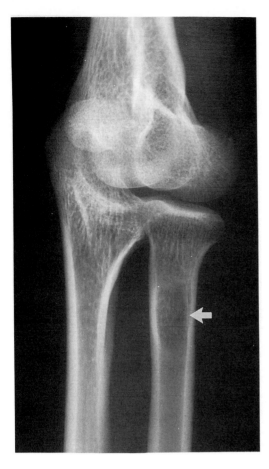

Figure 2-12. Pseudotumor (arrow) of the radius as a result of uniquely projected radial tuberosity.

SUGGESTED READINGS

FRACTURES OF THE PROXIMAL HUMERUS

1. Castagno AA, Shuman WP, Kilcoyne RF, Haynor DR, Morris ME, Matsen FA. Complex fractures of the proximal humerus: role of CT in treatment. Radiology 1987; 165:759–762
2. Neer CS II. Displaced proximal humeral fractures. I. Classification and evaluation. J Bone Joint Surg (Am) 1970; 52:1077–1089
3. Neer CS II, Rockwood CA. Fractures and dislocations of the shoulder. In: Rockwood CA, Green DP (eds), Fractures in adults. Philadelphia: JB Lippincott; 1984:675–707
4. Ross GJ, Love MB. Isolated avulsion fracture of the lesser tuberosity of the humerus: report of two cases. Radiology 1989; 172:833–834

TUMORS OF THE PROXIMAL HUMERUS

5. Dahlin DC. Giant cell tumor of bone: highlights of 407 cases. AJR 1955; 144:955–960

6. Hudson TM, Hawkins IF Jr. Radiological evaluation of chondroblastoma. Radiology 1981; 139:1–10

PSEUDOCYSTS

7. Helms CA. Pseudocysts of the humerus. AJR 1978; 131:287–288
8. Keats TE. Atlas of normal roentgen variants that may simulate disease, 5th ed. St. Louis: Mosby-Year Book; 1991
9. Resnick D, Cone RO III. The nature of humeral pseudocysts. Radiology 1984; 150:27–28

Notes

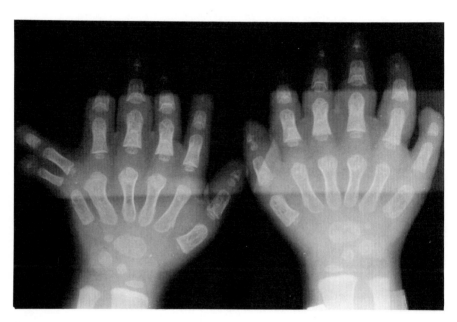

Figure 3-1. This 2-year-old child has a heart murmur. You are shown a posteroanterior radiograph of the hands.

Case 3:   Ellis-van Creveld Syndrome

Question 11

Which *one* of the following cardiac abnormalities is the MOST likely diagnosis?

    (A) Tetralogy of Fallot
    (B) Peripheral pulmonic stenosis
    (C) Septal defect
    (D) Patent ductus arteriosus
    (E) Coarctation of the aorta

The test image reveals several skeletal abnormalities, the most strik-ing of which is the presence of extra fingers on both hands (Figure 3-1). There are six metacarpal bones on each side; the right hand has six fin-gers, and the left has seven. The term used to describe the presence of extra digits is polydactyly. When the extra digits are on the ulnar side of the hand, as seen in the test image, the configuration is called postaxial polydactyly. When the extra digits are on the radial side of the hand, it is called preaxial polydactyly. Also evident in the test image are cone-shaped epiphyses at the bases of many of the phalanges, and large cen-tral carpal bones, which probably represent coalition of the capitate and hamate bones (Figure 3-2).

The radiologic findings in the test image are typical of the Ellis-van Creveld syndrome (chondroectodermal dysplasia). Between 50 and 60% of the children with this syndrome also have cardiovascular anomalies, most commonly septal defects **(Option (C) is correct).** Atrial septal defect (ASD) is the most common, although single-atrium and ventricu-lar septal defect (VSD) also occur in association with the Ellis-van Crev-eld syndrome.

Tetralogy of Fallot (Option (A)) is one of the most common cyanotic congenital heart anomalies. This complex anomaly includes right-ven-tricular outflow obstruction, a VSD with an overriding dextropositioned aorta, and right-ventricular hypertrophy. Tetralogy of Fallot is some-times an isolated anomaly, but it is often associated with other anomalies and syndromes, many of which include skeletal abnormalities. Perhaps

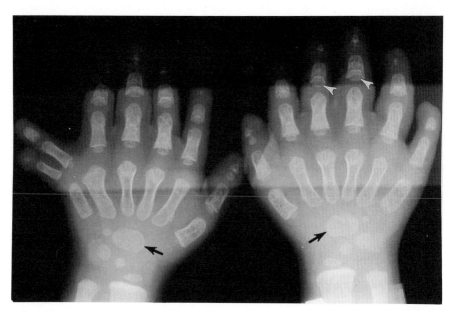

Figure 3-2 (Same as Figure 3-1). Chondroectodermal dysplasia (Ellis-van Creveld syndrome) in an infant. Note the postaxial polydactyly, cone-shaped epiphyses (arrowheads), and coalitions of the capitate and hamate bones (arrows).

the best known association of tetralogy of Fallot is with Down's syndrome (trisomy 21). Patients with Down's syndrome may have a wide variety of skeletal abnormalities, but they do not have polydactyly. Similarly, polydactyly does not have a known association with any other occurrence of tetralogy of Fallot. Therefore, tetralogy of Fallot would not be expected in the test patient.

Stenosis of the pulmonary arterial system may occur at one or more levels such as the pulmonic valve, the infundibulum, or the peripheral pulmonary arteries. Peripheral pulmonic stenosis (Option (B)) may manifest as narrowing of the central pulmonary artery, the left or right main pulmonary artery, or the more peripheral arterial branches. Peripheral pulmonic stenosis may complicate tetralogy of Fallot and may also occur in association with idiopathic hypercalcemia of infancy (Williams' syndrome) or with the congenital rubella syndrome. Children with these syndromes often have skeletal abnormalities, but polydactyly, cone epiphyses, and focal carpal abnormalities are not among the expected skeletal features.

The ductus arteriosus is patent throughout fetal life and is essential for the normal fetal shunting of blood from the pulmonary to the systemic circulation. Within the first few days of life, the ductus closes secondary to the physiologic changes that occur at birth. In some infants, however, the ductus fails to close and a left-to-right shunt develops. This is referred to as patent ductus arteriosus (PDA) (Option (D)), a short, tubular, valveless connection between the concavity of the aortic arch and the main pulmonary artery, usually located immediately below the origin of the left subclavian artery. PDA is commonly an isolated anomaly, but it can be found in a number of congenital syndromes that affect the skeleton. The most common syndromes that combine PDA and skeletal abnormalities are trisomy 18 and the congenital rubella syndrome. Less commonly, PDA is encountered in patients with trisomy 21, trisomy 13, chondrodysplasia punctata, cerebrohepatorenal syndrome, or Rubenstein-Taybi syndrome. None of these syndromes is associated with polydactyly.

Coarctation of the aorta (Option (E)) is a localized obstruction or stenosis of the aorta at or near the junction of the aorta and the ductus arteriosus, a location that correlates with the embryologic junction of the fourth branchial arch and the dorsal aorta. Two types of coarctation are described, preductal and postductal. Preductal coarctation is the less common form and is usually discovered in infancy. It varies from complete aortic atresia proximal to the brachiocephalic artery to localized aortic hypoplasia or stenosis proximal to the left subclavian artery. Postductal coarctation frequently presents during adult life and is commonly associated with a bicuspid aortic valve. Coarctation of the aorta is most often an isolated anomaly but may occur in association with Turner's syndrome (monosomy X), idiopathic hypercalcemia of infancy, neurofibromatosis type 1, and Sturge-Weber syndrome. None of these syndromes has a known association with the anomalies shown in the test image, excluding coarctation as a likely association.

Question 12

Concerning syndromes with combined skeletal and cardiac abnormalities,

    (A) lower-extremity skeletal abnormalities are more common than cardiac abnormalities in patients with the cardiomelic (Holt-Oram) syndrome

    (B) cardiac abnormalities are more common than skeletal abnormalities in patients with Turner's syndrome (monosomy X)

    (C) short stature is more common than septal defects in patients with Down's syndrome (trisomy 21)

    (D) skeletal abnormalities produce more important long-term sequelae than do cardiac anomalies in patients with congenital rubella syndrome

    (E) aortic root disorders are common in patients with Marfan's syndrome

Congenital and developmental anomalies of the skeleton are often associated with cardiac anomalies. These associations are fairly consistent and therefore generally predictable. Not all patients with a particular syndrome will have all possible manifestations or associations, but a careful assessment of the skeleton can be a reliable predictor of cardiac abnormalities and vice versa. Some of the more common associations between cardiovascular and skeletal anomalies are shown in Table 3-1.

In 1960, Holt and Oram described a syndrome of skeletal and cardiac anomalies that now bears their names. The Holt-Oram syndrome is also known as the cardiomelic syndrome, a term derived from the Greek words *kardia* and *melos*, meaning heart and limb, respectively. What is not apparent in this descriptive name is that the skeletal anomalies of this syndrome are confined to the upper extremities. The lower extremities are not involved **(Option (A) is false).**

Several cardiac abnormalities occur in patients with the cardiomelic syndrome. Rhythm disturbance is the most common and includes atrioventricular conduction defects, bradycardia, atrial fibrillation, and ventricular premature contraction. Of the morphologic cardiac abnormalities encountered, septal defects are the most common. Septal defects may be atrial, ventricular, or both. Persistence of the left superior vena cava may also occur.

The skeletal malformations of the cardiomelic syndrome, even though confined to the upper extremity, are diverse and variable. The anomalies are commonly confined to the distal portions of the upper extremities, but abnormalities of the shoulder joints, clavicles, and humeral epicondyles have been reported. These proximal abnormalities include thickening of the clavicle, abnormal clavicular processes that may articulate with the scapula, and abnormal positioning of the scapula. The radial head may be deformed, but absence of the radius is rare.

The hands are the most frequently affected musculoskeletal sites. The carpal scaphoid may be abnormally shaped; carpal coalitions may

Table 3-1: Some skeletal malformation syndromes with their associated cardiac anomalies[a]

Syndrome	ASD	VSD	PDA	TF	VPS	PPS	AC
Ellis-van Creveld (chondroectodermal dysplasia)	++	+					
Holt-Oram (cardiomelic)	++	++					
Down's (trisomy 21)	++	++	+	++			
Trisomy 18	+	++	++		+		
Trisomy 13	++	++	++				
Congenital rubella	+	+	++		+	++	
Idiopathic hypercalcemia of infancy (Williams' syndrome)		+	+			++	++
Turner's syndrome							++
Chondrodysplasia punctata	+	+	+				

[a] ASD = atrial septal defect; VSD = ventricular septal defect; PDA = patent ductus arteriosus; TF = Tetralogy of Fallot; VPS = valvular pulmonic stenosis; PPS = peripheral pulmonic stenosis; AC = aortic coarctation; ++ = common; + = occurs

occur, and an additional carpal bone, the os centrale, is often present (Figure 3-3). Occasionally, multiple additional bones form a middle carpal row. Involvement of the thumb is almost invariable, producing a fingerlike triphalangeal digit in some cases (Figure 3-4). At the other end of the spectrum, the first metacarpal or even the entire thumb may be hypoplastic or absent. Thumb enlargement is usually accompanied by abnormal curvature. Likewise, the little finger often has a short middle phalanx, which may be trapezoidal, creating a lateral curvature of the finger (clinodactyly). In rare cases, there is proximal shortening of the limb (phocomelia) (Figure 3-5). Other abnormalities include pectus excavatum and absence of the pectoralis major muscle.

The cardiomelic syndrome is inherited as an autosomal dominant trait with variable penetrance. Identical manifestations are not neces-

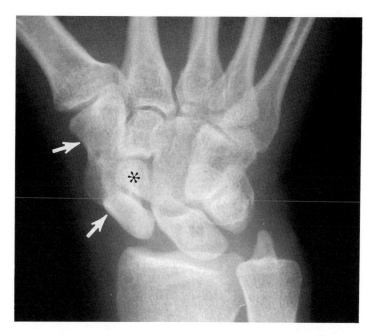

Figure 3-3. Cardiomelic syndrome. The wrist shows scaphotrapezial carpal coalition (arrows) and an extra carpal bone, the os centrale (✻). This patient also had an atrial septal defect and a triphalangeal thumb.

sarily encountered in affected relatives (Figures 3-4 and 3-5). In some families with the cardiomelic syndrome, individuals have been reported in whom upper-extremity defects were present without cardiac anomalies (Figure 3-6) and vice versa.

Turner's syndrome (monosomy X) is a common chromosomal malformation syndrome. Affected individuals have only 45 chromosomes, with a single X chromosome and no Y chromosome. They are phenotypically female and have a broad chest, wide nipple spacing, and often a webbed neck. All are short in stature, most have ovarian dysgenesis, and some are intellectually subnormal. More than 99% are sterile, and most have amenorrhea and sexual infantilism. Cardiovascular anomalies occur in only 20% of patients with Turner's syndrome; the most common are aortic coarctation and VSD. In contrast, skeletal abnormalities are almost invariably present **(Option (B) is false).** Unexplained hypertension may occur.

Shortening of the fourth metacarpal bone is the most common and also the best-known osseous abnormality in patients with Turner's syndrome (Figure 3-7), but it is not a universal feature, being present in less than 50% of cases. The third and fifth metacarpal bones may also be

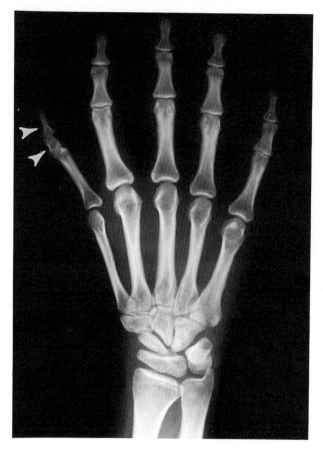

Figure 3-4. Cardiomelic syndrome. Scapholunate carpal coalition, trapeziotrapezoidal carpal coalition, os centrale, and triphalangeal thumb (arrowheads) are present.

short (Figure 3-8), and similar findings may be seen in the metatarsal bones of the feet. Carpal anomalies are relatively frequent, with a V-shaped proximal carpal row and a decreased carpal angle seen most frequently, at times producing the Madelung deformity. The distal phalanges may have a drum-stick appearance. The presence of enlarged medial femoral condyles and tibial exostoses in the lower extremities has been reported. The tibial condyles may develop abnormally, and a bowing pattern, similar to Blount's disease, may be present.

The skeletal manifestations of Turner's syndrome are not confined to the extremities. Generalized osteopenia (osteoporosis) and delayed skeletal maturation are both seen. Osteoporosis may respond to the cyclical estrogen therapy that is often used to treat amenorrhea and sexual

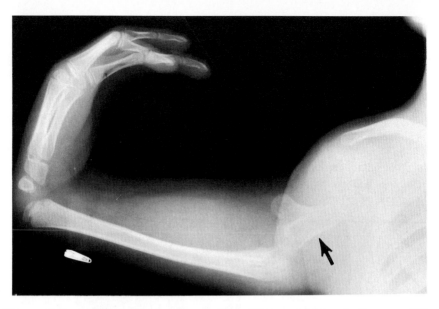

Figure 3-5. Cardiomelic syndrome. This 10-year-old boy is the son of the woman whose hand is shown in Figure 3-4. He has PDA as well as the extensive radial ray anomaly shown here. Note the severe shortening of his humerus (arrow).

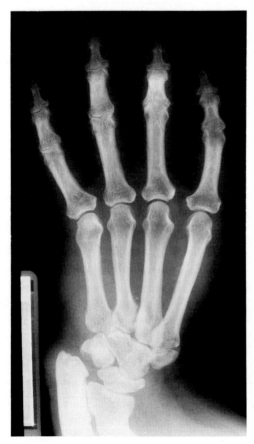

Figure 3-6. Cardiomelic syndrome. This 64-year-old man has several anomalies typical of the cardiomelic syndrome but has no family history of limb anomalies. His heart is normal. His hand radiograph shows shortening of the radius, absence of the thumb, and presence of carpal coalitions.

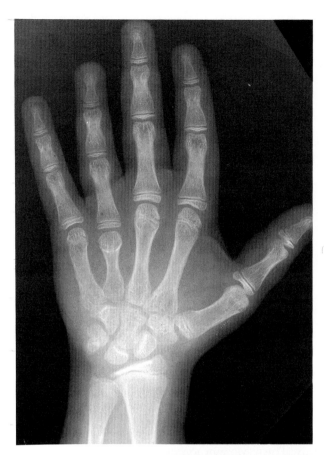

Figure 3-7 (left). Monosomy X (Turner's syndrome). This 12-year-old girl has marked shortening of her fourth metacarpal. There is also a decreased carpal angle and a V-shaped proximal carpal row.

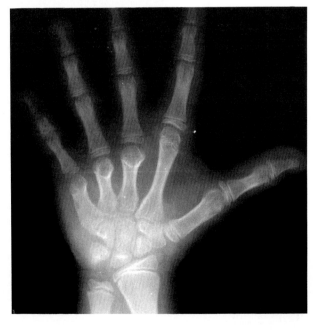

Figure 3-8 (right). Monosomy X (Turner's syndrome). The third, fourth, and fifth metacarpals are shortened in this 13-year-old girl. The carpal angle is decreased.

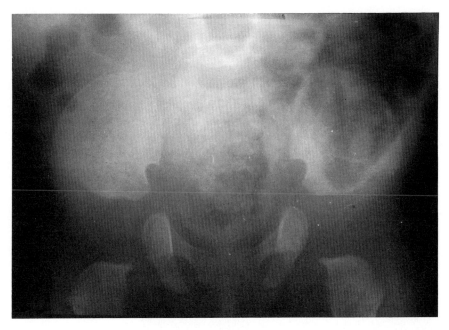

Figure 3-9. Trisomy 21 (Down's syndrome). This 3-month-old girl has the typical pelvic abnormalities seen in patients with this disorder. The iliac bones are flared and tapered, and the acetabular roofs are flattened.

infantilism. Vertebral anomalies occur, affecting the first two cervical vertebrae most commonly. These vertebrae may be hypoplastic, and the odontoid process may be abnormally shaped. Squaring of the lumbar vertebral bodies is sometimes present. Scoliosis and increased kyphosis may be seen. Involvement of the skull base includes basilar impression, flattening of the basal angle, and a small sella turcica. Some patients have brachycephaly, and craniosynostosis has been reported. Neurologic deficits are not a feature of Turner's syndrome. The mandible may be small, and the paranasal sinuses may be excessively pneumatized.

Down's syndrome (trisomy 21), another common chromosomal disorder, is easily recognized by the presence of short stature and characteristic facies, with prominent epicanthic folds. Abnormalities are seen throughout the skeleton. Flaring of the iliac wings, flattening of the acetabular roofs, and tapering of the ilia make up a classic pelvic triad that can be identified on a pelvic radiograph during the first year of life (Figures 3-9 and 3-10). Ninety percent of individuals with trisomy 21 have absent frontal sinuses, and a similar number have paired instead of single ossification centers for the manubrium. Brachycephaly, microcephaly, orbital hypotelorism, and delayed sutural closure also occur. Skeletal maturation may be delayed.

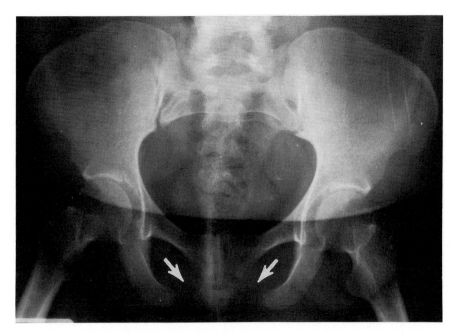

Figure 3-10. Trisomy 21 (Down's syndrome). In this 21-year-old woman the iliac wings are flared and the ischiopubic rami are deficient (arrows). Note the similarity between the pelvis in this adult and that in the infant in Figure 3-9.

The carpal angle is usually increased in patients with Down's syndrome, whereas it is typically decreased in patients with Turner's syndrome. Shortening of the middle phalanges (brachymesophalangy) and clinodactyly, producing short, stubby fingers, are seen in about 20% of patients with Down's syndrome. Severe soft tissue laxity about joints may lead to hip dislocation, patellofemoral instability, genu valgum, and deformities of the feet. Slipped capital femoral epiphyses may occur.

Anomalies of the craniocervical junction are common and may lead to subluxation and neurologic problems (Figure 3-11). Atlantoaxial instability has been found in up to 20% of patients with Down's syndrome. Routine radiographic screening of patients with Down's syndrome for upper cervical instability is recommended because some patients need surgical fusion to prevent serious injury to the cervical spinal cord. The lumbar and thoracic vertebral bodies typically appear squared, and there are usually only 11 pairs of ribs.

Approximately half the patients with Down's syndrome have cardiac manifestations, whereas all have short stature **(Option (C) is true).** The most common cardiac anomaly is an atrioventricular cushion defect. Many other serious cardiac defects also occur, the most common being

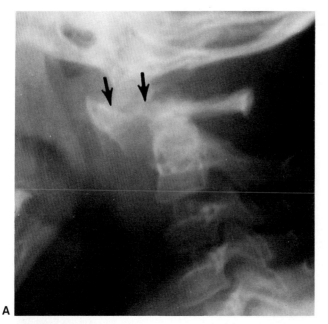

A

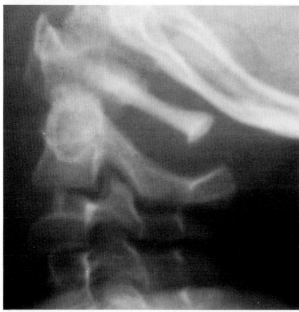

B

Figure 3-11. Tri-
somy 21 (Down's
syndrome). Lateral
radiographs of the
cervical spine in
flexion (A) and ex-
tension (B) show
marked instability
of the C1-C2 junc-
tion in this 7-year-
old boy. There is
wide subluxation
(arrows in panel A)
of the atlantoaxial
joint on flexion,
which reduces on ex-
tension.

VSD, PDA, and tetralogy of Fallot. These cardiac anomalies may cause
significant intracardiac shunting or decreased pulmonary blood flow,
leading to severe cardiovascular deficiency that necessitates surgical correction. Other cardiac anomalies of lesser clinical significance are also

encountered. Many asymptomatic adults with Down's syndrome have mitral valve prolapse, and anomalous right subclavian arteries are found in 10 to 20% of subjects with this disorder, a prevalence almost 20 times that in the normal population.

The congenital rubella syndrome is caused by intrauterine rubella virus infection. Eighty percent of affected fetuses develop serious malformations of the cardiovascular system. Almost half have ocular abnormalities, including cataracts and glaucoma. Many have thrombocytopenic purpura with hepatosplenomegaly, and about 25% are deaf. Osseous manifestations occur in approximately 60%, but these are a less frequent cause of important long-term sequelae than are the cardiac anomalies **(Option (D) is false).** Moreover, the skeletal manifestations frequently revert to normal soon after birth.

Almost half the infants with congenital rubella syndrome have PDA. Slightly less than half have peripheral pulmonary artery stenosis. Other common cardiac defects are pulmonic-valve-leaflet thickening and pulmonic insufficiency. Less common cardiac anomalies include septal defects, aortic coarctation, and aortic stenosis. Any one of these disorders can lead to significant cardiovascular malfunction, and many require surgical correction.

The skeletal features of the congenital rubella syndrome are found predominantly in the extremities. The abnormalities are typically metaphyseal and are similar in morphology to the osseous changes observed in patients with other congenital viral infections. These metaphyseal features are not due to osteomyelitis but result from altered osteoid deposition and impaired matrix mineralization. Typically the zone of provisional calcification is poorly defined. Metaphyseal trabeculae are coarsened, and metaphyseal margins are typically frayed and irregular, occasionally with beaklike projections (Figure 3-12). In infants who do well, these metaphyseal changes heal rapidly and the affected bones soon return to a normal appearance. In infants who do poorly, the morphologic alterations progress, and eventually alternating bands of sclerosis and lucency are produced. At times, these bands may be longitudinal, an osseous pattern termed the "celery stick" appearance (Figure 3-13). Diaphyseal involvement does not occur. The axial skeleton is largely unaffected, although the anterior fontanelle of the skull tends to be large.

Marfan's syndrome is an autosomal dominant disorder with variable expression and incomplete penetrance. Affected individuals tend to be tall with long fingers and toes (arachnodactyly) and high-arched palates. They have decreased subcutaneous fat, and their muscles are both hypoplastic and hypotonic. Their joints are hyperextensible, and they have either pectus carinatum or excavatum deformities. Kyphoscoliosis is

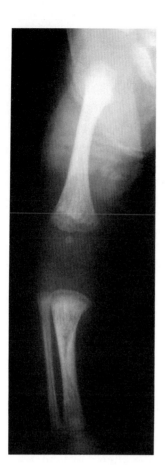

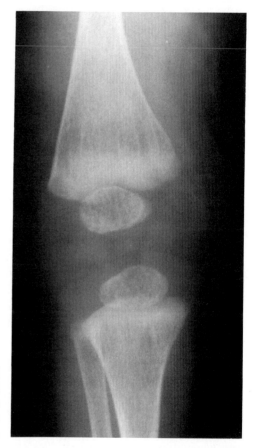

Figure 3-12 (left). Congenital rubella syndrome. Coarsened trabeculae and metaphyseal lucent bands characterize the lower-extremity long bones of this 5-day-old infant.

Figure 3-13 (right). Congenital rubella syndrome. The striated distal metaphyses in this 7-month-old child resemble a celery stick.

common. Lenticular subluxation occurs in the eyes of more than 50% of affected individuals.

Combined cardiovascular and skeletal problems are characteristic of Marfan's syndrome, and both are present to some degree in all patients. Cardiovascular problems include prolapse of the mitral valve, dilatation of the aortic root, insufficiency of both mitral and aortic valves, and narrowing of the coronary ostia. Aortic abnormalities, the most life threaten-

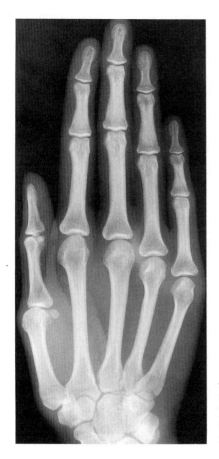

Figure 3-14. Marfan's syndrome. Elongation of the metacarpals and phalanges, typical of arachnodactyly, is seen in this 26-year-old woman. Her metacarpal index is 11.6.

ing of which are dissection and rupture of the proximal aorta, result from cystic medial degeneration of the vessel wall. These are the most frequent cardiovascular anomalies encountered in patients with Marfan's syndrome **(Option (E) is true).** Aortic dissection usually has an acute onset; 30% of patients die within 24 hours if untreated, and 50% die within a week. Only about 10% of aortic dissections are chronic. Cardiovascular disorders are so common in patients with Marfan's syndrome that 90% of patients die of them. The average age at death for persons with Marfan's syndrome is 30 years.

Arachnodactyly is present in all patients with Marfan's syndrome. Radiographic evaluation reveals elongation and narrowing of all of the tubular bones, particularly in the hands and feet (Figure 3-14). The measurement most commonly used to assess arachnodactyly is the metacarpal index, which is defined as the average of the ratios of length to breadth of the second through fifth metacarpals. In normal individuals this ratio is less than 7.9, and in patients with Marfan's syndrome it is greater than 8.4. Other skeletal abnormalities include clinodactyly, proximal positioning of the patella, and abnormal skull shape.

The major differential diagnosis for Marfan's syndrome is homocystinuria, which is due to cystathionine synthase deficiency. The absence of this enzyme leads to elevated levels of homocysteine and methionine in serum, with persistent urinary excretion of homocystine. Most of these patients have mental retardation, a feature not seen in patients with Marfan's syndrome. The presence of homocystine in the urine provides a simple diagnostic biochemical test that is usually positive within 48 hours of birth. The skeletal and ocular manifestations of this disorder are similar to those of Marfan's syndrome, but patients with Marfan's syndrome do not have homocystine in their urine.

Question 13

Congenital heart disease is associated with:

(A) clubbing
(B) articular erosions
(C) osteosclerosis
(D) premature fusion of sternal ossification centers
(E) accelerated bone age
(F) scoliosis
(G) rib notching

Clubbing refers to a proliferation of the soft tissues around the terminal phalanges of the fingers and toes. There may be no osseous abnormality at these sites. Fibroelastic tissue proliferates in and around the nail bed, elevating the nail base and decreasing the nail angle. The tips of the digits become relatively bulbous, and the tufts of the distal phalanges may enlarge. Clubbing is seen in patients with a wide variety of diseases, most commonly those of pulmonary origin. A number of these disorders have radiographic skeletal manifestations, the most common of which is hypertrophic osteoarthropathy. Clubbing may also be seen in patients with no demonstrable underlying disorder (Figure 3-15).

Hypertrophic osteoarthropathy is a clinical syndrome characterized by painful swelling of the extremities, at times mistaken for inflammatory arthritis, and clubbing of the fingers and toes. It was initially thought to be associated only with pulmonary disease but is now known to occur in conjunction with a variety of other disorders. Radiographs of patients with hypertrophic osteoarthropathy reveal metadiaphyseal periosteal new-bone formation and occasionally endosteal bone formation along the distal forearm and leg bones. Later these changes progress

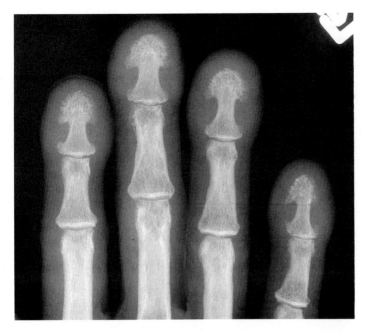

Figure 3-15. Clubbing. Posteroanterior radiograph of the fingers of this 55-year-old woman reveals clubbing of the tips. There was no known cause of the clubbing.

to involve the short tubular bones of the hands and feet, the femurs, and the humeri. At times, periarticular osteopenia is found.

Hypertrophic osteoarthropathy is encountered in patients with several different congenital cyanotic heart disorders, and these disorders are therefore associated with clubbing **(Option (A) is true)**. Clubbing may also be encountered in patients with thyroid acropachy and pachydermoperiostosis, in association with a wide variety of gastrointestinal disorders and several nonpulmonary neoplasms, and in an idiopathic form.

Congenital heart diseases are frequently associated with osseous anomalies, and some patients with hypertrophic osteoarthropathy complain of joint pain; however, there is no specific association between congenital heart diseases and joint diseases such as erosive arthropathy. Articular erosions are therefore not expected **(Option (B) is false)**.

Certain congenital malformation syndromes (e.g., Turner's syndrome) are commonly associated with generalized osteopenia, but osteosclerosis does not occur in association with congenital heart disease **(Option (C) is false)**.

Certain skeletal abnormalities commonly occur in conjunction with congenital heart disease, but these combinations do not necessarily rep-

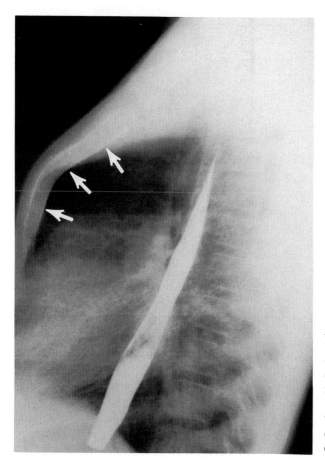

Figure 3-16. Premature fusion of the ossification centers of the sternum (arrows) is seen in this 14-year-old boy with Noonan's syndrome and an associated ASD.

resent a direct causative relationship attributable to a specific congenital malformation syndrome. These secondary associations represent inductions of osseous abnormalities as a result of underlying physiologic aberrations. Examples of such indirect skeletal responses include hypertrophic osteoarthropathy, as mentioned above, and premature fusion of the sternal ossification centers **(Option (D) is true)** (Figure 3-16).

The etiology of premature sternal fusion is unknown, but it can be seen in association with a number of different cyanotic heart disorders. One possible explanation is a response to right-sided cardiac enlargement. Another possibility is an intrauterine insult occurring at a critical time in the development of both the sternum and the heart. Other nonspecific but probably gene-controlled skeletal changes seen in association with congenital heart disease include cleft palate and facial anomalies. Delayed skeletal maturation is fairly common, but accelerated maturation does not occur **(Option (E) is false)**. Scoliosis and rib notching are

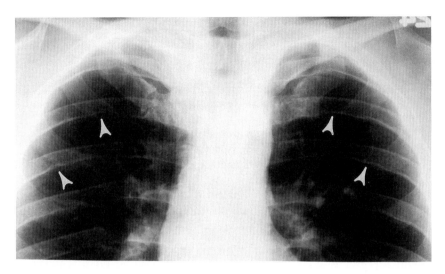

Figure 3-17. Rib notching (arrowheads) in a 39-year-old man with coarctation of the aorta.

also frequently associated with congenital heart disease **(Options (F) and (G) are true).** Scoliosis is more frequent in patients with congenital heart disease than in the normal population and is approximately twice as frequent in patients with cyanotic forms of congenital heart disease than it is in those with acyanotic forms. Moreover, it tends to be more severe in patients with cyanotic disease. Rib notching is seen most commonly in patients with aortic coarctation and is caused by enlarged, tortuous intercostal arteries (Figure 3-17). It also occurs in association with disorders causing decreased pulmonary blood flow, including tetralogy of Fallot, pulmonary atresia, pulmonic stenosis, and Epstein's anomaly.

Question 14

Concerning upper-extremity musculoskeletal anomalies,

(A) duplication of the little finger is an example of preaxial polydactyly
(B) failure of separation of the long and ring fingers is the most common form of syndactyly
(C) lunotriquetral carpal coalition is usually syndrome related
(D) the carpal angle is increased in patients with Madelung deformity
(E) the frequency of associated anomalies in patients with congenital radial defects is less than 10%

Polydactyly means simply that an individual has more than the normal complement of five digits on one or both hands or feet. This deformity has been known for a very long time, the first reference coming from the Old Testament (2 Samuel 21:18–22). Polydactyly is usually described as being preaxial or postaxial. Preaxial literally means "occurring before an axis." When referring to an extremity, preaxial means lateral to the midline of the extremity. Conversely, postaxial refers to the medial side of an extremity. Therefore, in the hand, preaxial refers to extra digits arising from the radial side, and postaxial refers to extra digits on the ulnar side **(Option (A) is false).** Duplications of the second, third, or fourth digit occur but are far less common than duplications of the first or fifth digit. Duplication of the third digit is usually referred to as either axial or central polydactyly.

Polydactyly is usually inherited. It may be an isolated finding (Figure 3-18), but it is commonly associated with other anomalies and should therefore stimulate a search for evidence of cardiovascular or other defects. A family history is therefore useful for diagnosis, management, and family genetic counseling.

Poznanski classifies polydactyly of the hand as follows:

1. Postaxial (from the ulnar side)
    a. Fully developed extra digits
    b. Rudimentary extra digits
2. Preaxial (from the radial side)
    a. Thumb polydactyly
    b. Polydactyly of a triphalangeal thumb
    c. Polydactyly of an index finger
    d. Polysyndactyly
3. High degrees of duplication of parts of the upper extremity

Syndactyly is defined as a lack of differentiation between two or more digits. This does not normally represent fusion of developing tis-

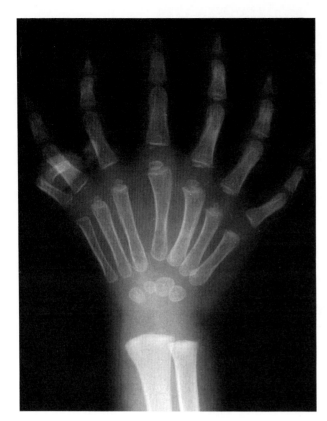

Figure 3-18. Sporadic polydactyly. This 4-year-old boy has a "mirror hand" deformity with 7 digits. This was an isolated unilateral anomaly in an otherwise healthy child.

sues but rather a failure of mesenchymal differentiation (segmentation) at an early stage of development. Syndactyly may involve only the soft tissues (Figure 3-19) or both bones and soft tissues. These two variants probably represent different degrees of the same failure of differentiation. Syndactyly can involve any of the fingers or toes, but the most common variety (also known as zygosyndactyly) involves the long and ring fingers of the hand **(Option (B) is true).** As with most congenital malformations, syndactyly is encountered both as an isolated finding and as part of a more generalized congenital malformation syndrome. Polysyndactyly refers to a combination of polydactyly and syndactyly in the same hand or foot (Figure 3-20).

Carpal coalition is similar to syndactyly in that it represents failure of complete differentiation (segmentation) between mesenchymal elements of the wrist. Carpal coalition may occur within the proximal or the distal carpal row or between the two rows. The latter is more typically seen in patients with generalized malformation syndromes, whereas carpal coalition within a row is more often an isolated anomaly. Union of the

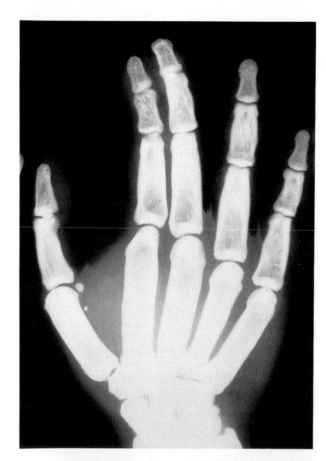

Figure 3-19. Syndactyly. This 40-year-old man with sclerosteosis not only has dense, malformed phalanges and metacarpals but also has soft tissue syndactyly of the index and long fingers.

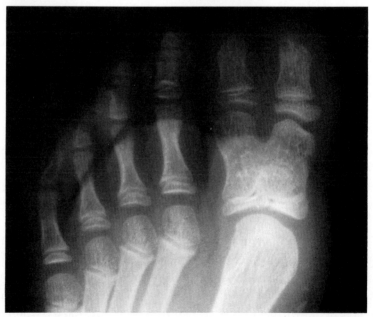

Figure 3-20. Sporadic polysyndactyly. Partial duplication of the great toe was present in an otherwise normal 14-year-old girl.

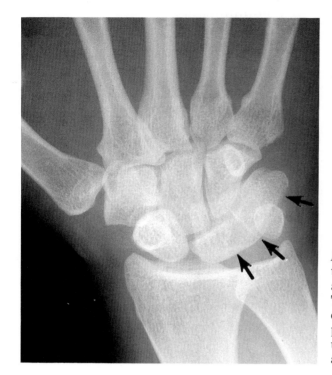

Figure 3-21. Luno-triquetral carpal coalition (arrows). This is the most common form of carpal coalition and is usually an isolated anomaly.

lunate and triquetrum (Figure 3-21) is the most common form of carpal coalition and is almost always an isolated anomaly **(Option (C) is false).** Capitohamate carpal coalition (Figure 3-22) is the second most common of the carpal coalitions. It may be a feature of certain malformation syndromes, such as chondroectodermal dysplasia, but it is an isolated anomaly in many instances. Coalitions between other carpal bones (Figures 3-23 and 3-24) are much less common.

Madelung deformity (Figure 3-25) is characterized by volar angulation of the radius, volar subluxation of the carpus, a V-shaped articulation between the carpus and distal forearm, and a decreased carpal angle **(Option (D) is false).** The carpal angle is the obtuse angle between a line drawn tangential to the proximal surfaces of the scaphoid and lunate and a line drawn tangential to the proximal surfaces of the lunate and triquetrum. In normal individuals, this angle is approximately 130°. Changes in this angle are associated with a wide variety of disorders, and the angle may be either increased or decreased, depending on the type of disorder.

Madelung deformity is a congenital or developmental wrist anomaly that is believed to be caused by premature partial fusion of the radial growth plate (physis). This deformity is a characteristic feature of a generalized bone dysplasia known as dyschondrosteosis, but it may also

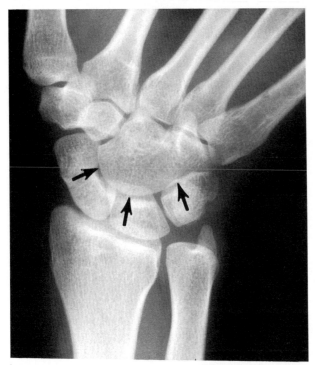

Figure 3-22 (left).
Capitohamate carpal coalition (arrows). This can be an isolated anomaly, as in this example, but it is also encountered in patients with congenital malformation syndromes.

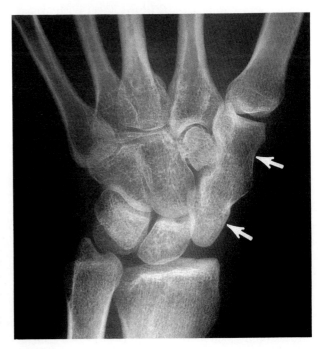

Figure 3-23 (right).
Scaphotrapezial carpal coalition (arrows) in a 30-year-old woman with an atrial septal defect. Her daughter had similar anomalies.

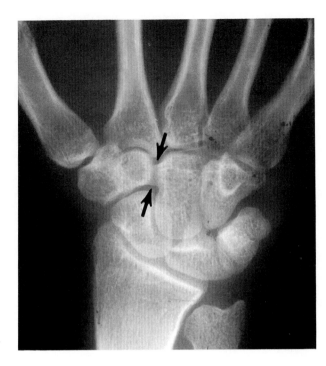

Figure 3-24. Capitotrapezoidal carpal coalition (arrows). This was discovered incidentally when the hand of this 18-year-old girl was radiographed following an injury.

occur as an isolated anomaly or as a part of other malformation syndromes. The most common syndrome associated with Madelung deformity is Turner's syndrome, but the Madelung deformity can also be seen in patients with multiple enchondromatosis and multiple osteochondromatosis. A distal radial injury during childhood can result in premature partial closure of the physis, leading to a posttraumatic Madelung deformity.

Congenital radial defects are uncommon, with an incidence of about 1 in 30,000 live births. Most of these anomalies are sporadic, although some appear to be inherited as autosomal dominant traits. The spectrum of radial ray disorders ranges from minimal thumb defects to complete absence of the radius and the radial half of the hand (Figure 3-26). Associated congenital abnormalities elsewhere in the body are present in approximately 40% of patients **(Option (E) is false);** the most common are congenital heart defects, which are present in greater than 10% of affected individuals. The cardiac anomalies include coarctation of the aorta, dextrocardia, septal defects (especially VSD), PDA, and pulmonic stenosis. Morphologic anomalies also affect the eyes, ears, face, skull, gastrointestinal tract, genitourinary tract, vertebral column, and other areas of the appendicular skeleton. Spina bifida, cleft palate or lip, and

A   B

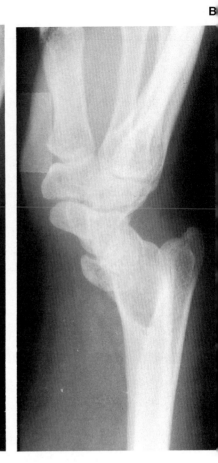

Figure 3-25. Madelung deformity. Anteroposterior (A) and lateral (B) radiographs of the wrist of this 35-year-old woman reveal typical changes including a V-shaped articulation between the carpus and distal forearm, a decreased carpal angle, volar angulation of the radius, and volar subluxation of the carpus.

renal defects are nearly as common as cardiac abnormalities in association with radial defects. Perhaps the best known syndrome involving both radial ray defects and cardiac anomalies is the Holt-Oram syndrome. Other syndromes involving this combination include the thrombocytopenia-absent radius (TAR) syndrome, Fanconi's anemia, thalidomide embryopathy, and the VATER association.

In patients with TAR syndrome, the thumb is present in spite of radial absence (Figure 3-27), the converse of most radial ray defects. In patients with Fanconi's anemia, duplications of the thumb are the most common radial ray abnormality. Thalidomide embryopathy tends to produce phocomelia and a triphalangeal thumb. The VATER association is

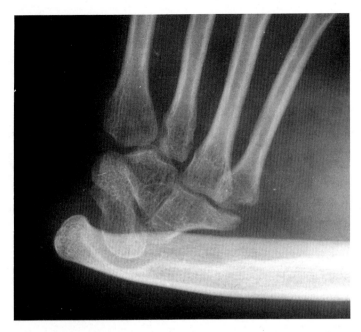

Figure 3-26. Radial agenesis. In this 19-year-old boy, radial agenesis is manifested as complete absence of the thumb and radius.

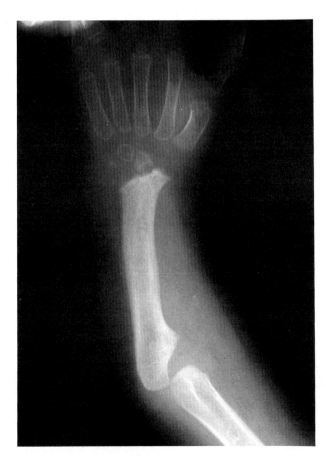

Figure 3-27. Thrombocytopenia-absent radius syndrome. This 16-month-old girl has a thumb but no radius.

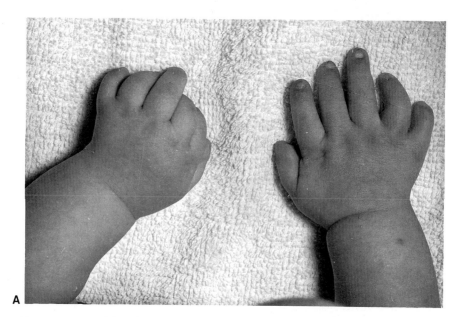

Figure 3-28. Chondroectodermal dysplasia. This infant has polydactyly of the hands (A) and the feet (B).

not really a syndrome but rather a collection of congenital abnormalities that have a strong tendency to coexist. The acronym "VATER" contains the first letter of each anomaly: "V" for vertebral anomalies, "A" for anorectal anomalies (e.g., atresia), "T" for tracheoesophageal fistula, "E" for esophageal atresia, and "R" for both radial and renal defects. The radial defects seen in patients with the VATER association are variable and may be bilateral or unilateral. The radius may be present or absent.

Discussion

The Ellis-van Creveld syndrome is not the most common malformation syndrome with both skeletal and cardiac abnormalities, but it is the syndrome most commonly associated with polydactyly. This syndrome consists of an autosomal recessive short-limbed dwarfism with variable expression. The extremities manifest progressive distalward shortening. Postaxial or central polydactyly of the hands is common (Figure 3-28A), and similar polydactyly may be seen in the feet (Figure 3-28B). The nails are hypoplastic (Figure 3-29), and the hair is sparse: hence the scientific

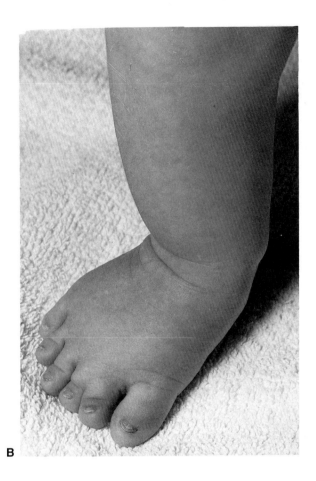

B

name chondroectodermal dysplasia. The upper lip is usually short and connected to the alveolar ridge by multiple frenula. Dental problems are common. Partial adontia or delayed eruption of the teeth may occur. The teeth have a high incidence of caries, premature loss, and malalignment (Figure 3-30). Cardiac defects are often present, but they are less common than the bone, nail, and tooth anomalies. A small thorax and knock-knee deformities are occasional findings. These individuals have normal intelligence.

The multisystem anomalies of the Ellis-van Creveld syndrome are all present at birth, with infant mortality approaching 50% if untreated. Most infant deaths are secondary to cardiac or pulmonary involvement. Cardiac failure due to the abnormal hemodynamics of a heart defect is often the terminal event. Lethal pulmonary insufficiency results primarily from the small rib cage, but malformations of the tracheobronchial tree may contribute. Prompt surgical correction of cardiac anomalies

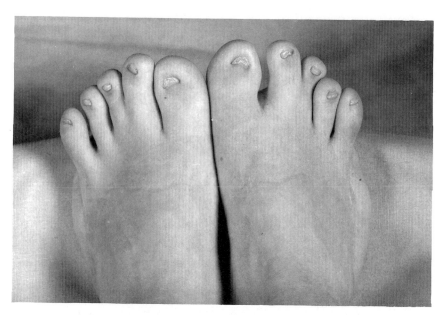

Figure 3-29. Chondroectodermal dysplasia. This young man has typical hypoplastic nails and evidence of previously excised extra toes laterally.

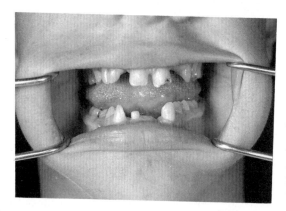

Figure 3-30. Chondroectodermal dysplasia. Note the absence of many teeth and the deformities and malalignments of those that remain.

may be necessary to prevent early death. Life expectancy is normal in the absence of cardiac or pulmonary problems.

The dominant radiographic feature of this disorder is postaxial or central polydactyly, sometimes associated with fusion of metacarpals or phalanges. Cone-shaped epiphyses are common in the middle and distal phalanges and may also be seen in the proximal phalanges (Figure 3-1). Pseudoepiphyses are often seen, as a result of incomplete physis-like

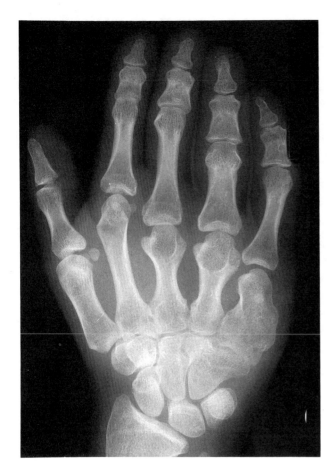

Figure 3-31. Chondroectodermal dysplasia. This 18-year-old girl has short third through fifth metacarpals. Her carpal hamate and fifth metacarpal are very broad, a residual deformity where her sixth digit was surgically removed. The phalanges become progressively shorter, giving a broad appearance to the middle phalanges.

clefts in the proximal metacarpals, where physes do not normally occur. There is progressive shortening of the tubular bones from proximal to distal, with broad middle phalanges and hypoplastic distal phalanges. Coalition, broadening, or overlapping of the capitate and hamate bones may occur (Figure 3-31). Extra carpal bones also occur but are less common (Figure 3-32).

The pelvis often appears abnormal early in life, with short iliac wings and hooklike processes at the medial and occasionally the lateral acetabular margins. The femoral capital epiphyses may ossify early. Slanting of the lateral aspect of the proximal tibial metaphyses may occur, with medial placement of the epiphyseal center. This is usually bilateral and can produce a marked valgus deformity at the knees (Figure 3-33). Conversely, a varus deformity may be seen if the slant is on the medial side of the tibia. The chest is narrow in some infants as a result of rib shortening. This may result in severe pulmonary insufficiency early

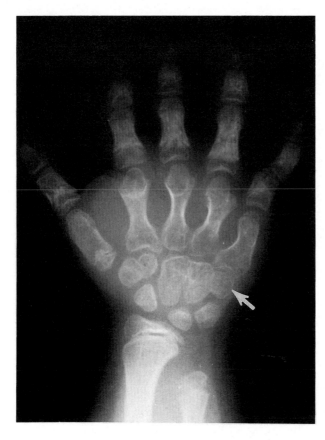

Figure 3-32. Chondroectodermal dysplasia. A supernumerary finger between the fourth and fifth digits was removed surgically. An extra bone is present in the distal carpal row (arrow), and cone-shaped epiphyses are present in all the phalanges.

in life. As these children mature, the thoracic and pelvic abnormalities tend to correct themselves, resulting in relatively normal adult pelvic and thoracic shapes.

The major differential diagnostic consideration for Ellis-van Creveld syndrome is asphyxiating thoracic dystrophy. Patients with this disorder also exhibit polydactyly, a narrow thorax, and an almost identical pelvic dysplasia. Some variant of polydactyly is always present in patients with Ellis-van Creveld syndrome, but it is an inconstant finding in those with asphyxiating thoracic dystrophy. Likewise, patients with asphyxiating thoracic dystrophy do not have the severe hypoplasia of the fingers and nails or the gingival abnormalities found in patients with Ellis-van Creveld syndrome. Asphyxiating thoracic dystrophy is not associated with congenital heart disease. Survivors of asphyxiating thoracic dystrophy develop hepatic fibrosis and progressive renal disease.

The presence of normal intelligence and the tendency for the thoracic and pelvic abnormalities to resolve provide an excellent long-term prog-

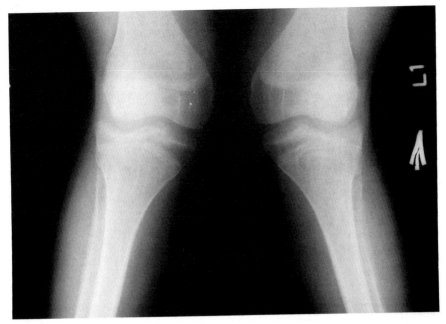

Figure 3-33. Chondroectodermal dysplasia. Typical knee deformity is present in this 15-year-old boy. The proximal tibial metaepiphyseal zones are slanted, with a lateral notch and relative enlargement of the medial aspects of the epiphyses, leading to a knock-knee deformity (genu valgum).

nosis for persons with Ellis-van Creveld syndrome. All patients have short stature, but many acquire an adult height close to 5 feet. If the cardiac anomalies are corrected and appropriate plastic surgical procedures are used for polydactyly, persons with Ellis-van Creveld syndrome are capable of leading an essentially normal life.

Anthony J. Wilson, M.B., Ch.B.
William A. Murphy, Jr., M.D.

SUGGESTED READINGS

ELLIS-VAN CREVELD SYNDROME (CHONDROECTODERMAL
DYSPLASIA)

1. Ellis RW, van Creveld S. A syndrome characterized by ectodermal dysplasia, polydactyly, chondro-dysplasia and congenital morbus cordis. Report of three cases. Arch Dis Child 1940; 15:65–84

2. McKusick VA, Egeland JA, Eldridge R, Krusen DE. Dwarfism in the Amish. I. The Ellis-van Creveld syndrome. Bull Hopkins Hosp 1964; 115:306–330

3. McKusick VA, Eldridge R, Hostetler JA, Egeland JA. Dwarfism in the Amish. Trans Assoc Am Physicians 1964; 77:151–168

HOLT-ORAM (CARDIOMELIC) SYNDROME

4. Holt M, Oram S. Familial heart disease with skeletal malformations. Br Heart J 1960; 22:236–242

5. Kaufman RL, Rimoin DL, McAlister WH, Hartmann AF. Variable expression of the Holt-Oram syndrome. Am J Dis Child 1974; 127:21–25

6. Poznanski AK, Gall JC Jr, Stern AM. Skeletal manifestations of the Holt-Oram syndrome. Radiology 1970; 94:45–53

TURNER'S SYNDROME (MONOSOMY X)

7. Keats TE, Burns TW. The radiographic manifestations of gonadal dysgenesis. Radiol Clin North Am 1964; 2:297–313

8. Levin B. Gonadal dysgenesis. Clinical and roentgenologic manifestations. AJR 1962; 87:1116–1127

9. Rainier-Pope CR, Cunningham RD, Nadas AS, Crigler JF Jr. Cardiovascular malformations in Turner's syndrome. Pediatrics 1964; 33:919–925

DOWN'S SYNDROME (TRISOMY 21)

10. Caffey J, Ross S. Pelvic bones in infantile mongoloidism. Roentgenographic features. AJR 1958; 80:458–467

11. Miller JD, Grace MG, Lampard R. Computed tomography of the upper cervical spine in Down syndrome. J Comput Assist Tomogr 1986; 10:589–592

12. Rosenbaum DM, Blumhagen JD, King HA. Atlantooccipital instability in Down syndrome. AJR 1986; 146:1269–1272

13. Stein SM, Kirchner SG, Horev G, Hernanz-Schulman M. Atlanto-occipital subluxation in Down syndrome. Pediatr Radiol 1991; 21:121–124

14. Warkany J, Passarge E, Smith LB. Congenital malformations in autosomal trisomy syndromes. Am J Dis Child 1966; 112:502–517

CONGENITAL RUBELLA INFECTION

15. Silverman FN. Virus diseases of bone. Do they exist? The Neuhauser Lecture. AJR 1976; 126:677–703

16. Singleton EB, Rudolph AJ, Rosenberg HS, Singer DB. The roentgenographic manifestations of the rubella syndrome in newborn infants. AJR 1966; 97:82–91

17. Whalen JP, Winchester P, Krook L, O'Donohue N, Dische R, Nunez E. Neonatal transplacental rubella syndrome. Its effect on normal maturation of the diaphysis. AJR 1974; 121:166–172

18. Williams HJ, Carey LS. Rubella embryopathy. Roentgenologic features. AJR 1966; 97:92–99

MARFAN'S SYNDROME

19. Beals RK, Mason L. The marfan skull. Radiology 1981; 140:723–725
20. Bianchine JW. The Marfan syndrome revisited. J Pediatr 1971; 79:717–718
21. Joseph KN, Kane HA, Milner RS, Steg NL, Williamson MB Jr, Bowen JR. Orthopedic aspects of the Marfan phenotype. Clin Orthop 1992; 277:251–261
22. Magid D, Pyeritz RE, Fishman EK. Musculoskeletal manifestations of the Marfan syndrome: radiologic features. AJR 1990; 155:99–104
23. Murdoch JL, Walker BA, Halpern BL, Kuzma JA, McKusick VA. Life expectancy and causes of death in the Marfan syndrome. N Engl J Med 1972; 286:804–808

CARDIO-OSTEO-ARTICULAR ASSOCIATIONS

24. Currarino G, Silverman FN. Premature obliteration of the sternal sutures and pigeon-breast deformity. Radiology 1958; 70:532–540
25. Danilowicz DA. Delay in bone age in children with cyanotic congenital heart disease. Radiology 1973; 108:655–658
26. Fischer KC, White RI Jr, Jordan CE, Dorst JP, Neill CA. Sternal abnormalities in patients with congenital heart disease. AJR 1973; 119:530–538
27. Gabrielsen TO, Ladyman GH. Early closure of the sternal sutures and congenital heart disease. AJR 1963; 89:975–983
28. Jordan CE, White RI Jr, Fischer KC, Neill C, Dorst JP. The scoliosis of congenital heart disease. Am Heart J 1972; 84:463–469
29. Katariya S, Prasad PJ, Marwaha RK, Chandra J. Hypertrophic osteoarthropathy in a young child with congenital cyanotic heart disease. Br J Radiol 1986; 59:75–76
30. White RI Jr, Jordan CE, Fischer KC, Lampton L, Neill CA, Dorst JP. Skeletal changes associated with adolescent congenital heart disease. AJR 1972; 116:531–538

UPPER-EXTREMITY ANOMALIES

31. Barnes JC, Smith WL. The VATER association. Radiology 1978; 126:445–449
32. Hall JG, Levin J, Kuhn JP, Ottenheimer EJ, van Berkum KA, McKusick VA. Thrombocytopenia with absent radius (TAR). Medicine 1969; 48:411–439
33. Lawhon SM, MacEwen GD, Bunnell WP. Orthopaedic aspects of the VATER association. J Bone Joint Surg (Am) 1986; 68:424–429
34. Simcha A. Congenital heart disease in radial clubbed hand syndrome. Arch Dis Child 1971; 46:345–349

OTHER ANOMALIES

35. Beuren AJ. Supravalvular aortic stenosis: a complex syndrome with and without mental retardation. Birth Defects 1972; 8:45–56
36. Mason RC, Kozlowski K. Chondrodysplasia punctata. A report of 10 cases. Radiology 1973; 109:145–150

37. Moseley JE, Wolf BS, Gottlieb MI. The trisomy 17-18 syndrome. Roentgen features. AJR 1963; 89:905–913
38. Smith DW. The 18 trisomy and the 13 trisomy syndromes. Birth Defects 1969; 5:67–71

GENERAL

39. Bergsma D (ed). Birth defects compendium, 2nd ed. New York: Alan R Liss; 1979
40. Poznanski AK. The hand in radiologic diagnosis, 2nd ed. Philadelphia: WB Saunders; 1984
41. Spranger JW, Langer LO, Wiedemann HR. Bone dysplasias. An atlas of constitutional disorders of skeletal development. Philadelphia: WB Saunders; 1974
42. Taybi H, Lachman RS. Radiology of syndromes, metabolic disorders, and skeletal dysplasias, 3rd ed. Chicago: Year Book; 1990

Notes

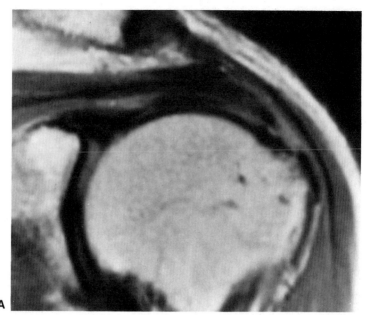

SE 1,800/20

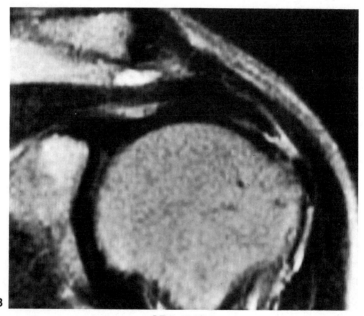

SE 1,800/80

Figure 4-1. This 55-year-old man has severe pain in his left shoulder. You are shown proton-density (A) and T2-weighted (B) coronal oblique MR images of the left shoulder.

Case 4:   Painful Shoulder

Question 15

The test images demonstrate abnormalities of the:

    (A) supraspinatus tendon
    (B) infraspinatus tendon
    (C) subscapularis tendon
    (D) subacromial bursa
    (E) long head of biceps tendon

    Proton-density (Figure 4-1A) and T2-weighted (Figure 4-1B) coronal oblique MR images of the left shoulder at the level of the acromioclavicular joint show abnormal signal intensity in the tendon of the supraspinatus muscle near its insertion on the greater tuberosity (see Figure 4-2) **(Option (A) is true).** The supraspinatus tendon is well visualized on these coronal oblique images, which are performed in a plane oriented along the long axis of the belly of the supraspinatus muscle. In all spin-echo images, the rotator cuff tendons should appear as a signal void or show low to intermediate signal intensity (Figure 4-3). In the proton-density and the T2-weighted images of the test patient, the focal intermediate signal intensity and the high signal intensity, respectively, within the tendon near its insertion represent fluid in a tear of the tendon.

    The rotator cuff is composed of four muscles and their respective tendons: the supraspinatus, infraspinatus, teres minor, and subscapularis. The tendons of the first three muscles insert on the greater tuberosity of the humerus, and the tendon of the subscapularis inserts on the lesser tuberosity (Figure 4-3B). The supraspinatus muscle arises from the dorsal aspect of the scapula superior to the spine of the scapula and inserts on the superior aspect of the greater tuberosity of the humerus. The supraspinatus tendon is the portion of the rotator cuff that is most frequently involved in impingement syndrome. Inflammation (tendinitis), degeneration, and tears of the supraspinatus tendon are all usually best visualized on coronal oblique images. With tendinitis and tendon degen-

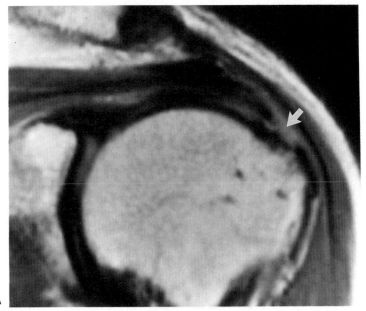

SE 1,800/20

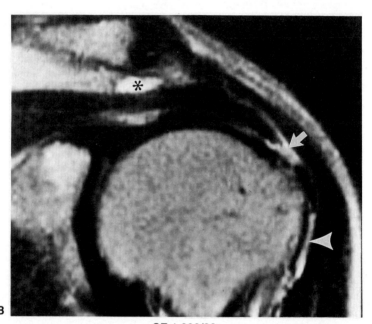

SE 1,800/80

Figure 4-2 (Same as Figure 4-1). Supraspinatus tendon rupture. Proton-density (A) and T2-weighted (B) coronal oblique MR images at the level of the acromioclavicular joint show abnormal signal intensity (arrow) in the tendon of the supraspinatus muscle near its insertion on the greater tuberosity of the humerus. The T2-weighted image shows high-intensity fluid in the subacromial bursa (✱) and in the subdeltoid bursa (arrowhead).

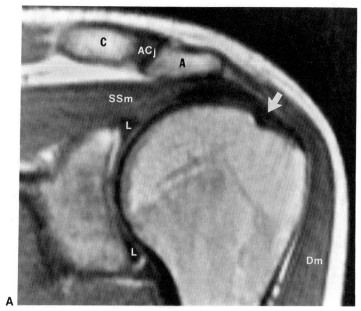

A

SE 700/15

Figure 4-3. Normal shoulder anatomy. MR images of the shoulder in a normal 25-year-old female volunteer. (A) Coronal oblique T1-weighted image shows low signal intensity of the normal supraspinatus tendon (arrow). A = acromion; ACj = acromioclavicular joint; C = clavicle; L = labrum; Dm = deltoid muscle; SSm = supraspinatus muscle. (B) Transaxial T1-weighted image shows low signal intensity of the normal subscapularis tendon (arrow). BG = bicipital groove; CBm = coracobrachialis muscle; Dm = deltoid muscle; L = labrum; ISm = infraspinatus muscle; SBm = subscapularis muscle; SDb = subdeltoid bursa. (C) The subdeltoid bursa (arrow) is identified on this T1-weighted coronal oblique image by a linear high-signal-intensity band thought to be due to a thin layer of fat which parallels the potential space of the bursa. (D) The biceps tendon (arrow) is identified on this T1-weighted transaxial image lying within the intertubercular groove of the humerus.

eration, increased water content within or surrounding the tendon results in increased signal intensity on the proton-density image (Figure 4-4A), but the signal intensity is neither as focal nor as bright on the T2-weighted image (Figure 4-4B), as is evident in the test images. With increasing severity and chronicity, rotator cuff tears can also show muscle retraction and atrophy, which are not present in the test case.

Tears of the infraspinatus, teres minor, and subscapularis tendons are much less common than tears of the supraspinatus tendon. The infraspinatus tendon lies posterior and inferior to the supraspinatus ten-

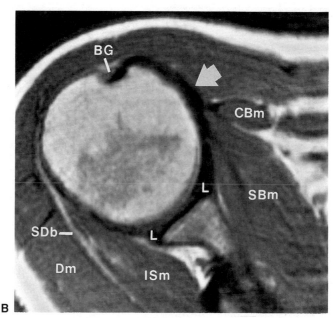

B

SE 700/15

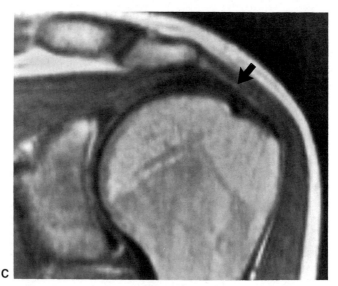

C

SE 700/15

don and is not shown in the test images **(Option (B) is false).** The teres minor tendon inserts immediately distal to the infraspinatus tendon. The subscapularis muscle is triangular and originates from the anterior aspect of the body of the scapula. Its tendon attaches to the lesser tuber-

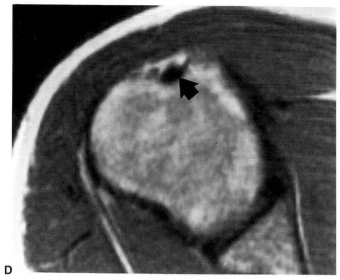

D

SE 700/15

osity. The tendon of the subscapularis is not shown in the test images **(Option (C) is false).** The infraspinatus and subscapularis muscles and tendons are seen to best advantage on axial images (Figure 4-3B).

The subacromial bursa is a potential space between the acromion and the supraspinatus muscle and tendon. It communicates with the subdeltoid bursa, which lies laterally and inferiorly between the deltoid muscle and the rotator cuff tendons and subjacent humeral head. In its normal state, the subacromial-subdeltoid bursal complex is often identified on T1-weighted images by a linear high-intensity band thought to be due to a thin layer of fat which parallels the potential space of the bursa (the subacromial-subdeltoid fat plane) (Figure 4-3C).

When there is a complete rotator cuff tear, the glenohumeral joint cavity communicates with the subacromial bursa and the bursa may contain joint fluid. The focus of high signal intensity just below the acromioclavicular joint on the T2-weighted test image (Figure 4-2B) represents an abnormal subacromial bursa containing joint fluid **(Option (D) is true).** Fluid is also seen within the subdeltoid bursa immediately lateral to the humeral head. The presence of fluid in the subacromial-subdeltoid bursa is often associated with a rotator cuff tear; however, fluid may be present in the absence of a tear, and a tear may be present without bursal fluid. Intrasubstance rotator cuff tears and inferior-surface partial incomplete tears do not of themselves result in a fluid-filled subacromial bursa.

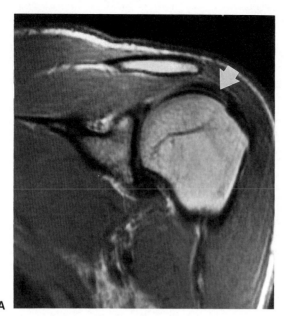

SE 1,800/15

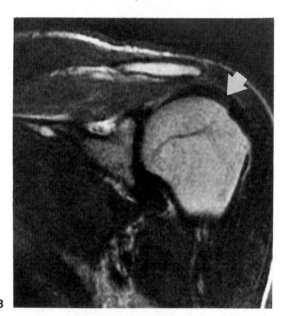

SE 1,800/70

Figure 4-4. Tendinitis in a 48-year-old woman with a painful left shoulder. (A) A coronal oblique proton-density image reveals a linear area of increased signal intensity (arrow) within the supraspinatus tendon near its insertion on the greater tuberosity. (B) Coronal oblique T2-weighted image. The signal in the tendon (arrow) does not increase in intensity. The diagnosis was tendinitis, and the patient responded to conservative therapy.

The tendon of the long head of the biceps muscle arises near the base of the superior glenoid labrum and passes within the joint to exit through the bicipital groove (Figure 4-3D). The biceps tendon is not seen in the test images **(Option (E) is false).**

Question 16

Concerning impingement syndrome of the shoulder,

    (A) it is the underlying cause of most rotator cuff tears
    (B) a low-lying acromion predisposes to this condition
    (C) early surgical intervention is required in most cases
    (D) radiographic changes occur early
    (E) arthrography is an effective method for early detection

Classic impingement syndrome of the shoulder is a painful condition in which the supraspinatus tendon and subacromial bursa are entrapped between the humeral head below and either the anterior acromion itself, spurs of the anterior acromion, degenerative changes of the acromioclavicular joint, or the coracoacromial ligament above (Figure 4-5). Occasionally, impingement involves the tendon of the long head of the biceps. Impingement syndrome affects people of all ages. Neer has reported that 95% of rotator cuff tears result from chronic impingement **(Option (A) is true)**.

Pain due to impingement syndrome is exacerbated when the arm is abducted and externally rotated or internally rotated and elevated. Impingement syndrome results most often from repetitive trauma caused by vigorous overhead occupational or athletic endeavors or degenerative exostoses. Repetitive trauma results in a reparative response with edema and an increase in volume of the bursa and tendon, which causes further relative reduction of the space within which the tendon and bursa must function. According to Neer, anatomic variations in the shape and slope of the acromion can predispose to impingement syndrome because a low-lying anterior acromion or down-sloping anterolateral acromion can compromise the acromiohumeral distance **(Option (B) is true)**.

Three progressive stages of shoulder impingement syndrome as found clinically and at surgery have been described. The early stages of the condition are usually reversible with conservative therapy, and surgery is necessary only when conservative treatment has failed or impingement has already progressed to a tear of the rotator cuff **(Option (C) is false)**. Stage I consists of edema and hemorrhage and is reversible with conservative therapy. Stage II implies fibrosis and thickening of the subacromial soft tissues and is manifested clinically by recurrent pain. Surgery is considered for stage II lesions only when symptoms have persisted despite conservative treatment, including rest, anti-inflammatory medications, and physical therapy. Stage III represents a tear of the rotator cuff and requires surgery for restoration of normal function (Figure 4-6).

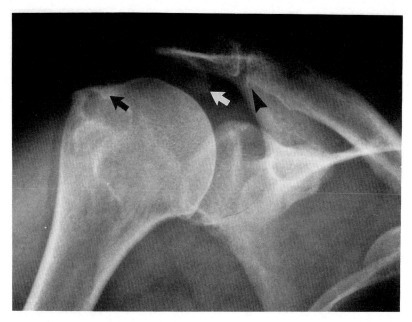

Figure 4-5. Impingement syndrome. An anteroposterior radiograph (with 30° caudal angulation) of the right shoulder of a 50-year-old man with a long history of shoulder pain is shown. Radiographic findings include sclerosis (black arrow) of the greater tuberosity of the humerus, a large spur (white arrow) off the anteroinferior surface of the acromion, and a smaller spur (arrowhead) at the inferior aspect of the acromioclavicular joint. These are all findings associated with classic impingement syndrome.

The MR appearance of soft tissue changes due to impingement reflects inflammatory and/or degenerative changes in the bursa and tendon. Subacromial bursitis resulting from impingement is evident as thickening of the normally thin subacromial bursal fat as a result of hypertrophic synovitis (Figure 4-7). Tendon inflammation and degeneration usually appear intermediate in signal intensity on T1-weighted images. With T2 weighting the signal may decrease or slightly increase, but it does not reach the high signal of a focal fluid collection, as is seen with a tear. This appearance may also be seen in asymptomatic individuals and must be interpreted in conjunction with clinical information and associated MR findings of impingement.

Several clinical tests have been devised to detect impingement syndrome, but the signs and symptoms may be nonspecific and the diagnosis is often delayed until a full-thickness tear of the rotator cuff has occurred. Similarly, radiography plays little or no role in early diagnosis, because radiographic changes are absent or occur only late in the course

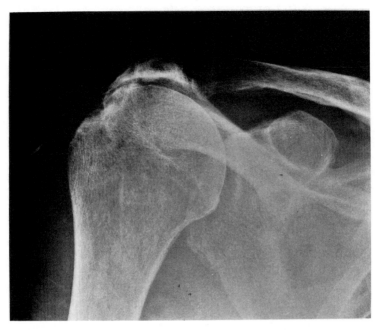

Figure 4-6. Advanced impingement syndrome in a 65-year-old man with cuff tear arthropathy. The anteroposterior view reveals that the humeral head has migrated superiorly to impinge on the acromion.

of the disease **(Option (D) is false).** When radiographic changes do occur, they include sclerosis of the greater tuberosity of the humerus and spurring of the anteroinferior surface of the acromion or acromioclavicular joint. As the disorder progresses, radiographs may show the typical bony changes associated with a chronic rotator cuff tear, including an acromiohumeral distance of less than 7 mm as a result of superior migration of the humeral head and a concave depression on the undersurface of the acromion. However, even in stage III disease, radiographs are frequently normal. Conversely, irregularity or apparent sclerosis of the greater tuberosity can be a normal variant, and spurs of the inferior margin of the acromion or acromioclavicular joint are not necessarily associated with soft tissue disease.

Arthrography provides little information in the early diagnosis of impingement syndrome **(Option (E) is false).** Even when arthrography is performed with CT, the arthrogram is usually normal in stage I disease and is sometimes normal in stage II disease. However, MRI offers an effective noninvasive means of evaluating the extent of soft tissue involvement and usually provides clinically useful information regarding the offending structures. This specific information assists in patient

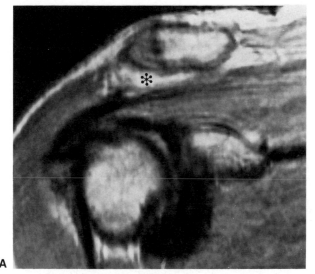

A

SE 2,000/15

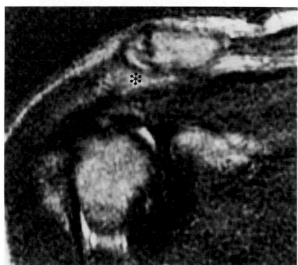

B

SE 2,000/80

Figure 4-7. Subacromial bursitis. Proton-density (A) and T2-weighted (B) coronal oblique MR images of a 21-year-old man with shoulder pain demonstrate marked thickening of the subacromial bursa (✻) but no excess fluid in the bursa. This reflects hypertrophic synovitis due to impingement. There is motion artifact.

counseling and preoperative planning. Impingement without rotator cuff tear due to an anterior acromial spur or down-sloping anterolateral acromion (Figure 4-8) may, for example, be treated with an arthroscopic subacromial decompression (acromioplasty). Impingement due to degenerative spurs and/or capsular hypertrophy of the acromioclavicular joint may require partial or complete excision of the acromioclavicular joint. If the cuff is torn, an open procedure may be necessary to restore function.

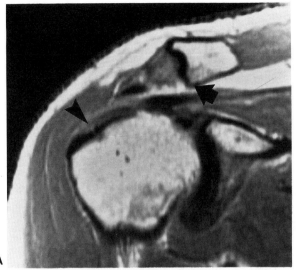

A

SE 1,000/15

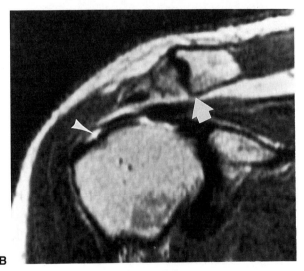

B

SE 1,800/70

Figure 4-8. Subacromial spur. MR images of a 38-year-old man with shoulder pain and decreased range of motion. Proton-density (A) and T2-weighted (B) coronal oblique images demonstrate a large spur (arrow) off the anterolateral aspect of the acromion. Fluid in the supraspinatus tendon indicates an associated tendon tear (arrowhead).

Massive chronic rotator cuff tears (Figure 4-9) may not be amenable to surgical repair, but debridement of the cuff, acromioplasty, and/or resection of acromioclavicular joint spurs may provide significant pain relief.

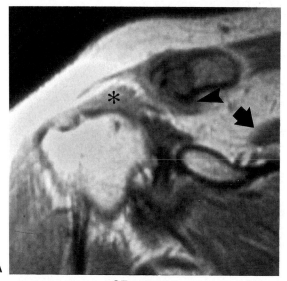

SE 1,000/15

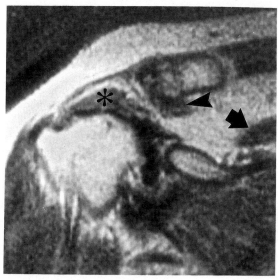

SE 1,800/70

Figure 4-9. Massive tear. MR images of a 79-year-old woman with a several-year history of shoulder pain. Proton-density (A) and T2-weighted (B) coronal oblique images demonstrate severe retraction of the supraspinatus muscle (arrow) due to a massive tear. A large spur is seen off the acromioclavicular joint (arrowhead), and the supraspinatus tendon has been replaced with fibrous scar tissue (*). Arthroscopic debridement and resection of the spur resulted in a marked reduction in pain and increased range of motion.

Question 17

Concerning glenohumeral joint stability,

(A) the glenoid labrum is the major soft tissue support for the glenohumeral joint
(B) CT arthrography is an effective method of evaluating the anatomic structures of the glenohumeral joint
(C) tears of the anterior labrum are more common than tears of the posterior labrum
(D) the presence of a labral tear implies a previous dislocation
(E) the term "Bankart lesion" is limited to osseous fractures of the glenoid rim

The shallow depression of the bony glenoid and the spherical surface of the humeral head permit a wide range of motion of the upper extremity, but the glenohumeral joint is also inherently unstable. Glenohumeral instability is a common cause of chronic shoulder pain and disability.

The fibrocartilaginous glenoid labrum, located at the circumference of the glenoid fossa, deepens the articular depression, but it is not believed to provide the major soft tissue support for the joint **(Option (A) is false).** A number of other soft tissue structures, including the fibrous capsule, glenohumeral ligaments, and rotator cuff muscles and tendons, contribute to the stability of the joint (Figure 4-10). Among these, the inferior glenohumeral ligament is considered the most effective of the anterior and inferior stabilizing structures.

Several problems are encountered in evaluating the unstable shoulder. For example, not all patients have a history of dislocation or subluxation, and many patients complain only of pain, fatigue, weakness, numbness, or diminished range of motion. The physical examination in these patients may be inconclusive, and some patients may have multidirectional instability. If only the more common anterior lesion is diagnosed and treated, patients may suffer persistent pain and disability from persistent posterior or inferior instability. Although a labrum tear is the most frequent pathologic finding, complex soft tissue lesions, often involving not only the glenoid labrum but also the joint capsule and occasionally the rotator cuff, may be present.

The anterior and posterior glenohumeral joint and glenoid labrum are best depicted on axial images. Both CT arthrography and MRI are currently used to evaluate shoulder instability and labral and capsular abnormalities. CT arthrography is superior to conventional arthrotomography for demonstrating the anatomic structures of the glenohumeral joint and is an effective method of evaluating the glenohumeral joint, including capsular structures **(Option (B) is true).** With CT arthrography, the differences between the anterior and posterior capsulolabral complexes are well demonstrated. Posteriorly, the joint capsule is

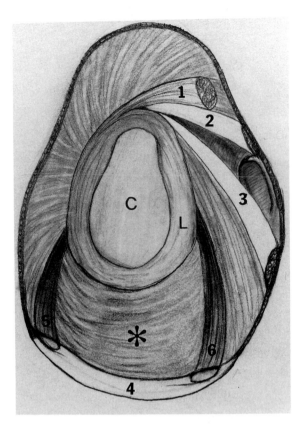

Figure 4-10 (left). Drawing of the glenoid and its surrounding structures. A fibrous capsule (✱) surrounds the glenoid labrum (L) and hyaline cartilage (C). The tendon of the biceps (1) arises at the superior aspect of the glenoid labrum and functions as a humeral head depressor. The superior (2), middle (3), and inferior (4) glenohumeral ligaments are three anterior thickenings of the capsule that act as static restraints during glenohumeral abduction. The most important of these is the inferior glenohumeral ligament with its posterior (5) and anterior (6) bands, which resists anterior migration of the humeral head and is avulsed from the glenoid rim in the Bankart lesion. (Adapted with permission from Fu et al. [2].)

Figure 4-11 (right). Normal labra. Double-contrast CT arthrogram of a 52-year-old man with chronic shoulder pain but no history of dislocation shows normal anterior (arrow) and posterior (arrowhead) glenoid labra.

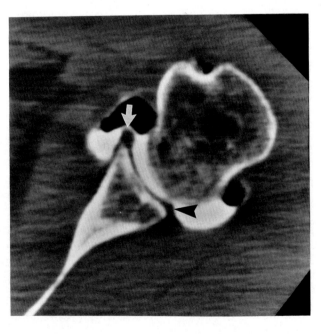

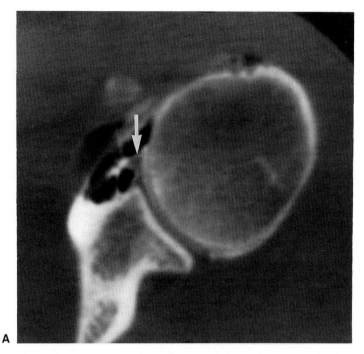

A

Figure 4-12. Normal variations of anterior capsulolabral complex. (A) CT arthrogram image at the level of the subscapularis bursa. A well-developed middle glenohumeral ligament is visualized along and apparently attached to the labrum (arrow). (B) The middle glenohumeral ligament is visualized adjacent to the labrum (arrow). (C) The middle glenohumeral ligament (thin arrow) runs parallel to the capsule (thick arrows), forming a bursa in between them. (Panels A and B are reprinted with permission from Rafii [24]. Panel C is reprinted with permission from Rafii et al. [21].)

attached to the glenoid margin and blends with the periphery of the labrum, which is usually smaller and more rounded than the anterior labrum (Figure 4-11). Anteriorly, considerable variations exist in the development of the glenohumeral ligaments and the glenoid site of attachment of the capsule and its ligaments, resulting in some variable morphology of the capsulolabral complex (Figures 4-12 and 4-13). Scapular attachment of the anterior joint capsule varies from near the glenoid margin to the scapular neck region (Figure 4-14).

Most dislocations and subluxations are anterior, and so anterior labral tears are more common than posterior tears **(Option (C) is true)**. Criteria for identifying labral tears on CT arthrography include air or positive contrast, or both, entering the substance of the labrum or the

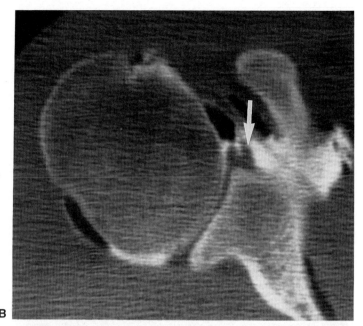

B

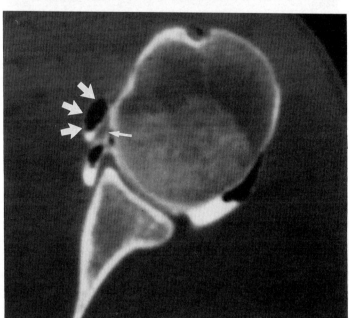

C

junction of the labrum with the glenoid (Figure 4-15); labral blunting; fragmentation (Figure 4-16); and segmental or complete absence of the labrum (Figure 4-17). In MR images, labral injury may appear as a line of increased signal intensity that completely traverses the normal low-

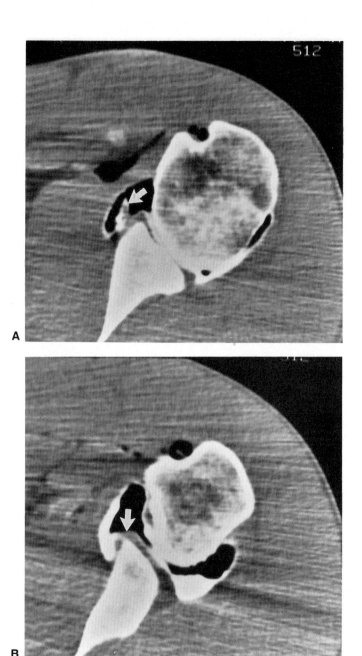

Figure 4-13. Normal variations of anterior capsulolabral complex. (A) The inferior glenohumeral ligament is frequently visualized in the vicinity of anteroinferior glenoid margin (arrow). (B) This ligament often becomes confluent with the inferior labrum, which in this region may show a truncated or flattened configuration (arrow).

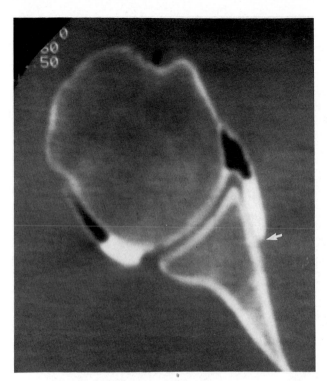

Figure 4-14. Normal variation, scapular neck insertion of anterior capsule. A CT arthrogram at mid glenohumeral level (below the subscapularis bursa) is shown. The remote capsular insertion from the glenoid margin is demonstrated (arrow). Note normal labrum and smooth reflection of the capsule over the scapular neck. (Reprinted with permission from Rafii et al. [21].)

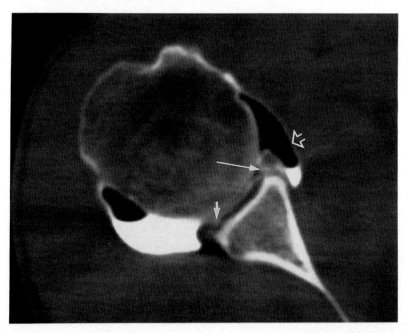

Figure 4-15. Anterior labrum tear in recurrent subluxation. A CT arthrogram at mid glenoid level shows tear and detachment of the labrum from the glenoid margin (long solid arrow). The anterior capsule is slightly expanded (open arrow). Also, a partial tear of the posterior labrum is present (short solid arrow). (Reprinted with permission from Rafii [20].)

122

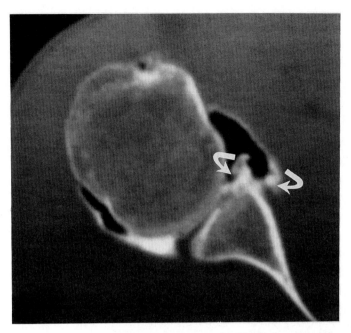

Figure 4-16. Recurrent anterior dislocation. A CT arthrogram below mid glenoid level shows marked irregularity and fragmentation of the anterior labrum and associated irregularity of the adjacent capsule (curved arrows). Note associated erosion and deficiency of the glenoid margin and glenoid articular surface. (Reprinted with permission from Rafii et al. [22].)

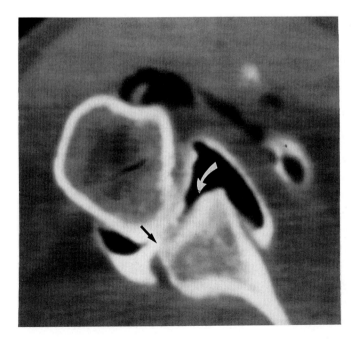

Figure 4-17. Recurrent anterior dislocation. There is absence of the anterior labrum with the osseous glenoid margin exposed (curved arrow). The joint capsule in this region is stripped away from the glenoid and as a result extends to the scapular neck, a pathologic finding unlike the normal variation demonstrated in Figure 4-12. The posterior glenoid labrum is also torn (black arrow). (Reprinted with permission from Rafii et al. [22].)

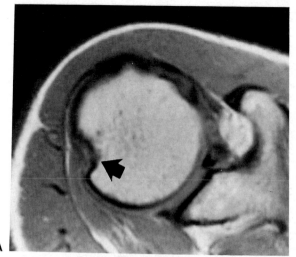

A

SE 1,500/20

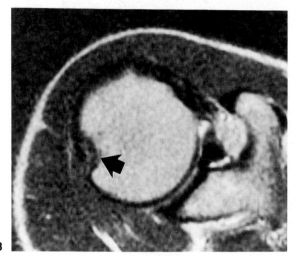

B

SE 1,500/80

Figure 4-18. Hill-Sachs lesion in a 31-year-old man. Proton-density (A) and T2-weighted (B) transaxial images at the level of the coracoid process. The patient had a previous anterior dislocation. The Hill-Sachs lesion (arrow) is evident as a depressed fracture of the posterolateral aspect of the superior humeral head. The absence of marrow edema indicates that this defect is not a recent injury.

intensity labral structure or as labral blunting, fragmentation, or absence. Labral abnormalities are often associated with previous dislocation but may also be seen following subluxation without frank dislocation or even in patients without clinically demonstrable instability **(Option (D) is false).** Hill-Sachs (Figure 4-18) and osseous Bankart lesions can be found in association with glenohumeral subluxation or dislocation and may be seen on either CT or MR examinations. A Bankart fracture is a fracture of the anteroinferior glenoid rim. The classic Bankart lesion is a soft tissue injury, which involves separation of the labrum from the

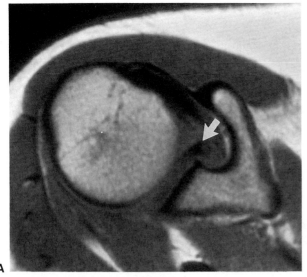

A

SE 1,500/15

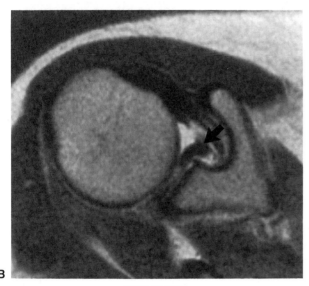

B

SE 1,500/70

Figure 4-19. Bankart lesion. MR images of a 17-year-old girl who sustained an anterior dislocation of the shoulder at the time of a motor vehicle accident. Proton-density (A) and T2-weighted (B) trans-axial images at the level of the coracoid process reveal the low signal intensity of the detached anterior glenoid labrum (arrow). On the T2-weighted image, the fragment is surrounded by high-signal-intensity joint fluid.

underlying bony glenoid and/or a tear of the joint capsule (Figures 4-19 and 4-20) **(Option (E) is false).**

Lawrence W. Bassett, M.D.
Mahvash Rafii, M.D.
Leanne L. Seeger, M.D.

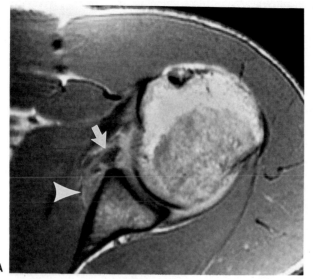

SE 1,500/15

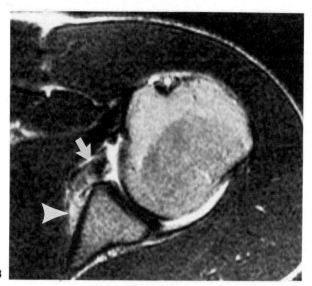

SE1,500/70

Figure 4-20. Bankart lesion. MR images of a 22-year-old male football player with a history of recent anterior dislocation of the shoulder are shown. Proton-density (A) and T2-weighted (B) transaxial images show the detached anterior labrum (arrow). Fluid dissecting along the anterior border of the scapula (arrowhead) indicates a tear of the capsule.

SUGGESTED READINGS

NORMAL ANATOMY

1. Deutsch AL, Resnick D, Mink JH, et al. Computed and conventional arthrotomography of the glenohumeral joint: normal anatomy and clinical experience. Radiology 1984; 153:603–609

2. Fu FH, Seel MJ, Berger RA. Relevant shoulder biomechanics. Op Tech Orthop 1991; 1:134–146

3. Huber DJ, Sauter R, Mueller E, Requardt H, Weber H. MR imaging of the normal shoulder. Radiology 1986; 158:405–408

4. Kieft GJ, Bloem JL, Obermann WR, Verbout AL, Rozing PM, Doornbos J. Normal shoulder: MR imaging. Radiology 1986; 159:741–745

5. Middleton WD, Kneeland JB, Carrera GF, et al. High-resolution MR imaging of the normal rotator cuff. AJR 1987; 148:559–564

6. Mitchell MJ, Causey G, Berthoty DP, Sartoris DJ, Resnick D. Peribursal fat plane of the shoulder: anatomic study and clinical experience. Radiology 1988; 168:699–704

7. Neumann CH, Holt RG, Steinbach LS, Jahnke AH Jr, Petersen SA. MR imaging of the shoulder: appearance of the supraspinatus tendon in asymptomatic volunteers. AJR 1992; 158:1281–1287

8. Seeger LL, Ruszkowski JT, Bassett LW, Kay SP, Kahmann RD, Ellman H. MR imaging of the normal shoulder: anatomic correlation. AJR 1987; 148:83–91

9. Zlatkin MB, Bjorkengren AG, Gylys-Morin V, Resnick D, Sartoris DJ. Cross-sectional imaging of the capsular mechanism of the glenohumeral joint. AJR 1988; 150:151–158

IMPINGEMENT SYNDROME

10. Burk DL Jr, Karasick D, Kurtz AB, et al. Rotator cuff tears: prospective comparison of MR imaging with arthrography, sonography, and surgery. AJR 1989; 153:87–92

11. Cone RO III, Resnick D, Danzig L. Shoulder impingement syndrome: radiographic evaluation. Radiology 1984; 150:29–33

12. Kieft GJ, Bloem JL, Rozing PM, Obermann WR. Rotator cuff impingement syndrome: MR imaging. Radiology 1988; 166:211–214

13. Kneeland JB, Middleton WD, Carrera GF, et al. MR imaging of the shoulder: diagnosis of rotator cuff tears. AJR 1987; 149:333–337

14. Neer CS II. Impingement lesions. Clin Orthop 1983; 173:70–77

15. Rafii M, Firooznia H, Sherman O, et al. Rotator cuff lesions: signal patterns at MR imaging. Radiology 1990; 177:817–823

16. Seeger LL, Gold RH, Bassett LW, Ellman H. Shoulder impingement syndrome: MR findings in 53 shoulders. AJR 1988; 150:343–347

17. Watson M. Rotator cuff function in the impingement syndrome. J Bone Joint Surg (Br) 1989; 71:361–366

18. Zlatkin MB, Iannotti JP, Roberts MC, et al. Rotator cuff tears: diagnostic performance of MR imaging. Radiology 1989; 172:223–229

SHOULDER INSTABILITY

19. Kieft GJ, Bloem JL, Rozing PM, Obermann WR. MR imaging of recurrent anterior dislocation of the shoulder: comparison with CT arthrography. AJR 1988; 150:1083–1087

20. Rafii M. Shoulder. In: Firooznia H, Golimbu CN, Rafii M, Rauschning W, Weinreb JC (eds), MRI and CT of the musculoskeletal system. St. Louis: Mosby-Year Book; 1992:465–549

Case 4 / 127

21. Rafii M, Firooznia H, Golimbu C, Minkoff J, Bonamo J. CT arthrography of capsular structures of the shoulder. AJR 1986; 146:361–367
22. Rafii M, Minkoff J, Destefano V. Diagnostic imaging of the shoulder. In: Nicholas JA, Hershman EB (eds), The upper extremity in sports medicine. St. Louis: Mosby-Year Book; 1990:91–158
23. Rowe CR, Zarins B. Recurrent transient subluxation of the shoulder. J Bone Joint Surg (Am) 1981; 63:863–872
24. Seeger LL, Gold RH, Bassett LW. Shoulder instability: evaluation with MR imaging. Radiology 1988; 168:695–697
25. Turkel SJ, Panio MW, Marshall JL, Girgis FG. Stabilizing mechanisms preventing anterior dislocation of the glenohumeral joint. J Bone Joint Surg (Am) 1981; 63:1208–1217

Notes

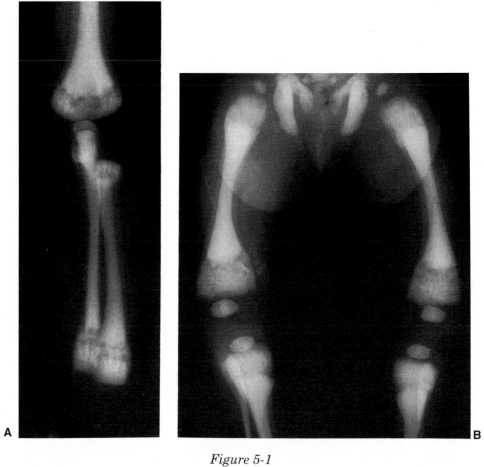

A

B

Figure 5-1

Figures 5-1 and 5-2. This 10-month-old chronically ill infant was anemic. You are shown anteroposterior radiographs of the left forearm (A) and both femora (B) taken at diagnosis (Figure 5-1), as well as similarly positioned radiographs obtained 6 months later (Figure 5-2).

Case 5: Tissue Transplantation

Question 18

Which *one* of the following is the MOST likely cause of the change in skeletal pattern?

- (A) Tissue transplantation
- (B) Radiation therapy
- (C) Steroid therapy
- (D) Antibiotic therapy
- (E) Withdrawal of noxious agent

The anteroposterior radiograph of the left forearm (Figure 5-1A) shows sclerotic diaphyses and metaphyses of the radius, ulna, and distal humerus. In addition, transverse alternating lucent and dense bands are present in all metaphyses. The texture of the osteosclerotic diaphyses is homogeneous, whereas the texture of the banded metaphyses is striated. The sclerotic segments of the bones are primarily the medullary cavities. The cortical bone is faintly seen (see Figure 5-3A).

The anteroposterior radiograph of the femora (Figure 5-1B) shows features identical to those seen in the left forearm. All visualized bones are involved and are sclerotic. This includes the pubic, ischial, tibial, and fibular bones, as well as the femora. Even the epiphyses are sclerotic. Again, the medullary portions are most sclerotic, the metaphyses are banded and striated, and the cortices are faint (see Figure 5-3B).

The first task in deciphering this test case is to determine the diagnosis at presentation as represented by the initial radiographs shown in Figure 5-1. Unfortunately, the differential diagnosis of sclerotic bones is a very long one. However, it can be shortened by division into localized and generalized osteosclerosis. The test case clearly is an example of generalized osteosclerosis since no bone shown in the radiographs is spared. Many diseases cause generalized osteosclerosis (Table 5-1), but only a

---

Figures 5-1 and 5-2 were provided courtesy of Phoebe A. Kaplan, M.D., University of Virginia, Charlottesville, Va.

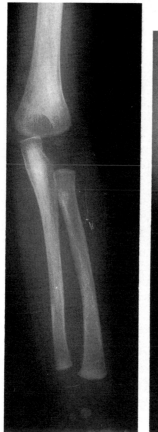
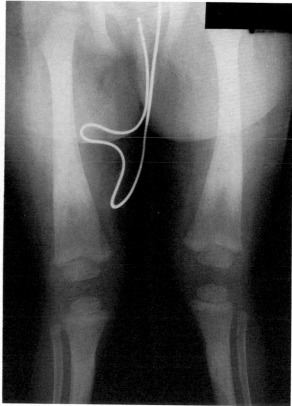

Figure 5-2

few do so in infants and are associated with chronic illness. Those conditions are heavy metal poisoning, hypervitaminoses A and D, and osteopetrosis.

When the radiographic features are considered, heavy metal poisoning and hypervitaminoses A and D can be eliminated. Lead, phosphorus, and bismuth poisoning can produce dense metaphyses. In these conditions, the zones of provisional calcification are involved and are typically homogeneously dense (Figure 5-4). The dense metaphyseal bands vary in width depending upon the duration of the poisoning. On occasion, alternating dense and lucent bands are encountered if the episodes of heavy metal intoxication were intermittent (Figure 5-5). The diaphyses, however, remain normal, and this feature excludes the heavy metals as causative agents in the test case.

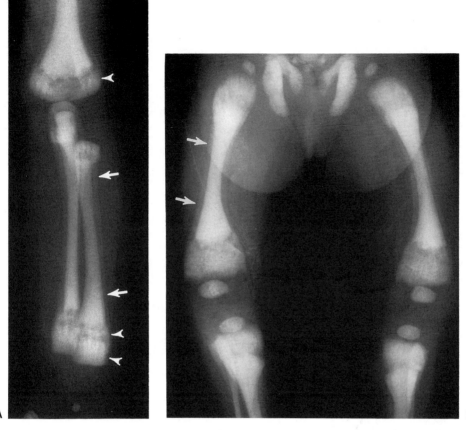

Figure 5-3 (Same as Figure 5-1). Osteopetrosis. (A) An anteroposterior radiograph of the left forearm shows generalized osteosclerosis, homogeneous density of the metadiaphyseal medullary space, faint cortices (arrows), and expanded, banded, and striated metaphyses (arrowheads). (B) An anteroposterior radiograph of the femora shows similar features. The faint cortices are more easily seen (arrows), and the femora are slightly bowed.

Hypervitaminosis A can occur in the first year of life due to overzealous nutritional supplementation. Its radiographic pattern is one of periosteal reaction without the dramatic sclerosis shown in the test case. Hypervitaminosis D can also develop as a result of too much nutritional supplementation. Dense metaphyseal bands can occur, and there can also be cortical thickening from periosteal bone apposition. Dense medullary osteosclerosis is not a feature of hypervitaminosis D. Metastatic calcification of blood vessels, periarticular tissues, and muscles occurs and

Table 5-1: Disorders That Cause Generalized Osteosclerosis

Dysplasias
    Craniodiaphyseal dysplasia
    Craniometaphyseal dysplasia
    Dysosteosclerosis
    Endosteal hyperostosis
    Frontometaphyseal dysplasia
    Infantile cortical hyperostosis
    Metaphyseal dysplasia
    Mixed sclerosing bone dystrophy
    Osteopathia striata
    Osteopetrosis
    Osteopoikilosis
    Progressive diaphyseal dysplasia
    Pyknodysostosis

Metabolic Disorders
    Fluorosis
    Heavy metal poisoning
    Hypervitaminosis A
    Hypervitaminosis D
    Renal osteodystrophy

Other Disorders
    Axial osteomalacia
    Fibrogenesis imperfecta ossium
    Mastocytosis
    Myelofibrosis
    Plasma cell myeloma
    Skeletal metastases

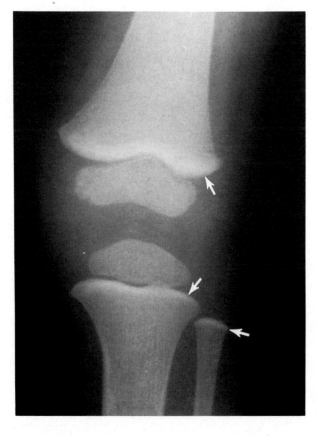

Figure 5-4. Lead poisoning. An anteroposterior radiograph of the left knee shows thin, dense bands of sclerosis abutting the metaphyseal edge of the physes (arrows). This represents failure to absorb excess mineral deposited in the zone of provisional calcification. Note that the medullary cavity is of normal bone density.

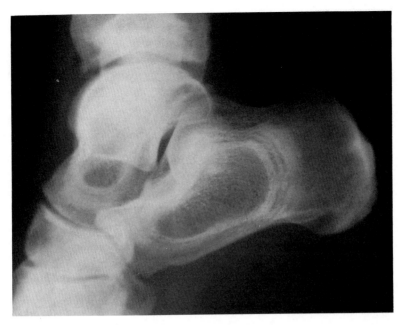

Figure 5-5. Phosphorus poisoning. A lateral radiograph of the ankle shows concentric rings of sclerosis in the calcaneus, talus, and cuboid. This patient had been treated in infancy and childhood with large doses of phosphorized cod-liver oil. The intermittent nature of the rings is evidence of the several treatments the patient underwent. The pattern is also termed "bone in bone" or endobone appearance.

is a prominent feature, but these findings are not present in the test images. Thus, these hypervitaminoses are excluded as causes of the features shown in Figure 5-1.

Therefore, the best diagnosis for the condition displayed in the test images is osteopetrosis. Generalized osteosclerosis is the principal feature of osteopetrosis. The skeleton can be homogeneously dense, as shown in the diaphyses, or there can be alternating dense and lucent bands, as evident in the metaphyses. Vertebrae, and at times other bones, can show a "bone-in-bone" or endobone appearance.

Whenever osteopetrosis is considered as a potential diagnosis, pyknodysostosis should also be considered because it shares many of the same radiologic features. However, infants and children with pyknodysostosis are generally healthy. Thus pyknodysostosis is also excluded.

Once the condition of osteopetrosis has been determined, one still must explain the change in skeletal pattern exhibited in Figure 5-2, a change that occurred within only 6 months. This change is a dramatic, but incomplete, normalization of the bone density and configuration. The

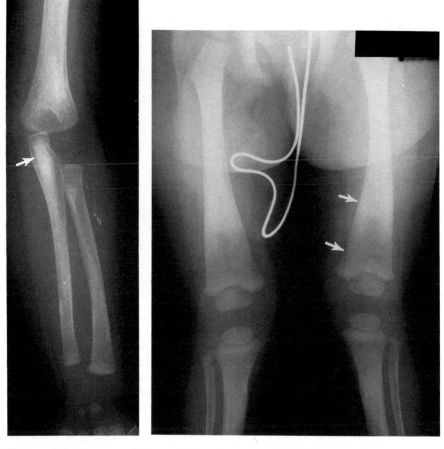

A

B

Figure 5-6 (Same as Figure 5-2). Osteopetrosis following bone marrow transplantation. (A) An anteroposterior radiograph of the left forearm shows remarkable normalization of bone density and shape. Only mild sclerosis remains in the proximal ulna (arrow) and distal humerus. (B) An anteroposterior radiograph of the femora shows similar normalization compared with Figure 5-1B. Although the femora are less bowed, there is residual flaring of the distal femoral metaphyses (arrows).

long bones show remarkable loss of the osteosclerosis, particularly of the medullary cavities, with a return to an almost normal medullary bone density (Figure 5-6A). The metaphyses have remodeled with loss of the banded and striated pattern. The shape of the metaphyses has become more normal, but the distal femoral metaphyses remain mildly flared (Figure 5-6B). The femora are less bowed. The cortices are more normal in both thickness and density and have a more normal appearance in relationship to the medullary cavities. Overall, it is difficult to believe the radiographs in Figure 5-2 are of the same patient as those in Figure 5-1, since the change is so striking.

Which of the situations posed in Question 18 is most likely to have caused this unexpected and extraordinary resolution of bone density in this infant? Since analysis of Figure 5-1 has led to a diagnosis of osteopetrosis, the task is simplified. Osteopetrosis, first described in 1904 by Albers-Schönberg, is often subdivided into two principal forms, an autosomal-dominant type with few symptoms and an autosomal-recessive type that can be fatal in infancy. Other, less common types exist such as an intermediate, less serious autosomal-recessive form found in older children and a form found in adults and characterized by a deficiency of the carbonic anhydrase II isoenzyme. The pathogenesis of these several forms of osteopetrosis is defective osteoclast function, wherein skeletal tissue is improperly resorbed. There is no known noxious agent involved in the causation of osteopetrosis. Therefore, the withdrawal of a noxious agent (Option (E)) could not lead to the changes evident in the test patient.

In general, therapy for the dominant form of osteopetrosis is unnecessary and therapy for the recessive infantile form is unsuccessful. Certainly, radiation therapy (Option (B)) and antibiotic therapy (Option (D)) do not alter the fundamental osteoclast malfunction and would not be expected to induce the normalization demonstrated in the test patient. Large doses of glucocorticoids may have some beneficial effect in the autosomal-recessive infantile form, particularly in stabilizing symptoms. Steroid therapy (Option (C)) would not dramatically alter the underlying cellular dysfunction or result in such remarkable radiographic resolution.

Pharmacologic doses of calcitriol (1,25-dihydroxyvitamin D_3) supplemented by a calcium-deficient diet can dramatically improve the clinical expression of the infantile form of osteopetrosis. This effect is probably mediated through calcitriol stimulation of osteoclast activity. The treatment regimen can result in hypocalcemia and rickets, however. Dramatic resolution of radiographic features has not been demonstrated.

Transplantation of allogeneic bone marrow in several infants with autosomal-recessive osteopetrosis has led to striking clinical improvement. Symptomatic, hematologic, histologic, and radiographic improvement and normalization have occurred. Tests of these infants have shown that donor osteoclasts have repopulated the host bone marrow. This observation also supports the concept that osteoclasts are derived from stem-cell precursors in the marrow. Therefore, tissue transplantation is the most likely cause of the change in skeletal pattern **(Option (A) is correct).** Unfortunately, bone marrow transplantation does not result in such dramatic results in all patients with osteopetrosis as it did in the test patient. The outcome is complicated by many host, donor, and technical factors.

Among the clinical problems of autosomal-recessive infantile osteopetrosis are hematologic, neurologic, musculoskeletal, and immunologic dysfunctions. The major hematologic manifestations are anemia, thrombocytopenia, and hepatosplenomegaly. The most serious neurologic problem is bone encroachment upon the neural foramina of the skull with resultant cranial nerve deficits. This bone overgrowth leads to blindness, deafness, facial and oculomotor nerve palsies, and hydrocephalus. The significant musculoskeletal complication is fracture of the brittle bone. Osteomyelitis also occurs, particularly in the mandible. Due to immunologic compromise, all infections are more frequent and serious. Successful bone marrow transplantation reverses these clinical features.

Bone marrow transplantation is now an accepted therapeutic technique for treating hematologic neoplasms and other conditions of bone marrow origin. The transplant is preceded by ablation of the recipient's marrow by high-dose chemotherapy (with or without additional whole-body irradiation). The donor must be as closely matched to the recipient as possible for human lymphocyte antigens. Syngeneic transplants come from identical twin donors, allogeneic transplants from genetically different but closely matched donors, and autologous transplants from the patient's own previously stored bone marrow. In the test patient, the transplant came from the infant's father and therefore was categorized as allogeneic. Pretransplant immunosuppression was accomplished with systemic chemotherapy and splenic irradiation. Recovery following transplantation was uneventful. The infant was female, and post-transplant bone marrow evaluation of the patient demonstrated Y chromosomes, indicating successful establishment of the tissue transplant.

Question 19

Effects of radiotherapy on the skeleton include:

    (A) arrest of epiphyseal chondrogenesis
    (B) periosteal reaction
    (C) asymptomatic fractures
    (D) formation of exostoses
    (E) induction of chondrosarcoma more frequently than osteosarcoma

Growing bone is sensitive to radiation, and the region about the physis is the most sensitive. Early dystrophic effects of radiation are at the zone of provisional calcification. The number of chondrocytes is diminished, and the columnar arrangement of cartilage cells is disturbed.

Chondrocytes then degenerate. These events result in an arrest of epiphyseal chondrogenesis **(Option (A) is true).**

The growing physis is sensitive to doses of radiation as low as 300 rads (3 Gy), and damage is roughly proportional to the amount of radiation received and the growth potential of the particular anatomic structure. In general, growth disturbance is inversely proportional to the child's age. Decreased growth can become evident at doses as small as 400 rads (4 Gy) and is essentially always present at doses of 2,000 rads (20 Gy) or greater.

Radiographic changes consisting of metaphyseal sclerosis and fraying accompanied by physeal-plate widening have been observed in irradiated epiphyseal regions of long bones. These changes are reminiscent of rickets. In some patients, a dense metaphyseal band can develop following resumption of growth after irradiation. Both the rickets-like alterations and the metaphyseal bands disappear as normal bone remodeling resumes.

The diaphyses of bones are relatively resistant to radiation even during childhood. The periosteum can be affected and so result in modeling disturbances, but periosteal reaction is not a feature of skeletal response to irradiation **(Option (B) is false).** Radiation of a diaphyseal segment can lead to a diminished cross-sectional diameter, but it does not result in thickening of the bone. Mature bone and cartilage are very radioresistant.

The most important site of growth disturbance is the spine. The earliest changes occur in the zone of provisional calcification, and the associated deformities become evident as growth resumes. The manifestations of growth disturbance in the spine are the development of sclerotic bands parallel to vertebral body end plates, the endobone appearance, irregular and scalloped end plates, deformed vertebral bodies, and scoliosis (Figure 5-7). These changes can follow radiation therapy for abdominal, retroperitoneal, or truncal malignant neoplasms. Over the years, radiation-induced scoliosis has been most commonly associated with treatment of Wilms' tumor. Inclusion of the iliac crest in a radiation port contributes to the severity of scoliosis. Asymmetric spinal radiation leads to more frequent deformities and more severe scoliotic curves.

Strategies to diminish the frequency of occurrence and the severity of radiation-induced scoliosis have been routinely used for many years. These protective measures include restriction of the radiation field and of the total radiation dose, respectively, to the smallest size and lowest amount necessary for adequate therapy; inclusion of entire vertebrae rather than portions of vertebrae in the radiation field; and exclusion of the iliac crests when possible. These approaches help to reduce the frequency of radiation-induced scoliosis. At doses above 2,000 rads (20 Gy),

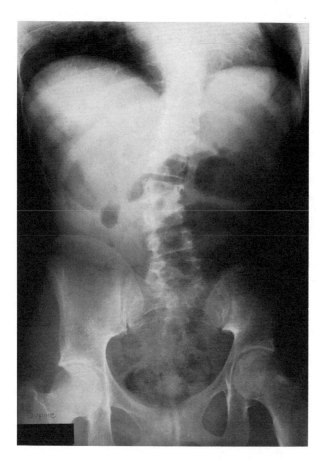

Figure 5-7. Radiation-induced scoliosis. This 23-year-old woman had undergone a left nephrectomy at age 2 for Wilms' tumor. Radiation therapy to the left flank followed the surgery. The anteroposterior radiograph of the abdomen shows a dextroscoliosis with the concave curve centered at the site of radiation to the tumor bed on the left. The affected vertebrae and left ilium are hypoplastic and deformed. Even the lower left ribs are small.

irreversible spinal changes can still occur. At doses below 1,000 rads (10 Gy), there are no observable radiographic changes.

Radiation-induced osteonecrosis is a result of a combined effect of the death of osteoblasts and of vascular damage. This condition is dependent upon dose (generally occurring at doses above 5,000 rads [50 Gy]), the quality of the radiation beam, the schedule of fractionation, the specific anatomic site, and the duration of time following therapy. Osteonecrosis is most prevalent in the mandible, but it also occurs in the clavicle, pelvis and sacrum, ribs, shoulders, and knees. The typical radiographic features are ill-defined osteopenia, subtle sclerosis, and eventually a disintegration of the affected bone. The devascularized, dead bone is subject to fracture and infection. Often, these fractures are initially asymptomatic **(Option (C) is true).** Common sites of fracture are weight-bearing areas such as the pelvis and femoral neck or load-bearing areas such as the long bones, shoulders, and ribs. Pubic fractures can be asymptomatic for long periods of time (Figure 5-8).

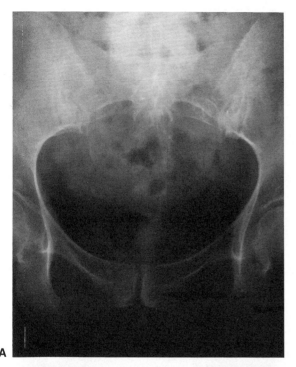

A

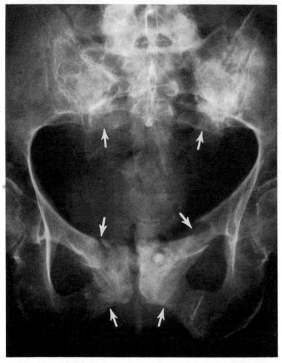

B

Figure 5-8. Radiation-induced osteonecrosis. This 79-year-old woman underwent postoperative radium-implant radiotherapy for poorly differentiated endometrial adenocarcinoma. (A) An anteroposterior radiograph of the pelvis obtained prior to radiotherapy shows osteopenia, but otherwise normal bone. (B) A similarly positioned anteroposterior radiograph obtained 17 months later shows osteonecrosis of the sacrum and pubis. Spontaneous fractures developed in the sacrum and pubis (arrows). The sacral fractures were symptomatic, whereas the pubic fractures were not.

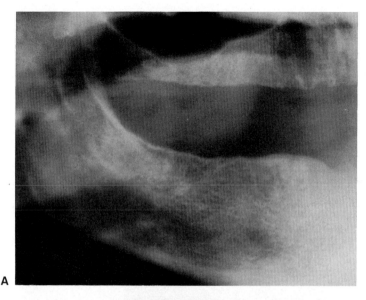

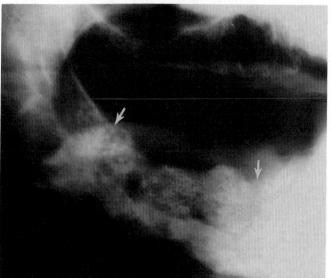

Figure 5-9. Radiation-induced osteonecrosis. This 68-year-old man underwent radiotherapy for squamous cell carcinoma of the tongue. Details from panoramic images show the mandible prior to radiotherapy (A) and following development of osteonecrosis (B). Note the osteosclerotic change and the pathologic fractures (arrows).

Osteonecrosis of the mandible (Figure 5-9) is particularly common, due to the mandible's superficial location and sparse blood supply, as well

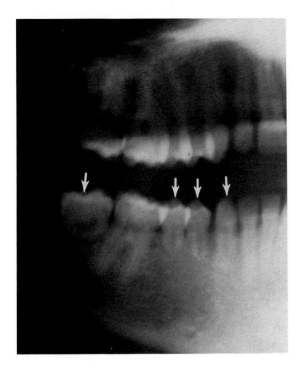

Figure 5-10. Radiation-induced dental hypoplasia. This young man received radiation therapy for rhabdomyosarcoma of the tongue when he was 9 years old. As a result, several teeth remain hypoplastic (arrows).

as the high doses of radiation (7,000 rads [70 Gy] or greater) necessary to control or cure cancers of the region. This complication is more common when a local tumor invades the mandible. Mandibular osteonecrosis, when focal, can be transient. It can also be complicated by fractures and by infection. Recurrent tumor can be difficult to differentiate from osteonecrosis on the basis of clinical or radiographic criteria, and a biopsy is often necessary to make the distinction. Other complications of radiation to the oral cavity include oral mucosal atrophy (painful mucositis), salivary gland damage (xerostomia), loss of taste (ageusia) due to taste bud injury, accelerated development of dental caries, and growth disturbances of mandibular or dental structures (Figure 5-10).

Radiation therapy can induce both benign and malignant neoplasms. Osteocartilaginous exostoses are the most frequent benign type (Figure 5-11) **(Option (D) is true).** They develop in childhood and in any irradiated bone. Typically, a radiation-induced exostosis becomes apparent within 5 years of the radiation therapy. The radiographic and histologic characteristics are indistinguishable from spontaneously occurring exostoses. Malignant transformation does not appear to occur in radiation-induced exostoses.

Radiation induction of sarcoma in bone is a well-known phenomenon. A radiation-induced sarcoma can develop after doses as low as 800 rads

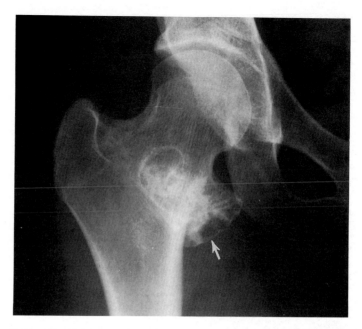

Figure 5-11. Radiation-induced exostosis. This 22-year-old woman received radiation therapy to the pelvis in an inverted-Y configuration for Hodgkin's disease when she was 11 years old. She now has an asymptomatic exostosis arising from the right femoral neck (arrow); this was discovered incidentally when bone scintigraphy was performed for an unrelated reason.

(8 Gy), but it usually requires a dose in excess of 3,000 rads (30 Gy). Such sarcomas always develop within the radiation field, but they can occur in normal bone or in bone that harbored a neoplasm. A latent period of about 10 years is typical, but this can be as short as 4 years. Osteosarcoma is the most common radiation-induced sarcoma; malignant fibrous histiocytoma is also frequently encountered. Chondrosarcomas are uncommon, accounting for less than 10% of radiation-induced sarcomas, and are certainly less common than osteosarcomas **(Option (E) is false).** Radiation-induced sarcomas have a radiographic appearance similar to that of their spontaneous counterparts, but they have a worse prognosis.

Questions 20 through 23

For each numbered medication listed below (Questions 20 through 23), select the *one* lettered musculoskeletal manifestation (A, B, C, D, or E) that is MOST closely associated with it. Each lettered musculoskeletal manifestation may be used once, more than once, or not at all.

20. Isotretinoin
21. Phenytoin
22. Sodium fluoride
23. Prostaglandin E$_1$

    (A) Growth arrest lines
    (B) Osteomalacia
    (C) Periostitis
    (D) Intra-articular calcification
    (E) Hyperostosis

Retinoids are synthetic derivatives of vitamin A. The agent that has found greatest clinical efficacy is 13-*cis*-retinoic acid or isotretinoin. This retinoid is used to treat and control severe dermatologic conditions such as cystic and conglobate acne and lamellar ichthyosis. The treatment is systemic, often high dose, and usually long-term. Such regimens have caused a mineralization diathesis of the spine and entheses, commonly referred to as hyperostosis **(Option (E) is the correct answer to Question 20).** Typically, anterior osteophyte formation occurs at vertebral-body end-plate margins. This progresses to ossification of the anterior longitudinal ligament (Figure 5-12A). The cervical spine is affected more frequently and more severely than is the thoracolumbar spine. The posterior longitudinal ligament can also ossify, but this is a less common outcome. In the appendicular skeleton, ossification of the entheses occurs about the major joints. This pattern is particularly common in the pelvis (Figure 5-12B) and at the quadriceps and Achilles tendon insertions. About half of affected patients complain of musculoskeletal pain, but they generally choose to continue the therapy in order to control the skin condition. Retinoid therapy can also cause osteopenia and premature epiphyseal closure. Severe fluorosis may cause a limited periosteal reaction, but not a pronounced hyperostosis.

Phenytoin (Dilantin®) is a widely used anticonvulsant agent with several known side effects, primarily the induction of a mineral metabolism imbalance. Intestinal absorption of calcium diminishes, serum alkaline phosphatase activity increases, and histologic evidence of osteomalacia develops **(Option (B) is the correct answer to Question 21).** Rickets or osteomalacia occurs in about 20% of patients who are on long-term treatment. The exact cause of the osteomalacia is uncertain, but it

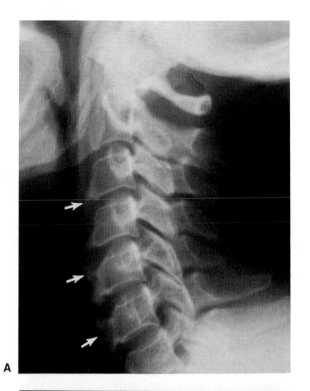

A

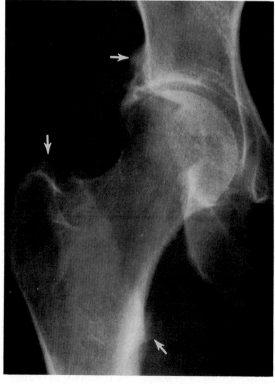

B

Figure 5-12. Isotretin-
oin-induced hyperosto-
sis. This 40-year-old
woman with Darier's
disease, an inherited
pigmented papular skin
disorder, was treated
with isotretinoin at
6-month intervals for 5
years. (A) A lateral ra-
diograph of the cervical
spine shows hyperos-
tosis of the anterior
longitudinal ligament
(arrows). (B) An antero-
posterior radiograph of
the pelvis shows ossifi-
cation at many entheses
(arrows).

146 / *Musculoskeletal Disease*

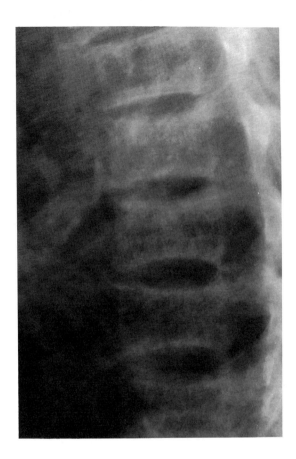

Figure 5-13. Fluoride-induced osteomalacia. This 87-year-old woman had been treated with sodium fluoride for 5 years in an effort to control postmenopausal osteoporosis. Detail of the thoracic spine from a lateral radiograph shows mild osteosclerosis and coarse trabeculae, findings consistent with fluorosis and osteomalacia.

seems to be hepatic in origin and is probably related to the induction of microsomal enzymes that deactivate 25-hydroxyvitamin D_3. Long-term phenytoin administration can also cause thickening of the diploic space and the heel fat pad.

Sodium fluoride has been used for more than 20 years to treat osteoporosis. Prolonged therapy can lead to fluorosis. Affected patients tend to develop osteosclerosis, primarily of cancellous bone and often evident in the spine (Figure 5-13). Trabeculae and cortices become thickened, and the medullary space seems to diminish. These features are consistent with osteomalacia **(Option (B) is the correct answer to Question 22).** The mechanism is stimulation of osteoid synthesis and impairment of mineral deposition in the osteoid. If the condition becomes severe, lower extremity stress fractures develop. Aluminum intoxication, excessive use of antacids, and Thorotrast in the bone marrow can also induce osteomalacia.

Prostaglandin E_1 has been used to maintain the patency of the ductus arteriosus in infants with severe cyanotic congenital heart disease until they are able to undergo corrective heart surgery. If long periods of treatment are required, periostitis can develop **(Option (C) is the correct answer to Question 23).** The periosteal reaction is diaphyseal and can be extensive. Once the medication is stopped, the periosteal reaction mineralizes and incorporates into a normal-appearing bone. The phenomenon is rare because prostaglandin E_1 is usually used for short periods. The mechanism of periostitis induction is unknown.

Prominent but thin transverse bands of trabeculae located in metaphyses parallel to physes are termed growth arrest lines (Option (A)). These lines are most frequently found in areas characterized by rapid growth such as the knee. While the pathogenesis of these lines is uncertain, no drug is known to induce them. Development of osteopenia can unmask growth arrest lines, and hence they can become apparent during systemic steroid therapy. Traditionally, growth arrest lines have been attributed to episodes of stress, either nutritional or disease related. Conceptually, these lines are more properly considered post-stress recovery lines rather than arrest lines.

Intra-articular calcification (Option (D)) occurs in the calcium pyrophosphate dihydrate and hydroxyapatite deposition diseases, as well as occasionally with chronic granulomatous infections such as tuberculosis. It is a well-known manifestation of synovial chondromatosis. The one medication capable of producing intra-articular calcification is a steroid when injected directly into a joint. This situation occurs most frequently in small joints of the hand following multiple sequential steroid injections into a selected joint.

William A. Murphy, Jr., M.D.

SUGGESTED READINGS

TISSUE TRANSPLANTATION AND OSTEOPETROSIS

1. Coccia PF, Krivit W, Cervenka J, et al. Successful bone-marrow transplantation for infantile malignant osteopetrosis. N Engl J Med 1980; 302:701–708
2. Kaplan FS, August CS, Fallon MD, Dalinka M, Axel L, Haddad JG. Successful treatment of infantile malignant osteopetrosis by bone-marrow transplantation. A case report. J Bone Joint Surg (Am) 1988; 70:617–623
3. Key L, Carnes D, Cole S, et al. Treatment of congenital osteopetrosis with high-dose calcitriol. N Engl J Med 1984; 310:409–415
4. Patzik SB, Smith C, Kubicka RA, Kaizer H. Bone marrow transplantation: clinical and radiologic aspects. RadioGraphics 1991; 11:601–610

5. Shapiro F, Glimcher MJ, Holtrop ME, Tashjian AH Jr, Brickley-Parsons D, Kenzora JE. Human osteopetrosis: a histological, ultrastructural, and biochemical study. J Bone Joint Surg (Am) 1980; 62:384–399

6. Whyte MP, Murphy WA. Osteopetrosis and other sclerosing bone disorders. In: Avioli LV, Krane SM (eds), Metabolic bone disease, 2nd ed. Philadelphia: WB Saunders; 1990:616–658

RADIATION-INDUCED CONDITIONS

7. Butler MS, Robertson WW Jr, Rate W, D'Angio GJ, Drummond DS. Skeletal sequelae of radiation therapy for malignant childhood tumors. Clin Orthop 1990; 251:235–240

8. De Smet AA, Kuhns LR, Fayos JV, Holt JF. Effects of radiation therapy on growing long bones. AJR 1976; 127:935–939

9. Goldwein JW. Effects of radiation therapy on skeletal growth in childhood. Clin Orthop 1991; 262:101–107

10. Herman TE, McAlister WH, Rosenthal D, Dehner LP. Case report 691. Radiation-induced osteochondromas (RIO) arising from the neural arch and producing compression of the spinal cord. Skeletal Radiol 1991; 20:472–476

11. Lorigan JG, Libshitz HI, Peuchot M. Radiation-induced sarcoma of bone: CT findings in 19 cases. AJR 1989; 153:791–794

12. Probert JC, Parker BR. The effects of radiation therapy on bone growth. Radiology 1975; 114:155–162

13. Weatherby RP, Dahlin DC, Ivins JC. Postradiation sarcoma of bone: review of 78 Mayo Clinic cases. Mayo Clin Proc 1981; 56:294–306

DRUG-INDUCED CONDITIONS

14. Dravaric DM, Parks WJ, Wyly JB, Dooley KJ, Plauth WH Jr, Schmitt EW. Prostaglandin-induced hyperostosis. A case report. Clin Orthop 1989; 246:300–304

15. El-Khoury GY, Moore TE, Albright JP, Huang HK, Martin RK. Sodium fluoride treatment of osteoporosis: radiologic findings. AJR 1982; 139:39–43

16. Lawson JP. Drug-induced lesions of the musculoskeletal system. Radiol Clin North Am 1990; 28:233–246

17. McCrea ES, Rao CV, Diaconis JN. Roentgenographic changes during long-term diphenylhydantoin therapy. South Med J 1980; 73:312–317

18. Pennes DR, Martel W, Ellis CN, Voorhees JJ. Evolution of skeletal hyperostoses caused by 13-cis-retinoic acid therapy. AJR 1988; 151:967–973

19. Rowley RF, Lawson JP. Case report 701: Prostaglandin E_1 (PGE_1) periostitis. Skeletal Radiol 1991; 20:617–619

20. Schnitzler CM, Wing JR, Gear KA, Robson HJ. Bone fragility of the peripheral skeleton during fluoride therapy for osteoporosis. Clin Orthop 1990; 261:268–275

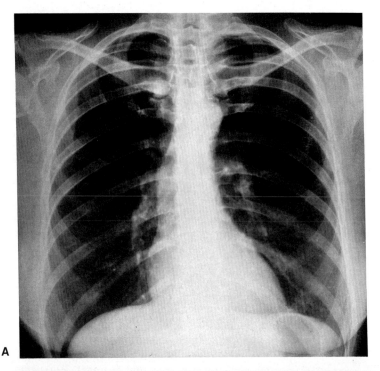

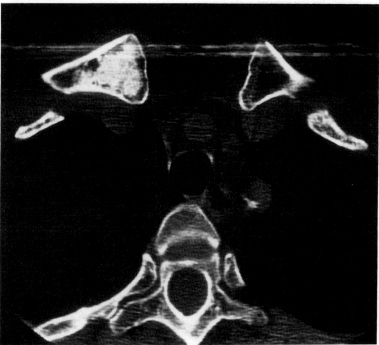

Figure 6-1. This 54-year-old woman complained of pain in the right sternoclavicular region. You are shown a posteroanterior chest radiograph (A) and a CT scan (B) through the region of the sternoclavicular joint.

Case 6: Osteitis Condensans of the Clavicle

Question 24

Which *one* of the following is the MOST likely diagnosis?

(A) Sternocostoclavicular hyperostosis
(B) Osteitis condensans
(C) Osteomyelitis
(D) Paget's disease
(E) Osteosarcoma

The chest radiograph (Figure 6-1A) and CT scan (Figure 6-1B) through the sternal ends of the clavicles demonstrate unilateral sclerosis of the medial portion of the right clavicle (Figure 6-2). The sternoclavicular joint appears normal on the chest radiograph, and the soft tissues about the medial clavicle are normal on the CT section. These are the typical features of osteitis condensans of the clavicle (**Option (B) is correct**).

In contrast to osteitis condensans of the clavicle, which is usually unilateral, sternocostoclavicular hyperostosis (Option (A)) is usually bilateral. In addition, whereas osteitis condensans of the clavicle involves only the one bone, patients with sternocostoclavicular hyperostosis also demonstrate radiographic changes of hyperostosis of the sternum, upper anterior ribs, and intervening soft tissues. Interposed joints are also abnormal. Therefore, sternocostoclavicular hyperostosis is an unlikely diagnosis in the test case.

In patients with osteomyelitis (Option (C)) of the clavicle, the radiographs may initially be normal. However, as the condition progresses, radiographic evidence of soft tissue swelling, demineralization, bony destruction, periosteal reaction, and joint space narrowing becomes apparent. All of these findings are absent in the test images.

The clavicle is an uncommon site of involvement for Paget's disease (Option (D)). Paget's disease typically affects men aged 50 and older.

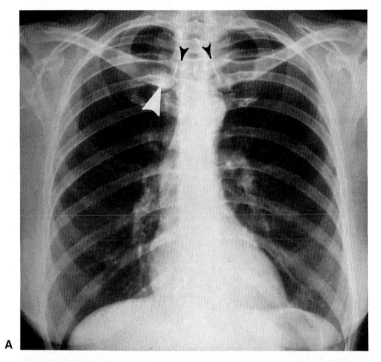

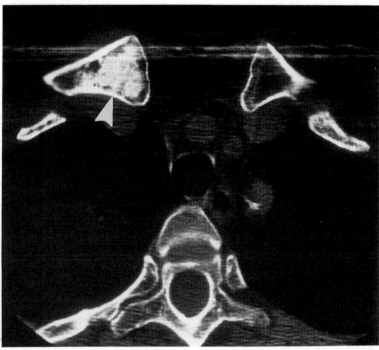

Figure 6-2 (Same as Figure 6-1). Osteitis condensans of the clavicle. (A) The posteroanterior chest radiograph is normal except for focal sclerosis of the sternal end of the right clavicle (white arrowhead). The sternoclavicular joints also appear normal (black arrowheads). (B) The CT scan shows amorphous sclerosis of the right clavicular bone marrow (arrowhead) with no evidence of cortical or soft tissue abnormality.

152

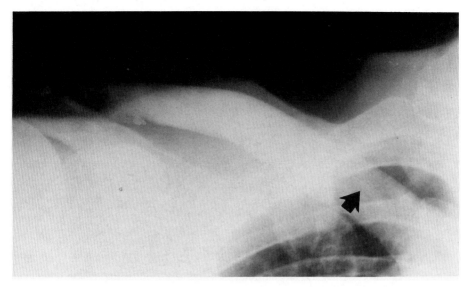

Figure 6-3. Paget's disease of the clavicle. A 60-year-old man with Paget's disease involving several bones. There is overall enlargement of the clavicle. The thickened trabeculae (arrow) are most obvious proximally. All but the distal end of the bone is involved.

Radiographically, in addition to trabecular thickening, there should be cortical thickening and overall bone enlargement (Figure 6-3), findings that are absent in the test images. Careful inspection of the pattern of sclerosis shows an amorphous mineralization of the marrow rather than the typical coarsened trabeculae expected in Paget's disease. For these reasons, Paget's disease is an unlikely diagnosis.

Osteosarcoma (Option (E)) rarely involves the clavicle, and this malignant bone tumor most commonly affects males from 10 to 30 years old. It is associated with cloudlike new bone formation (Figure 6-4), cortical destruction, and periosteal elevation, findings that are not present in the test images. Osteosarcoma may complicate Paget's disease as a result of malignant transformation of cells in an affected bone. However, as indicated above, there is no evidence of Paget's disease in the test patient. Therefore, neither primary nor secondary osteosarcoma is a likely diagnosis.

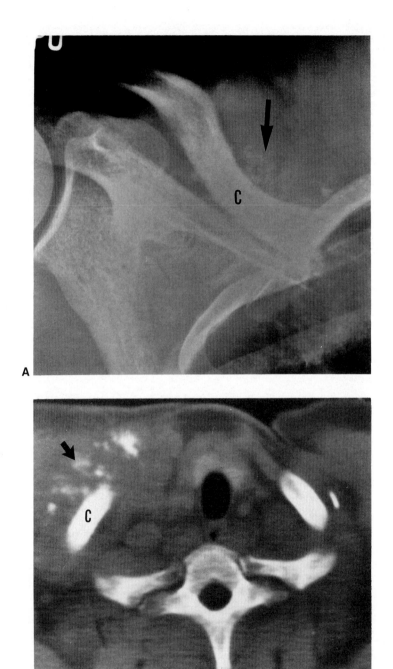

Figure 6-4. Anteroposterior radiograph (A) and CT scan (B) of osteogenic sarcoma of the right clavicle manifested by sclerosis of the proximal clavicle (C) and cloudlike new bone formation (arrow) extending into
the surrounding soft tissues.

Question 25

Concerning sternocostoclavicular hyperostosis,

    (A) it is more common in women than in men
    (B) it is associated with pustular lesions of the palms and soles
    (C) an associated spondyloarthropathy is common
    (D) histocompatibility antigen HLA B27 is usually present
    (E) histologically it is identical to osteitis condensans

Sternocostoclavicular hyperostosis was initially recognized as a distinct clinical entity in 1974 in Japan. The disease affects men more often than women and typically affects men from 30 to 50 years of age **(Option (A) is false).** Patients experience bilateral pain, swelling, and heat in the anterior upper chest; these symptoms may be long standing and may be aggravated by cold, damp weather and recurrent infections. Patients may also complain of upper-extremity edema, which may result from impingement on the subclavian vein by a hyperostotic clavicle. Pustular eruptions may be present on the volar surfaces of the hands and feet **(Option (B) is true).** In one study, sternocostoclavicular hyperostosis was identified in more than 9% of all patients with pustulosis palmaris et plantaris.

Radiographic findings of sternocostoclavicular hyperostosis are distinctive. They include hyperostosis and soft tissue ossification between the anterior portions of the upper ribs (most often the second, third, and fourth ribs) and the clavicles (Figure 6-5). The condition can be staged on the basis of the radiographic findings. In stage 1, ossification is mild and is confined to the region of the costoclavicular ligaments. In stage 2, an ossific mass is interposed between the clavicle and first rib and is accompanied by extensive bone formation in the costoclavicular ligaments and adjacent soft tissues. In stage 3, the hyperostosis involves both superior and inferior borders of the clavicles and first ribs.

An associated spondyloarthropathy is common **(Option (C) is true).** Approximately one-third of patients with sternocostoclavicular hyperostosis have associated radiographic changes of ankylosing spondylitis, sacroiliitis, or diffuse idiopathic skeletal hyperostosis. About 32% of patients have inflammatory arthritis of the peripheral joints. Involvement of the manubrosternal articulation is common. Bone scintigrams are positive before the onset of the radiographic findings, and bone scintigraphy is useful in identifying the extent of the disease (Figure 6-6).

Serologic tests in patients with sternocostoclavicular hyperostosis may reveal an abnormally elevated erythrocyte sedimentation rate and alpha-2 globulin level, as well as a positive test for C-reactive protein. However, leukocytosis is absent and tests for rheumatoid factor and his-

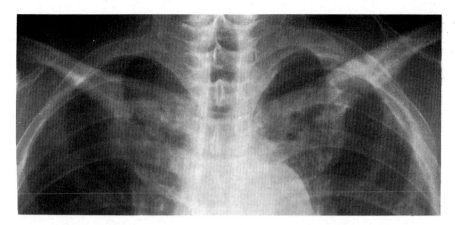

Figure 6-5. Sternocostoclavicular hyperostosis. This detail from a posteroanterior chest radiograph shows bilaterally symmetric hyperostosis of the clavicles and anterior aspects of the upper ribs. Soft tissue ossification between the clavicles, first ribs, and sternum has obliterated the sternoclavicular joints.

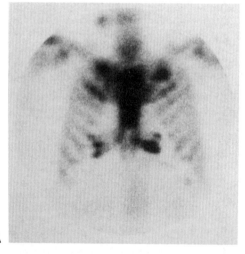

A

Figure 6-6. Sternocostoclavicular hyperostosis. (A) An anterior Tc-99m MDP scintigram shows increased tracer uptake in the sternum and symmetrically in several ribs and costal cartilages. Posteroanterior (B) and lateral (C) chest radiographs show hyperostosis of the anterior aspects of the first and second ribs and sternum (arrowheads). The lateral radiograph also shows diffuse hyperostosis of the thoracic spine (arrows in panel C). (D) A CT scan at the level of the first costal cartilages shows hyperostosis of the sternum and ossification of the costal cartilages. (Reprinted with permission from Dehdashti F, Siegel BA. General diagnosis case of the day. Sternocostoclavicular hyperostosis. AJR 1989; 152:1319–1321.)

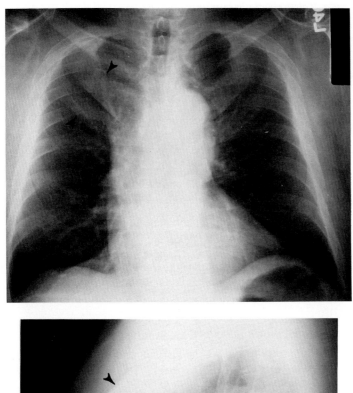

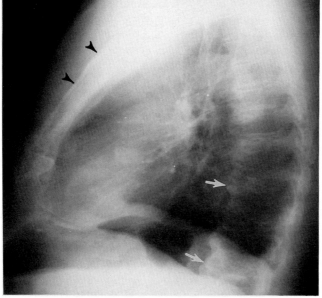

tocompatibility antigen HLA B27 are negative in patients with this condition **(Option (D) is false).**

Biopsies of affected tissues have revealed evidence of an inflammatory condition with marked new bone formation, fibrosis with mild granulation tissue, and round cell infiltration. These findings are readily dis-

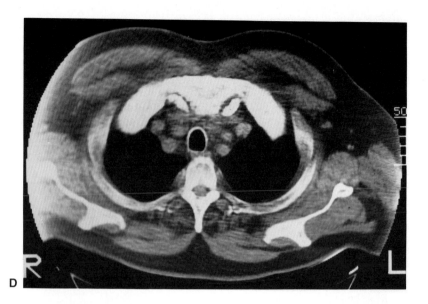

D

tinguishable from those of osteitis condensans of the clavicle, which shows trabecular thickening and spurs consistent with a response to mechanical stress **(Option (E) is false).** Examination of tissues from regions of sternocostoclavicular hyperostosis have thus far failed to identify a causative infectious agent.

Question 26

Concerning osteitis condensans of the clavicle,

    (A) it is a response to mechanical stress
    (B) histologically the lesion consists of thickened trabeculae
    (C) the width of the sternoclavicular joint is normal
    (D) bone scintigraphy is usually normal
    (E) treatment with anti-inflammatory medications usually relieves symptoms

Osteitis condensans of the clavicle is a rare disease that affects women, and the average age at diagnosis is 40 years. This condition is frequently misdiagnosed by radiologists and clinicians; as a result, extensive unnecessary radiologic and clinical investigations may be performed to rule out a suspected blastic metastasis or osteosarcoma of the clavicle.

    Osteitis condensans of the clavicle is believed to be caused by mechanical stress **(Option (A) is true).** Some patients with osteitis condensans of the clavicle report a specific antecedent history of mechanical stress to the sternoclavicular region, usually from occupational heavy lifting or sports activities. Therefore, the designation "posttraumatic clavicular sclerosis" has been suggested for this abnormality. When the condition is symptomatic, patients experience local swelling and tenderness and ipsilateral shoulder pain, which is accentuated by abduction or forward elevation of the shoulder. Physical examination may reveal a palpable fullness over the medial aspect of the clavicle, but there should be no overlying skin changes that would suggest infection or inflammation.

The radiographic hallmark of osteitis condensans of the clavicle is unilateral increased density of the medial aspect of the clavicle without involvement of the sternoclavicular joint or other surrounding structures (Figures 6-1 and 6-2). The increased bone density may be confined to the inferior margin of the medial aspect of the clavicle. The involved portion of the clavicle may be slightly expanded, but neither bone destruction nor periosteal reaction should be present. Occasionally, an osteophyte is observed arising from the inferomedial aspect of the sternal end of the clavicle.

In patients who have undergone excisional biopsy, specimen radiography has demonstrated thickened trabeculae. Histologic examination confirms an increase in the thickness of cancellous bone, with resultant obliteration of the marrow space **(Option (B) is true).** Although the bone density is increased as a result of trabecular proliferation and thickening, the sternoclavicular joint space maintains its normal width and appearance **(Option (C) is true).** Bone scintigraphy shows abnormally increased uptake of the tracer in the region of bone sclerosis (Figure 6-7) **(Option (D) is false).** However, although bone scintigraphy is sensitive, it is a relatively nonspecific indicator of pathologic changes. Therefore, correlation of bone scintigraphic findings with the radiographs is required for the correct diagnosis of this benign disorder. Clinical laboratory tests are normal, and cultures of biopsy specimens are negative.

If symptoms attributable to osteitis condensans of the clavicle are present, they are often not relieved by treatment with anti-inflammatory medications **(Option (E) is false).** When conservative management is unsuccessful, patients may have to undergo excision of the medial clavicle to relieve pain.

The differential diagnosis of osteitis condensans of the clavicle includes ischemic necrosis of the medial end of the clavicle (Friedrich disease), bone island (enostosis), osteoid osteoma, fibrous dysplasia, osteosarcoma, metastasis, osteoarthritis of the sternoclavicular joint, infection, and sternocostoclavicular hyperostosis.

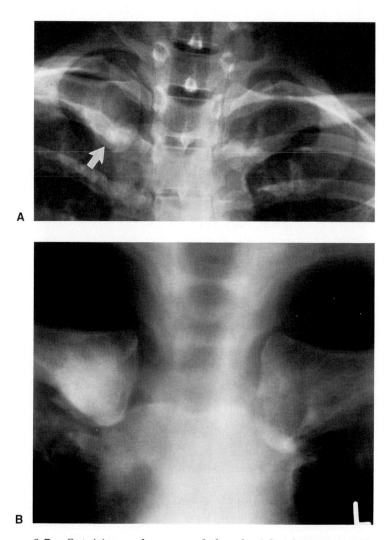

Figure 6-7. Osteitis condensans of the clavicle. A 30-year-old woman had severe pain in the right sternoclavicular joint. (A) An anteroposterior radiograph shows a sclerotic lesion (arrow) in the right distal clavicle. (B) A trispiral tomogram shows sclerosis of the inferior aspect of the right clavicular head. (C) A CT scan shows sclerosis of the clavicular head and adjacent soft tissue swelling (arrow). (D) Bone scintigraphy shows increased uptake of tracer at the sternal end of the right clavicle. Diagnosis of osteitis condensans of the clavicle was confirmed by excisional biopsy. (Reprinted with permission from Greenspan et al. [4].)

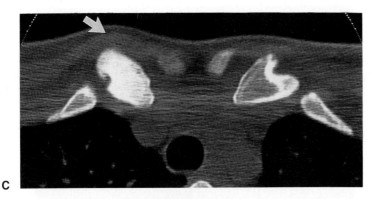

C

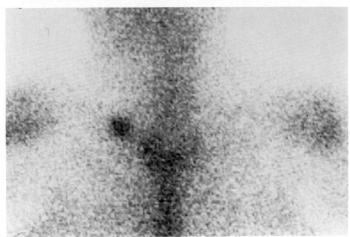

D

Question 27

Concerning the sternoclavicular joint,

    (A) it is a synovial joint
    (B) posterior dislocations are more common than anterior ones
    (C) it is involved in about 5% of patients with rheumatoid arthritis
    (D) it is a common site of septic arthritis in drug abusers

The sternoclavicular joint is formed by the medial end of the clavicle, the clavicular notch of the sternum, and the cartilage of the first rib. The medial end of the clavicle is enlarged and is directed inferiorly, anteriorly, and medially to articulate with the clavicular notch of the manubrium and the first rib (Figure 6-8). The sternoclavicular joint is lined with synovial membrane and is freely movable **(Option (A) is true).** It

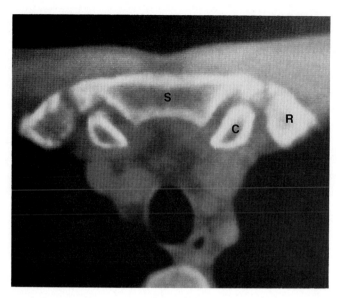

Figure 6-8. Normal sternoclavicular joint. CT scan shows the relationships of the sternum (S), first rib (R), and medial clavicle (C) with respect to one another and to the adjacent mediastinal structures.

is surrounded by a fibrous capsule and is divided into two separate articular spaces by an intra-articular fibrous disk. This disk attaches superiorly to the posterior border of the clavicle and inferiorly to the first rib; it also has attachments to the fibrous capsule of the joint. The disk acts to prevent displacement of the sternal end of the clavicle. The sternoclavicular joint is reinforced by anterior and posterior sternoclavicular, interclavicular, and costoclavicular ligaments.

Radiographic evaluation of the sternoclavicular joint is challenging because of the following impediments: (1) the oblique orientation of the joint prevents symmetric viewing of right and left joints for comparison purposes; (2) the overlying ribs, spine, and soft tissues obscure the joint; and (3) the relatively thin cortices and low osseous density of the adjacent bones contribute to its poor visualization. CT is often required to depict the joint optimally.

Dislocations at the sternoclavicular joint are rare, representing only 2 to 3% of the dislocations that occur about the shoulder. Anterior dislocations are more common than posterior ones **(Option (B) is false).** However, posterior dislocations are more serious (Figure 6-9), since the displaced clavicle may impinge on the neurovascular or visceral structures of the mediastinum. Although there have been reports of congenital or spontaneous displacements, dislocations are usually produced by a

162 / *Musculoskeletal Disease*

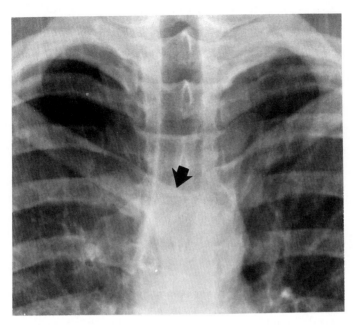

Figure 6-9. Sternoclavicular joint dislocation. The patient was in an automobile accident, which resulted in posteroinferior dislocation of the proximal right clavicle (arrow). The left clavicle is in its normal position.

traumatic force of great magnitude. CT is the most sensitive modality for demonstrating dislocations of the sternoclavicular joint (Figures 6-10 and 6-11).

Patients seldom present with an arthritis limited to the sternoclavicular joint. Nonetheless, the joint may be involved in several types of arthritis, including rheumatoid arthritis, osteoarthritis, and ankylosing spondylitis. Radiographic manifestations of arthritis at the sternoclavicular joint are difficult to depict on routine radiographic projections. However, using conventional tomography, some investigators have reported that this joint is involved in up to 30% of patients with rheumatoid arthritis **(Option (C) is false).** The radiographic manifestations of rheumatoid arthritis of the sternoclavicular joint include osteoporosis and subchondral and marginal erosions. Rheumatoid arthritis usually involves the sternoclavicular joint late in the course of the disease, when abnormalities at more commonly involved joints have already been documented. Osteoarthritis may also involve the sternoclavicular joint, and it is characterized by joint space narrowing, osteophyte formation, subchondral cysts, and subluxation (Figure 6-12).

Intravenous-drug abusers have a high incidence of septic arthritis. These joint infections tend to occur at unusual locations. Common sites

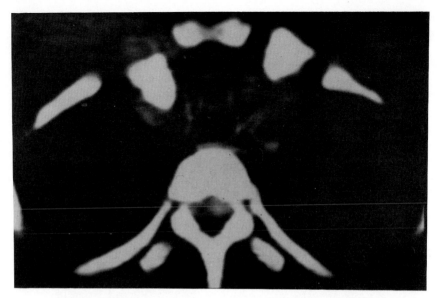

Figure 6-10. A CT scan reveals posterior sternoclavicular dislocation. Posterior dislocation may be difficult to diagnose clinically. The posteriorly dislocated clavicle can have significant consequences as a result of impingement on brachiocephalic vessels, the trachea, or neural structures. Absence of a significant hematoma on the CT examination ruled out major vascular injury in this case. (Reprinted with permission from Stark and Jaramillo [18].)

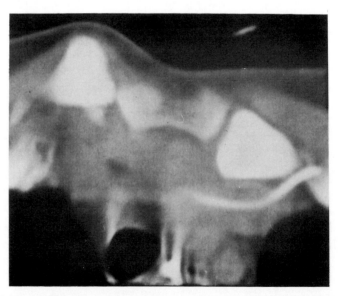

Figure 6-11. A CT scan shows anterior dislocation of the right clavicle. Anterior dislocation is more common than posterior dislocation, and CT is rarely necessary because of obvious clinical findings. (Reprinted with permission from Stark and Jaramillo [18].)

164

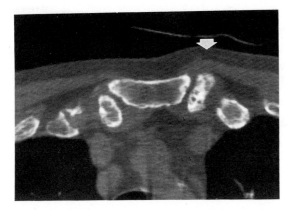

Figure 6-12. Sternoclavicular joint osteoarthritis. A 70-year-old man complained of a hard "bump" and pain over the left sternoclavicular joint. A CT scan shows narrowing, sclerosis, and multiple cysts involving the left sternoclavicular joint. The palpable bump (arrow) was secondary to anterior subluxation of the underlying sternal end of the left clavicle. The right sternoclavicular joint is involved to a lesser extent.

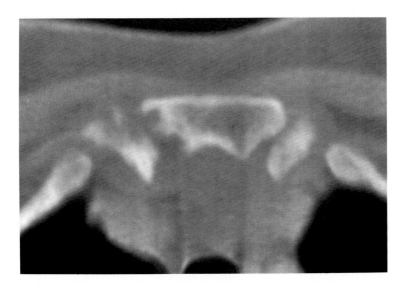

Figure 6-13. Sternoclavicular joint osteomyelitis. A CT scan shows erosions and widening of the right sternoclavicular joint. The patient was an intravenous-drug abuser. (Courtesy of William A. Murphy, Jr., M.D., Mallinckrodt Institute of Radiology, St. Louis, Mo.)

of septic arthritis in intravenous-drug abusers include the spine, sacroiliac joints, and sternoclavicular joints (Figure 6-13) **(Option (D) is true).** In addition, infections in intravenous-drug abusers are frequently caused by unusual types of organisms, particularly *Pseudomonas, Klebsiella,* and *Serratia* species. Infections of the sternoclavicular joint may also occur after surgery or radiation therapy. Patients with infective endocarditis or adjacent mediastinal infections are also susceptible to infections of the sternoclavicular joints.

Sternoclavicular joint septic arthritis and clavicular osteomyelitis are very similar processes. The only difference is where the infection seems to have begun, because the natural history of both conditions is to involve both bone and joint. The radiographic findings are soft tissue swelling, bone dissolution, and joint destruction. When the infection is eradicated and healing is complete, a chronic secondary osteoarthritis commonly results.

Vijay P. Chandnani, M.D.
Lawrence W. Bassett, M.D.

SUGGESTED READINGS

OSTEITIS CONDENSANS OF THE CLAVICLE

1. Appell RG, Oppermann HC, Becker W, Kratzat R, Brandeis WE, Willich E. Condensing osteitis of the clavicle in childhood: a rare sclerotic bone lesion. Review of literature and report of seven patients. Pediatr Radiol 1983; 13:301–306
2. Brower AC, Sweet DE, Keats TE. Condensing osteitis of the clavicle: a new entity. AJR 1974; 121:17–21
3. Cone RO, Resnick D, Goergen TG, Robinson C, Vint V, Haghighi P. Condensing osteitis of the clavicle. AJR 1983; 141:387–388
4. Greenspan A, Gerscovich E, Szabo RM, Matthews JG II. Condensing osteitis of the clavicle: a rare but frequently misdiagnosed condition. AJR 1991; 156:1011–1015
5. Teates CD, Brower AC, Williamson BR, Keats TE. Bone scans in condensing osteitis of the clavicle. South Med J 1978; 71:736–738

STERNOCOSTOCLAVICULAR HYPEROSTOSIS

6. Resnick D. Sternocostoclavicular hyperostosis. AJR 1980; 135:1278–1280
7. Sartoris DJ, Schreiman JS, Kerr R, Resnick CS, Resnick D. Sternocostoclavicular hyperostosis: a review and report of 11 cases. Radiology 1986; 158:125–128
8. Sonozaki H, Azuma A, Okai K, et al. Clinical features of 22 cases with "inter-sterno-costo-clavicular ossification." A new rheumatic syndrome. Arch Orthop Trauma Surg 1979; 95:13–22
9. Sonozaki H, Furusawa S, Seki H, Kurokawa T, Tateishi A, Kabata K. Four cases with symmetrical ossifications between the clavicles and the first ribs on both sides. Kanto J Orthop Trauma 1974; 5:244–247

10. Sonozaki H, Kawashima M, Hongo O, et al. Incidence of arthro-osteitis in patients with pustulosis palmaris et plantaris. Ann Rheum Dis 1981; 40:554–557

11. Sonozaki H, Mitsui H, Miyanaga Y, et al. Clinical features of 53 cases with pustulotic arthro-osteitis. Ann Rheum Dis 1981; 40:547–553

STERNOCLAVICULAR JOINT

12. Destouet JM, Gilula LA, Murphy WA, Sagel S. Computed tomography of the sternoclavicular joint and sternum. Radiology 1981; 138:123–128

13. Goldin RH, Chow AW, Edwards JE Jr, Louie JS, Guze LB. Sternoarticular septic arthritis in heroin users. N Engl J Med 1973; 289:616–618

14. Kalliomäki JL, Viitanen SM, Virtama P. Radiological findings of sternoclavicular joints in rheumatoid arthritis. Acta Rheumatol Scand 1968; 14:233–240

15. Levinsohn EM, Bunnell WP, Yuan HA. Computed tomography in the diagnosis of dislocations of the sternoclavicular joint. Clin Orthop 1979; 140:12–16

16. Resnick D, Niwayama G. Anatomy of individual joints. In: Resnick D, Niwayama G (eds), Diagnosis of bone and joint disorders. Philadelphia: WB Saunders; 1988:647–777

17. Sokoloff L, Gleason IO. The sternoclavicular articulation in rheumatic diseases. Am J Clin Pathol 1954; 24:406–414

18. Stark P, Jaramillo D. CT of the sternum. AJR 1986; 147:72–77

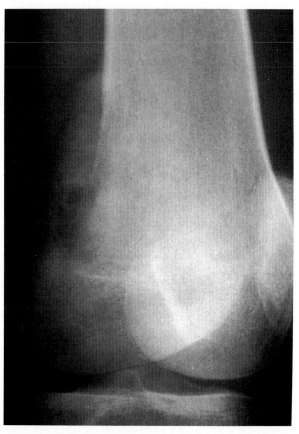

Figure 7-1. You are shown an oblique radiograph of the right knee in a 16-year-old athlete with right knee pain.

Case 7: Osteosarcoma

Question 28

Which *one* of the following is the MOST likely diagnosis?

(A) Well-differentiated osteosarcoma
(B) Osteoblastoma
(C) Aneurysmal bone cyst
(D) Nonossifying fibroma
(E) Chondrosarcoma

The oblique radiograph of the distal femur (Figure 7-1) of this young athlete shows an expansile lesion in the lateral aspect of the metaphysis. The lesion has both a lytic area and a cloudlike matrix, without definite chondroid elements such as punctate lucencies or curvilinear calcifications. The lesion margins are not well defined, and there is no evidence of a sclerotic border. The thin rim of bone defining the lateral margin of the expansile portion is indistinct and irregular (Figure 7-2), suggesting a possible soft tissue component. There is no periosteal reaction associated with the lesion. This set of radiographic features is most consistent with a well-differentiated osteosarcoma **(Option (A) is correct).** These features are confirmed in the test patient's anteroposterior radiograph (Figure 7-3), and cortical thinning and disruption can also be seen.

Well-differentiated osteosarcoma accounts for approximately 1% of all osteosarcomas and occurs most frequently in the distal femur. Although these tumors are rare, knowledge of their radiographic appearance is important since they are frequently misdiagnosed as benign lesions such as enchondroma or chondroblastoma. Radiographically, the margins of this tumor can be either poorly or well defined. Cortical thinning and discontinuity are typical, as is extraosseous involvement of the soft tissues. The medullary tumor can be purely lytic but is more often mixed lytic and blastic. CT and MRI (Figure 7-4) are useful in evaluating these lesions since any soft tissue mass associated with the lesion will be revealed, allowing appropriate exclusion of more-benign processes and increasing the level of suspicion for well-differentiated osteosarcoma. In

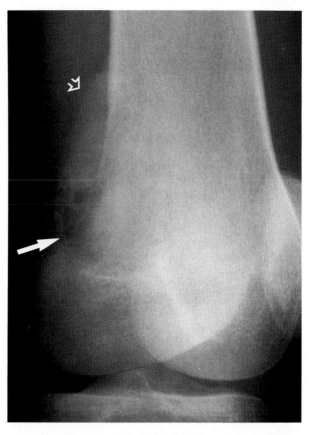

Figure 7-2 (Same as Figure 7-1). Well-differentiated osteosarcoma. An oblique radiograph of the distal right femur shows an expansile lesion of the lateral femoral metaphysis with a cloudlike matrix containing faint lytic areas inferiorly (solid arrow). The lesion margin is irregular superiorly (open arrow).

addition, cortical erosion, which may not be apparent on the radiograph, can be seen on both CT and MRI.

An osteoblastoma (Option (B)), a vascular lesion consisting of osteoblasts, osteoid, and trabeculae, rarely exceeds 8 cm in greatest dimension when found in the long bones. Osteoblastomas are usually well-marginated, mostly lytic lesions, and thus an osteoblastoma is not the most likely diagnosis in the test patient. A centrally placed sclerotic area can result in the appearance of a giant nidus, but there is rarely reactive sclerosis to suggest an osteoid osteoma. A narrow band of condensed bone may give a distinct margin to the lesion. While central osteoblastomas result in fusiform bony enlargement, eccentrically positioned lesions

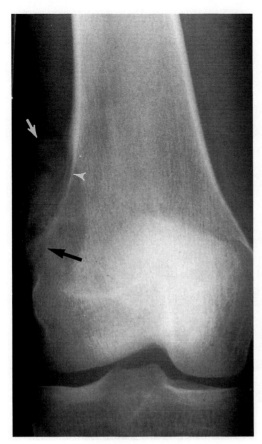

Figure 7-3. Same patient as in Figure 7-1. Well-differentiated osteosarcoma. An anteroposterior radiograph of the distal femur confirms the cloudlike lesion matrix and the irregular superior border (white arrow). There is some preservation of cortical bone superiorly (arrowhead) but disruption of cortical bone inferiorly (black arrow).

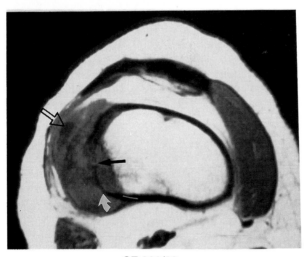

SE 800/20

Figure 7-4. Same patient as in Figure 7-1. Well-differentiated osteosarcoma. A T1-weighted transaxial MR image through the superior aspect of the osteosarcoma shows cortical penetration (solid black arrow) and infiltration of tumor through the cortex (curved arrow). A soft tissue mass lies outside the confines of the pseudocapsule (open arrow). The intermediate-intensity tumor matrix is heterogeneous. (Reprinted with permission from Moore [7].)

171

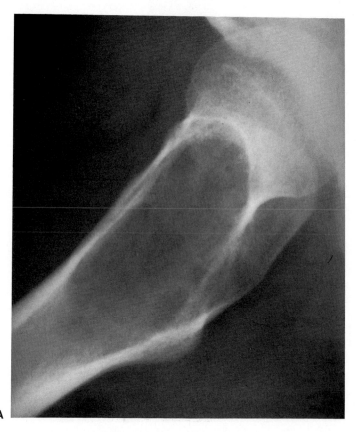

A

Figure 7-5. Aneurysmal bone cyst. (A) A frog-leg lateral radiograph of the proximal right femur in a 15-year-old girl shows an expansile lytic lesion with limited internal bony architecture. Transaxial proton-density (B) and T2-weighted (C) images through the lesion show fluid-fluid levels. The higher-intensity fluid evident on the proton-density image (arrow) is consistent with hemorrhage. (Reprinted with permission from Moore et al. [8].)

will expand, thin, and sometimes destroy the cortex. A very thin rim of calcific bone or a margin of periosteum typically separates the mass from the surrounding soft tissues. There is no evidence of periosteal reaction.

Aneurysmal bone cyst (Option (C)) is a non-neoplastic solitary lesion of bone seen most frequently during adolescence. About 75% of cases occur in the first two decades of life, and there is a slight female predominance. Aneurysmal bone cysts are either asymptomatic or cause vague pain, swelling, and limitation of motion. They occur in every bone of the skeleton, although nearly 50% occur in the long bones and about 30% in the spine.

Grossly, aneurysmal bone cysts are well-circumscribed cavities or cavernous spaces within bone. These cavities are not lined with endothe-

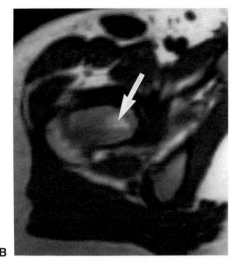 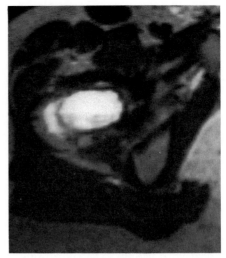

B

SE 2,000/20

SE 2,000/80

C

lial cells and are frequently filled with blood. They also can be primarily fluid filled, can contain thick connective tissue septa filled with blood, or can be predominantly fibrous.

Radiographically, aneurysmal bone cysts have four stages of development. (1) The initial, or lytic, phase is indicated by a well-circumscribed ovoid area of rarefaction, which can be central, eccentric, or parosteal. (2) The active growth phase is characterized by rapid destruction of bone and a subperiosteal "blowout" pattern (Figure 7-5). (3) The mature stage, or stage of stabilization, is manifested by formation of a distinct peripheral bony shell and internal bony septa and trabeculations, producing the characteristic radiographic "soap bubble" appearance. (4) In the healing phase, there is progressive calcification and ossification of the cyst with eventual transformation into a dense bony mass. The cyst size will be directly proportional to the lesion age, with the greatest dimension along the long axis of the bone.

Four discrete types of aneurysmal bone cysts occur in the long bones: diaphyseal, metadiaphyseal, parosteal, and central. The rare parosteal aneurysmal bone cyst appears to arise from the periosteum, with minimal erosion of the outer cortex and extension into the surrounding soft tissues. In the long bones, most aneurysmal bone cysts are eccentric, osteolytic, and metaphyseal in location. The inner margin of the lesion is well defined, and there may be a rim of sclerosis. Although the expansile nature of the lesion can lead to disruption of the cortex, an intact thin rim of cortical bone is frequently seen. In the test patient, the destruction of the inferior aspect of the cortex, the cloudlike lesion matrix, and the extension of these vague calcific densities into the soft tissues do not support the diagnosis of aneurysmal bone cyst.

The presence of multiple serous and hemorrhagic fluid-fluid levels within cystlike cavities is characteristic of aneurysmal bone cyst on CT and MR examination. CT is also useful in delineating the intraosseous and extraosseous extent of the lesion, which may be difficult to evaluate on conventional radiographs, especially in the spine, pelvis, and skull. Aneurysmal bone cysts are typically multiloculated and expansile on MRI and may have a prominent "soft tissue" component. On T1-weighted MR images, aneurysmal bone cysts are usually well demarcated from the surrounding high-signal-intensity fatty marrow. The lesion's internal signal intensity can be heterogeneous and can include areas of low, intermediate, and high signal intensity. The low signal intensity correlates best with the presence of fibrous tissue, internal osseous architecture, or hemosiderin. The intermediate signal intensity may represent fluid, hemorrhage at various ages, or soft tissue. The increased signal intensity is usually the result of subacute hemorrhage. On T2-weighted images, prominent heterogeneity is also seen, but the lesion will typically have more areas of increased signal intensity since reactive fibrous tissue and fluid will increase in signal intensity. The lesion remains well demarcated from surrounding normal marrow, and there is usually no evidence of marrow edema. Surrounding soft tissue edema has been reported.

The variable MR appearance of fluid-fluid levels in aneurysmal bone cysts reflects the type of fluid within cystic spaces. The fluid in one cavernous space can have high signal intensity on both T1- and T2-weighted images, whereas the fluid in an adjacent cavernous space can have a low signal intensity on T1-weighted images and a high signal intensity on T2-weighted images. Layers within the same cyst can vary in signal intensity, displaying either low signal intensity on T1-weighted images and high signal intensity on T2-weighted images or else high signal intensity on both T1- and T2-weighted images. Occasionally, fluid levels of widely differing signal intensity are seen on T1-weighted images, and the dependent layer often has bright signal intensity. This is presumably secondary to T1 shortening by methemoglobin in the more dense, dependent blood layer. Since both hemorrhage and fluid increase in signal intensity on T2-weighted images, fluid-fluid levels are often less conspicuous. The age of the blood, the presence of proteinaceous fluid, and the amount of solid tissue will all affect the MR appearance of the lesion.

A low-signal-intensity rim is sometimes seen surrounding an aneurysmal bone cyst. This corresponds to a rim of reactive bone. Often, the thin rim of cortex surrounding the expansile portion of the lesion is not seen on MRI, and it can be difficult to distinguish an aneurysmal bone cyst from a tumor with a soft tissue mass without the benefit of conventional radiographs. The differential diagnosis of aneurysmal bone cyst based on the CT and MR appearance includes complicated unicameral bone cyst, giant cell tumor, chondroblastoma, hemangioma, and telangiectatic osteogenic sarcoma, all of which can present with hemorrhagic fluid-fluid levels.

Nonossifying fibroma (Option (D)) and the related fibrous cortical defect are commonly found in the distal femur. Recently, the histologic classification of these lesions was reviewed by investigators at the Armed Forces Institutes of Pathology; they suggested using the term fibroxanthoma to describe these benign lesions of connective tissue. Others prefer to maintain the distinction between the smaller fibrous cortical defect and the larger, primarily intramedullary nonossifying fibroma, and frequently these terms (fibroxanthoma, nonossifying fibroma, and fibrous cortical defect) are used interchangeably. Histologically, fibroxanthomas are composed of uniform, benign-appearing, spindle-shaped fibroblasts that are arranged in intersecting bands. This creates a whorled pattern. Within a fibroxanthoma one can find multinucleated giant cells, foam cells, cholesterol crystals, and hemosiderin pigment. Little or no mitotic activity can be detected, although occasionally foci of metaplastic bone or osteoid will be seen. Radiographically, fibroxanthomas are circular or oval and are well delineated, with smooth or lobulated edges (Figure 7-6). They arise in the metaphysis, a short distance from the physis or, less commonly, adjacent to the physeal plate. As bone growth occurs, the lesions will migrate to a central location. There may be sclerosis within a portion of the lesion, and sclerosis of adjacent bone is typical. Larger lesions can have a multiloculated appearance, and there are usually well-delineated, smooth, or lobulated edges. In the test patient, the lesion does not have a sharply demarcated border, nor is there adjacent sclerosis. Therefore, nonossifying fibroma is an unlikely diagnosis.

Chondosarcoma (Option (E)) is a malignant tumor of connective tissue origin that can arise either *de novo* within the medullary cavity or as a result of malignant transformation of a preexisting lesion (enchondroma, osteochrondroma, chondroblastoma, chondromyxoid fibroma, and unicameral bone cyst). They can arise in any bone preformed in cartilage, although about 50% are found in the pelvis and upper femur. Chondrosarcomas are categorized by the precise location within bone (central, peripheral, or juxtacortical) and by the degree of cellular differentiation (low, medium, or high grade). Lesions that arise *de novo* typically occur in the medullary cavity; secondary lesions will occur centrally when arising from an enchondroma or peripherally when arising from an osteochondroma. Chondrosarcomas arising *de novo* from the periosteal mem-

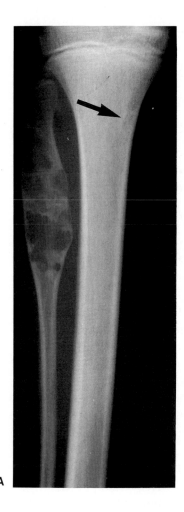

A

Figure 7-6. Nonossifying fibroma. Anteroposterior radiographs of the proximal right tibia and fibula show the natural history of a nonossifying fibroma of the proximal fibula for the patient at 10 years of age (A), at 13 years of age (B), and at 17 years of age (C). (A) At age 10, the lesion is expansile, oval, well demarcated from the surrounding marrow, and lobulated in contour. A fibrous cortical defect is identified in the medial proximal tibial metaphysis (arrow). (B) At age 13, the lesion is smaller and less expansile and shows partial mineralization consistent with regression. (C) At age 17, the lesion is almost healed.

brane (juxtacortical or periosteal chondrosarcoma) are typically detected in the long bones (particularly the femur).

Chondrosarcoma occurs more frequently in men than in women by a ratio of 3:2. While it can be diagnosed at any age, it is most frequently discovered in the fourth through seventh decades. Patients with peripheral, as opposed to central, chondrosarcomas tend to be slightly younger. Clinically, patients present with pain, which may be associated with a soft tissue mass. Pathologic fractures are seen in approximately 3% of patients at presentation, and in most cases symptoms have been present for 1 to 2 years.

Most chondrosarcomas occur in the long bones (45%), with the femur being most commonly affected (25%). Tumors also occur in the innomi-

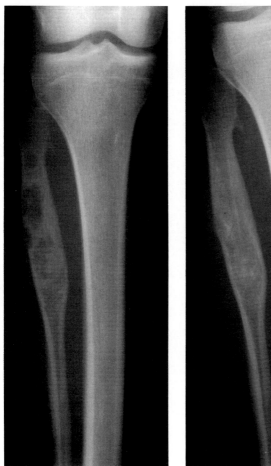

B   C

nate bone (25%) and ribs (8%). Vertebrae and other flat bones are less
frequently affected. Most chondrosarcomas develop within the metaphysis, with extension into the epiphysis. In the long bones, involvement of
the proximal portion of the bone is more frequent than involvement of
the distal portion. When arising in the ribs or sternum, chondrosarcomas
are typically encountered at or near the costochondral junction.

Radiographically, chondrosarcomas are typically radiolucent with a
calcified chondroid matrix characterized by dense calcific rings, floccules,
or pinpoint calcifications. Identification of chondrosarcoma tumor matrix
is important both for diagnosis and for assessment of lesion aggressiveness. Well-organized calcific rings within cartilage are usually indicative
of a low-grade tumor (Figure 7-7), whereas high-grade tumors often contain various amounts of myxoid materials and have large areas of non-

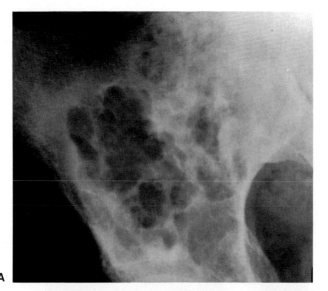

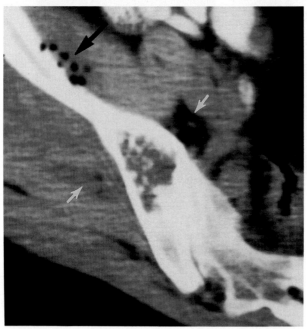

Figure 7-7. Chondrosarcoma. An anteroposterior radiograph (A) and a CT scan (B) of the right ilium in a 32-year-old woman with multiple echondromas show a radiolucent lesion with a calcified chondroid matrix. A soft tissue mass can be seen on the CT scan as a low-attenuation region both anterior and posterior to the ilium (white arrows). Air in the soft tissues (black arrow) is secondary to a biopsy.

calcified tumor matrix (Figure 7-8). When calcification does occur in high-grade chondrosarcomas, it is typically amorphous, punctate, or irregular. Tumor margins commonly are ill-defined with a large zone of transition between the tumor and normal portions of bone, although low-grade tumors can have a well-defined margin with the surrounding bone

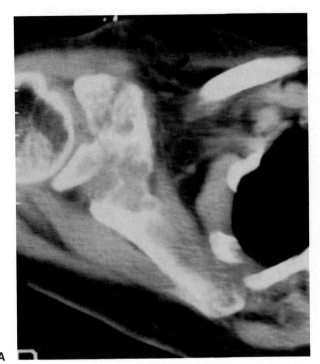

A

Figure 7-8. Poorly differentiated chondrosarcoma. This 59-year-old woman had pain in the right scapula. (A) A CT scan shows a destructive, lytic lesion of the glenoid and scapular wing with little calcified tumor matrix. The cortex is disrupted in many places. Coronal proton-density (B) and T2-weighted (C) MR images show intermediate- and high-intensity tumor, respectively. Note the region where the tumor invades the muscle (arrows).

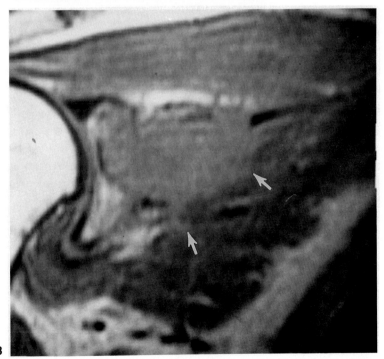

B

SE 1,900/20

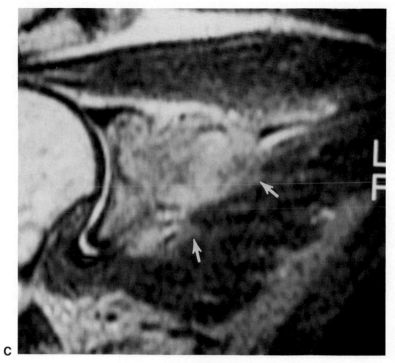

C

SE 1,900/80

marrow. The bone cortex often bulges outward, and there may be endosteal thinning at the tumor site.

The radiographic features of chondrosarcoma are influenced by the anatomic location of the tumor. A peripheral chondrosarcoma similar in position to the lesion in Figure 7-1 would most commonly arise from a pre-existing exostosis or, rarely, from the periosteal membrane (juxtacortical chondrosarcoma). Such a lesion would typically show cartilaginous tumor matrix, as well as an underlying exostosis. Therefore, chondrosarcoma is not a likely diagnosis on the basis of the test images.

Evidence of malignant transformation in a case of exostosis includes the presence of a bulky cartilaginous cap, an irregular indistinct bony surface beneath the cartilaginous cap, scattered calcification in the cartilaginous (soft tissue) portion of the tumor, focal areas of radiolucency in the interior of the exostosis, significant soft tissue mass, and destruction or pressure erosion of the adjacent bone. The long axis of the tumor is parallel to the long axis of the bone, and the subjacent cortex may be partially eroded. Typically, the medullary cavity appears normal.

Central chondrosarcoma, on the other hand, has an abnormal medullary cavity and is typically found in a long bone such as the proximal femur. Typically, it is an elongated, slightly expansile, lobulated osteolytic lesion. Often, there is periosteal bone formation, cortical thickening, and scattered spicules or irregular calcifications. In instances of aggressive central chondrosarcoma, cortical destruction and soft tissue mass can be identified.

Question 29

Concerning well-differentiated osteosarcoma,

    (A) the distal femur is the most common site
    (B) it is most commonly a lytic lesion
    (C) it is often expansile
    (D) it is histologically similar to parosteal osteosarcoma
    (E) it is commonly misdiagnosed as a benign lesion

Well-differentiated osteosarcoma was first described by Unni et al. in 1977. Histologically, this tumor resembles low-grade parosteal osteosarcoma, although radiographically its appearance mimics that of many benign lesions. This tumor, although malignant, has a fairly good prognosis if diagnosed in a timely fashion. Most patients present during the second, third, or fourth decade of life. Symptoms are relatively mild at the time of presentation, consisting of pain or swelling in the region of a palpable mass. The average duration of symptoms prior to diagnosis is 9 months.

Most well-differentiated osteosarcomas occur in the appendicular skeleton, most frequently in the distal femur **(Option (A) is true)**. The proximal tibia, proximal humerus, and distal fibula are also affected. These tumors are primarily intramedullary and central in location rather than eccentric. They arise most frequently in the metaphysis but can spread to the diaphysis or epiphysis. Only rarely are lesions solely diaphyseal.

Radiographically, the pattern of mineralization in well-differentiated osteosarcoma is almost always mixed lytic and blastic. Only rarely is the lesion purely lytic **(Option (B) is false)**. Lesions are typically poorly defined, although they can be well defined, but there is no associated sclerotic rim. The tumor matrix is most frequently homogeneous and cloudlike (Figure 7-9), although it can appear trabeculated or mixed.

The tumor expands the host bone in approximately 50% of cases **(Option (C) is true)**. In almost all cases, cortical thinning and discontinuity are visible on the radiographs and, in all cases reported to date, cortical thinning and discontinuity have been demonstrated by CT. There is frequently an extraosseous soft tissue mass. Reactive periosteal

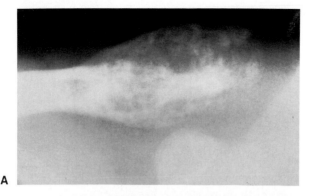

A

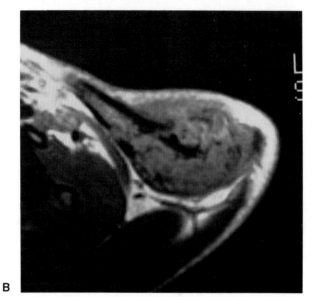

B

SE 2,000/20

Figure 7-9. Well-differentiated osteosarcoma. (A) An anteroposterior radiograph of the distal left clavicle shows an expansile lesion with a cloudlike matrix and disruption of the bone margins. (B) A transaxial proton-density MR image shows cortical disruption and a soft tissue mass. (Reprinted with permission from Moore et al. [8].)

bone is seen in only 25% of cases, with a rare Codman's triangle or lamellated periosteal bone. There is increased tracer uptake on bone scintigraphy. Angiograms show hypervascularity and neovascularity. MR examination accurately delineates the intraosseous, as well as the extraosseous, extent of the tumor.

Histologically, well-differentiated osteosarcoma resembles low-grade parosteal osteosarcoma, even though the tumors have different radiographic characteristics (Figure 7-10) **(Option (D) is true).** These lesions are characterized by proliferating trabecular bone, well-differentiated cartilage cells showing some enchondromal ossification, and unremarkable fibrous stroma. Well-differentiated osteosarcoma can also resemble

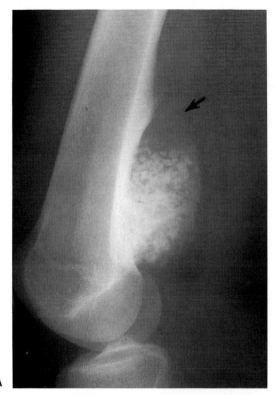

A

Figure 7-10. Parosteal osteosarcoma. (A) A lateral radiograph of the knee shows cortical thickening and a large mineralized mass attached to the dorsal aspect of the distal femoral metaphysis. There is very little calcification in the superior aspect of the mass (arrow). (B) A T1-weighted sagittal MR image shows the typical heterogeneous mineralization of the otherwise confined soft tissue mass. F = femur. (Reprinted with permission from Moore [7].)

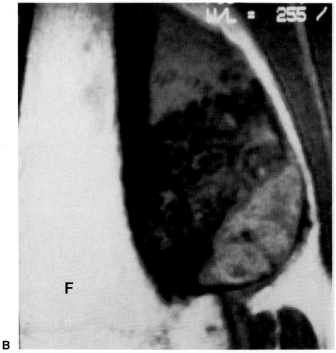

B

SE 700/30

other, more benign, lesions; for this reason the clinical, pathologic, and radiographic findings must be considered together to arrive at the correct diagnosis. A progression of well-differentiated osteosarcoma to a higher histologic grade can occur in patients with recurrence. While metastasis is uncommon in well-differentiated osteosarcoma, it can occur, most commonly to the lungs. Well-differentiated osteosarcomas can be misdiagnosed radiographically as ossifying fibroma, fibroma, desmoplastic fibroma, nonossifying fibroma, aneurysmal bone cyst, fibroxanthoma, chondromyxoid fibroma, and fibrous dysplasia **(Option (E) is true).**

Some studies suggest that the radiographic pattern of the tumor matrix is related to lesion aggressiveness. Low-grade lesions appear to have a more heavily trabeculated pattern, either because they produce trabecular bone or, more likely, because they grow slowly and result in incomplete destruction of residual normal trabecular bone. Higher-grade lesions progress more rapidly and seem to produce an osteoid-rich tumor bone that replaces the normal trabecular bone.

Question 30

Concerning osteoblastoma,

    (A) there is a male predominance
    (B) recurrence is common following surgical resection
    (C) about 30% occur in the vertebrae
    (D) epidural extension occurs with vertebral lesions
    (E) appendicular lesions are usually lytic

Osteoblastoma is an uncommon primary neoplasm of bone, with a male predominance of 2:1 **(Option (A) is true).** Although osteoblastoma can occur at any age, most lesions are diagnosed in individuals less than 30 years of age, with 70% of cases appearing in the second or third decade of life. Pain and mild local tenderness are the most common presenting complaints, and surgical excision is required for treatment. Recurrence is rare **(Option (B) is false).** There have been a few reports of malignant sarcomatous transformation.

About 30% of osteoblastomas occur in the vertebrae and are frequently confined to the neural arch **(Option (C) is true).** Another 35% occur in the long bones. Lesions can be central, cortical, or periosteal. Pathologically, lesions are vascular and consist of a loosely fibrillar and highly vascular matrix rich in osteoblasts. The histology is heterogeneous; sheets of osteoblasts can be seen in one area, whereas osteoid and trabeculae predominate in another. Lesions can be difficult to differentiate from osteoid osteoma, although the number of osteoblasts tends to be

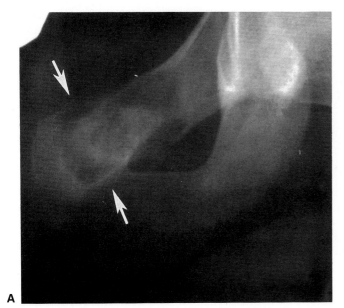

A

Figure 7-11.
Osteoblastoma.
(A) An anteropos-
terior radiograph
of the pubis
shows a lytic le-
sion of the left su-
perior pubic ra-
mus (arrows)
with a miner-
alized center sim-
ulating a button
sequestrum.
(B) The CT scan
confirms these
features.

greater in osteoid osteoma than in osteoblastoma. In general, both the location and the size of the lesion can help to separate the two entities; a lesion of more than 2 cm in size occurring in a region typical for osteo-blastoma is considered indicative of osteoblastoma. The clinical presen-tation of osteoblastoma differs somewhat from that of osteoid osteoma; the pain in osteoblastoma is a nagging pain that does not respond to aspirin nor does it awaken the patient. Lesions in the spine are similar in behavior to osteoid osteoma because both may be accompanied by pain, muscle spasm, scoliosis, and neurologic symptoms.

Radiographically, osteoblastomas are lytic lesions and are less dense than normal surrounding bone, although various degrees of bone produc-tion can be present (Figure 7-11). When present, this osteosclerosis can be accompanied by exuberant periostitis. Pathologic fractures are a rare feature. The expanding lesion can eventually thin and ultimately erode the cortical bone, destroying the cortex and resulting in a soft tissue mass. An internal pattern of equal-sized flecks of calcification is common. This internal pattern constitutes one of the more characteristic features of osteoblastoma, although occasionally a few larger irregular calcific deposits can be present, giving the lesion the appearance of a cartilagi-nous tumor. These lesions maintain distinct borders with the medullary cavity and often display a thin calcific shell on high-quality radiographs. Lesions show increased activity on scintigraphy.

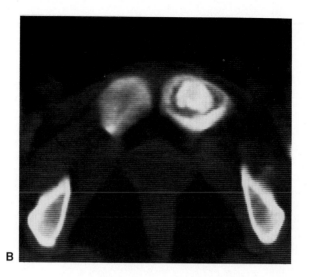

B

In the skull, osteoblastoma typically appears as a circumscribed, radiolucent oval defect with marginal sclerosis. A smoothly mineralized mass can occupy much of the defect centrally, giving the appearance of a sequestrum or button of bone. The inner and outer tables of the skull may be expanded.

In the spine, tumors originate from the posterior elements, may involve the vertebral body, and may extend into the epidural space causing cord compression **(Option (D) is true).** Lesions are typically lytic and expansile, although they frequently show some bone-forming activity and may become heavily ossified when fully mature. Initially, a spinal osteoblastoma can present as an enlargement of the transverse process, with focal areas of calcification centrally and an uninterrupted calcific shell peripherally. Conversion to an aneurysmal bone cyst has been reported.

About 75% of long-bone osteoblastomas occur in the diaphysis, while the remainder occur in the metaphysis. Lesions are only rarely seen in the epiphysis. Long bone osteoblastomas usually are lytic lesions **(Option (E) is true).** Central diaphyseal lesions are predominantly lytic, have clearly defined borders, and expand the shaft in a fusiform shape, whereas peripheral diaphyseal lesions are seen as sharply outlined destructive lesions within thickened cortical bone (Figure 7-12). Lesions sometimes arise within the periosteum and may project from the cortical surface with a thin shell, simulating cortical aneurysmal bone cyst.

In the metaphysis, osteoblasts can also be central or peripheral. Central metaphyseal lesions tend to be purely lytic, with symmetrical expan-

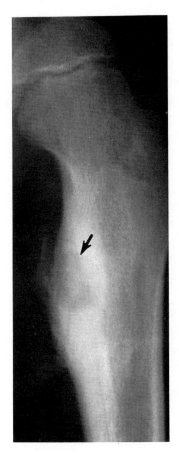

Figure 7-12. Osteoblastoma. An anteroposterior radiograph of the femur shows an ovoid lytic lesion (arrow) surrounded by thickened cortical bone.

sion of the cortex on either side. The demarcation between normal and abnormal bone is sharp. There is typically no evidence of surrounding sclerosis. Peripheral lesions are also radiolucent, but early destruction is usually incomplete and a sharply delineated sclerotic border will be present. Cortical margins are typically thinned and can be interrupted, with extension of the osteoblastoma into the soft tissues. Both central and peripheral lesions in the epiphyses also present as large lytic lesions with sharp demarcation from surrounding bone.

Osteoblastoma of the small bones of the hands and feet can result in either a focal fusiform expansion of bone or a replacement of the entire bone by a mixed type of lytic and sclerotic lesion. Lesions in the flat bones are lytic, but they typically have bony sclerosis and cortical thickening exceeding that of lesions at other locations. Characteristic intralesional clusters of calcifications are typical.

The MR appearance of osteoblastoma is variable and reflects the degree of bone destruction and sclerosis. Predominantly lytic osteoblastomas tend to be vascular and cellular, with intermediate signal intensity on T1-weighted images and homogeneous or heterogeneous high signal intensity on T2-weighted images. Cortical lesions are usually accompanied by thickened cortical bone of low signal intensity and various degrees of internal ossification. The lytic component of these lesions will again show intermediate signal intensity on T1-weighted images and heterogeneous high signal intensity on T2-weighted images. Marrow and soft tissue edema are usually not seen.

Question 31

Concerning nonossifying fibromas,

(A) they most often occur in the metadiaphyseal region
(B) they are most common about the knee
(C) the inner boundary is usually poorly defined
(D) there is associated marrow edema on MR images
(E) most lesions show homogeneous high signal intensity on T2-weighted MR images

Nonossifying fibroma, fibroxanthoma, and fibrous cortical defect are all terms used to describe histologically similar lesions that occur in the metaphyseal or metadiaphyseal region of the bones in the developing skeleton **(Option (A) is true).** Fibroxanthoma is the term preferred by the Armed Forces Institute of Pathology because it more accurately reflects the underlying histology. The spectrum of fibroxanthoma ranges from small cortical lesions (traditionally termed fibrous cortical defect) to larger intramedullary lesions (traditionally termed nonossifying fibroma). Pathologically, these lesions contain foci of fibrous tissue consisting of whorled bundles of spindle-shaped connective tissue cells. Each focus may be surrounded by a thin shell of reactive bone or sclerotic spongiosa. These lesions frequently contain multinucleated giant cells, cholesterol crystals, hemorrhage, and hemosiderin.

The smaller fibroxanthomas (fibrous cortical defects) occur primarily in children between the ages of 4 and 8 years. These fibroxanthomas are usually less than 2 cm in diameter, are eccentrically located within the metaphysis, and have a predilection for the medial femoral condyle. They do not require treatment. Radiographically, they are seen within the metaphyseal cortex. The margin is usually poorly defined. In older, regressing lesions the margin may be well defined with a thin rim of reactive bone. Spontaneous regression or extrusion of the defect through the cortex will eventually occur.

The larger, medullary fibroxanthomas (nonossifying fibromas) are asymptomatic, well-defined osteolytic lesions that involve the cortex and medullary cavity of the metaphysis and adjacent diaphysis of the long bone. The lesions are usually at least 4 cm in diameter and can be the result of a "fibrous cortical defect" that has persisted. About 75% of these lesions occur in children between the ages of 10 and 15 years, with most occurring about the knee, in the medial and posterior aspect of the distal femur and proximal tibia **(Option (B) is true).** They also occur in the lateral and posterior aspects of the distal tibia. Most lesions heal spontaneously (Figure 7-6). Radiographically, medullary fibroxanthomas are eccentrically located within the metaphyseal region of bone. The inner boundary is usually well demarcated by a scalloped sclerotic border **(Option (C) is false),** and the cortex can be either thin or else thickened and sclerotic. Pathologic fractures are uncommon but do occur.

Fibroxanthomas are easily recognized on MR images, and familiarity with the MR appearance is important since the lesions are so common in the pediatric population. The cortical lesions lie within the cortex and, when large, extend into the medullary space. The surrounding low-signal-intensity cortical bone can be either normal or thickened. Fibrous cortical defects have low to intermediate signal intensity on T1-weighted images, although foci with high signal intensity on T1-weighted images will sometimes be seen in hemorrhagic lesions. Occasionally, lesions will have very low signal intensity on both T1- and T2-weighted images, reflecting a combination of hemosiderin deposition, osteosclerosis, and dense fibrous connective tissue (Figure 7-13).

The larger, intramedullary lesions (nonossifying fibromas) have a lobulated contour (Figure 7-14). They are sharply demarcated from the surrounding normal bone marrow, and there is a lack of surrounding marrow or soft tissue edema **(Option (D) is false).** There should be no soft tissue component. On T2-weighted images, most lesions are heterogeneous but primarily of low to intermediate signal intensity **(Option (E) is false).** Lesions can have high signal intensity on T2-weighted images, but this is an infrequent occurrence. The central portion of the nonossifying fibroma can be either homogeneous or heterogeneous and may be delimited by a zone of high signal intensity. The fibroxanthomas apparently have a relatively long T2 relaxation time, since their signal intensity increases at TE values over 150 msec.

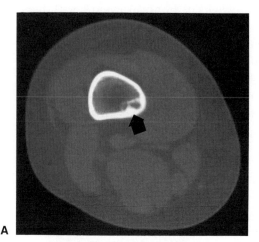

A

Figure 7-13. Fibrous cortical defect. A CT scan (A) and coronal T1-weighted (B) and T2-weighted (C) MR images through the distal femur in a 17-year-old boy show a resolving fibrous cortical defect (arrow). Low signal intensity on both T1- and T2-weighted images reflects the combined effects of hemosiderin deposition, sclerotic bone, and possibly dense fibrous elements. (Reprinted with permission from Moore [7].)

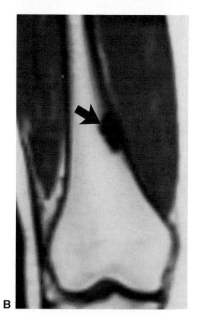

B

SE 300/15

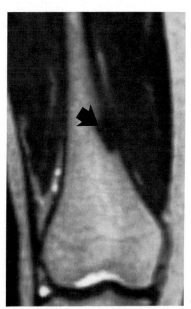

C

SE 2,500/80

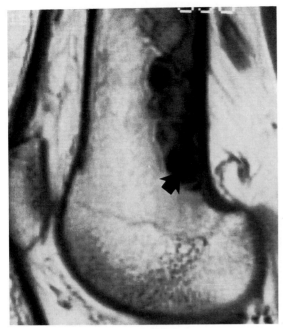

Figure 7-14. Nonossifying fibroma. A T1-weighted sagittal MR image through the distal femur in an 18-year-old girl shows a lobulated and sharply demarcated tumor. Focal regions of very low signal intensity most likely represent hemosiderin deposition (arrow). (Reprinted with permission from Moore [7].)

SE 800/20

Question 32

Concerning benign neoplasms of bone,

(A) periosteal reaction distal to the lesion is often seen with chondroblastoma

(B) intra-articular osteoid osteoma of the elbow is usually predominantly osteolytic

(C) marrow edema is seen on T2-weighted MR images of osteoid osteoma

(D) the perichondrium has low signal intensity on both T1- and T2-weighted MR images of osteochondroma

(E) aneurysmal bone cysts rarely occur in a subperiosteal location

Chondroblastoma is a rare benign chondrogenic primary bone tumor seen in children before epiphyseal closure. These lesions are thought to derive from cartilage "germ cells" or cells of the epiphyseal cartilage. Treatment is conservative, consisting of lesion curettage and packing with cancellous bone chips. Most chondroblastomas occur about the knee or in the proximal femur; the proximal humerus is the third most common site. Recurrence occurs in 10 to 25% of patients but does not necessarily herald malignant transformation.

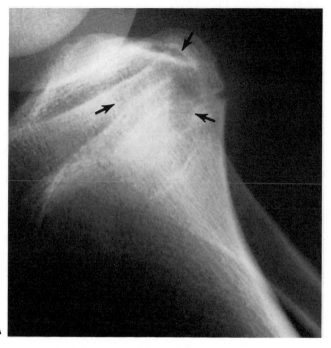

A

Figure 7-15. Chondroblastoma. (A) A lateral radiograph of the knee in a child shows a lucent, well-defined epiphyseal lesion with sclerotic margins (arrows). T1-weighted coronal (B) and T2-weighted sagittal (C) MR images show a well-defined intermediate-intensity lesion on the T1-weighted image that increases in intensity on the T2-weighted image. Note that the tumor perforates the physis (arrow in panel B).

Radiographically, these epiphyseal lesions are eccentric and uniformly lucent, with faint bony septa and a well-defined sclerotic margin (Figure 7-15). Lamellated or buttressed periosteal reaction is a recognized manifestation of chondroblastoma. In a study by Brower et al., periostitis was present in 47% of 214 chondroblastomas. Of long-bone chondroblastomas, 57% of cases showed periostitis and, notably, 73% of cases in the proximal humerus demonstrated periostitis. The periosteal reaction was always diametaphyseal and distant from the actual chondroblastoma **(Option (A) is true).** Both single- and multiple-lamellar ("onion-skin") types of periostitis are seen. Regardless of the number of actual layers of periosteal reactions, the reaction is always thick and solid. Soft tissue swelling is detected in up to 50% of patients; however, identification of an actual soft tissue mass is rare.

On MR examination, chondroblastomas appear as well-defined areas of intermediate to low signal intensity on T1-weighted images and have

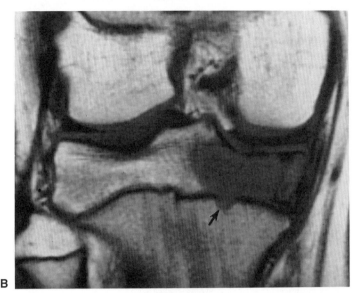

B

SE 300/15

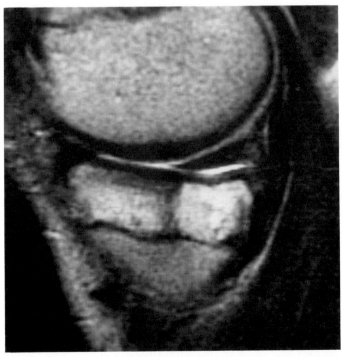

C

SE 2,000/80

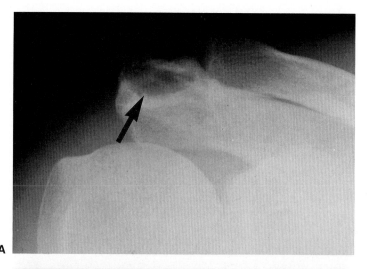

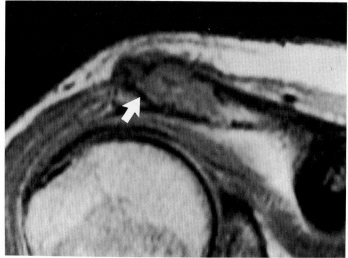

SE 300/15

Figure 7-16. Chondroblastoma of the acromion. (A) An anteroposterior radiograph shows well-defined lytic lesion (arrow). (B) A T1-weighted coronal MR image shows an intermediate-intensity lesion with a low-intensity sclerotic margin (arrow).

either intermediate or increased signal intensity on T2-weighted images (Figure 7-15). Trabeculations within the lesion can be seen as bands of low signal intensity on both T1- and T2-weighted images. A low-signal-intensity rim, corresponding to a sclerotic margin, can also be seen (Figure 7-16).

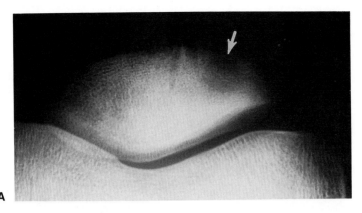

A

Figure 7-17. Osteoid osteoma. (A) An axial radiograph of the patella shows a round radiolucent lesion surrounded by sclerotic bone in the lateral aspect of the patella (arrow). (B) The lesion is shown more clearly on the CT scan, where the radiolucent nidus and surrounding sclerotic bone are clearly visible. A central calcification is also seen.

Osteoid osteoma is a benign osteoblastic bone tumor requiring surgical removal for cure. It is commonly found in the femur and tibia but occurs in every bone except the sternum and clavicle. About 75% of affected patients are between 5 and 25 years of age, and there is a 3:1 male predominance. Clinical symptoms are characterized by nocturnal bone pain that is relieved by aspirin. Soft tissue swelling and limitation of joint motion can occur. Scoliosis will occur as a result of osteoid osteoma of the spine. Pathologically, osteoid osteoma is characterized by a reddish-brown nidus less than 1 cm in diameter that is composed of highly vascular osteogenic connective tissue, with variable amounts of osteoid and well-differentiated osteoblasts encased within surrounding reactive bone.

Radiographically, osteoid osteomas are oval or round radiolucent lesions surrounded by a wide zone of sclerotic bone (Figure 7-17). The nidus can be lytic or dense, is eccentric, and does not invade the soft tissues. Three types of osteoid osteoma have been described. (1) Cortical osteoid osteoma is the most common type and typically demonstrates fusiform sclerotic cortical thickening of the long bone shaft. The nidus is radiolucent and is located centrally within an area of osteosclerosis. (2) Cancellous osteoid osteoma is less common and tends to occur in either the femoral neck or small bones of the hand or foot. The nidus typically fails to stimulate osteosclerosis, and therefore accompanying sclerosis may not be seen. (3) Subperiosteal osteoid osteoma is the least common type. It arises immediately adjacent to the affected bone, typically in the medial aspect of the femoral neck.

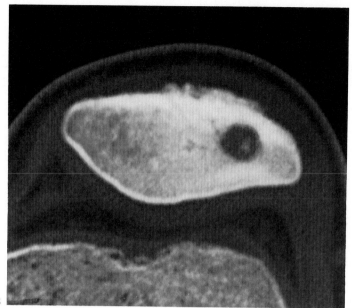

B

Osteoid osteoma of the elbow (Figure 7-18) is associated with abundant osteosclerosis **(Option (B) is false).** The diagnosis can be difficult but can be made once a nidus is identified on radiography or CT. In general, a reasonable work-up of the patient with elbow pain resembling that of osteoid osteoma should include conventional radiographs and, if necessary, scintigraphy and CT with bone windows. Increased activity on bone scintigraphy reflects osteoblastic tissue. The radiographs and CT images should be carefully scrutinized for the presence of joint effusion and coexistent periosteal reaction of the affected or adjacent bone, as well as identification of the nidus. Periosteal reaction frequently accompanies osteoid osteoma of the elbow and may be found on both sides of the elbow joint. The periosteal reaction can be adjacent to the osteosclerosis or else separated from the osteosclerosis that envelops the nidus. Joint effusion will be present in at least half of all cases. Increased density in the nidus is found more commonly late in the disease. The lesion can be associated with intense cortical thickening.

On MR examination, osteoid osteoma is typically accompanied by extensive marrow edema (Figure 7-19), which can be diffuse and seen as decreased marrow signal intensity on T1-weighted images and increased signal intensity on T2-weighted and STIR images **(Option (C) is true).** The nidus lies within this marrow edema, and since the lesion can be

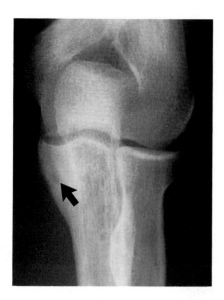

Figure 7-18 (left). Osteoid osteoma. An anteroposterior radiograph of the elbow in a patient with nocturnal pain is shown. The findings are characteristic of osteoid osteoma of the ulna, with a radiolucent nidus (arrow) and surrounding osteosclerosis. (Case courtesy of Robert D. Katz, M.D., Cedars-Sinai Medical Center, Los Angeles, Calif.)

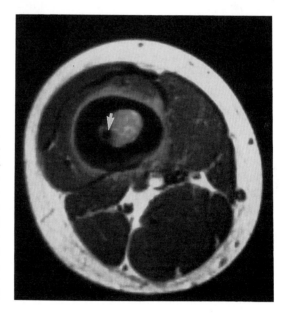

Figure 7-19 (right). Osteoid osteoma. A T1-weighted transaxial MR image through the right femur is shown. Intermediate-intensity marrow reflects marrow edema. The nidus (arrow) has low signal intensity, as does the thickened cortical bone. (Reprinted with permission from Moore [7].)

found in either the spongiosa or the cortex, the nidus is identified either centrally or peripherally. A variable MR appearance of the nidus has been reported; a primarily cellular (lytic) nidus is seen as an area of intermediate signal intensity on T1-weighted images and increased signal intensity on T2-weighted images. A densely sclerotic nidus has low to intermediate signal intensity on both T1- and T2-weighted images. If the osteoid osteoma is near a joint, and particularly if the lesion is intracapsular, an associated joint effusion can be identified.

Sclerotic bone surrounding the nidus will exhibit low signal intensity on both T1- and T2-weighted images. The cortex should be carefully examined for marked thickening in cases of suspected osteoid osteoma. This thickening of cortical bone is reactive, may be especially prominent in intramedullary lesions, and tends to exhibit low signal intensity, although intermediate cortical signal intensity can occur. The significance of increased cortical bone signal is uncertain, but it may represent cortical "edema."

Osteocartilaginous exostosis (osteochondroma) is a common tumor in the growing skeleton. It is a benign bone tumor characterized by cartilage-capped bony growths that appear in a variety of sizes and shapes: from slender and bulky to pointed and blunt to sessile and pedunculated. The perichondrium covers the lesion. Osteochondromas can be found in any bone that is preformed in cartilage but most frequently occur in the metaphyseal portion of a long bone. Approximately one-third are located in the distal femur, and another third are divided equally between the proximal humerus and proximal tibia. Clinical symptoms will occur if there is trauma, malignant transformation, or pressure on surrounding nerves or vessels. The onset of pain (even if inconstant and mild) and a sudden spurt of tumor growth (especially when bone growth has stopped) constitute reliable evidence that sarcomatous transformation has occurred. Lesions most frequently transform to chondrosarcoma, although osteosarcoma has been reported arising in the bone adjacent to an osteochondroma.

On MRI, osteochondromas are seen as bony growths, extending from the metaphyseal region, with marrow signal intensity that is the same as that of the shaft. The low-signal-intensity osteochondral cortex should be continuous with the cortex of the host bone. The cartilaginous cap, which typically ossifies with skeletal maturation and marks the end of exostotic growth, is the most characteristic feature of osteochondroma, and remnants of a quiescent cartilage cap can persist into adult life. The cartilage cap has intermediate signal intensity (equal to muscle) on T1-weighted images and increased signal intensity on T2-weighted images. A low-signal-intensity zone overlying the cartilaginous cap seen on both T1- and T2-weighted images represents an intact perichondrium **(Option (D) is true)**. Identification of the cartilaginous cap and perichondrium is important to confirm that the lesion is an osteochondroma and to distinguish it from other juxtacortical lesions such as juxtacortical chondroma or ossifying hematoma. Identification of a smooth and contiguous cartilaginous cap and intact perichondrium are consistent with a benign lesion.

Aneurysmal bone cysts are usually located centrally or eccentrically within the medullary cavity, although rarely aneurysmal bone cyst can have a subperiosteal location **(Option (E) is true).** The radiographic appearance of these rare subperiosteal or parosteal aneurysmal bone cysts can be indeterminate. CT examination is helpful in identifying both the thin cortical shell of the aneurysmal bone cyst and the fluid-fluid levels. MR is also useful in identifying fluid-fluid levels, as well as benign (low-signal-intensity) reactive cortical bone abutting the parosteal lesion. Hemorrhagic fluid-fluid levels within the lesion are often sufficient to make the diagnosis.

Discussion

Osteosarcoma, the most common primary bone tumor in children and young adults, occurs primarily between the ages of 10 and 25 years. It arises from undifferentiated connective tissue of bone and, depending on the predominant type of tumor tissue found, can be classified as osteoblastic, fibroblastic, chondroblastic, or telangiectatic. Pain and swelling of the affected region and rapid tumor growth can be accompanied by systemic symptoms such as weight loss and anemia. Osteosarcoma metastasizes relatively early, primarily to the lungs and long bones.

Radiographically, osteosarcomas are characterized by enlargement and destruction of bone. Soft tissue invasion is frequent. Lesions produce neoplastic osteoid, which mineralizes to a variable degree. There may be cortical thickening and periosteal reaction; complex periosteal reactions (e.g., sunburst or spiculated) and Codman's triangles are characteristic of these aggressive lesions. Tumors can be lytic, mixed, or blastic; in the case of telangiectatic osteosarcoma they may have a complex lytic appearance with multiple septations and cortical destruction. Lesions are located either centrally (diaphyseal, metaphyseal, or epiphyseal) or peripherally (juxtacortical). The majority (86%) of osteosarcomas are found in the long bones; 52% percent of these are solely metaphyseal, 30% are both metaphyseal and epiphyseal, 8% are both metaphyseal and diaphyseal, 8% are solely diaphyseal, and 2% are peripheral.

Localized cortical penetration by tumor can raise the periosteum and form a limiting membrane or barrier to the extraosseous tumor. This limiting membrane can frequently be identified on MRI. The intraosseous portion of tumor will extend deep into the medullary cavity and often terminates in a more or less dome-shaped plug that represents the advancing edge of tumor. The interface with normal marrow is usually well defined. A moderate-to-large soft tissue mass is almost always present and usually has intermediate intensity on T1-weighted images and heterogeneous high intensity on T2-weighted images. Discrete intercalation of tumor through the cortical bone is appreciated as focal areas of intermediate signal intensity within the cortex. At pathologic examination, the intramedullary spread of tumor is often equal in length to the extraosseous extent of tumor, which may eventually encircle the bone. Extension through the physis and into the epiphysis is seen in almost one-third of cases, although penetration of the joint capsule is unusual. Intact, low-signal-intensity cortex may be interposed between much of the intramedullary and extramedullary extent of tumor.

The MR appearance of osteosarcoma reflects the underlying histology. Osteosclerotic tumors contain areas of low signal intensity on both T1- and T2-weighted images, since sclerotic bone has a low proton density and a short T2 relaxation time. Osteolytic tumors are generally seen as lesions with low to intermediate intensity on T1-weighted images and high signal intensity on T2-weighted images. Osteosarcomas have a homogeneous to markedly heterogeneous appearance on MR images, depending on the relative predominance of the underlying cell types, as well as the presence of necrosis, hemorrhage, and sclerotic bone. Telangiectatic osteosarcomas can have a fairly characteristic MR appearance consisting of multiple cavities and hemorrhagic fluid-fluid levels. Low-signal-intensity septations can usually be seen separating the large blood-filled cavities. This appearance can also be seen in several other lesions, including aneurysmal bone cyst and giant cell tumor.

Multicentric osteosarcoma, or osteosarcomatosis, is characterized by multiple lesions at multiple sites of involvement. Osteosarcomatosis was previously felt to represent multiple primary osteosarcomas, but recent evidence supports the view that osteosarcomatosis is not a primary entity but is a diffuse skeletal metastatic disease. Osteosarcomatosis tends to affect patients younger than those who develop other types of osteosarcoma. Most patients will have a dominant lesion, both radiographically and clinically, and there is a tendency for this lesion to occur in a metaphysis within a lower extremity. The secondary lesions are either uniformly sclerotic (type I) or mixed lytic/sclerotic (type II) and occur predominantly at locations distant from the dominant lesion. Determination of the number and location of lesions is probably best achieved by scintigraphy. Pulmonary metastatic disease is seen in more than half of the patients.

Sheila G. Moore, M.D.

SUGGESTED READINGS

OSTEOSARCOMA

1. Aisen AM, Martel W, Braunstein EM, McMillin KI, Phillips WA, Kling TF. MRI and CT evaluation of primary bone and soft-tissue tumors. AJR 1986; 146:749–756
2. Bloem JL, Bluemm RG, Taminiau AH, van Oosterom AT, Stolk J, Doornbos J. Magnetic resonance imaging of primary malignant bone tumors. RadioGraphics 1987; 7:425–445
3. Boyko OB, Cory DA, Cohen MD, Provisor A, Mirkin D, DeRosa GP. MR imaging of osteogenic and Ewing's sarcoma. AJR 1987; 148:317–322
4. Ellis JH, Siegel CL, Martel W, Weatherbee L, Dorfman H. Radiologic features of well-differentiated osteosarcoma. AJR 1988; 151:739–742
5. Harms SE, Greenway G. Musculoskeletal tumors. In: Stark DD, Bradley WG Jr (eds), Magnetic resonance imaging, 2nd ed. St. Louis: Mosby-Year Book; 1992:2107–2222
6. Hopper KD, Moser RP Jr, Haseman DB, Sweet DE, Madewell JE, Kransdorf MJ. Osteosarcomatosis. Radiology 1990; 175:233–239
7. Moore SG. Pediatric musculoskeletal imaging. In: Stark DD, Bradley WG Jr (eds), Magnetic resonance imaging, 2nd ed. St. Louis: Mosby-Year Book; 1992:2223–2330
8. Moore SG, Dawson KL. Tumors of the musculoskeletal system. In: Cohen MD, Edwards MK (eds), Magnetic resonance imaging of children. Philadelphia: BC Decker; 1990:825–911
9. Sundaram M, McGuire MH, Herbold DR. Magnetic resonance imaging of osteosarcoma. Skeletal Radiol 1987; 16:23–29
10. Unni KK, Dahlin DC, McLeod RA, Pritchard DJ. Intraosseous well-differentiated osteosarcoma. Cancer 1977; 40:1337–1347

OSTEOBLASTOMA

11. McLeod RA, Dahlin DC, Beabout JW. The spectrum of osteoblastoma. AJR 1976; 126:321–325
12. Tonai M, Campbell CJ, Ahn GH, Schiller AL, Mankin HJ. Osteoblastoma: classification and report of 16 patients. Clin Orthop 1982; 167:222–235
13. Wilner D. Benign osteoblastoma. In: Wilner D (ed), Radiology of bone tumors and allied disorders. Philadelphia: WB Saunders; 1982:217–270

ANEURYSMAL BONE CYST

14. Beltran J, Simon DC, Levy M, Herman L, Weis L, Mueller CF. Aneurysmal bone cysts: MR imaging at 1.5 T. Radiology 1986; 158:689–690
15. Burnstein MI, DeSmet AA, Hafez GR, Heiner JP. Case report 611: Subperiosteal aneurysmal bone cyst of tibia. Skeletal Radiol 1990; 19:294–297
16. Capanna R, Van Horn JR, Biagini R, Ruggieri P. Aneurysmal bone cyst of the sacrum. Skeletal Radiol 1989; 18:109–113
17. Cory DA, Fritsch SA, Cohen MD, et al. Aneurysmal bone cysts: imaging findings and embolotherapy. AJR 1989; 153:369–373

18. de Santos L, Murray JA. The value of arteriography in the management of aneurysmal bone cyst. Skeletal Radiol 1978; 2:137

19. Moore SG, Stoller DW. Pediatric musculoskeletal magnetic resonance imaging. In: Stoller DW (ed), Magnetic resonance imaging in orthopaedics and rheumatology. Philadelphia: JB Lippincott; 1989:23–61

20. Munk PL, Helms CA, Holt RG, Johnston J, Steinbach L, Neumann C. MR imaging of aneurysmal bone cysts. AJR 1989; 153:99–101

21. Wilner D. Aneurysmal bone cyst. In: Wilner D (ed), Radiology of bone tumors and allied disorders. Philadelphia: WB Saunders; 1982:1003–1103

NONOSSIFYING FIBROMA (FIBROXANTHOMA)

22. Bohndorf K, Reiser M, Lochner B, Feaux de Lacroix W, Steinbrich W. Magnetic resonance imaging of primary tumours and tumour-like lesions of bone. Skeletal Radiol 1986; 15:511–517

23. Kransdorf MJ, Utz JA, Gilkey FW, Berrey BH. MR appearance of fibroxanthoma. J Comput Assist Tomogr 1988; 12:612–615

24. Resnick D, Kyriakos M, Greenway GD. Tumors and tumor-like lesions of bone: imaging and pathology of specific lesions. In: Resnick D, Niwayama G (eds), Diagnosis of bone and joint disorders. Philadelphia: WB Saunders; 1988:3616–3888

25. Wilner D. Fibrous defects of bone. In: Wilner D (ed), Radiology of bone tumors and allied disorders. Philadelphia: WB Saunders; 1982:551–611

CHONDROSARCOMA

26. Cohen EK, Kressel HY, Frank TS, et al. Hyaline cartilage-origin bone and soft tissue neoplasms: MR appearance and histologic correlation. Radiology 1988; 167:477–481

27. Evans HL, Ayala AG, Romsdahl MM. Prognostic factors in chondrosarcoma of bone: a clinicopathologic analysis with emphasis on histologic grading. Cancer 1977; 40:818–831

28. Henderson ED, Dahlin DC. Chondrosarcoma of bone—a study of two hundred and eighty-eight cases. J Bone Joint Surg (Am) 1963; 45:1450–1458

29. Mankin HJ, Cantley KP, Lippiello L, Schiller AL, Campbell CJ. The biology of human chondrosarcoma. I. Description of the cases, grading, and biochemical analyses. J Bone Joint Surg (Am) 1980; 62:160–176

30. Norman A, Sissons HA. Radiographic hallmarks of peripheral chondrosarcoma. Radiology 1984; 151:589–596

31. Sanerkin NG, Gallagher P. A review of the behaviour of chondrosarcoma of bone. J Bone Joint Surg (Br) 1979; 61:395–400

32. Wilner D. Chondrosarcoma. In: Wilner D (ed), Radiology of bone tumors and allied disorders. Philadelphia: WB Saunders; 1982:2170–2280

CHRONDROBLASTOMA

33. Bloem JL, Mulder JD. Chondroblastoma: a clinical and radiological study of 104 cases. Skeletal Radiol 1985; 14:1–9

34. Brower AC, Moser RP, Kransdorf MJ. The frequency and diagnostic significance of periostitis in chondroblastoma. AJR 1990; 154:309–314
35. Wilner D. Benign chondroblastoma. In: Wilner D (ed), Radiology of bone tumors and allied disorders. Philadelphia: WB Saunders; 1982:453–510

OSTEOID OSTEOMA

36. Glass RB, Poznanski AK, Fisher MR, Shkolnik A, Dias L. MR imaging of osteoid osteoma. J Comput Assist Tomogr 1986; 10:1065–1067
37. Moser RP Jr, Kransdorf MJ, Brower AC, et al. Osteoid osteoma of the elbow. A review of six cases. Skeletal Radiol 1990; 19:181–186
38. Wilner D. Osteoid osteoma. In: Wilner D (ed), Radiology of bone tumors and allied disorders. Philadelphia: WB Saunders; 1982:144–216

OSTEOCHONDROMA

39. Lee JK, Yao L, Wirth CR. MR imaging of solitary osteochondromas: report of eight cases. AJR 1987; 149:557–560

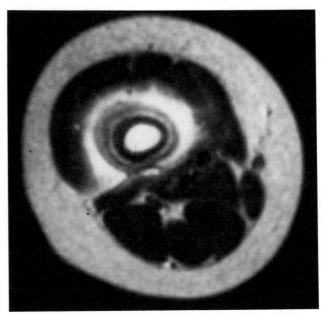

SE 2,500/80

Figure 8-1. This 3-year-old girl presented with a tumor of the right femur. You are shown a transaxial T2-weighted MR image of the right femur.

Case 8: Tumor Staging

Question 33

The test image demonstrates:

(A) "onion skin" periosteal reaction
(B) tumor within the medullary cavity of the femur
(C) edema of the vastus intermedius muscle
(D) cortical penetration by tumor
(E) sparing of the femoral neurovascular bundle

The transaxial T2-weighted MR image (Figure 8-1) shows that abnormal high-intensity cellular marrow has replaced normal lower-intensity femoral diaphyseal fatty and hematopoietic marrow. Low-intensity diaphyseal cortical bone is surrounded by alternating concentric intermediate- and high-intensity rings (Figure 8-2). A zone of high signal intensity is interposed between the femur and the vastus intermedius and biceps femoris muscles. The zone has a feathery periphery as it extends into these muscles. The remaining muscles are normal. This child has Ewing's sarcoma of the femur and underwent MR examination for tumor staging.

The concentric rings of intermediate and high signal intensity that surround the femur represent alternating zones of lamellated periosteal reaction and tumor. This is the "onion skin" pattern of periosteal reaction that has long been recognized on conventional radiographs (Figure 8-3) **(Option (A) is true).** Onion skin periosteal reaction is created by concentric planes of ossification elevated beyond the cortex. Initially, the zones between the lamellated bone are occupied by prominent dilated vessels within loose connective tissue. These spaces are ultimately colonized by tumor cells. At first, this colonization may be focal, but with time, tumor cells occupy most of the space between the layers of lamellated periosteal reaction. Onion skin periosteal reaction also occurs in bones of patients with nonneoplastic conditions, including osteomyelitis, stress fracture, and hypertrophic pulmonary osteoarthropathy.

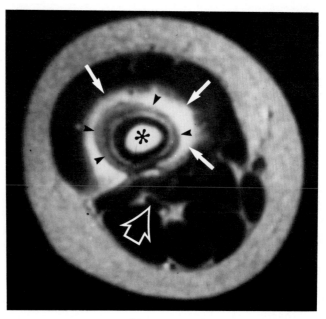

SE 2,500/80

Figure 8-2 (Same as Figure 8-1). Ewing's sarcoma. The diaphyseal medullary cavity (✳) exhibits high signal intensity (higher than that of subcutaneous fat). The very low intensity femoral cortex is surrounded by concentric rings of periosteal reaction (arrowheads). High-intensity edema extends beyond the periosteal reaction to involve the surrounding muscles (arrows). The neurovascular bundle is spared (open arrow).

In a 3-year-old child, the femoral diaphysis is composed primarily of red marrow with some yellow marrow. On T1-weighted MR images, the signal intensity of femoral diaphyseal marrow is usually higher than that of muscle but lower than that of fat. Typically, such marrow exhibits a slight increase in signal intensity on T2-weighted images. Normal marrow does not exhibit the markedly increased signal intensity evident in the test image. Therefore, this feature represents tumor within the medullary cavity (Figure 8-4) **(Option (B) is true).**

The abnormally increased signal intensity seen in the vastus intermedius muscle has a feathery periphery but conforms to soft tissue planes. It does not distort the muscle contour or have a masslike appearance. The absence of a mass is an important feature. It means that the high-intensity zone beyond the bone most probably represents edema of the vastus musculature **(Option (C) is true).**

On MR images, normal cortical bone appears black because of a lack of mobile protons. Increased signal intensity is encountered within corti-

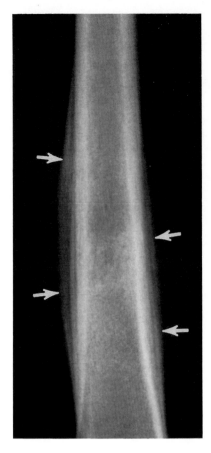

Figure 8-3. Same patient as in Figures 8-1 and 8-2. Ewing's sarcoma with onion skin periosteal reaction. A lateral radiograph of the femur shows layered or lamellated structure of onion skin periosteal reaction (arrows). (Reprinted with permission from Moore [10].)

cal bone that has been invaded by an adjacent soft tissue lesion or an intramedullary lesion. This abnormally increased signal intensity reflects mobile water protons from edema or tumor (Figure 8-5). Tumor spread into the cortex may or may not cause cortical destruction. No abnormal signal is seen within the cortical bone in the test image, and so cortical invasion or penetration by tumor is not demonstrated **(Option (D) is false)**.

The femoral neurovascular bundle is readily identified in the test image and is not in the region of the tumor. There is no abnormal signal within or surrounding the neurovascular bundle, it is not displaced, and normal fat separates these structures from adjacent muscle. Therefore, the femoral neurovascular bundle is spared **(Option (E) is true)**.

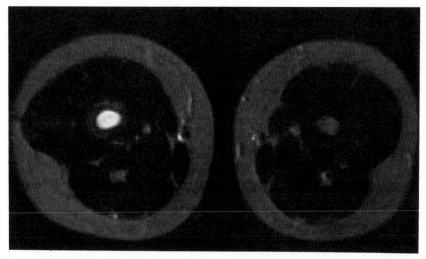

SE 2,500/80

Figure 8-4. Same patient as in Figures 8-1 through 8-3. Ewing's sarcoma versus normal diaphyseal marrow signal. A transaxial T2-weighted image of the test patient's femora at a more proximal level shows high medullary signal intensity on the involved right side and normal medullary signal intensity on the uninvolved left side. The signal intensity of the left femoral marrow appears similar to that of subcutaneous fat. This image was obtained with the use of window settings different from those used for the test image and was obtained at an anatomic location beyond the peritumoral edema. (Reprinted with permission from Moore and Dawson [11].)

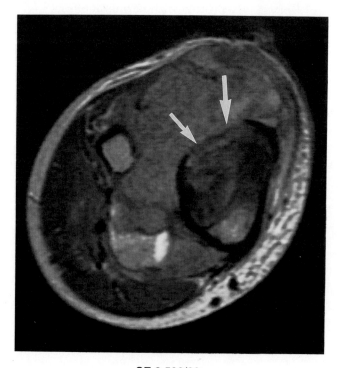

Figure 8-5 (left). Tumor spread through cortical bone. A transaxial proton-density image through the calf in an 18-year-old boy with osteosarcoma shows low-intensity tibial cortical bone except anterolaterally, where intermediate-intensity tumor has disrupted the cortex (arrows).

SE 2,500/20

Discussion

Comparison of MRI with other imaging modalities generally supports the use of MRI for pretherapeutic staging of musculoskeletal neoplasms. The advantages of MRI include superior tissue contrast between normal and pathologic soft tissue processes, increased sensitivity for definition of normal and abnormal marrow, only an occasional need for administration of an intravenous contrast agent, and a lack of ionizing radiation or known deleterious biologic effect.

Conventional radiography is currently the least expensive and most reliable imaging method for prediction of the histologic nature of a musculoskeletal neoplasm and should be performed before any more sophisticated imaging study. MRI (preferably performed before biopsy) is generally the imaging modality of choice when further tumor definition is needed, but specific indications exist for the use of CT, scintigraphy, and angiography. These include the identification of lesion calcification, the evaluation of subtle cortical or periosteal changes, screening for skeletal metastases, intravascular therapy, and the evaluation of vascular anatomy or physiology not adequately delineated by MR examination.

There have been several studies comparing MRI and CT in the evaluation of musculoskeletal tumors. One study, by Bloem et al., that evaluated the extent of disease in primary bone sarcoma showed that measurements of intraosseous tumor length from the MR images were better correlated with measurements made by pathologic/morphologic examination ($r = 0.99$) than were measurements made by CT ($r = 0.86$). For soft tissue extent of tumor and involvement of specific muscle groups, CT has a reported sensitivity of 71% and specificity of 93%, compared with a reported sensitivity of 96% and specificity of 99% for MRI. For the evaluation of cortical invasion and periosteal reaction, recent reports suggest that as MR techniques and interpretive skills have improved, the sensitivity and specificity of MRI in the evaluation of these features have approached or even exceeded those of CT.

A typical protocol used for MR examination of musculoskeletal tumors includes an initial T1-weighted "localizer" sagittal or coronal scan of the entire affected bone or soft tissue compartment followed by transaxial T1-weighted, proton-density, and T2-weighted images of the entire neoplasm. These images are acquired at the same anatomic levels so that specific tissue signal characteristics and morphologic features can be compared from image to image and among the pulse sequences. Sagittal or coronal images are used to evaluate the long axis of the anatomic compartments to detect skip lesions and to exclude partial-volume effects, as well as to determine tumor length, physeal or epiphyseal involvement, and joint involvement.

MR evaluation of musculoskeletal neoplasms should be performed before biopsy whenever possible, since post-biopsy hemorrhage and edema can obscure tumor margins or mimic tumor spread. Accurate pretherapeutic staging of soft tissue or bone lesions requires evaluation of the following parameters:

- Lesion origin (bone or soft tissue) and size
- Lesion characteristics
- Extent of tumor and/or edema within marrow
- Physeal and/or epiphyseal involvement
- Cortical bone involvement (including penetration)
- Periosteal reaction
- Joint involvement
- Size and extent of soft tissue mass and edema
- Neurovascular involvement
- Presence of lymphadenopathy
- Presence of skip lesions
- Estimate of stage

Most malignant musculoskeletal neoplasms have elongated T1 and T2 relaxation times. Therefore, the cellular components of most musculoskeletal neoplasms generally exhibit intermediate signal intensity on T1-weighted and proton-density images and high signal intensity on T2-weighted, fat-saturation, and short-T1 inversion recovery (STIR) images (Figure 8-6). Fat has high signal intensity on T1-weighted images and becomes progressively less bright on proton-density and T2-weighted images. Chronic fibrosis, sclerotic bone, and reactive bone formation have low signal intensity on all sequences.

Zones of intermediate signal intensity on T1-weighted images that increase in intensity on T2-weighted images are characteristic not only of tumors but also of edema, fluid collections, tumor necrosis, granulation tissue, and early fibrosis. A region with relatively high signal intensity on both T1- and T2-weighted images may represent fat, subacute hemorrhage, mucus, or the effect of contrast agents such as gadolinium DTPA.

The signal intensity of hemorrhage is variable and depends on the age of the hemorrhage, but signal intensity that is intermediate on T1-weighted images but becomes decreased on T2-weighted images may represent acute hemorrhage, whereas high signal intensity on both T1- and T2-weighted images may represent subacute hemorrhage. When evidence of blood is identified, hemorrhage into a neoplasm, recent biopsy,

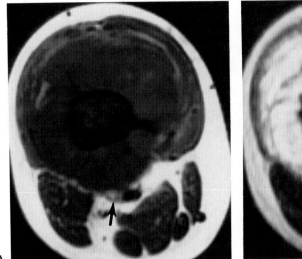 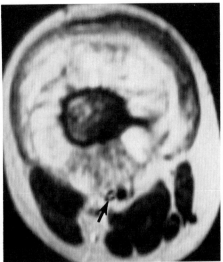

A   B

SE 300/15   SE 2,500/80

Figure 8-6. Osteoblastic osteosarcoma. Transaxial MR images through the distal femur in a 17-year-old boy with osteoblastic osteosarcoma. T1-weighted (A) and T2-weighted (B) images show low-intensity marrow on both sequences, indicative of densely mineralized tumor matrix. A large soft tissue mass surrounds the femur, and its cellular component has intermediate signal intensity on the T1-weighted image and high signal intensity on the T2-weighted image. The radiating low-intensity streaks within the soft tissue mass, most prominent on the T2-weighted image, represent spiculated tumor new bone formation. The tumor abuts the neurovascular bundle (arrow).

or a primary hemorrhagic tumor (such as telangiectatic osteosarcoma) should be considered (Figure 8-7).

Masses with a large fraction of mature collagen may have a distinct low-intensity appearance on both T1- and T2-weighted images. This pattern reflects the lack of mobile protons in relatively acellular fibrous lesions. Dense mineralized osteoid as encountered in some osteoid-producing tumors such as osteoblastic osteosarcoma also produces low-intensity regions on both T1- and T2-weighted images.

The extent of marrow involvement by neoplasia can usually be determined on T1-weighted coronal or sagittal images, because these optimize contrast between fat and other tissues and give the best visualization of the long axis of most bones. Low- or intermediate-intensity tumor is easily distinguished from the high-intensity fatty marrow in bones with predominantly yellow marrow (Figure 8-8). In bones with predominantly red marrow, such as are found in infants, young children, and patients

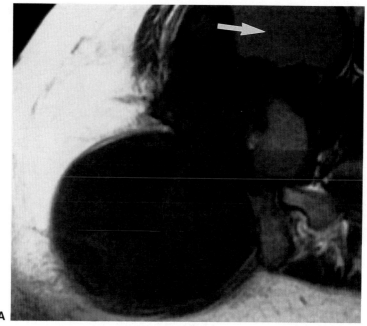

A

SE 300/15

Figure 8-7. Hemorrhage into telangiectatic osteosarcoma. This 30-year-old woman presented with right sciatic pain. (A and B) Transaxial MR images through the pelvis show a large tumor extending both anterior and posterior to the right ilium. T1-weighted (A) and proton-density (B) images show a slightly heterogeneous, intermediate-intensity tumor with evidence of subacute hemorrhage in its anterior aspect (straight arrow). Note the fluid-fluid level within the hemorrhage (curved arrow, panel B). (C) A gradient-echo image shows heterogeneity of the posterior tumor cellularity. The tumor abuts the iliac artery and vein. There is normal flow in the right iliac artery (arrow) but decreased flow in the iliac vein (arrowhead).

with chronic hematopoietic disorders or red marrow hyperplasia, intermediate-intensity tumor can be difficult to distinguish from intermediate-intensity red marrow on T1-weighted images (Figure 8-9). In these cases, the use of T2-weighted fat-suppression or STIR images may increase lesion conspicuity and facilitate assessment of tumor extent.

Distinguishing "marrow edema" from tumor infiltration of marrow is sometimes difficult. Often, marrow edema appears feathery with low- to intermediate-intensity strands on T1-weighted images. These edematous zones exhibit increased signal intensity on T2-weighted images and commonly appear more homogeneous. Marrow edema can also be homogeneous on T1-weighted images and can therefore be difficult to distin-

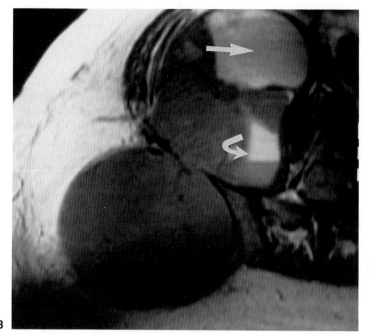

B

SE 2,500/20

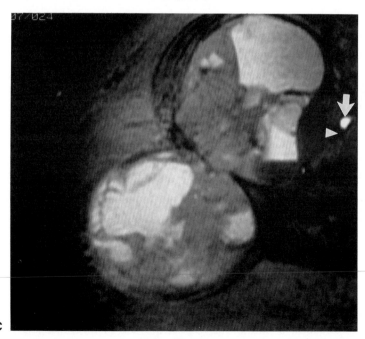

C

GRE 22/13/30°

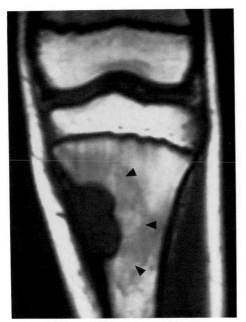

SE 300/20

Figure 8-8 (left). Intramedullary tumor extent. A coronal T1-weighted image through the left knee in an 11-year-old boy with a proximal tibial osteosarcoma shows that the intramedullary extent of the tumor is easily estimated. The subtle low-intensity zone (arrowheads) surrounding the intramedullary lesion represents reactive bone and bone marrow. The physis has low signal intensity and shows no evidence of tumor involvement.

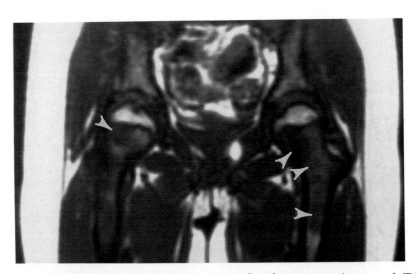

Figure 8-9. Osteosarcomatosis in sites of red marrow. A coronal T1-weighted MR image through the proximal femora in a child with multiple foci of osteosarcoma shows that the intermediate-intensity normal red marrow of the proximal femora obscures the multiple slightly lower intensity deposits of tumor (arrowheads). (Reprinted with permission from Moore [10].)

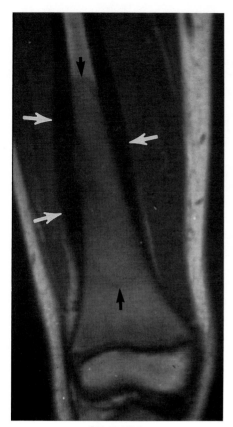

SE 800/20

Figure 8-10. Marrow edema. A coronal T1-weighted image through the right femur in an 8-year-old girl with an osteoid osteoma shows low-intensity cortical thickening (white arrows). Extensive intermediate-intensity marrow edema is sharply demarcated from the normal marrow (black arrows). (Reprinted with permission from Moore and Sebag [12].)

guish from medullary tumor. Typically, primary bone tumors are not accompanied by much marrow edema, whereas metastases, infections, trauma, and osteoid osteoma can be accompanied by extensive marrow edema (Figure 8-10).

Coronal or sagittal images are optimal for assessment of physeal and epiphyseal anatomy and involvement by tumor. The physis is normally seen as an undulating low-intensity line on T1-weighted images. The physis decreases in thickness with maturation, and a thin physeal remnant is sometimes seen in a mature bone. In children, the normal intermediate-intensity cartilaginous epiphysis seen on T1-weighted images increases in signal intensity on T2-weighted images. The ossifying epiphysis is characterized by high-intensity fatty marrow and can be identified within the cartilaginous epiphysis (Figure 8-11). The epiphysis eventually attains a mature size and shape, and, except in the first few

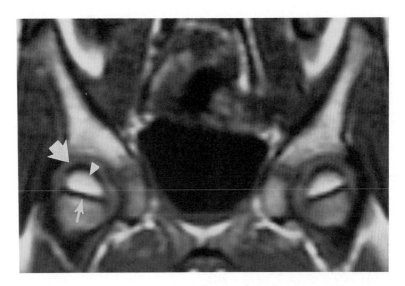

SE 300/15

Figure 8-11. Ossifying epiphyses. A coronal T1-weighted images through the hips in a 4-year-old girl show intermediate-intensity cartilaginous epiphyses (thick arrow) and high-intensity fat within the ossifying epiphyses (arrowhead). Note also the low-intensity physis (thin arrow).

months of life, normal marrow in the ossified epiphysis is always seen on MR images as high-intensity yellow marrow.

If intramedullary (diaphyseal or metaphyseal) tumor stops short of the physis, with normal yellow or red marrow interposed between the physis and tumor, physeal involvement by tumor can be excluded (Figure 8-8 shows an example of this situation). If tumor abuts the physis but there is no change of physeal morphology or signal intensity, microscopic invasion cannot be confirmed or excluded. In these cases, intermediate signal intensity within the physis juxtaposed to the metaphyseal tumor makes invasion of the physis more likely, whereas normal physeal signal intensity makes physeal invasion less likely. Abnormal physeal signal intensity accompanied by signal abnormality in the adjacent epiphysis corresponds to physeal penetration by tumor (Figure 8-12). Epiphyseal tumor typically has intermediate signal intensity and is surrounded by high-intensity fatty marrow on T1-weighted images.

Cortical bone of long bones is usually best evaluated on transaxial images, since this gives the least partial-volume averaging and best demonstrates the radial extent of tumor. Intermediate signal intensity within otherwise normal low-intensity cortical bone on T1-weighted, proton-density, T2-weighted, fat-saturation, and STIR images is indicative

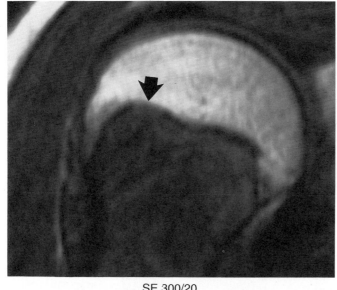

SE 300/20

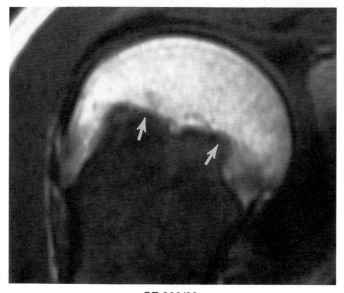

SE 300/20

Figure 8-12. Ewing's sarcoma penetrating the physis. Coronal T1-weighted images through the proximal humerus in a 10-year-old girl with metaphyseal Ewing's sarcoma. The signal intensity of the proximal metaphyseal marrow is abnormally low. (A) The tumor abuts and appears to invade the physis (arrow), with focal intermediate signal intensity seen within the otherwise low-intensity physis. (B) An image 5 mm anterior to that in panel A shows penetration of tumor into the high-intensity (fatty marrow) epiphysis, obliterating the low-intensity physeal line centrally (arrows).

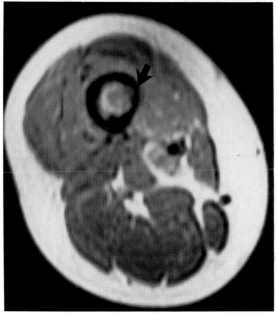

Figure 8-13. Endosteal erosion. A transaxial proton-density image through the femur shows an intramedullary tumor with endosteal erosion of medial cortex (arrow).

SE 2,500/20

of either edema or tumor within the cortex. Endosteal erosion is seen on MRI as thinning of the very low intensity (black) cortical bone (Figure 8-13). Permeation of tumor through cortical haversian canals with expansion of the canals is manifest as intermediate signal intensity extending either partially or completely through the affected cortical bone. Tumor eventually extends through the cortex and into the soft tissues as a solid mass (Figure 8-14). Identification of cortical disruption is important since spread of tumor cells associated with cortical penetration or its complications, pathologic fracture and hematoma formation, may necessitate more aggressive therapy. Also, many surgeons prefer to perform biopsies through a preexisting cortical defect, if present, and MRI can help localize the biopsy site.

Intermediate signal intensity within cortical bone can also be a manifestation of aggressive osteoporosis, osteoid osteoma, infection, and other inflammatory processes.

Chemical-shift artifacts can be a problem in the evaluation of cortical bone. Chemical shift in the frequency-encoding direction causes thickening of the cortex on one side and thinning on the opposite side, giving the appearance of cortical erosion by tumor (Figure 8-15). By reversing the frequency-encoding direction of the MR examination, cortical bone adjacent to the tumor can be accurately evaluated.

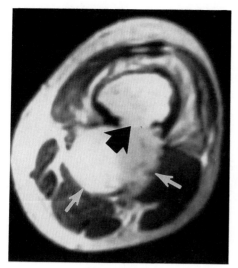

SE 2,000/40

Figure 8-14. Cortical disruption by chondrosarcoma. A transverse proton-density image through the distal femur shows high-intensity chondrosarcoma with endosteal erosion and expansion of the marrow cavity. Cortical penetration has occurred (black arrow). A large, posterior soft tissue mass (white arrows) is contiguous with the medullary tumor. (Reprinted with permission from Moore [10].)

An understanding of the pathophysiology of periosteal reaction is essential to the interpretation of periosteal reaction on all imaging studies. "Periosteal reaction" is a term used to describe vigorous deposition of juxtacortical soft tissue and bone in disease processes. The magnitude of periosteal reaction depends on the degree of periosteal elevation as well as the level of activity of the process stimulating the reaction. The periosteum is composed of an outer fibrous layer and an inner cellular, or cambium, layer, which surrounds the cortical bone and separates it from the surrounding soft tissue. In adults this periosteum is primarily fibrous. During reaction to injury, or in children during normal growth, two distinct and thickened layers of periosteum can be distinguished histologically. There is a zone of transition between the two layers in which modulation of fibroblasts into preosteoblasts through nuclear enlargement and acquisition of cytoplasm occurs. Subsequent mitosis and cell enlargement create the cambium layer, within which osteoid-secreting cells emerge.

Mineralization of periosteal reaction is necessary before it can be identified on a radiograph or CT scan. This usually requires 10 days to 3 weeks following the initial stimulus. The configuration of periosteal reaction reflects the rate of production and the manner in which the new bone is laid down. Periosteal reaction can be classified as continuous, interrupted, or complex (Figure 8-16). Continuous periosteal reaction can be accompanied by destruction of the underlying endosteal cortex, giving a "shell" appearance, or it can be accompanied by deposition of

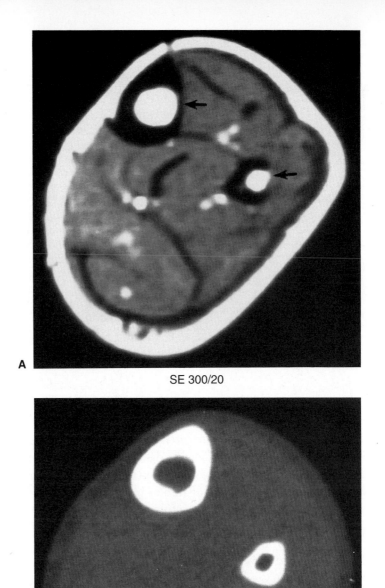

SE 300/20

Figure 8-15. Chemical-shift artifact. (A) A transaxial T1-weighted MR image shows a chemical-shift artifact in the frequency-encoding direction. The cortex appears thinned on the lateral (arrows) and thickened on the medial aspects of the tibia and fibula. Reversal of the frequency-encoding gradient could be used to exclude erosion of cortical bone by tumor if the tumor abutted the cortex. (B) A CT scan confirms the normal thickness of the cortex. (Reprinted with permission from Moore [10].)

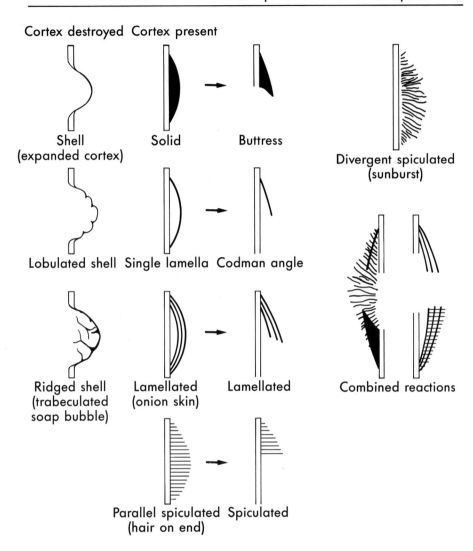

Continuous	Interrupted	Complex

Cortex destroyed Cortex present

Shell
(expanded cortex)

Solid

Buttress

Divergent spiculated
(sunburst)

Lobulated shell Single lamella Codman angle

Ridged shell
(trabeculated
soap bubble)

Lamellated
(onion skin)

Lamellated

Combined reactions

Parallel spiculated Spiculated
(hair on end)

Figure 8-16. Periosteal reaction. Continuous periosteal reaction can occur with destruction of cortex (column 1) or preservation of cortex (column 2). The lamellated bone laid down with continuous periosteal reaction is organized and has a structure identical to that of cortical bone. The type of interrupted periosteal reaction (column 3) depends on the underlying continuous periosteal reaction. Complex periosteal reaction (column 4) is also shown. (Reprinted with permission from Ragsdale et al. [22].)

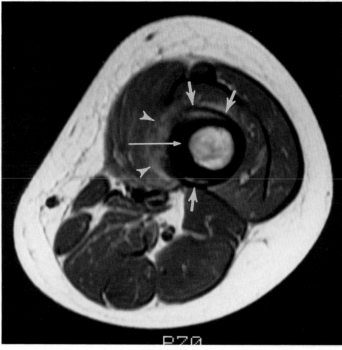

SE 2,500/20

Figure 8-17. Lamellated periosteal reaction. A transverse proton-density image through the distal femur in a 17-year-old boy with an osteosarcoma shows single lamellar periosteal reaction as a curvilinear low-intensity line surrounding the bone (short arrows). Increased-intensity tumor (arrowheads) is seen adjacent to the thickened medial cortex (long arrow).

cortical bone, resulting in cortical thickening. Continuous periosteal reaction of the solid, single lamellar, lamellated, or parallel spiculated ("hair on end") types can be found and is often associated with cortical penetration by abnormal marrow processes. Interrupted periosteal reaction is encountered when an aggressive process breaches a preformed continuous periosteal reaction. The appearance depends on the type of underlying periosteal reaction. The most common complex periosteal reaction encountered in musculoskeletal tumors is the "sunburst" variety.

Periosteal reactions are visible on both transaxial and longitudinal MR images, although subtle periosteal alterations are more readily seen on transaxial images. Solid periosteal reaction indicates a chronic indolent lesion such as an osteoid osteoma, eosinophilic granuloma, or large enchondroma. On MR examination this is seen as thickened, low-intensity cortical bone (Figure 8-17). As a general rule, thickened cortex without internal signal most probably represents "benign" cortical thickening. However, an example of a Ewing's sarcoma treated by preoperative therapy and with black, thickened, cortical bone shown by MRI but proven to have viable intracortical tumor at pathologic examination has been reported by Bloem et al.

Single lamellar periosteal reactions appear as thin, curvilinear, low-intensity lines on spin-echo MR images (Figure 8-17). These layers can surround either part or all of the involved bone. Single lamellar periosteal reaction is characteristic of acute osteomyelitis and early phases of neoplasms. "Onion skin" periosteal reaction is seen as alternating bands of intermediate and low signal intensity on T1-weighted images and alternating bands of high and low signal intensity on T2-weighted images (Figure 8-1). The concentric rings of low signal intensity on both T1- and T2-weighted images correspond grossly to organized lamellar bone, and the interposed intermediate- or high-intensity rings correspond grossly to cellular components. This lamellated periosteal reaction is characteristic of malignant tumors (especially Ewing's sarcoma) but also occurs in patients with nonneoplastic diseases such as osteomyelitis, hypertrophic pulmonary osteoarthropathy, and stress fracture.

Parallel spiculated "hair-on-end" periosteal reaction is seen most commonly in patients with Ewing's sarcoma and in those with the calvarial reaction associated with severe anemia such as that characteristic of thalassemia major. On T1-weighted MR images, this type of periosteal reaction manifests as alternating bands of low and intermediate signal intensity extending outward from cortical bone (Figure 8-18). In other cases, the spiculated periosteal reaction is not readily apparent on MR images because the very thin lamellar bone is not of sufficient volume to be resolved. "Hair-on-end" periosteal reaction has also been found in patients with syphilis, myositis, or Caffey's disease.

"Interrupted" periosteal reaction is the result of tumor involvement of the soft tissue space within an already formed periosteal reaction. The MR appearance of these interrupted reactions reflects the pattern of the underlying continuous periosteal reaction, with abrupt termination of this periosteal reaction by the invasive pathologic process. Interrupted periosteal reaction is usually seen at the edges of a lesion and is best demonstrated on coronal or sagittal images (Figure 8-19).

Complex periosteal reaction is common in bone tumors, especially osteosarcoma. The divergent spiculated pattern, or sunburst pattern, is a sign of malignant osteoid production. Histologically, the individual "rays" of ossification seen on radiographs, CT, or MRI represent either a combination of sarcoma bone and reactive bone or sarcoma bone alone. The space between individual rays is usually occupied by cellular tumor and

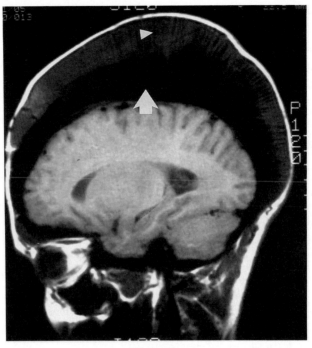

SE 600/20

Figure 8-18. Osteopetrosis with "hair-on-end" periosteal reaction. A sagittal T1-weighted image of the skull in a 14-year-old girl with osteopetrosis shows a thickened osteopetrotic skull (arrow) and radiating, lamellated spicules of periosteal reaction with the "hair-on-end" appearance (arrowhead). (Reprinted with permission from Cook PF, Moore SG. Case report 746. Osteopetrosis. Skeletal Radiol 1992; 21:396–398.)

tumor products, often chondroid or myxoid. The reactive bone is oldest and most mature adjacent to the cortex. On MR examination, the "sunburst" calcification pattern seen on conventional radiographs is commonly obscured and only a soft tissue mass is seen.

The MR features of periosteal reactions reflect the underlying histology. Cortex is compact, well-organized, mineralized bone with haversian spaces. The structure of this lamellar bone is such that its protons do not resonate during clinical proton MRI. Therefore, cortical bone appears as a black or very low intensity structure on MR images. Similarly, compact, well-organized lamellar periosteal reaction exhibits low signal intensity on T1- and T2-weighted images. By comparison, complex periosteal reactions tend to be structurally disorganized and enveloped by protein matrix. Their protons are therefore more free to precess, and their signal intensity is intermediate and even increased on spin-echo

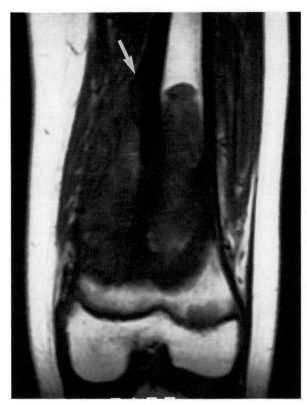

SE 300/15

Figure 8-19. Interrupted periosteal reaction. A coronal T1-weighted image of the distal femur in a patient with osteosarcoma shows low-intensity periosteal reaction with an interrupted lamellated pattern and a Codman's angle (arrow).

images. Recognition of periosteal reaction on an MR image is important, but the MR examination should never be interpreted without the benefit of recent radiographs.

In studies comparing MRI and CT for the evaluation of musculoskeletal tumors, MRI has generally been shown to be superior in assessing joint involvement by tumor. Coronal or sagittal MR images of the joint are usually best for evaluating tumor as it abuts the joint surface. Gross joint involvement by tumor can be appreciated on MR images, but subtle or microscopic involvement can be difficult to diagnose. Thin sections (3 mm) through the joint can aid in this assessment. When gross extension of tumor into the joint space is not clearly evident, the presence of tumor within the epiphysis, soft tissue tumor juxtaposed to the joint, or joint fluid can be used as adjunctive findings to suggest the possibility of joint invasion. Sympathetic joint effusions do occur, and so inspection of the joint during surgery is necessary in any patient in whom joint involvement is suspected. A clear margin of normal marrow between epiphyseal

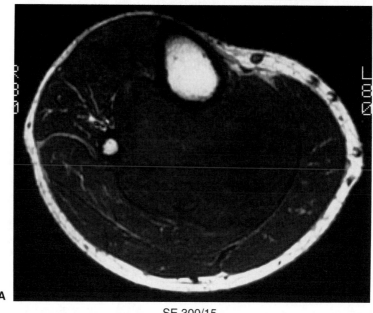

SE 300/15

Figure 8-20. Malignant fibrous histiocytoma. Transaxial T1-weighted (A) and T2-weighted (B) images through the midcalf in a 50-year-old man with soft tissue sarcoma of the posterior compartment. Note the fairly homogeneous intermediate signal intensity of the tumor on the T1-weighted image, which makes differentiation from muscle difficult. On the T2-weighted image, there is heterogeneity of both morphologic and signal intensity patterns.

tumor and the joint space, with no evidence of joint effusion, essentially excludes joint involvement. If the tumor abuts the joint surface and the (normally black) cortical bone shows foci of intermediate signal intensity or is not clearly intact, microscopic joint involvement should be considered. Knowledge of the specific anatomic confines of each joint capsule is essential, since some capsules extend above the level of the physis. Metaphyseal tumor can therefore theoretically break through the cortex and involve the joint space even when the epiphysis, physis, and epiphyseal cortex are normal.

There are several studies comparing MRI and CT in the evaluation of soft tissue tumors. In general, these studies show that MRI is superior to CT in defining lesion extent. Sharp, clearly defined margins and a homogeneous signal intensity on T2-weighted images suggest a less aggressive process. Less well-defined lesions with heterogeneous signal intensity on T2-weighted images are frequently associated with a more

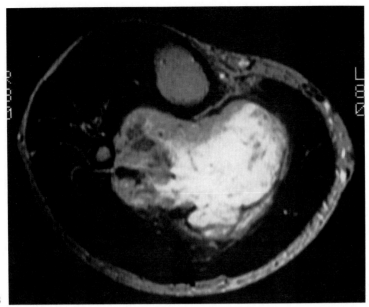

B

SE 2,000/80

aggressive process (Figure 8-20). Bone involvement by soft tissue masses and invasion of the neurovascular bundle are additional criteria that suggest malignancy.

Signal intensity and morphologic patterns are important in distinguishing a soft tissue mass from soft tissue edema. A region that is mass-like, has a nodular or irregular contour, displaces normal structures, or distorts soft tissue planes is likely to represent tumor. Tissue that shows intermediate signal intensity on T1-weighted images and high signal intensity on T2-weighted images but is feathery in appearance, conforms to soft tissue planes, and does not distort surrounding normal structures or musculature is more likely to represent soft tissue edema or post-therapeutic tissue changes. Edematous muscle can swell, but its overall contour remains relatively normal. The more removed the affected muscle is from the primary mass, the more likely it is that feathery signal intensity changes in the muscle represent edema and not tumor infiltration.

Neurovascular involvement is most accurately assessed by pulse sequences that emphasize blood flow, such as gradient-recalled-echo (GRE) images. When a soft tissue mass is anatomically separate from the neurovascular bundle and the fascial planes surrounding the neurovascular bundle are normal, neurovascular involvement can be confidently excluded. If the soft tissue mass is anatomically separate from the neurovascular bundle but there is decreased signal intensity on T1-weighted images and increased signal intensity on T2-weighted images in the fascial planes surrounding the neurovascular bundle, microscopic tumor invasion of the neurovascular bundle must be considered. Displacement, encasement, and slow or absent flow in the neurovascular bundle are also abnormal.

Lymph nodes exhibit intermediate signal intensity on T1-weighted images and increased signal intensity on T2-weighted, fat-saturation, and STIR images. GRE images are useful in differentiating vessels from lymph nodes, since flow has high signal intensity and nodes have intermediate signal intensity. There are no criteria for differentiating malignant from hyperplastic nodes on MRI, and nodes greater than 1 cm in diameter are considered suspicious for malignancy.

The characteristics of musculoskeletal tumors as derived from imaging studies, particularly MRI, should be synthesized into a description that predicts the surgical stage of the tumor. An accurate description is required for planning successful surgical treatment. The staging system is based on the histologic grade of the tumor, the extent of the tumor, and the presence or absence of metastases.

Benign tumors are classified as grade 0. Malignant tumors are grade 1 if their histologic features indicate little risk of metastases and grade 2 if there is a significant risk of metastases. Conventional radiographs provide an excellent approximation of grade for bone tumors, and MRI provides a similar assessment for soft tissue masses.

The anatomic extent of tumor depends on an understanding of the concept of anatomic compartments. The human body is divided into many anatomic compartments separated by barriers to tumor spread. For example, each bone, with its enveloping periosteum and articular cartilage, is an individual compartment. Likewise, muscle groups are separated by fascial planes and have unique blood supplies. They, too, are considered individual compartments. The anatomic extent of a tumor is either intracompartmental or extracompartmental. Extracompartmental tumors are usually those that have crossed a natural barrier; these require more extensive therapy and have a poorer prognosis.

Sheila G. Moore, M.D.

SUGGESTED READINGS

TUMOR STAGING

1. Aisen AM, Martel W, Braunstein EM, McMillin KI, Phillips WA, Kling TF. MRI and CT evaluation of primary bone and soft-tissue tumors. AJR 1986; 146:749–756

2. Bloem JL, Taminiau AH, Eulderink F, Hermans J, Pauwels EK. Radiologic staging of primary bone sarcoma: MR imaging, scintigraphy, angiography, and CT correlated with pathologic examination. Radiology 1988; 169:805–810

3. Bohndorf K, Reiser M, Lochner B, Féaux de Lacroix W, Steinbrich W. Magnetic resonance imaging of primary tumours and tumour-like lesions of bone. Skeletal Radiol 1986; 15:511–517

4. Boyko OB, Cory DA, Cohen MD, Provisor A, Mirkin D, DeRosa GP. MR imaging of osteogenic and Ewing's sarcoma. AJR 1987; 148:317–322

5. Cohen EK, Kressel HY, Frank TS, et al. Hyaline cartilage-origin bone and soft-tissue neoplasms: MR appearance and histologic correlation. Radiology 1988; 167:477–481

6. Demas BE, Heelan RT, Lane J, Marcove R, Hajdu S, Brennan MF. Soft-tissue sarcomas of the extremities: comparison of MR and CT in determining the extent of disease. AJR 1988; 150:615–620

7. Frank JA, Ling A, Patronas NJ, et al. Detection of malignant bone tumors: MR imaging vs scintigraphy. AJR 1990; 155:1043–1048

8. Gillespy T III, Manfrini M, Ruggieri P, Spanier SS, Pettersson H, Springfield DS. Staging of intraosseous extent of osteosarcoma: correlation of preoperative CT and MR imaging with pathologic macroslides. Radiology 1988; 167:765–767

9. Harms SE, Greenway G. Musculoskeletal tumors. In: Stark DD, Bradley WG Jr (eds), Magnetic resonance imaging, 2nd ed. St. Louis: Mosby-Year Book; 1992:2107–2222

10. Moore SG. Pediatric musculoskeletal imaging. In: Stark DD, Bradley WG Jr (eds), Magnetic resonance imaging, 2nd ed. St. Louis: Mosby-Year Book; 1992:2223–2330

11. Moore SG, Dawson KL. Tumors of the musculoskeletal system. In: Cohen MD, Edwards MK (eds), Magnetic resonance imaging of children. Philadelphia: BC Decker; 1990:825–911

12. Moore SG, Sebag GH. Primary disorders of bone marrow. In: Cohen MD, Edwards MK (eds), Magnetic resonance imaging of children. Philadelphia: BC Decker; 1990:765–824

13. Pettersson H, Gillespy T III, Hamlin DJ, et al. Primary musculoskeletal tumors: examination with MR imaging compared with conventional modalities. Radiology 1987; 164:237–241

14. Sundaram M, McGuire MH. Computed tomography or magnetic resonance for evaluating the solitary tumor or tumor-like lesion of bone? Skeletal Radiol 1988; 17:393–401

15. Sundaram M, McLeod RA. MR imaging of tumor and tumorlike lesions of bone and soft tissue. AJR 1990; 155:817–824

16. Totty WG, Murphy WA, Lee JK. Soft-tissue tumors: MR imaging. Radiology 1986; 160:135–141

17. Wetzel LH, Levine E, Murphey MD. A comparison of MR imaging and CT in the evaluation of musculoskeletal masses. RadioGraphics 1987; 7: 851–874
18. Zimmer WD, Berquist TH, McLeod RA, et al. Bone tumors: magnetic resonance imaging versus computed tomography. Radiology 1985; 155:709–718

CORTEX AND PERIOSTEAL REACTION

19. Dick BW, Mitchell DG, Burk DL, Levy DW, Vinitski S, Rifkin M. The effect of chemical shift misrepresentation on cortical bone thickness on MR imaging. AJR 1988; 151:537–538
20. Greenfield GB, Warren DL, Clark RA. MR imaging of periosteal and cortical changes of bone. RadioGraphics 1991; 11:611–623
21. Moore SG. Magnetic resonance imaging and computed tomography of cortical bone. In: Bloeme JL, Sartoris DJ (eds), MRI and CT of the musculoskeletal system. A text atlas. Baltimore: Williams & Wilkins; 1992: 139–152
22. Ragsdale BD, Madewell JE, Sweet DE. Radiologic and pathologic analysis of solitary bone lesions. Part II: periosteal reactions. Radiol Clin North Am 1981; 19:749–783

Notes

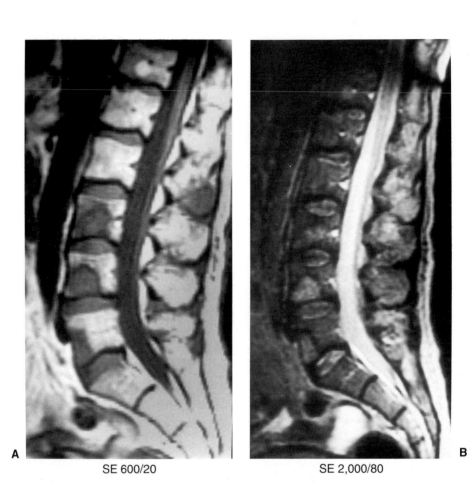

SE 600/20   SE 2,000/80

Figure 9-1. This 58-year-old man has adenocarcinoma of the lung. Bone scintigrams and radiographs of the lumbar spine were normal. You are shown sagittal T1-weighted (A) and T2-weighted (B) MR images of the lumbar spine.

Case 9:   Bone Biopsy

Question 34

Which *one* of the following statements concerning bone biopsy of this patient is correct?

- (A) It is not indicated because the negative results of bone scintigraphy make metastatic disease highly unlikely.
- (B) Percutaneous biopsy is feasible even though the lesions cannot be seen on radiographs.
- (C) It is not indicated because the diagnosis is obvious on the MR images.
- (D) Biopsy of the L3 body is inappropriate because of the high risk of vertebral collapse.
- (E) Open biopsy would be safer than percutaneous biopsy.

Sagittal T1- and T2-weighted spin-echo MR images of the lumbar spine (Figure 9-1) demonstrate multiple focal marrow-replacing lesions involving vertebral bodies and posterior elements (Figure 9-2). The presence of these lesions in a patient with or without a known malignancy makes metastatic disease statistically the most likely diagnosis. A fluoroscopically guided percutaneous needle biopsy of the L3 vertebral-body lesion confirmed the presence of metastatic lung cancer in the test patient.

As demonstrated in the test patient, bone lesions can be diagnosed by percutaneous biopsy even though they are not seen on radiographs **(Option (B) is correct).** Before the biopsy, lesions must be identified and accurately localized by some imaging technique. This was accomplished by MRI of the lumbar spine in the test patient. In other instances, the lesion could have been localized by using conventional radiography, bone scintigraphy, or CT. Once an abnormality is accurately localized, a biopsy can be performed even if the lesion is occult on one of the imaging modalities. For example, lesions not evident on conventional radiographs may be identified and localized by CT, MRI, or bone scintigraphy; this allows a biopsy needle to be properly placed under fluoroscopic or CT guidance.

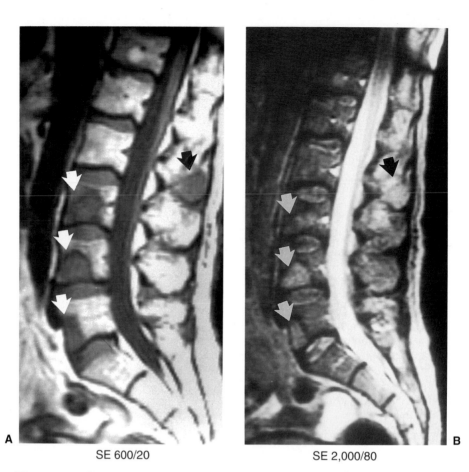

SE 600/20   SE 2,000/80

Figure 9-2 (Same as Figure 9-1). Metastases. Sagittal T1-weighted (A) and T2-weighted (B) MR images of the lumbar spine show multiple focal lesions involving vertebral bodies and posterior elements. The lesions have replaced the normal high-intensity yellow marrow on the T1-weighted image, where they are seen as regions of low signal intensity (arrows). The corresponding areas exhibit high signal intensity (arrows) on the T2-weighted image. Percutaneous biopsy diagnosed metastatic lung cancer.

The choice of imaging modality for biopsy guidance depends primarily on the location of the lesion. Fluoroscopy is relatively fast, simple, and inexpensive and is readily available. Therefore, it is frequently used. CT provides better visualization of surrounding soft tissue structures, allowing determination of the precise path for needle placement. CT is advantageous when a lesion is not evident on the conventional radiograph, when it is small, or when it is located deeply or in a particularly complex anatomic site. MRI also provides an excellent display of anatomy, but it is rarely used for biopsy guidance because of severely restricted access inherent in the bore of superconductive magnets and because of the limitations on the use of ferromagnetic materials during the biopsy.

Negative bone scintigraphy is generally a good indicator of the absence of metastatic disease; however, the identification of lesions by MRI, as in the test patient, indicates that bone scintigraphy can be falsely negative. Bone scintigraphy represents a very useful method for detection of metastatic disease, is much more sensitive than conventional radiography, and still represents the best survey technique available for detecting skeletal metastases. However, in the presence of negative or equivocal bone scintigrams, MRI is often useful because it is, in fact, more sensitive to marrow replacement than is bone scintigraphy. The scintigraphic examination is performed with a Tc-99m phosphate analog, typically methylene diphosphonate; localization of the agent depends on local blood flow and bone turnover. Certain neoplastic processes within bone marrow, notably multiple myeloma, neuroblastoma, and highly anaplastic tumors, can result in a negative bone scintigram, primarily because of a lack of osseous metabolic response to the tumors. The distinctly abnormal MR findings in the test patient warrant biopsy despite the negative results of scintigraphy.

The discovery of metastases commonly results in an altered treatment protocol. Therefore, the initial finding of metastasis is usually verified by biopsy and histologic documentation even if metastatic disease is strongly suspected and even when more than one abnormal focus has been identified on an imaging study. Moreover, not every suspected metastasis is truly a metastasis. Corcoran et al. reported benign causes of 36% of solitary abnormalities on bone scintigrams in patients with known extraosseous malignancies. Mink corroborated this finding by showing that, in patients with a known malignancy, 18% of multiple and 31% of single abnormalities on bone scintigrams had benign causes.

Potential complications of the bone biopsy procedure depend largely on the location of the lesion and the type of biopsy needle used. Some complications are generic, the risks occurring with either closed or open biopsy, and include pain, bleeding, infection, pathologic fracture, and the potential (albeit very low) for spread of disease. Other complications such as pneumothorax and neurologic damage are more site specific but again may follow both closed and open procedures. Percutaneous biopsy has the advantages over open surgical procedures of being less expensive, of obviating general anesthesia, and of avoiding the morbidity of the surgical exposure needed to perform an open biopsy. Murphy et al. reported 2 complications, both pneumothoraces, in a series of 169 percutaneous

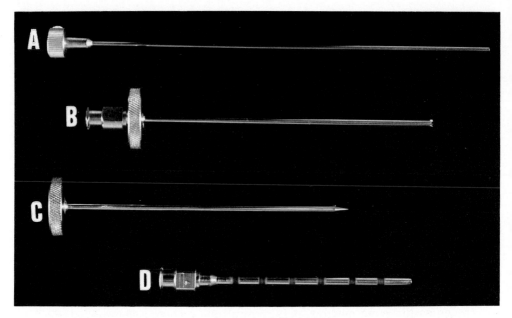

Figure 9-3. Ackermann biopsy set includes blunt obturator used to express the sample (A), trephine cutting needle (B), pointed obturator or guide (C), and sheath or cannula (D). After insertion of the sheath and pointed obturator as a single unit, the pointed obturator is removed, leaving the sheath in place. The trephine needle can then be passed coaxially through the sheath. Multiple samples can be obtained without replacing the sheath.

biopsies. They also reviewed the English-language literature and found 20 reported complications in at least 9,500 procedures performed over the previous 50 years. These included seven pneumothoraces, four cases of permanent neurologic sequelae, and two deaths, for an overall complication rate of 0.2% and a mortality rate of 0.02%. A higher complication rate (about 10%) has been reported for the subset of percutaneous vertebral-body biopsies. Complications of vertebral-body biopsy are mainly neurologic. Tumor seeding along the needle track and pathologic fracture are extremely rare occurrences in any location.

A variety of biopsy needles have been devised for various applications. These can generally be divided into aspiration needles and trephine needles. Trephine needles are large-gauge needles with a serrated cutting edge and are generally used for bone biopsies. Examples of trephine and cutting needles are the Ackermann (Cook Inc., Bloomington, IN) (Figure 9-3), the Craig (Becton-Dickinson, Rutherford, NJ), the Turkel (Turkel Instruments, Inc., Southfield, MI), and the Jamshidi (Baxter

Health Care Corporation, Pharmaseal® Division, Valencia, CA). All these needles are used in a similar fashion. A sheath (cannula) and guide are initially placed through soft tissues until the bone surface is contacted. The trephine or cutting needle is passed through the sheath coaxially after the guide is removed. The sheath protects the surrounding tissues, allowing multiple biopsy passes with the trephine or cutting needle.

Percutaneous biopsy procedures can obtain samples suitable for both cytologic and histologic analysis. The reported accuracy from these procedures has varied from 11 to 95%. Early work was done without radiographic guidance and yielded poor results. However, more recent reports have shown a definite trend toward better results, with peak accuracies exceeding 90%. Murphy et al. and Mink reported accuracies of 94 and 95.4%, respectively. In their review of the literature, Murphy et al. detected an average overall accuracy of approximately 80%. The reported results are influenced by the types of lesions subjected to biopsy; accuracy rates are higher with metastatic lesions than with primary bone tumors because primary bone tumors are difficult to diagnose without large tissue samples. In addition, variation in cell type from one area to another within a primary tumor means that a percutaneous biopsy sample of a suspected primary bone tumor may not be representative of all important cell types within the tumor. However, percutaneous bone biopsy is unquestionably highly accurate and cost effective for diagnosing suspected metastatic deposits and infections of bone.

Most metastases occur in the regions of greatest concentration of hematopoietic (red) marrow and blood flow. Therefore, the axial skeleton, particularly the spine and pelvis, is where most lesions are found and where most biopsies are performed. Biopsies of the osseous pelvis are relatively straightforward and involve little risk. Vertebral biopsies can be more challenging because of the necessity to avoid adjacent structures such as the lungs, aorta, spinal cord, and nerves. Several approaches to thoracic and lumbar vertebral-body lesions have been described. The choice of approach is influenced largely by the location of the lesion. The posterolateral approach (Figure 9-4) represents the traditional approach to vertebral-body lesions. The biopsy needle is typically inserted approximately 6 cm from the midline for thoracic spine biopsies and approximately 10 cm from the midline for lumbar spine biopsies. It is angled toward the vertebral body and passes lateral to the transverse process. Other options include the transpedicular or transcostovertebral approaches.

The transpedicular approach (Figure 9-5) can be useful for lesions located adjacent to the pedicle or in the posterocentral aspect of the vertebral body, where access by a standard posterolateral approach is difficult. Needle placement for sampling of thoracic vertebral-body lesions by

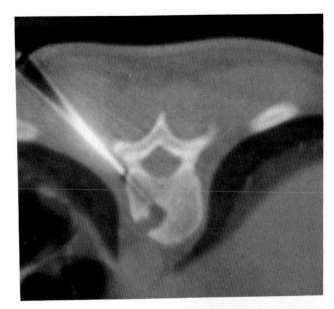

Figure 9-4 (left). Posterolateral biopsy approach. CT-guided vertebral biopsy with an Ackermann needle directed from a posterolateral insertion site to an anteriorly located lytic thoracic vertebral-body lesion (eosinophilic granuloma).

Figure 9-5 (right). Transpedicular biopsy approach. CT-guided vertebral biopsy with a 20-gauge aspiration needle through the right pedicle of a lower thoracic vertebra. Metastasis was confirmed. (Courtesy of Donald Renfrew, M.D., Rush Presbyterian St. Luke's Medical Center, Chicago, Ill.)

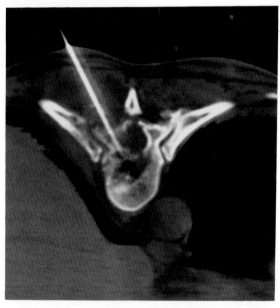

a posterolateral approach can be difficult because ribs and transverse processes can obstruct needle placement, especially if there has been compression of the vertebral body. In these cases, a transpedicular or transcostovertebral approach (Figure 9-6) may be useful. Biopsies of lesions involving cervical vertebral bodies are usually performed from an anterior approach, with the needle passing between the pharynx and carotid sheath.

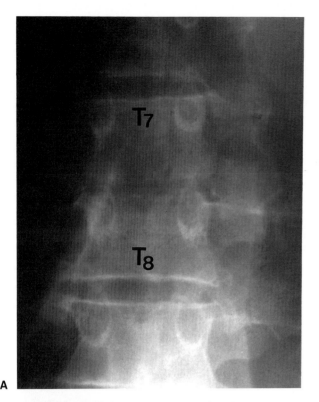

T7

T8

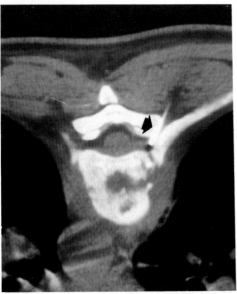

Figure 9-6. Transcostovertebral biopsy approach. (A) An anteroposterior radiograph of the thoracic spine shows disc space narrowing with destruction of the adjacent vertebral-body end-plates at the T7-T8 level. (B) CT-guided vertebral biopsy, using the transcostovertebral approach, with a 20-gauge spinal needle (arrow). A culture of the biopsy specimen was positive for gram-negative bacteria.

Consultation with the orthopedic surgeon and pathologist is important to ensure a successful outcome. Collaboration with the orthopedic surgeon is important for biopsies of primary bone tumors because the biopsy needle track must be resected; proper planning of the biopsy site is therefore critical. If a long bone or vertebral body contains a suspected metastatic lesion that is large, creates marked cortical thinning, or otherwise has features that are suspicious for an impending pathologic fracture, the lesion should be evaluated in conjunction with an orthopedic surgeon or neurosurgeon prior to percutaneous biopsy. If the orthopedic surgeon believes that the lesion should be operatively stabilized, a specimen for histology can be obtained at the time of surgery and the patient will be spared the risk and expense of an unnecessary percutaneous biopsy. Likewise, if the spinal cord is at risk, the neurosurgeon may wish to perform a surgical decompression, also obviating percutaneous biopsy. The pathologist will determine the adequacy of the specimen and ensure that it is handled appropriately. This may require special coordination for best results.

Craig W. Walker, M.D.
Phoebe A. Kaplan, M.D.

SUGGESTED READINGS

1. Ayala AG, Zornosa J. Primary bone tumors: percutaneous needle biopsy. Radiologic-pathologic study of 222 biopsies. Radiology 1983; 149:675–679

2. Brugieres P, Gaston A, Heran F, Voisin MC, Marsault C. Percutaneous biopsies of the thoracic spine under CT guidance: transcostovertebral approach. J Comput Assist Tomogr 1990; 14:446–448

3. Collins JD, Bassett L, Main GD, Kagan C. Percutaneous biopsy following positive bone scans. Radiology 1979; 132:439–442

4. Corcoran RJ, Thrall JH, Kyle RW, Kaminski RJ, Johnson MC. Solitary abnormalities in bone scans of patients with extraosseous malignancies. Radiology 1976; 121:663–667

5. Debnam JW, Staple TW. Trephine bone biopsy by radiologists. Radiology 1975; 116:607–609

6. DeSantos LA, Murray JA, Ayala AG. The value of percutaneous needle biopsy in the management of primary bone tumors. Cancer 1979; 43:735–744

7. Fyfe IS, Henry AP, Mulholland RC. Closed vertebral biopsy. J Bone Joint Surg (Br) 1983; 65:140–143

8. Kattapuram SV, Rosenthal DI. Percutaneous biopsy of the cervical spine using CT guidance. AJR 1987; 149:539–541

9. Kattapuram SV, Rosenthal DI. Percutaneous biopsy of skeletal lesions. AJR 1991; 157:935–942

10. Larédo JD, Bard M. Thoracic spine: percutaneous trephine biopsy. Radiology 1986; 160:485–489
11. Mink J. Percutaneous bone biopsy in the patient with known or suspected osseous metastasis. Radiology 1986; 161:191–194
12. Moore TM, Meyers MH, Patzakis MJ, Terry R, Harvey JP Jr. Closed biopsy of musculoskeletal lesions. J Bone Joint Surg (Am) 1979; 61:375–380
13. Murphy WA, Destouet JM, Gilula LA. Percutaneous skeletal biopsy 1981: a procedure for radiologists—results, review, and recommendations. Radiology 1981; 139:545–549
14. Renfrew DL, Whitten CG, Wiese JA, el-Khoury GY, Harris KG. CT-guided percutaneous transpedicular biopsy of the spine. Radiology 1991; 180:574–576
15. Tehranzadeh J, Freiberger RH, Ghelman B. Closed skeletal needle biopsy: review of 120 cases. AJR 1983; 140:113–115

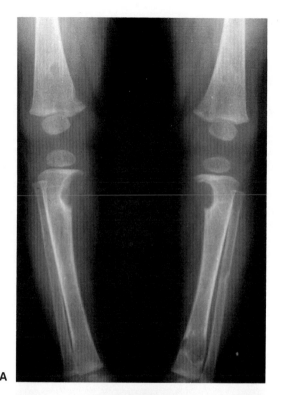

A

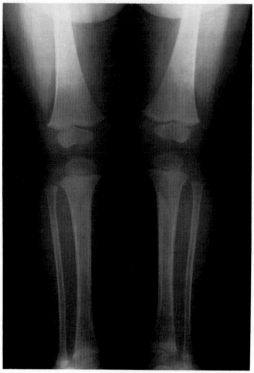

B

Figure 10-1. You are shown radiographs obtained at 7 (A) and 18 (B) months of age. The patient received no treatment between these studies.

Case 10: Fibromatosis

Question 35

Which *one* of the following is the MOST likely diagnosis?

(A) Fibrous dysplasia
(B) Congenital multiple fibromatosis
(C) Neurofibromatosis type 1
(D) Cystic angiomatosis
(E) Multiple hemangioma of bone

The radiograph at 7 months of age (Figure 10-1A) shows lytic lesions in the distal right femur, proximal tibiae, distal left tibia, and left fibula (Figure 10-2). The lesions involve cortex and medullary bone, are well defined, and have a sclerotic margin. There is no matrix calcification and no radiographic evidence of soft tissue mass or phlebolith. No additional bone deformities are associated nor is there evidence of periostitis. The follow-up radiograph obtained 11 months later is normal (Figure 10-1B). The lytic lesions have totally resolved. Again, there is no evidence of soft tissue mass, phlebolith, or osteosclerosis. The lesions seen at 7 months of age and their regression without intervening treatment are typical of congenital multiple fibromatosis **(Option (B) is correct).**

Congenital multiple fibromatosis is a disorder of the subcutaneous tissues and bone and consists of multiple benign fibrous tumors, usually diagnosed at birth or within the first few months of life. Clinically, these fibrous tumors typically grow for 3 to 4 months and then regress or remain stable. Radiographically, the bone lesions are cystic, well-demarcated lesions with smooth and sclerotic borders. The sclerotic border can be pronounced or subtle. The lesions typically involve both the medullary and cortical portions of bone and usually extend into the soft tissues. Pathologic fractures and expansion of bone have been described. Matrix calcification is not seen. The osseous fibromas usually increase in size and then regress spontaneously, leaving either normal bone or a mild residual scarring defect. The radiographic features of these lesions are very similar to those of neurofibromatosis, lymphangiomatosis, and lipo-

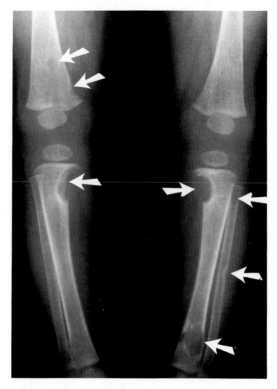

Figure 10-2 (Same as Figure 10-1A). Congenital multiple fibromatosis. A radiograph shows several well-defined cystic or lytic lesions involving cortex and medullary bone (arrows).

matosis. However, these other disorders do not typically resolve, and lipomatosis frequently calcifies. Metastatic neuroblastoma can occasionally cause medullary and cortical lytic lesions similar in appearance to those seen in the test images.

Skeletal changes seen in fibrous dysplasia (Option (A)) can be either solitary or multiple and can occur in one or more than one bone, although 70 to 80% are monostotic. Polyostotic fibrous dysplasia can be unilateral or bilateral and can affect several bones of a single limb or more than one limb. Long bone lesions are usually intramedullary, occur predominantly in the diaphysis, and only rarely occur in the epiphysis or metaphysis. They are most frequently radiolucent, as in the test patient, but contain a hazy matrix giving the lesion a "ground glass" appearance. The lesions are well defined and may be bordered by a zone of reactive sclerosis or thickened cortex. In most instances, the size and number of skeletal lesions do not increase, although lesions occasionally extend or new lesions may appear in additional bones after initial diagnosis. This is particularly true when extensive fibrous dysplasia occurs early in life. Fibrous dysplasia tends to become quiescent at puberty and is not associated with spontaneous regression. This lack of spontaneous regression, as well as the appearance and location of the lesions, makes fibrous dysplasia an unlikely diagnosis in the test patient.

Neurofibromatosis is one of the most common genetic disorders. This autosomal-dominant trait occurs in approximately 1 in 3,000 births. Many cases are the result of spontaneous mutations; fathers over the age of 35 years have a twofold risk of producing offspring with a new mutation for the disorder, whereas maternal age appears to have no effect on the spontaneous mutation rate.

Two distinct forms of neurofibromatosis have been described. Neurofibromatosis type 1 (NF1) (Option (C)) occurs approximately 17 times more frequently than neurofibromatosis type 2 (NF2). The genetic lesion of NF1 is located on chromosome 17. The diagnosis is made when any two of the following criteria are present: café-au-lait spots; at least two neurofibromas or one plexiform neurofibroma; optic nerve glioma; two or more iris nodules; characteristic bone lesions with or without pseudarthrosis; and a parent, sibling, or offspring with NF1. NF2 is rare, and the genetic defect is associated with chromosome 22. It is characterized primarily by the presence of bilateral acoustic neuromas. It can also be diagnosed in a patient having a first-degree relative with NF2 and either unilateral acoustic neuroma or two of the following: cutaneous neurofibromas, plexiform neurofibromas, schwannoma, meningioma, or presenile cataracts.

NF1 can involve all three embryologic cell layers but more typically involves both mesodermal and neuroectodermal elements. The bone abnormalities seen in NF1 are the result of a mesodermal dysplasia caused by the disorder. In the long bones, bowing, pathologic fracture, and pseudarthrosis are particularly common. Anterolateral bowing of the tibia, the most commonly affected bone, is characteristic and may be accompanied by fibular abnormalities consisting of hypoplasia or gracile shape (Figure 10-3).

The pathophysiology of lytic bone lesions in NF1 is somewhat controversial. Two types of lytic lesions, subperiosteal and intraosseous, have been described. The subperiosteal form, appearing as caves or notches in the cortical surface, could be caused by mechanical pressure from adjacent neurofibromas or possibly by focal hemorrhage from dysplastic periosteum. These lesions could be considered erosive defects and are regarded as one of the more characteristic bone changes in NF1.

Intraosseous lytic lesions, however, may not be a part of NF1. Initially, intraosseous lytic lesions were attributed to direct invasion of the

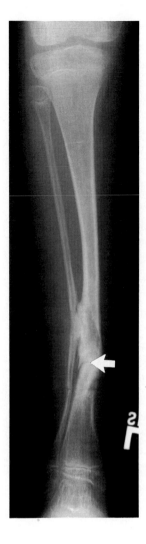

Figure 10-3. Neurofibromatosis type 1. An anteroposterior radiograph of the left leg in a 10-year-old girl shows anterolateral bowing of the tibia and fibula. Pseudarthroses of the tibia (arrow) and fibula are also present.

bone by adjacent 'neurofibromatous tissue or to neurofibromas arising within the marrow cavity. The possibility of neurofibromas arising within the medullary cavity seems unlikely. Most investigations recognize a periosteal nerve supply but do not confirm the presence of nerve fibers entering the medullary cavity. Regardless of the origin of the osseous lesions in NF1, whether secondary to mesodermal dysplasia or erosive changes from adjacent neurofibromas, these lesions do not regress spontaneously and NF1 is not a consideration in this case.

Peripheral nerve tumors most frequently result from proliferation of neural supporting tissues. Most commonly, these benign tumors are solitary or multiple and histologically are either neurofibromas or neurilem-

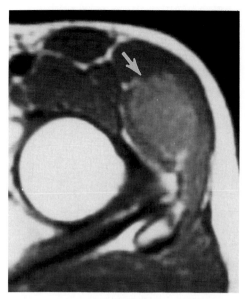

SE 800/20

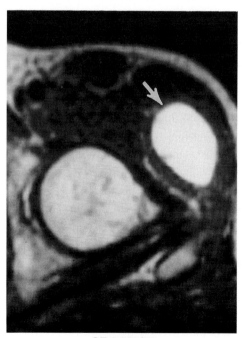

SE 2,000/70

Figure 10-4. Schwannoma. T1- and T2-weighted transaxial MR images of the pelvis of a 44-year-old man with NF1 show a soft tissue schwannoma (arrow) in the lateral left thigh. It has intermediate signal intensity (slightly higher than muscle) on the T1-weighted image and high signal intensity on the T2-weighted image. The smooth-margined tumor displaces the normal surrounding muscle.

momas (schwannomas) (Figure 10-4). Neurofibromas include Schwann cells, nerve fibers, and fibroblasts and result in diffuse enlargement of the nerve itself. Neurilemmomas are encapsulated lesions that lie on the

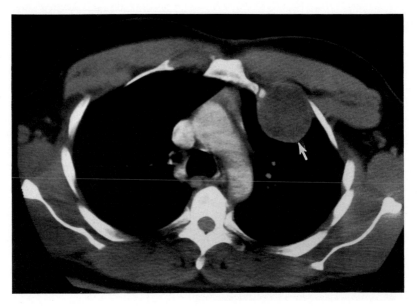

Figure 10-5. Malignant transformation of a neurofibroma to a malignant schwannoma. A postcontrast CT scan of the chest in a 30-year-old man shows a large soft tissue mass extending through the left anterior chest wall (arrow).

surface of the nerve, and the nerve enlargement can therefore be focal or diffuse, fusiform or multinodular. Plexiform neurofibromas result from proliferation and interdigitation of neurogenic tissue with fat and muscle. They tend to recur after resection and have a potential for malignant transformation.

Malignant transformation within neurogenic tumors has been estimated to occur in 2 to 29% of patients, but 5% can be used as an average estimate. Clinical symptoms include a new or enlarging mass or pain in an existing lesion. Malignant transformation can result in either soft tissue or bone sarcoma. Soft tissue sarcomas complicating NF1 are usually of nerve trunk origin and uniform in composition (malignant schwannoma and neurofibrosarcoma) (Figure 10-5). Rarely, a soft tissue sarcoma can show pleomorphism attributed to multipotential neurilemmal cells that produce cartilage, osteoid, fat, and striated muscle. Rhabdomyosarcoma, liposarcoma, or soft tissue osteosarcoma occasionally occurs in these patients. Intraosseous sarcoma is rare and is likely to be malignant fibrous histiocytoma or fibrosarcoma. Malignancies not arising from neural or neural-supporting tissues also occur at a higher frequency in patients with NF1 than they do in the general population. These include lesions of neural crest origin (neuroblastoma, pheochromocytoma, melanoma, and medullary thyroid carcinoma). Other tumors thought to occur more frequently in patients with neurofibromatosis include Wilms' tumor, rhabdomyosarcoma, and leukemia.

There are several vascular lesions commonly associated with NF1. Arterial abnormalities, including stenoses, aneurysms, and arterial wall thickening, are seen. Renal artery stenosis is the most likely cause of hypertension in a child with NF1, whereas in adults hypertension is more frequently caused by the presence of a pheochromocytoma. While 1% of patients with NF1 have pheochromocytomas, 5 to 25% of patients with pheochromocytomas have NF1. Coarctations of both the thoracic and abdominal aorta, congenital heart disease (primarily ventricular and atrial septal defects and pulmonary valvular stenosis), and stenosis or occlusion of cerebral arteries are also frequently observed. The pathophysiology of these vascular lesions is incompletely understood.

Early diagnosis of malignant transformation in NF1 is essential, since prognosis is generally poor for such patients. There is a known increase in occurrence of neurofibrosarcoma at sites of previous radiation, and therefore imaging techniques that utilize ionizing radiation in the evaluation of NF1 should be kept to a minimum. Biopsy is often required to distinguish between benign and malignant lesions. Almost all lesions associated with NF1 can be highly vascular, and therefore biopsy can be associated with hemorrhage. The hypervascularity and location of many of these lesions make surgical removal difficult if not impossible, and treatment often consists of radiation therapy or chemotherapy.

Imaging evaluation of both benign and malignant tumors associated with NF1 frequently requires the use of CT or MRI. These imaging modalities are not specific in differentiating among benign tumor types; however, there are several criteria that can be useful in distinguishing benign from malignant lesions.

CT characteristics of benign neural tumors include lower attenuation values than those of muscle, although neurofibromas can be isodense with muscle. This low attenuation is thought to be secondary to increased amounts of water and endoneural myxoid. Benign lesions are typically rounded or elliptical, smoothly marginated masses with homogeneously low attenuation values. Malignant lesions, on the other hand, tend to have irregular contours and to be heterogeneous. The heterogeneities are nonspecific and may represent hemorrhage, necrosis, or cystic degeneration. While these criteria are useful, they are not always reliable; benign lesions, particularly plexiform neurofibromas, can have an irregular contour, whereas malignant lesions can have a smooth and well-defined contour. Size cannot be used to distinguish malignant from benign lesions; benign tumors can grow to a large size. Both benign and malignant lesions can have calcifications and heterogeneous low- and high-density areas and exhibit contrast enhancement.

MRI is now the preferred method for imaging NF1. On T1-weighted images, most lesions of NF1 have intermediate intensity and distort the surrounding normal anatomy. These neural tumors enhance markedly after intravenous administration of gadolinium DTPA. On T2-weighted images, tumors have increased signal intensity and are frequently homogeneous. Lesions can also have a heterogeneous appearance on T2-weighted images, with some of the heterogeneity resulting from intralesional hemorrhage and necrosis. MR signs of malignant transformation include an irregular contour, surrounding edema, and heterogeneity of the lesion on T2-weighted images. Heterogeneous enhancement with gadolinium DTPA can also be seen. As with CT, these criteria cannot be used with complete confidence to separate benign from malignant lesions, since there is some overlap in their characteristics.

Cystic angiomatosis (Option (D)) is a rare skeletal disorder that can occasionally show spontaneous regression. It is characterized by widespread cystic lesions of bone. Visceral involvement occurs in 60 to 70% of cases and accounts for most symptoms. Patients typically present in the first three decades of life, and the clinical course depends to a large extent on the presence and degree of visceral involvement. In the absence of visceral involvement, patients can be asymptomatic or complain of soft tissue swelling and localized pain related to pathologic fracture. Patients with visceral involvement often die at an early age, consequent to involvement of liver, lungs, kidneys, and pericardium. Rendu-Osler-Weber disease (hereditary hemorrhagic telangiectasia) may be associated with this disorder.

Bone lesions associated with cystic angiomatosis can occur anywhere within the skeleton. In the skull, multiple grouped punched-out areas of bone destruction and bulging of the inner and outer tables are seen. In the ribs, the lesions cause expansion with cortical thinning and pathologic fractures can occur. Radiolucent lesions can be found in the bodies, pedicles, and transverse processes of vertebrae. In the long bones, the condition is often found near the nutrient foramina. The lucencies are primarily oval, well-defined, oriented in the long axis of the bone, and surrounded by a rim of sclerotic bone (Figure 10-6). Involvement is centered in the medullary cavity; cortical invasion, osseous expansion, and periostitis are uncommon. CT examination confirms that the lytic lesions are oriented in the long axis of the bone and surrounded by a sclerotic rim. On MRI, lesions have intermediate signal intensity on T1-weighted images and high signal intensity on T2-weighted images (Figure 10-7).

Although most cases of cystic angiomatosis present radiographically as widespread lytic or cystic lesions, these lesions can also be osteoblastic

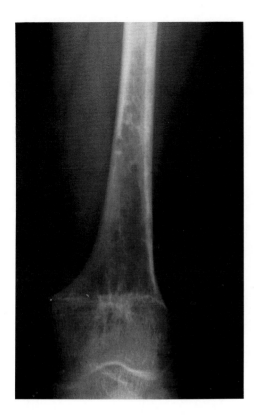

Figure 10-6. Cystic angiomatosis. An anteroposterior radiograph of the left femur shows oval radiolucent lesions bounded by sclerotic borders and oriented along the long axis of the bone.

with dense sclerotic masses in multiple bones. Alternatively, the disorder can present with mixed osteolytic and osteoblastic lesions. The radiographic finding typical for solitary hemangioma of bone, a striated "honeycomb" or "soap bubble" appearance, is rarely seen in cystic angiomatosis but has been reported.

Pathologically, cystic angiomatosis can resemble either a simple bone cyst or multiple communicating cysts of various sizes. Histologically, the lesions are similar to cavernous or capillary hemangiomas with numerous dilated thin-walled vascular channels filling the intertrabecular spaces. These cystic lesions are often filled with blood or serous fluid, and, for this reason, cystic angiomatosis is occasionally difficult to distinguish from lymphangiomatosis. The lesions of cystic angiomatosis rarely resolve spontaneously, tend to be intramedullary and not cortical, and are usually elongated in appearance. Therefore, the test patient is unlikely to have cystic angiomatosis.

Most hemangiomas of bone are singular, but cases of multiple hemangioma of bone (Option (E)) have been reported. Osseous hemangiomas are seen most frequently in the fourth and fifth decades of life, with

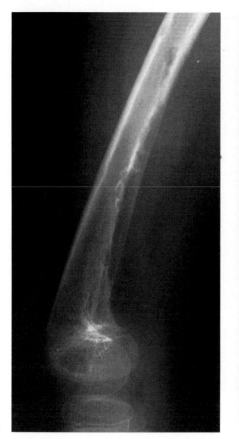
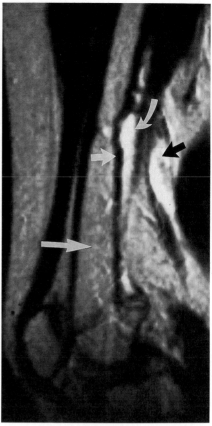

SE 2,000/80

Figure 10-7. Cystic angiomatosis. (A) A lateral radiograph shows well-defined longitudinal lucent lesions in the posterior aspect of the right femur. (B) A T2-weighted sagittal MR image shows normal fatty marrow (large white arrow) contrasted with the high-intensity angiomatous lesion (curved arrow). The low-intensity sclerotic lesion rim is easily recognized (small white arrow). The focal high intensity in the posterior thigh represents a second lesion (black arrow).

a predominance in women of approximately 2:1. While most multiple hemangiomas are asymptomatic, they can be symptomatic as a result of trauma or fracture. Additionally, vertebral hemangiomas can lead to compression fractures of bone or compression of the spinal cord secondary to expansion of bone by the hemangioma. Both single and multiple osseous hemangiomas, with or without soft tissue hemangiomas, can lead to hemihypertrophy.

Pathologically, hemangiomas of bone are cavernous, capillary, or venous. This histologic composition is identical to that found in soft tissue hemangioma. The cavernous variety is composed of large, thin-walled vessels lined by flat epithelial cells filled with fresh blood. Capillary hemangiomas are composed of similar but smaller vessels that are densely packed. Mixed hemangiomas containing both cavernous and capillary elements are encountered. Hemangiomas that contain thick-walled vessels composed of smooth muscle are referred to as venous hemangiomas. The vascular channels will either lie adjacent to trabecular bone or be separated from trabecular bone by fibrous connective tissue. Whereas most osseous hemangiomas are cavernous, hemangiomas seen in the vertebral bodies are most frequently capillary. These lesions can slowly increase in size or, rarely, undergo spontaneous regression.

Multiple hemangiomas can occur in one bone or multiple bones; they can occur in the skull, trunk, one extremity, or multiple extremities. The most common sites of involvement are the calvarium, facial bones, and spine. At autopsy up to 10% of spines contain hemangiomas; these are most frequently found in the thoracic region, although the cervical and lumbar regions can be affected. In the skull, the frontal and parietal bones are most frequently affected. In the long bones, the epiphyseal and metaphyseal regions are most frequently affected. Radiographically, hemangiomas result in a coarse, vertical trabecular pattern, particularly in the vertebral bodies. Additionally, focal radiolucent lesions with coarse trabeculae arranged in a honeycomb or cartwheel configuration surrounding the lesion can be seen. Vertebral fractures are uncommon.

In the long bones, radiographs typically show a radiolucent, slightly expansile, well-defined intraosseous lesion with latticelike or weblike trabecular bone surrounding the lytic lesion. While cortical thinning and osseous expansion are not uncommon, periostitis and adjacent soft tissue mass are rare. The characteristic trabecular pattern, which is not present in the test case, makes hemangioma of bone an unlikely diagnosis for the test patient.

Intracortical and periosteal hemangiomas, while rare, are typically found in the diaphyseal region, especially in the tibia and fibula. Radiographically, intracortical hemangiomas are characterized as well-defined, osteolytic lesions with or without cortical thickening and periostitis. Differential diagnosis includes osteoid osteoma, fibrous dysplasia, ossifying fibroma, or Brodie's abscess. This coarse trabecular pattern can be seen on CT. On MRI, vertebral hemangiomas are detected as focal or diffuse replacement of the vertebral body marrow with a lesion of high signal intensity on both T1- and T2-weighted images (Figure 10-8).

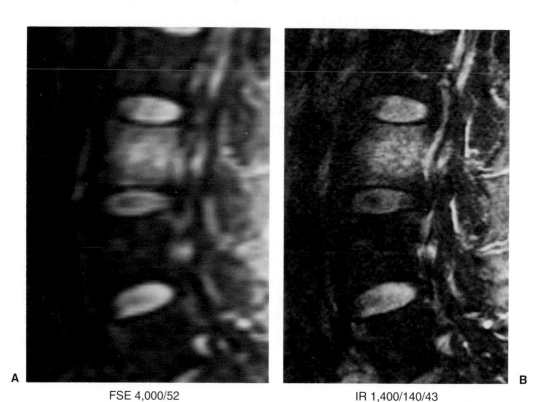

A   B

FSE 4,000/52   IR 1,400/140/43

Figure 10-8. Hemangioma. Fast spin-echo T2-weighted (A) and inversion-recovery (B) sagittal MR images of the lumbar spine show high-intensity tissue replacing the entire L3 vertebral body.

Questions 36 through 40

For each of the following clinical features (Questions 36 through 40), indicate whether it is more closely associated with the monostotic or polyostotic forms of fibrous dysplasia, equally associated with both, or associated with neither (A, B, C, or D). Each option may be used once, more than once, or not at all.

36. Soft tissue myxoma
37. Frequent resolution of the lesion
38. High signal intensity on T2-weighted images
39. Involvement of the spine
40. Malignant transformation

   (A) Monostotic
   (B) Polyostotic
   (C) Both
   (D) Neither

Fibrous dysplasia, a congenital abnormality of the bone-forming mesenchyma, is characterized by fibrous displacement of portions of the medullary cavity. Approximately 70 to 80% of cases are monostotic, while 20 to 30% are polyostotic; 2 to 3% are associated with endocrinopathies. Any bone can be affected, but monostotic fibrous dysplasia typically involves the rib, femur, tibia, mandible, and calvarium in decreasing frequency. The skull and facial bones, pelvis, spine, and shoulder girdle are more frequently involved in cases of polyostotic fibrous dysplasia. Axial skeletal involvement may be present. While most patients with monostotic fibrous dysplasia are asymptomatic, local swelling, especially in superficial bones such as the tibia or clavicle, does occur.

Radiographically, fibrous dysplasia has a variable appearance as it replaces the medullary cavity (Figure 10-9). It can be radiolucent or of homogeneous "ground glass" density, depending on the amount of fibrous or osseous tissue deposited within the medullary cavity. It can also be osteosclerotic, particularly in the skull and face. The cortex can be thin or thickened and may show endosteal irregularity. Long-bone lesions are primarily metaphyseal, although the diaphysis and, rarely, the entire bone length can be affected.

An association of soft tissue myxoma with polyostotic fibrous dysplasia has been reported **(Option (B) is the correct answer to Question 36).** Soft tissue myxomas occur in the vicinity of the most severely affected bones. They are usually multiple and intramuscular, and they often abut the cortex. Myxomas are rare, often invasive connective tissue tumors that can calcify. On MRI, they are seen as smooth, well-defined intramuscular lesions of intermediate intensity on T1-weighted images and of homogeneous, high intensity on T2-weighted images. MRI is valu-

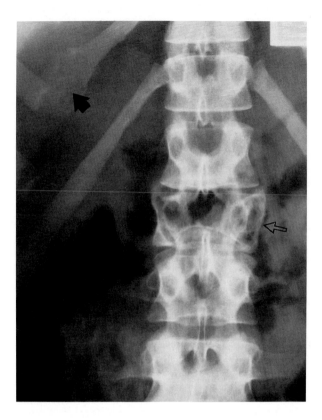

Figure 10-9. Polyostotic fibrous dysplasia. An anteroposterior radiograph of the thoracolumbar spine reveals expansion and a ground-glass appearance of the right 11th rib (solid arrow). The L2 vertebral body (open arrow) is demineralized and deformed.

able for defining lesion extent and for identifying normal cortex between the osseous changes of fibrous dysplasia and the soft tissue myxoma. This confirms that the myxoma is an associated, not contiguous, lesion. Surgical removal of a myxoma is recommended since it can be invasive and since the potential for malignant transformation to a myxosarcoma exists.

Fibrous dysplasia is most frequently diagnosed in the second and third decades of life. The age at diagnosis for polyostotic fibrous dysplasia is considerably younger than that for monostotic fibrous dysplasia, since the clinical and radiographic abnormalities are more severe.

Two-thirds of patients are symptomatic before the age of 10 years, and while it is thought that polyostotic disease favors one side of the body, the disease is frequently associated with generalized, bilateral, but asymmetric involvement. Polyostotic disease is frequently limited to a few osseous sites, with only one-fourth of the patients presenting with more than 50% of the skeleton involved. There have been no well-documented instances of conversion from monostotic to polyostotic disease. It is therefore thought that these two entities represent two independent forms of fibrous dysplasia. The prognosis depends on the extent and degree of initial skeletal involvement and whether there is involvement of extraskeletal sites. Rarely do existing lesions extend or new lesions appear.

Both polyostotic and monostotic fibrous dysplasia become quiescent at puberty and will remain so throughout life. Occasionally, progressive deformity will occur, particularly in the more severe cases of fibrous dysplasia. In these cases, fractures lead to bone deformity and some morbidity can be expected. On the other hand, disease that is initially limited is usually associated with little progression and a favorable prognosis independent of the age at diagnosis. Reactivation of fibrous dysplasia has been noted during pregnancy and estrogen therapy. The lesions of fibrous dysplasia do not resolve in either the polyostotic or monostotic forms **(Option (D) is the correct answer to Question 37).**

On MR examination, the signal intensity of fibrous dysplasia is generally intermediate (equal to muscle) on T1-weighted images unless there is a pathologic fracture, at which time foci of high intensity caused by subacute hemorrhage can be seen. On T2-weighted images, very high signal intensity (greater than that of subcutaneous fat) is characteristic of both monostotic and polyostotic lesions **(Option (C) is the correct answer to Question 38)** (Figure 10-10). While about 60% of lesions have high signal intensity, about 20% have signal intensity similar to that of subcutaneous fat, and another 20% have signal intensity similar to that of skeletal muscle on T2-weighted images. The variability of signal intensity on T2-weighted images probably reflects the underlying variability of lesion histology. A lesion composed primarily of quiescent fibrous tissue, reactive bone, or sclerotic bone can exhibit intermediate to low intensity on both T1- and T2-weighted images, whereas a lesion with a large cellular or reactive tissue component containing a large fraction of unbound water can have intermediate intensity on T1-weighted images and increased intensity on T2-weighted images. Heterogeneity and linear septations are not uncommon. There typically is a sharp demarcation between the lesion and the surrounding marrow, with no evidence of marrow edema. There should normally be no associated soft tissue mass, although a thin, curvilinear rim of intermediate (T1-weighted images) and increased (T2-weighted and fat-saturation images) intensity surrounding the bone may represent a thin layer of "cellular" periosteal reaction occurring as a result of bone remodeling and widening of the medullary space. Endosteal scalloping and involvement of the endosteal surface of the cortical bone can be seen.

Involvement of the spine is frequent in polyostotic fibrous dysplasia but occurs only very rarely in monostotic disease **(Option (B) is the**

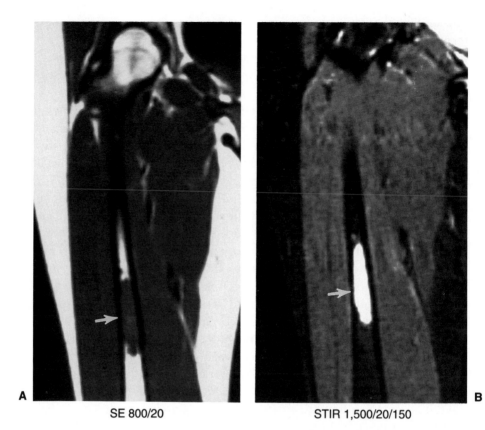

SE 800/20   STIR 1,500/20/150

Figure 10-10. Monostotic fibrous dysplasia. T1-weighted (A) and STIR
(B) coronal MR images of the left femur show a lesion (arrow) of intermediate intensity on the T1-weighted image and high intensity on the T2-
weighted image. (Reprinted with permission from Moore [8].)

correct answer to Question 39). Radiographic characteristics of spinal involvement include well-defined, expansile, radiolucent lesions with
multiple internal septations or striations of the vertebral body (Figure
10-11). Occasionally, the pedicles and transverse processes can be
affected. Paraspinal soft tissue extension and vertebral collapse have
been described and can lead to angular deformity and spinal cord compression. In these instances, MR imaging is the preferred method of evaluation so that the degree of spinal cord compression, if present, can be
determined without the need for intrathecal instillation of contrast
agent.

Polyostotic fibrous dysplasia is frequently associated with clinical
symptoms. Extremity pain can be secondary to spontaneous fracture.
Severe deformities, such as bowing, angular and curvilinear distortion,

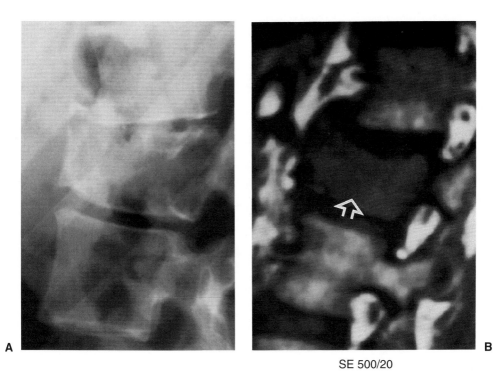

A

B

SE 500/20

Figure 10-11. Vertebral involvement in polyostotic fibrous dysplasia. A lateral radiograph (A) and a sagittal T1-weighted MR image (B) of the spine show expansion of the L2 vertebral body and angulation of the spine at this level. On the T1-weighted image, the replaced marrow is homogeneous and of intermediate intensity (arrow).

fusiform expansion, and linear growth discrepancies are more frequently associated with polyostotic than with monostotic disease. Malignant transformation in fibrous dysplasia is rare but occurs in both the polyostotic and monostotic forms **(Option (C) is the correct answer to Question 40).** The estimated frequency of malignant transformation ranges from 0.4 to 1%. In some cases, prior radiation therapy to the involved site has complicated the determination of spontaneous malignant transformation. In monostotic forms of the disease, malignant transformation occurs most frequently in the skull and facial bones, whereas malignant transformation in the polyostotic form of the disease occurs in the femur and facial bones. Sarcomatous transformation to osteosarcoma or fibrosarcoma is most common, although chondrosarcoma and giant cell tumor can also develop. The latency between diagnosis of fibrous dysplasia and the occurrence of malignant transformation varies but is most often measured in years or even decades. Symptoms and signs associated with malignant transformation include pain and swelling, osteolysis, cortical destruction, and soft tissue mass.

Question 41

Concerning congenital multiple fibromatosis,

    (A) lesions occur primarily in the soft tissues
    (B) osseous lesions are typically metaphyseal in location
    (C) lesions are usually similar in size
    (D) there is an association with pathologic fractures
    (E) the lesions resolve spontaneously in nearly all patients

Congenital multiple fibromatosis is a disorder usually diagnosed at birth, consisting of multiple benign musculoskeletal fibrous tumors. While most lesions occur in the soft tissues **(Option (A) is true)**, those that do arise in bone are typically metaphyseal and cortical in location **(Option (B) is true)**. Radiographically, the disorder is characterized by multiple bone and soft tissue masses; the soft tissue component may be recognized on conventional radiographs. Bone lesions are cystic and well demarcated, and the borders are smooth and sclerotic. Lesion size varies greatly **(Option (C) is false)**, from small cortical lesions to large medullary lesions. Lesions can be asymptomatic but frequently become symptomatic as a result of associated pathologic fracture **(Option (D) is true)**. The lesions of congenital multiple fibromatosis typically grow for several months and then regress and remain stable. Following the typical spontaneous regression, either normal bone or mild residual scarring will be seen on radiographs **(Option (E) is true)**.

Pathologically, the lesions of congenital multiple fibromatosis are well developed at the time of their discovery in the newborn. Fibrous tumors appear to arise from multiple sites *in utero,* and the rubbery grayish-white nodules removed in the neonatal period consist of interwoven strands of spindle-shaped maturing fibroblasts. Mitoses are rare, and there are no neural elements. The lesions do not metastasize, although they can be infiltrative and therefore histologically and clinically resemble low-grade fibrosarcoma. This entity does not result in long-term morbidity or death. One report describes a case of congenital fibromatosis involving both the kidney and musculoskeletal system that eventuated in complete spontaneous regression. This patient had a total of 31 bone tumors and 1 renal tumor. The renal tumor was surgically removed, and there was spontaneous regression of the bone tumors 6 months after diagnosis. This suggests that while congenital multiple fibromatosis with spontaneous regression is thought to occur almost exclusively in the musculoskeletal system, there can rarely be visceral involvement.

Congenital multiple fibromatosis differs from congenital generalized fibromatosis, a rare entity first described in 1952 as fibrosarcoma. Congenital generalized fibromatosis is characterized by multiple benign fibrous tumors that can involve not only the subcutaneous tissues and bone, but also the lungs, muscles, intestines, liver, pancreas, and kidneys. The lesions are frequently noted at birth or within the first month of life and are characterized by progressive growth and an 80% death rate resulting from complications of organ involvement.

Question 42

Concerning juvenile fibromatosis,

(A) it causes pressure erosions of the bone
(B) nearly all lesions have low signal intensity on T2-weighted MR images
(C) recurrence after surgical resection is uncommon
(D) aponeurotic lesions tend to calcify
(E) the foot is a common site of occurrence

Juvenile fibromatosis is a subset of a class of disorders comprising benign fibrous tumors. The fibrous tumors, or fibromas, are composed of normal fibrous elements covered by epidermis. When this benign proliferation of fibrous tissue becomes an infiltrating process, it is referred to as fibromatosis. These benign but potentially aggressive fibrous proliferations can occur in infancy, childhood, adolescence, or adulthood. Radiographically, the lesions may be recognized as soft tissue masses. However, when they are adjacent to bone, one may see pressure erosions of bone, cortical destruction, and lamellated periosteal reaction (**Option (A) is true**) (Figure 10-12).

The MR appearance of fibromatosis varies. Lesions are frequently both masslike and infiltrating. The MR signal characteristics appear to reflect the underlying histologic composition of interlacing bundles of proliferating spindle cells and various amounts of collagen. Lesions can be primarily acellular, with dense collagen tissue, or primarily cellular. Low signal intensity on both T1- and T2-weighted images is seen in lesions composed of primarily acellular collagenous tissue (Figure 10-13). Lesions with less collagen and increased cellularity show intermediate intensity on T1-weighted images and high intensity on T2-weighted (Figure 10-14) and short-tau inversion-recovery (STIR) images. Since most growing lesions will have a large component of cellular tumor, most will

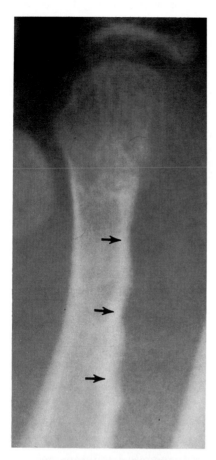

Figure 10-12 (left). Juvenile fibromatosis. An anteroposterior radiograph of the second metatarsal in an 18-year-old boy shows pressure erosion (arrows) of the bone from the adjacent fibromatosis.

Figure 10-13 (below). Aggressive juvenile fibromatosis. A proton-density transaxial MR image through the pelvis of a 21-year-old man shows a low-intensity lesion (arrow) that consists of mature fibrosis. The signal intensity remained low on the T2-weighted image. (Reprinted with permission from Moore [8].)

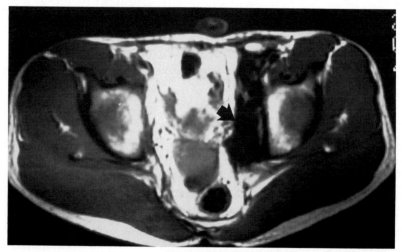

SE 2,000/20

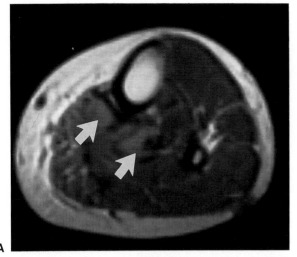

SE 2,000/20

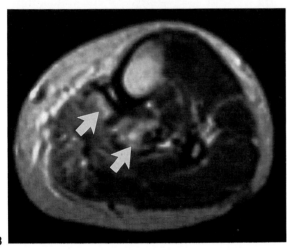

SE 2,000/80

Figure 10-14. Aggressive juvenile fibromatosis. Proton-density (A) and T2-weighted (B) transaxial MR images through the left calf of a 17-year-old girl show masslike lesions (arrows) posterior to the tibia. The higher signal intensity evident on the T2-weighted image indicates a greater cellularity. (Reprinted with permission from Moore [8].)

show heterogeneous intermediate and high signal intensity on T2-weighted images **(Option (B) is false)**.

Juvenile fibromatosis, an often relentless variety of fibrous proliferation, has an aggressive histologic appearance and is characterized by frequent recurrence after both surgery and radiation therapy **(Option (C) is false)** (Figure 10-15). The aggressive histologic appearance combined with the frequent recurrence has resulted in some question as to whether this disorder actually represents a low-grade malignancy in some patients. However, these lesions do not metastasize and therefore

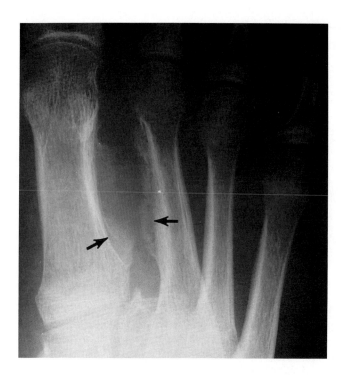

Figure 10-15. Recurrent juvenile fibromatosis. An anteroposterior radiograph of the left foot in a 14-year-old boy with recurrent tumor shows absence of the second metatarsal from resection 2 years earlier. Note the immature periostitis (arrows) of both the 1st and 3rd metatarsals, indicating a response of these bones to the locally recurrent tumor.

are not considered malignant. They do tend to calcify **(Option (D) is true),** especially in the aponeurotic tissues, and will infiltrate adjacent tissues (Figure 10-16). While the aponeurotic variety of fibromatosis tends to occur in the hands and feet, most cases of fibromatosis in young children and adolescents occur in the extremities, with the calf and posterior thigh as the most frequent sites of occurrence. With the exception of aponeurotic fibromatosis, the hands and feet are not often affected **(Option (E) is false).**

Discussion

The fibromatoses are rare disorders of fibroelastic derivation manifested by locally infiltrating fibrous lesions. They can occur at any age—infancy, childhood, adolescence, and adulthood—and there is a spectrum of disease characteristics that frequently reflects patient age. The congenital form is usually diagnosed in the first month of life. Generalized fibromatosis consists of widespread and locally infiltrating fibrous

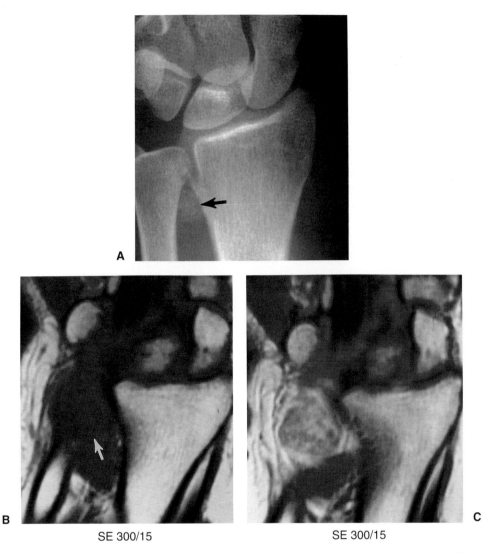

A

B

C

SE 300/15   SE 300/15

Figure 10-16. Aponeurotic fibroma. (A) An anteroposterior radiograph of
the right wrist in a 53-year-old woman shows a calcific mass (arrow)
adjacent to the distal radius. T1-weighted coronal MR images obtained
before (B) and after (C) gadolinium DTPA contrast enhancement show an
intermediate-intensity mass (arrow) that enhances with gadolinium
DTPA. The persistent intermediate (rather than high) signal intensity
within the mass on the postcontrast image likely reflects tissue calcium.

lesions involving both visceral organs and bones. Eighty percent of
patients die within the first 4 months of life secondary to involvement of
vital organs. Congenital multiple fibromatosis is a disorder characterized

by musculoskeletal, not visceral, involvement. Histologically maturing fibroblasts form rubbery grayish-white nodules that arise within bone and soft tissue and can result in the presence of multiple well-defined cystic bone lesions at birth. The lesions can grow initially, but many ultimately regress spontaneously, with complete healing or minimal residual bony scar. Aggressive fibromatosis exhibits a less-malignant behavior than does congenital generalized fibromatosis. Confined to the musculoskeletal system, there is no evidence of visceral involvement. The fibrous tumors of aggressive fibromatosis can grow for 3 to 4 months and then regress or remain stable. However, lesion growth can also be relentless, resulting in death from invasion of vascular structures and normal tissue. Recurrence is common, and amputation may be required to control disease spread in the extremities. The factors that determine the clinical course and lesion aggressiveness are unknown.

Sheila G. Moore, M.D.

SUGGESTED READINGS

CONGENITAL MULTIPLE FIBROMATOSIS

1. Baer JW, Radkowski MA. Congenital multiple fibromatosis. A case report with review of the world literature. AJR 1973; 118:200–205
2. Madewell JE, Sweet DE. Tumors and tumor-like lesions in or about joints. In: Resnick D, Niwayama G (eds), Diagnosis of bone and joint disorders, 2nd ed. Philadelphia: WB Saunders; 1988:3889–3943
3. Schaffzin EA, Chung SM, Kaye R. Congenital generalized fibromatosis with complete spontaneous regression. A case report. J Bone Joint Surg (Am) 1972; 54:657–662
4. Teng P, Warden MJ, Cohn WL. Congenital generalized fibromatosis (renal and skeletal) with complete spontaneous regression. J Pediatr 1963; 62:748–753

FIBROUS DYSPLASIA

5. Feldman F. Tuberous sclerosis, neurofibromatosis, and fibrous dysplasia. In: Resnick D, Niwayama G (eds), Diagnosis of bone and joint disorders, 2nd ed. Philadelphia: WB Saunders; 1988:4033–4072
6. Glass-Royal MC, Nelson MC, Albert F, Lack EE, Bogumill GP. Case report 557: Solitary intramuscular myxoma in a patient with polyostotic fibrous dysplasia. Skeletal Radiol 1989; 18:392–398
7. Kransdorf MJ, Moser RP Jr, Gilkey FW. Fibrous dysplasia. RadioGraphics 1990; 10:519–537
8. Moore SG. Pediatric musculoskeletal imaging. In: Stark DD, Bradley WG Jr (eds), Magnetic resonance imaging, 2nd ed. St Louis: Mosby-Year Book; 1992:2223–2330

9. Sundaram M, McDonald DJ, Merenda G. Intramuscular myxoma: a rare but important association with fibrous dysplasia of bone. AJR 1989; 153:107–108

10. Utz JA, Kransdorf MJ, Jelinek JS, Moser RP Jr, Berrey BH. MR appearance of fibrous dysplasia. J Comput Assist Tomogr 1989; 13:845–851

11. Wilner D. Fibrous dysplasia of bone. In: Wilner D (ed), Radiology of bone tumors and allied disorders. Philadelphia: WB Saunders; 1982:1443–1580

NEUROFIBROMATOSIS

12. Coleman B, Arger PH, Dalinka MK, Obringer AC, Raney BR, Meadows AT. CT of sarcomatous degeneration in neurofibromatosis. AJR 1983; 140: 383–387

13. Hunt JC, Pugh DG. Skeletal lesions in neurofibromatosis. Radiology 1961; 76:1–19

14. Sack GH Jr. Malignant complications of neurofibromatosis. Clin Oncol 1983; 9:17–23

CYSTIC ANGIOMATOSIS

15. Boyle WJ. Cystic angiomatosis of bone. A report of three cases and review of the literature. J Bone Joint Surg (Br) 1972; 54:626–636

16. Jacobs JE, Kimmelstiel P. Cystic angiomatosis of the skeletal system. J Bone Joint Surg (Am) 1953; 35:409–420

17. Resnick D, Kyriakos M, Greenway GD. Tumor and tumor-like lesions of bone: imaging and pathology of specific lesions. In: Resnick D, Niwayama G (eds), Diagnosis of bone and joint disorders, 2nd ed. Philadelphia: WB Saunders; 1988:3616–3888

18. Wallis LA, Asch T, Maisel BW. Diffuse skeletal hemangiomatosis: report of two cases and review of literature. Am J Med 1964; 37:545–563

19. Wilner D. Benign vascular tumors and allied disorders of bone. In: Wilner D (ed), Radiology of bone tumors and allied disorders. Philadelphia: WB Saunders; 1982:660–782

HEMANGIOMA OF BONE

20. Cohen J, Cashman WF. Hemihypertrophy of lower extremity associated with multifocal intraosseous hemangioma. Clin Orthop 1975; 109:155–165

21. Karlin CA, Brower AC. Multiple primary hemangiomas of bone. AJR 1977; 129:162–164

JUVENILE FIBROMATOSIS

22. Aisen AM, Martel W, Braunstein EM, McMillin KI, Phillips WA, Kling TF. MRI and CT evaluation of primary bone and soft-tissue tumors. AJR 1986; 146:749–756

23. Feld R, Burk DL Jr, McCue P, Mitchell DG, Lackman R, Rifkin RD. MRI of aggressive fibromatosis: frequent appearance of high signal intensity on T2-weighted images. Magn Reson Imaging 1990; 8:583–588

24. Moore SG, Dawson KL. Tumors of the musculoskeletal system. In: Cohen MD, Edwards MK (eds), Magnetic resonance imaging of children. Philadelphia: BC Decker; 1990:825–911

25. Sundaram M, McGuire MH, Schajowicz F. Soft-tissue masses: histologic basis for decreased signal (short T2) on T2-weighted MR images. AJR 1987; 148:1247–1250

Notes

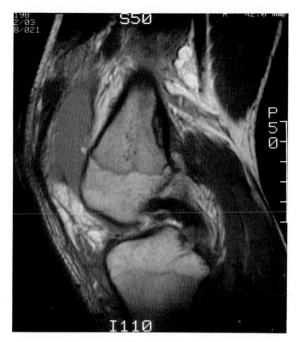

SE 600/20

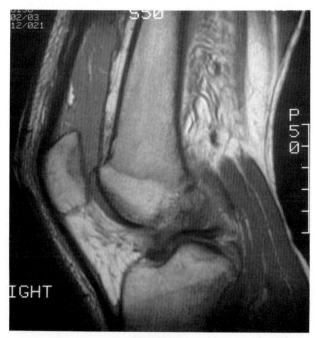

SE 600/20

Figure 11-1

Figures 11-1 through 11-3. This 17-year-old jogger was hit in the knee by a moving car. You are shown T1-weighted sagittal (Figure 11-1), gradient-echo sagittal (Figure 11-2), and T1-weighted coronal (Figure 11-3) MR images of the knee.

270

Case 11: Knee Injuries

Question 43

Abnormalities demonstrated in the test images include:

    (A) anterior cruciate ligament tear
    (B) posterior cruciate ligament tear
    (C) medial collateral ligament tear
    (D) lateral collateral ligament tear
    (E) quadriceps tendon tear
    (F) patellar tendon tear
    (G) medial meniscus tear
    (H) lateral meniscus tear
    (I)   bone marrow contusion
    (J) lipohemarthrosis

The direct blow to the posterolateral aspect of the test patient's knee resulted in major soft tissue and osseous injuries (Figures 11-1 through 11-3). In the medial side of the intercondylar notch, the posterior cruciate ligament is well delineated. There is abnormally increased signal intensity in the ligament near its attachment to the tibia, and the distal half of the ligament is abnormally thickened (Figure 11-4A). These findings are diagnostic of a ruptured posterior cruciate ligament **(Option (B) is true).** An image obtained from the lateral side of the intercondylar notch (Figure 11-4B) shows an angulated and wavy low-intensity band that represents a completely torn anterior cruciate ligament **(Option (A) is true).** The ligament rests against the tibia instead of following the normal straight-line course to an attachment on the lateral femoral condyle. Intermediate-intensity edema is present in the soft tissues surrounding the ruptured proximal aspect of the ligament.

The focal subcortical areas of low-intensity bone marrow on the T1-weighted image (Figure 11-4C) that become high-intensity regions on the corresponding gradient-echo image (Figure 11-5) are diagnostic of bone marrow contusion **(Option (I) is true).** The contusions are located in

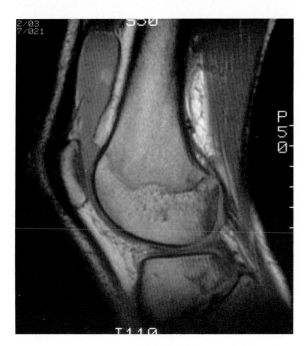

SE 600/20

Figure 11-1 (Continued)

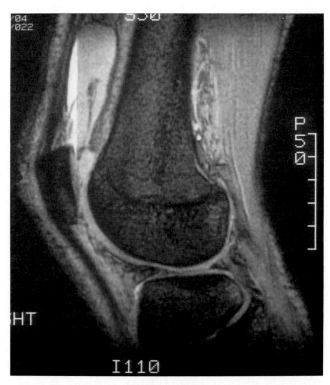

GRE 480/20/30°

Figure 11-2

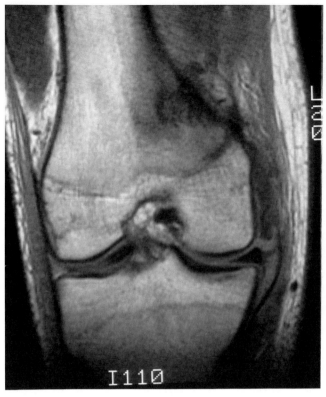

SE 600/20

Figure 11-3

the posterior aspects of the lateral femoral condyle and lateral tibial plateau, as well as in the fibular head (Figures 11-4C and 11-5).

Figures 11-4C and 11-5 demonstrate a large knee joint effusion with two layers of different fluids. The layers developed within a hemarthrosis, and the figures demonstrate the effect of separation of the blood cells, which settled in the dependent portion of the suprapatellar pouch, from blood serum, which floats on top of the cellular component. The serum exhibits intermediate signal intensity on the T1-weighted image (Figure 11-4C) and very high signal intensity on the gradient-echo image (Figure 11-5). This differs from the MR appearance of a lipohemarthrosis **(Option (J) is false)**, in which fat from the marrow cavity enters the joint via a fracture and floats on top of blood in the joint. Fat has high signal intensity on T1-weighted images (Figure 11-6) and lower signal intensity on gradient-echo and T2-weighted images. Therefore, the relative signal intensities of layering fluids in a hemarthrosis are opposite

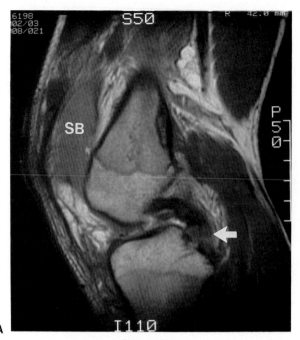

SE 600/20

Figure 11-4 (Same as Figure 11-1). Multiple knee injuries depicted on a series of T1-weighted sagittal MR images. (A) An image through the medial portion of the intercondylar notch shows a torn posterior cruciate ligament at its tibial attachment (arrow). At the tear, the ligament diameter is thickened and its substance has abnormally high signal intensity. A joint effusion is present in the suprapatellar bursa (SB). (B) An image through the lateral portion of the intercondylar notch shows that the anterior cruciate ligament has ruptured proximally and separated from its femoral attachment (black arrow). The wavy, lax anterior cruciate ligament drapes over the tibia (white arrows). Note the edema and hemorrhage surrounding the torn ligament. (C) An image further laterally shows bone marrow contusions of the fibular head and of the posterior aspects of the lateral tibial plateau and lateral femoral condyle (straight arrows). These are low-intensity regions in otherwise higher-intensity bone marrow. Intermediate-intensity hemarthrosis is visible in the suprapatellar pouch; also note the thin, subtle layering (curved arrows). Abnormal signal intensity and lack of morphologic definition of the lateral meniscus indicate a tear.

from those in a lipohemarthrosis. It is, however, possible for three layers to form: the cellular component, the blood serum, and the fat.

Figures 11-4C and 11-5 also show abnormally high signal intensity in the lateral meniscus; this is caused by a meniscal tear **(Option (H) is true).** The quadriceps and patellar tendons shown in Figures 11-4C and 11-5 are intact and normal **(Options (E) and (F) are false).**

The coronal T1-weighted image (Figure 11-7) confirms the lateral meniscus tear. Its also demonstrates absence in the intercondylar notch of the anterior cruciate ligament, which would normally reside immediately adjacent to the posterior cruciate ligament. The medial meniscus is

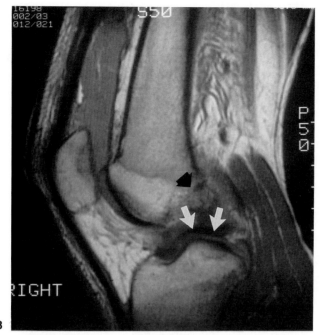

B

SE 600/20

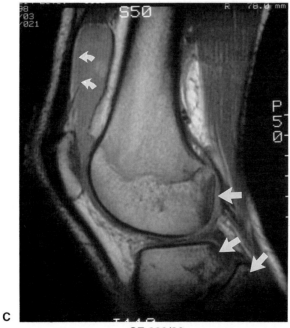

C

SE 600/20

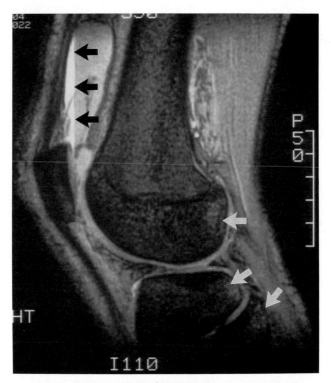

GRE 480/20/30°

Figure 11-5 (Same as Figure 11-2). Multiple knee injuries. Gradient-echo sagittal MR image from same section as Figure 11-4C shows bone marrow contusions as high-intensity regions (white arrows). Layering of the hemarthrosis components within the suprapatellar pouch is now conspicuous. The serum is very bright on this image (black arrows), whereas the dependent cellular elements remain intermediate in signal intensity.

also demonstrated and shows no abnormalities in this image **(Option (G) is false).**

The lateral collateral ligament is not fully demonstrated on any of the images shown **(Option (D) is false).** It would be optimally imaged and evaluated in the coronal plane at the level of the fibula, posteriorly. The torn medial collateral ligament is clearly seen on the coronal image (Figure 11-7). The medial meniscus is separated from the overlying linear low-intensity medial collateral ligament. Just above the level of the meniscus, the medial collateral ligament loses its normal morphology, becomes separated from the femoral condyle, is markedly thickened, and

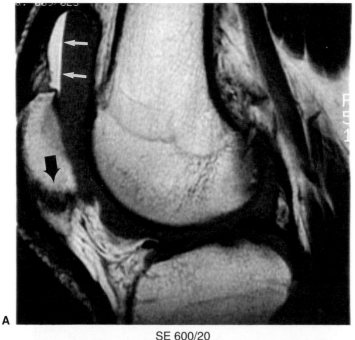

A

SE 600/20

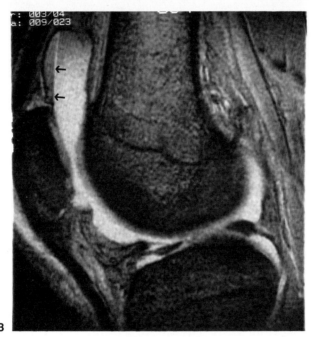

B

GRE 480/20/30°

Figure 11-6. Lipohemarthrosis. T1-weighted (A) and gradient-echo (B) sagittal MR images of the knee show fat (white arrows in panel A and black arrows in panel B) layered on blood. Fat has high signal intensity on T1-weighted images and intermediate signal intensity on T2-weighted images (the opposite signal characteristics of layered serum in a hemarthrosis—see Figures 11-4C and 11-5). In this case, the lipohemarthrosis is secondary to a patellar fracture (black arrow in panel A).

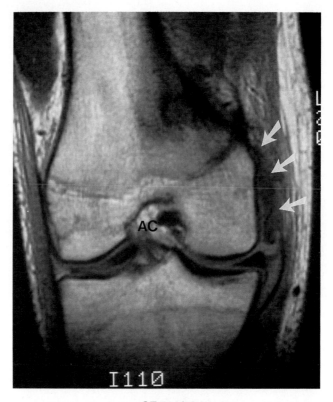

SE 600/20

Figure 11-7 (Same as Figure 11-3). Multiple knee injuries. A coronal
T1-weighted MR image shows a markedly thickened proximal medial
collateral ligament, separation of the ligament from the femoral condyle,
and loss of its normal morphologic definition (arrows), indicating that it
is torn. The lateral meniscus has abnormally increased signal intensity
and loss of morphologic configuration, also indicating an extensive tear.
The anterior cruciate ligament cannot be identified in the intercondylar
notch, where it would normally reside next to the posterior cruciate ligament (AC indicates the expected position of the anterior cruciate ligament).

is surrounded by soft tissue hemorrhage and edema, features diagnostic
of a rupture **(Option (C) is true).**

Question 44

Concerning MRI of meniscal injuries of the knee,

    (A) a "double cruciate" sign indicates a horizontal cleavage tear

    (B) meniscal tears are simulated by the ligament of Humphry

    (C) tears in the periphery of the meniscus are treated differently from those on the free edge

    (D) following conservative management of meniscal tear, persistent high signal intensity indicates failure to heal

    (E) a tear is present when the anterior horn of the medial meniscus is smaller than the posterior horn

The sagittal MR image is generally the most valuable for evaluation of the knee menisci. Coronal images should also be examined carefully for supportive evidence of meniscal tears initially identified on sagittal images and to locate displaced meniscal fragments. Normal menisci are composed of fibrocartilage (type I collagen with few mobile protons) and therefore demonstrate low signal intensity on all pulse sequences.

The MR appearance of the medial and lateral aspects of the knee joint differs in the sagittal plane. The posterior horn of the normal medial meniscus is approximately twice as long as the anterior horn when measured in the anteroposterior dimension **(Option (E) is false)** (Figure 11-8A). The anterior and posterior horns of the lateral meniscus are of equal size (Figure 11-8B). The substances of the menisci otherwise have very similar characteristics on MRI.

Sagittal images obtained in the periphery of a meniscus show a "bow-tie" appearance, which is formed by the triangular anterior and posterior horns connected by the intervening body of the meniscus (Figure 11-9). This bow-tie configuration should be evident on two adjacent sagittal sections when 4- or 5-mm-thick sections are obtained. If fewer than two consecutive sections show bow-ties, the finding is suggestive of a bucket-handle tear, whereas if more than two sections contain a meniscal bow-tie configuration, the finding is indicative of a discoid meniscus. In either situation, confirmatory evidence must be sought on coronal images (Figure 11-10). Sections toward the center of the knee and therefore near the free edge of a meniscus in the sagittal plane show the anterior and posterior horns without interconnecting meniscal tissue. Thus, two independent anterior and posterior triangular structures are evident, rather than the bow-tie configuration.

Several normal anatomic structures can simulate meniscal abnormalities when imaged in the sagittal plane. The appearance of a meniscal tear is created when a normal structure of low signal intensity similar to that of a meniscus is closely juxtaposed to an adjacent meniscus. The relatively high-intensity line formed at the junction between the two

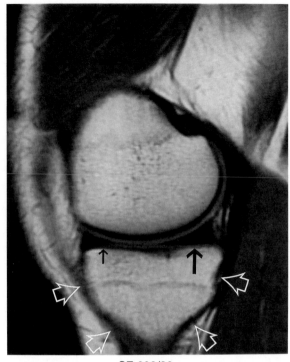

Figure 11-8. Normal knee. T1-weighted sagittal MR images of a normal knee show that medially (A) the tibia has a symmetric shape with a champagne-glass configuration (arrowheads). The low-intensity meniscus is asymmetric, with the posterior horn (large arrow) approximately twice the size of the anterior horn (small arrow). This is in contrast with the lateral aspect of the knee (B), wherein the tibia has an asymmetric shape because of a posteriorly projecting tuberosity that articulates with the fibular head. The anterior and posterior horns of the lateral meniscus are of nearly equal size (arrows). F = femur; T = tibia; f = fibula.

low-intensity structures mimics a meniscal tear. Normal anatomic structures that may cause this interpretive pitfall are the transverse geniculate ligament, the popliteus tendon, and the meniscofemoral ligaments of Humphry and Wrisberg.

The transverse geniculate ligament extends horizontally from the anterior horn of the medial meniscus to the anterior horn of the lateral meniscus. The thin space between the ligament and adjacent meniscus appears as a high-intensity line that may simulate a tear (Figure 11-11). This appearance can be encountered on both the medial and lateral sides of the joint, with the latter finding being far more common. The ligament is displayed in cross-section on sagittal images, and so the true nature of

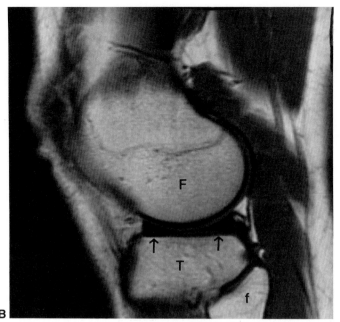

SE 600/20

the structure can be determined by following its course through adjacent sagittal images.

The popliteus tendon with its bursa is located posterolaterally within the joint capsule and is closely associated with a portion of the posterior horn of the lateral meniscus (Figure 11-12). Misinterpretation of this normal relationship as a meniscal tear can be avoided by knowing the location and appearance of the tendon. It is often useful to follow the tendon through a set of adjacent images.

The meniscofemoral ligaments of Humphry and Wrisberg (Figure 11-13) course from the posterior aspect of the lateral meniscus to the lateral surface of the medial femoral condyle. The branch of the ligament that passes ventral to the posterior cruciate ligament is named the ligament of Humphry; the branch dorsal to the posterior cruciate ligament is termed the ligament of Wrisberg. These ligaments are inconstant; either one, both, or neither may exist in any particular knee joint. The structures are imaged in the transverse plane on sagittal images, and in the intercondylar notch they may be misdiagnosed as an osteochondral loose body or a meniscal fragment. The ligaments may also simulate a meniscal tear near the attachment to the posterior horn of the lateral meniscus **(Option (B) is true).**

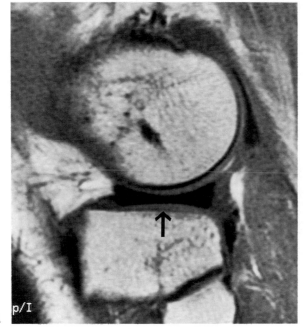

SE 600/20

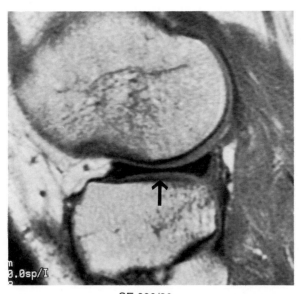

SE 600/20

Figure 11-9. "Bow-tie" appearance of the lateral meniscus. T1-weighted sagittal MR images through the lateral compartment of the knee joint. Both sections, toward the joint line (A) and toward the intercondylar notch (B), show low-signal-intensity lateral meniscus (arrow) with the bow-tie configuration where the anterior and posterior horns are connected by the body of the meniscus.

Meniscal tears may be diagnosed on MR images by recognition of departures from normal meniscal signal intensity, size, and configuration or by detection of displaced meniscal fragments. An intrameniscal

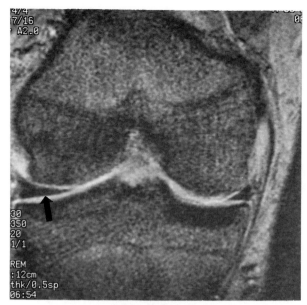

GRE 350/20/30°

Figure 11-10. Discoid meniscus. A gradient-echo coronal MR image shows an elongated lateral meniscus (arrow) as compared with the normal-length medial meniscus.

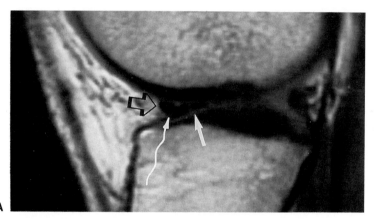

A

SE 600/20

Figure 11-11. Transverse geniculate ligament. (A) Lateral to the midline, a sagittal T1-weighted MR image shows what appears to be two linear high-intensity tears of the anterior horn of the lateral meniscus. However, the more anterior line (wavy white arrow) is a pseudotear formed by a thin layer of tissue trapped between the meniscus and the closely juxtaposed lateral geniculate ligament (open arrow). Only the more posterior linear high-intensity zone (straight white arrow) is a true tear of the lateral meniscus. (B) An adjacent section through the intercondylar notch of the same knee confirms the presence of the transverse geniculate ligament (open arrow).

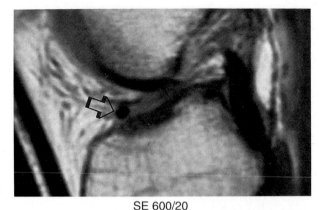

B

SE 600/20

Figure 11-11 (Continued)

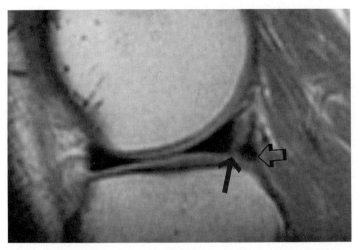

SE 600/20

Figure 11-12. Popliteus tendon. A sagittal T1-weighted MR image through the posterior horn of the lateral meniscus shows a pseudotear (solid arrow) where the popliteus tendon (open arrow) and bursa lie adjacent to the meniscus.

intermediate- or high-intensity focus evident on a T1-weighted MR image is the hallmark of a meniscal abnormality. However, menisci with focal high signal intensity confined within their substance typically are not associated with tears at arthroscopy. These abnormal intrameniscal signal patterns have been divided into two grades: focal round areas

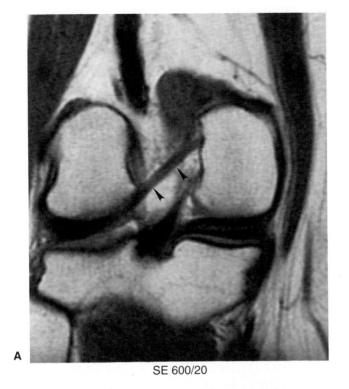

SE 600/20

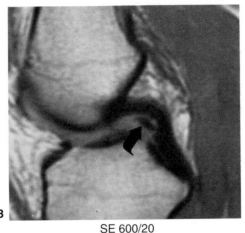

SE 600/20

Figure 11-13. Meniscofemoral ligaments. (A) A T1-weighted coronal MR image shows the meniscofemoral ligament of Wrisberg as a low-intensity band running obliquely from the posterior horn of the lateral meniscus to the medial femoral condyle (arrowheads). (B) A T1-weighted sagittal MR image shows the meniscofemoral ligament of Humphry ventral to the posterior cruciate ligament (arrow). (C) A T1-weighted sagittal MR image shows a pseudotear (white arrow) of the posterior horn of the lateral meniscus where the ligament (black arrow) lies closely juxtaposed to the more anterior meniscus.

285

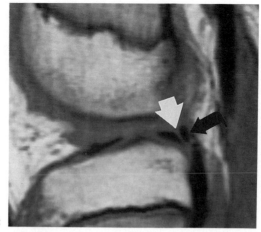

c

SE 600/20

(grade I) and focal linear areas (grade II). Grading intrameniscal focal signal patterns has little practical significance since both grade I and grade II signal patterns represent surgically undetectable lesions. Moreover, intrameniscal focal abnormalities are common in asymptomatic individuals, and the prevalence of such findings increases with increasing age. Histologically, the intrameniscal abnormal signal patterns correlate with focal mucinous degeneration of the meniscal substance. It has been postulated that these structural changes may diminish the elasticity of menisci and predispose the patient to complete meniscal tears. However, little change in grade II signal pattern has been shown at up to 3 years follow-up.

Extension of linear abnormal signal through one or more surfaces of a meniscus (grade III signal pattern) corresponds to arthroscopically detectable meniscal tears in over 90% of patients. Meniscal tears are demonstrated well on T1-weighted spin-echo and T2* gradient-echo images. T2-weighted spin-echo images commonly do not adequately demonstrate meniscal tears. Therefore, the correct diagnosis is usually based on the other pulse sequences.

Of all meniscal tears, diagnosis of small tears along the free edge of a meniscus is least accurate. Fortunately, many tears of this type have no clinical significance. The horizontal cleavage tear is the most common meniscal tear and is readily detected as an oblique high-intensity line extending to either an inferior or a superior meniscal surface (Figure 11-14). The posterior horn of the medial meniscus is the most frequently torn. Meniscal injuries may be complex, with more than one tear evident.

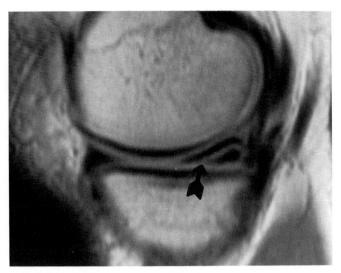

SE 600/20

Figure 11-14. Horizontal cleavage tear of the medial meniscus posterior horn. T1-weighted sagittal MR image shows the tear (arrow) extending to the inferior meniscal surface.

Meniscocapsular separations typically occur during an acute athletic injury. They are often difficult to diagnose by MRI because either a distinct meniscal tear is not evident or the meniscal tissue is only minimally displaced (Figure 11-15). If the knee is imaged shortly after the injury, joint effusion interposed between the meniscus and the capsule or edema in the immediately adjacent soft tissues may suggest the diagnosis. Detection of tears involving the periphery of the meniscus is critical because these injuries can be treated with a suture instead of requiring a partial meniscectomy. Meniscocapsular tears can be expected to heal because of the peripheral perimeniscal capillary plexus that supports ingrowth of fibrovascular connective tissue. Such a response does not exist in the avascular central and inner portions of the meniscus, and healing is not expected in these sites.

Bucket-handle meniscal tears usually involve the medial meniscus in young athletes and often present with locking of the knee as a result of displacement of the inner portion of the meniscus into the intercondylar notch, where the meniscal fragment obstructs the free range of motion. A bucket-handle tear is a vertical tear with longitudinal extension from the posterior to the anterior horn; the peripheral portion of the meniscus is the bucket, and the inner portion is the handle of the bucket. The inner meniscal fragment is termed an unstable fragment. Bucket-handle tears

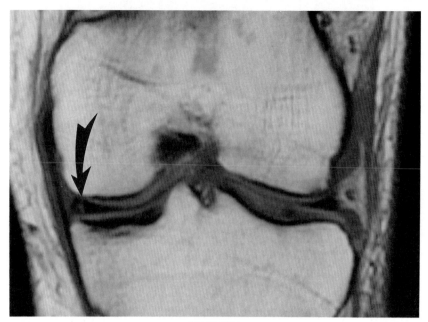

SE 600/20

Figure 11-15. Meniscocapsular separation. Coronal T1-weighted MR image shows a meniscal tear at the meniscocapsular junction (arrow). The tear is located in the vascularized zone of the meniscus and therefore may heal when stabilized with suture fixation.

may not present with linear high-signal regions like other meniscal tears and therefore may be missed if only sagittal images are analyzed. Coronal images are nearly always necessary to confirm the diagnosis and demonstrate the location of the displaced unstable fragment.

Bucket-handle tears of either meniscus may be detected on sagittal images as an abnormality in the absolute or relative size of the anterior and posterior horns (Figure 11-16A). For example, involvement of the medial meniscus may cause the posterior horn to appear the same size as or smaller than the anterior horn, although normally the posterior horn is larger. Conversely, the meniscal horns may be different sizes if a bucket-handle tear occurs in the lateral meniscus, as opposed to the normal situation in which the horns are almost the same size. The triangular configuration and signal of the menisci may be maintained even when they are torn. Subtle blunting or irregularity of the free internal edge of the meniscus will indicate the presence of the tear.

Sagittal images through the intercondylar notch (Figure 11-16B) may show a low-intensity band inferior and parallel to the posterior cru-

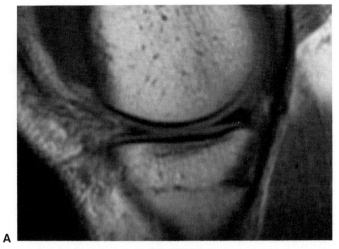

A

SE 600/20

Figure 11-16. Bucket-handle tear of the medial meniscus. (A) A T1-weighted sagittal MR image through the periphery of the medial compartment shows small anterior and posterior horns. Also, the horns are nearly equal in size, whereas normally the posterior horn is twice as large as the anterior horn. Note the absence of the body of the meniscus (no bow-tie appearance); it would normally be present this far peripherally in the joint. (B) A T1-weighted sagittal MR image through the intercondylar notch shows the "double posterior cruciate" sign. The displaced inner fragment of the bucket-handle tear (arrowheads) parallels the posterior cruciate ligament (arrows). (C) A T1-weighted coronal MR image confirms the displaced fragment (arrowhead) beneath the posterior cruciate ligament (arrow). The medial meniscus is much too small, indicating the presence of a tear.

ciate ligament. This "double cruciate" sign is caused by the displaced inner meniscal fragment **(Option (A) is false).** Coronal images may reveal both the peripheral fragment (the bucket) and the location of the displaced central fragment (the handle), which appears as a rounded structure just inferior to the posterior cruciate ligament (Figure 11-16C). However, the unstable bucket-handle fragment may become lodged in other locations such as within the capsular recess between the femoral condyle and the joint capsule just superior to the attached peripheral fragment (Figure 11-17). It is very important to identify the location of a displaced fragment during interpretation of an MR image so that the arthroscopist knows where to search for it, particularly if the location is atypical.

Meniscal tears may be treated conservatively or by arthroscopic surgery. Tears of the relatively avascular mid-portions and inner portions of

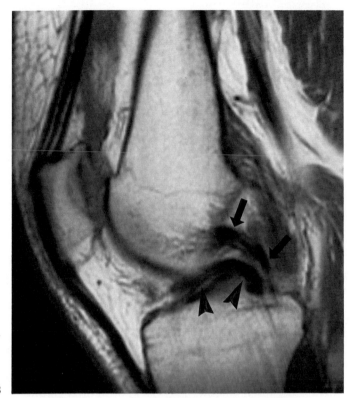

B

SE 600/20

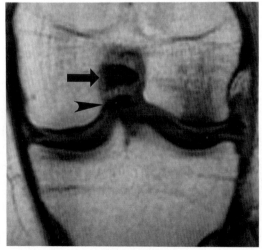

C

SE 600/20

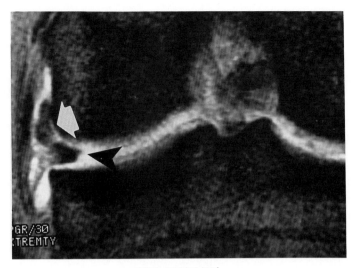

GRE 480/20/30°

Figure 11-17. Bucket-handle tear of a lateral meniscus. A gradient-echo coronal MR image shows a truncated, blunted, lateral meniscus (arrowhead) and a displaced inner fragment lodged between the lateral femoral condyle and the joint capsule (arrow). This pulse sequence imparts a high signal intensity to joint fluid, resulting in a large contrast difference between the low-intensity meniscal fragments and the enveloping effusion.

the menisci are usually treated arthroscopically by partial meniscectomy with removal of meniscal fragments. Tears in the outermost vascularized peripheral portions of the menisci may be treated with a stabilizing suture, leaving the meniscus in place and theoretically reducing the risk of an early onset of degenerative joint disease **(Option (C) is true).**

Follow-up MR examinations of meniscal tears that were left in place may be confusing because various signal patterns may be encountered. For example, the tear may heal and fill in with low-intensity fibrous tissue so that it is no longer evident. Alternatively, it may heal and fill in with regenerative chondrocytes instead of fibrous tissue. With chondrous repair, the old tear may show linear high signal intensity (similar to articular hyaline cartilage) and thus may be indistinguishable from a persistent or recurrent meniscal tear **(Option (D) is false).** Of course, a tear that is left in place may not heal. In any of these situations, the patient may become asymptomatic.

Question 45

Concerning tendons and ligaments of the knee,

(A) patellar tendon ruptures generally occur in the mid-substance of the tendon rather than at either end

(B) quadriceps tendon ruptures occur in an older population than do patellar tendon ruptures

(C) lateral collateral ligament tears are more common than medial collateral ligament tears

(D) the most common MR sign of a complete anterior cruciate ligament tear is inability to identify the ligament

(E) on MRI, alternating bands of high and low signal intensity are normally seen in the anterior cruciate ligament

The quadriceps and patellar tendons are the two most frequently injured or diseased tendons about the knee. These tendons are particularly well evaluated by MRI in the sagittal plane; supplementary axial images may give additional information.

Repetitive stresses across the knee joint may cause patellar tendinitis, tendon degeneration, and partial or complete tears of the tendon. Tendinitis and tendon degeneration both cause focal or diffuse enlargement of the tendon, with or without associated increased signal intensity within the tendon (Figure 11-18A). Diffuse thickening of the patellar tendon is a less common finding than are focal abnormalities such as regions of thickening, thinning, or alterations in signal pattern. Focal abnormalities usually occur at either end of the tendon. Osgood-Schlatter disease occurs at the distal attachment of the tendon (Figure 11-18B), whereas "jumper's knee" occurs at the proximal end of the tendon (Figure 11-18C). Both are manifested as regions of enlargement or increased signal intensity near the tibial or patellar attachments of the tendon.

Complete rupture of the patellar tendon is unusual, but when it occurs it is usually at either the proximal or distal end of the tendon rather than in its mid-portion **(Option (A) is false).** Patellar tendon tears usually occur through areas weakened by preexisting patellar tendinitis. Steroid injections and inflammatory arthritides also weaken the tendon and increase the likelihood of rupture. Finally, lacerations may cause or contribute to disruption of the patellar tendon. Most patellar tendon ruptures occur in people under 40 years of age.

The typical MR features of patellar tendon rupture are discontinuity of the tendon with interposition of hemorrhage and edema between the tendon fragments. MRI also shows the extent of separation of tendon fragments, any residual intact fibers within the torn tendon, and any associated underlying articular abnormalities (Figure 11-18D).

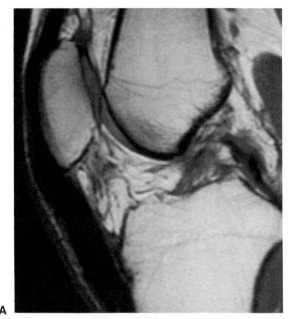

A

SE 600/20

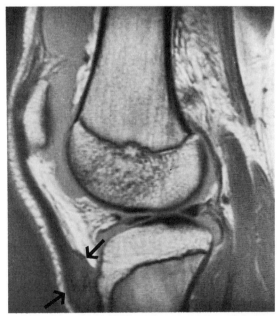

B

SE 800/20

Figure 11-18. Patellar tendon injuries depicted on T1-weighted sagittal MR images in four different patients. (A) Chronic tendinitis is manifested as diffuse thickening of the patellar tendon. (B) Osgood-Schlatter disease is manifested as a thickened patellar tendon at its tibial attachment (arrows). A knee joint effusion is also present. (C) A partial tendon tear, possibly with tendinitis ("jumper's knee"), is manifested as focal thickening with increased signal intensity within the tendon (arrow). The distal two-thirds of the patellar tendon is of normal thickness, configuration, and signal intensity. (D) A full-thickness rupture of the proximal patellar tendon (arrow) with associated soft tissue hemorrhage and edema.

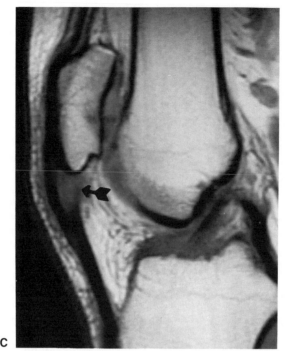

C

SE 600/20

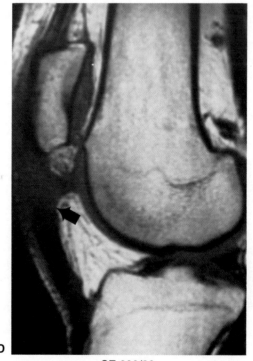

D

SE 600/20

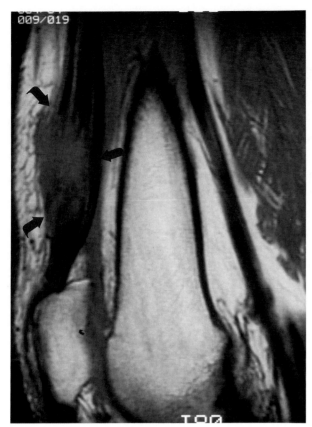

009/019

SE 600/20

Figure 11-19. Quadriceps tendon rupture. A T1-weighted sagittal MR image shows focal thickening and increased signal intensity within the distal quadriceps tendon (arrows). The thin intermediate-intensity lines in the tendon above the tear are normal. The MR appearance of a normal quadriceps tendon is shown in Figure 11-14B.

Quadriceps tendon tears or ruptures are uncommon and almost always occur in people over 40 years of age **(Option (B) is true).** They generally occur just proximal to the patella. Ruptures (partial or complete) tend to occur through regions of preexisting tendon degeneration, which significantly weakens the tendon so that only moderate forces are necessary to cause injury. Partial tears are difficult to diagnose clinically because they present with symptoms of internal derangement of the knee, sprain, or bruise. Complete ruptures may be mistaken for a neuropathy because they present with lack of extensor function. If a tear extends through the inner layers of the tendon to communicate with the suprapatellar pouch, a large knee hemarthrosis develops.

MRI of partial quadriceps tendon tears typically shows a focally thick tendon with increased signal intensity (Figure 11-19). Within the quadriceps tendon, it is important not to misdiagnose as tears the normal parallel lines of increased signal intensity that are sandwiched between the coarse fascicles of collagenous tendon. A complete rupture of this tendon requires transverse discontinuity, as with any other tendon rupture.

The lateral and medial (or fibular and tibial) collateral ligaments of the knee are important for joint stability and are often partially or completely torn during trauma. The lateral collateral ligament is smaller than the medial collateral ligament, but tears of the medial ligament are far more common **(Option (C) is false).** The mechanism of injury consists of a valgus stress across the knee, which places traction and stretching forces on the medial collateral ligament. When the inherent elasticity of the ligament is exceeded, the ligament tears.

The structures that provide stability to the lateral side of the knee include the lateral collateral ligament, the lateral capsular ligament, the arcuate ligament, the popliteus tendon, and the iliotibial band. The lateral collateral ligament runs obliquely in the anteroposterior direction but is commonly detected on a single MR image, where it appears as a low-intensity band extending from the lateral femoral condyle to the proximal fibula. It is a separate structure from the joint capsule and is not attached to the lateral meniscus. MRI shows fat separating the lateral collateral ligament from the lateral capsular ligament (Figure 11-20A).

The medial collateral ligament consists of superficial and deep (capsular) layers with an intervening interligamentous potential space. The deep layer is continuous with the joint capsule and the medial meniscus. The medial collateral ligament extends from the medial femoral condyle to the diametaphyseal region of the proximal tibia.

The collateral ligaments of the knee are best imaged in the coronal plane, where they appear as low-intensity bands of uniform thickness. The lateral collateral ligament is independent of and separated from the lateral meniscus, whereas the medial collateral ligament is closely associated with the adjacent medial meniscus. Injury may cause partial or complete tears of these ligaments. Complete tears are characterized on MRI as disruption and discontinuity of the ligament, and sometimes the ligament acquires a wavy configuration because it is no longer held taut. Intraligamentous focal increased signal intensity may result from hemorrhage and edema, which may also be found in the soft tissues around the injured ligament (Figure 11-20B). Other signs of a collateral ligament tear include separation of the medial collateral ligament from the medial meniscus (Figure 11-20C) and a widened medial or lateral joint space. Partial-thickness tears of the medial collateral ligament cause focal thickening of the ligament with or without increased signal intensity within the substance of the ligament.

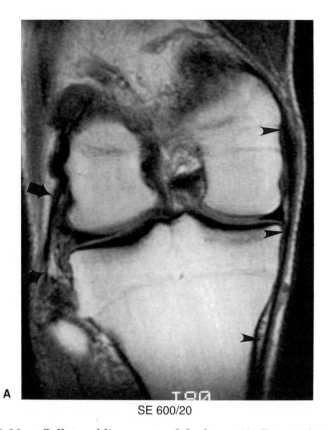

A

SE 600/20

Figure 11-20. Collateral ligaments of the knee. (A) T1-weighted coronal MR image shows the normal lateral collateral ligament (arrows) almost in its entirety coursing from the lateral femoral condyle to the fibular head, widely separated from the lateral joint capsule. The normal medial collateral ligament is a thin low-intensity band (arrowheads) extending from the medial femoral condyle, along the capsule of the knee joint, to attach to the proximal tibial diametaphysis. (B) T1-weighted coronal MR image in a different patient shows complete disruption of the midportion of the lateral collateral ligament (arrow). Surrounding soft tissue edema and hemorrhage obliterate the normal fat plane. (C) T1-weighted coronal MR image in a third patient demonstrates a tear of the distal medial collateral ligament, which is retracted, wavy, and lax instead of straight and taut (arrows). Proximally, the ligament is intact but displaced from the underlying bone by hemorrhage and edema.

When a tear of the medial collateral ligament is identified, a search for associated injuries must begin. The classic combination of injuries, known as O'Donahue's triad, consists of a tear of the medial collateral ligament, a tear of the medial meniscus, and a tear of the anterior cruciate ligament. Injury to bone must also be evaluated.

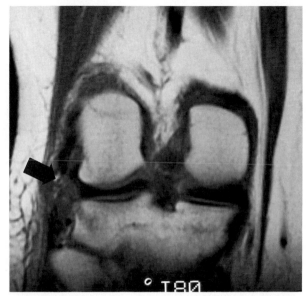

B

SE 600/20

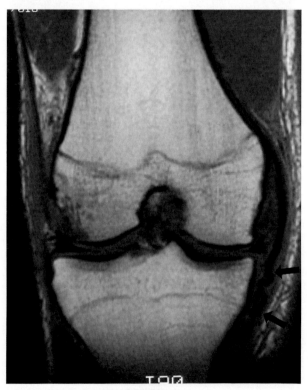

C

SE 600/20

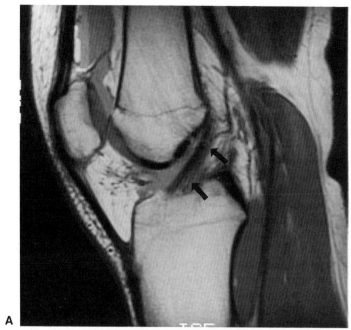

A

SE 600/20

Figure 11-21. Anterior cruciate ligament. (A) A T1-weighted sagittal MR image shows normal, straight anterior cruciate ligament (arrows). Note the normal alternating high- and low-intensity striations in the ligament. Also present is a three-layer lipohemarthrosis, with the highest-intensity fat directly beneath the quadriceps tendon, then intermediate-intensity serum, and finally low-intensity cellular elements of blood in the most dependent portion of the suprapatellar bursa. (B) A T1-weighted sagittal MR image in a different patient through the lateral portion of the intercondylar notch shows absent anterior cruciate ligament and cloudlike region of hemorrhage and edema (arrows). (C) A T2*-weighted sagittal MR image through the lateral notch in the same patient as in panel B shows replacement of the ligament with hyperintense tissue (arrows). (D) A T1-weighted sagittal MR image in a third patient shows a low-intensity band paralleling the expected course of the anterior cruciate ligament (open arrows). However, the course of the ligament should be slightly steeper than the roof of the intercondylar notch (arrowheads); in this case it is abnormally horizontal. This is a chronic anterior cruciate ligament tear. The proximal portion of the ligament is scarred down to the posterior cruciate ligament (solid arrow) instead of extending to the lateral femoral condyle.

The anterior cruciate ligament is best evaluated in the sagittal plane (Figure 11-21A). It runs obliquely within the lateral aspect of the intercondylar notch at a slightly steeper angle than that of the roof of the intercondylar notch. It attaches to the inner aspect of the lateral femoral

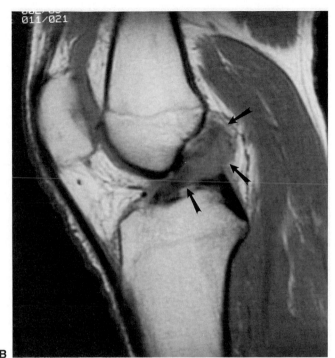

B

SE 600/20

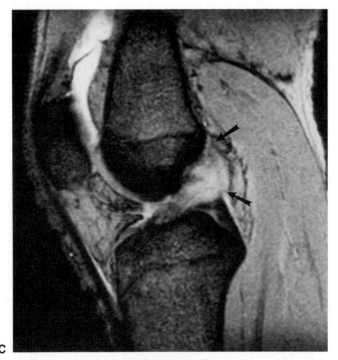

C

GRE 480/20/30°

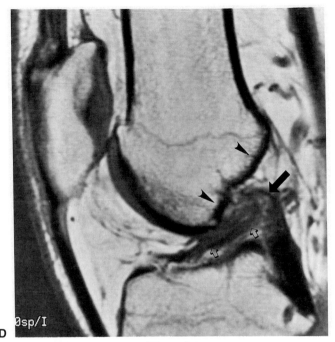

D

SE 600/20

condyle proximally and to the anterior aspect of the intercondylar eminence of the tibia distally. In a sagittal image, the anterior cruciate ligament is a straight, low-intensity band. Often, the ligament is composed of alternating bands of high and low signal intensity that course along its long axis **(Option (E) is true).** The latter appearance is similar to the striations seen in the quadriceps tendon and is an accurate representation of the normal anatomy. The anterior cruciate ligament is surrounded by a synovial sheath, which cannot be detected in an MR image.

MRI is highly accurate (95 to 100%) for diagnosing anterior cruciate ligament tears. Ligamentous laxity from injury is manifested as a sagging, inferiorly bowed ligament configuration but with fibers that remain in continuity. Partial ligament tears may be detected by focal increased signal zones within the ligament. Absence of the ligament (Figure 11-21B) is the most common manifestation of a complete tear **(Option (D) is true).** Many acute tears have a cloudlike edematous mass with well-defined margins running along the expected course of the absent ligament. The edematous mass has intermediate signal intensity on T1-weighted images (Figure 11-21B) and is mildly hyperintense on T2-weighted images (Figure 11-21C). Fragments of the low-intensity ligament are occasionally identified and appear angled, curved, or undulating instead of straight and taut.

Chronic anterior cruciate ligament tears may be diagnosed by absence of the ligament or identification of ligamentous fragments without associated edema. Scar tissue within the intercondylar notch occasionally creates a confusing appearance. The low-intensity scar parallels the expected course of the anterior cruciate ligament and can be mistaken for an intact ligament. A similar situation occurs when the anterior cruciate ligament ruptures proximally and the torn fragments scar down to the lateral aspect of the posterior cruciate ligament, close to the normal femoral insertion site of the anterior cruciate ligament. This creates a low-intensity straight band, with the orientation of a normal anterior cruciate ligament, that may be difficult or impossible to distinguish from an intact ligament (Figure 11-21D). Any angulation of the low-intensity band should alert the interpreter to the possibility of a chronic anterior cruciate ligament tear with scarring.

Additional signs that may aid in the diagnosis of an anterior cruciate ligament tear are bone marrow contusions, buckling of the posterior cruciate ligament, anterior subluxation of the tibia on the femur, and inability to identify the ligament in the intercondylar notch on coronal images.

The normal posterior cruciate ligament (Figure 11-22) is typically of homogeneous low signal intensity, of uniform thickness (about 4 mm thick), and of an arcuate configuration. Injuries to the posterior cruciate ligament may result in posterior instability of the knee. This is recognized as a feeling of unsteadiness and discomfort when the knee is partially flexed.

The posterior cruciate ligament may tear or rupture anywhere within its substance. A complete tear (Figure 11-23) typically causes a discrete disruption of the fibers of the ligament accompanied by focal or diffuse increased signal intensity and thickness of the ligament. Residual ligament fragments may retain low signal intensity. The ligament may be completely absent. Partial tears of the posterior cruciate ligament produce focal areas of increased signal intensity within the ligament. These are indistinguishable from asymptomatic foci of mucoid or eosinophilic degeneration that develop as an age-related phenomenon.

The posterior cruciate ligament may avulse along with an attached tibial bone fragment (Figure 11-24). Loss of tautness of the posterior cruciate ligament from avulsion or complete rupture may cause a wavy or redundant appearance of the ligament. The tibia may also sublux dorsally with respect to the femur. This results in a wavy appearance of an otherwise intact anterior cruciate ligament.

Bone marrow contusions are evident in over half of all acute anterior cruciate ligament tears. They occur in two predictable locations: the mid-

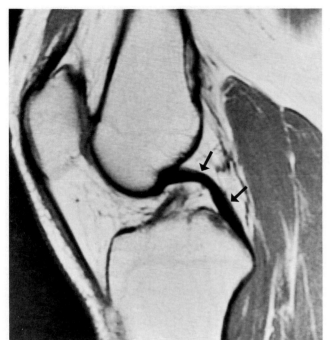

Figure 11-22 (left). Normal posterior cruciate ligament. A T1-weighted sagittal MR image shows a homogeneous low-signal-intensity ligament of uniform thickness and an arcuate shape (arrows).

SE 800/20

Figure 11-23 (right). Complete tear of posterior cruciate ligament. A T1-weighted sagittal MR image shows focally increased signal intensity and thickness of the ligament (arrowheads). Remnants of the intact ligament at proximal and distal attachments remain of low signal intensity (arrows).

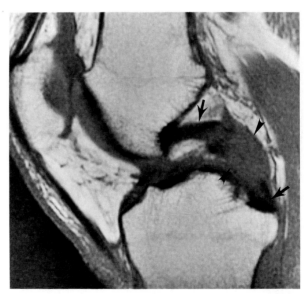

SE 600/14

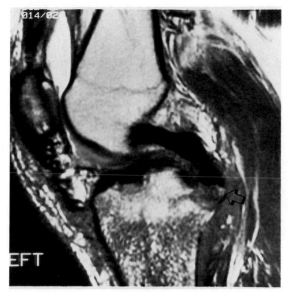

SE 800/20

Figure 11-24. Avulsion of posterior cruciate ligament from tibia. A T1-weighted sagittal MR image shows an avulsion fracture (open arrow) at the tibial attachment of the ligament. Subtle foci of increased signal intensity within the substance of the ligament are evidence of partial tears of the ligament. Other features shown in this image are a lipohemoarthrosis and a tibial bone marrow contusion.

portion of the lateral femoral condyle just above the anterior horn of the lateral meniscus and the posterior aspect of the lateral tibial plateau (Figure 11-25).

An anterior cruciate ligament-deficient knee allows the tibia to undergo subluxation anteriorly relative to the femur. This is the MR equivalent of the anterior drawer sign detected on physical examination. This abnormal tibial displacement causes buckling or acute angulation of the posterior cruciate ligament, which normally has a smooth, curved appearance when the knee is extended. A lax but still intact anterior cruciate ligament can also cause anterior tibial subluxation and buckling of the posterior cruciate ligament.

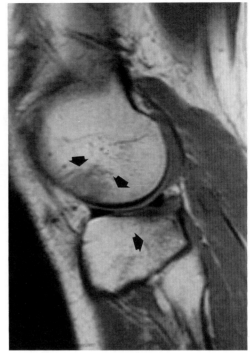

Figure 11-25. Bone marrow contusions. A T1-weighted sagittal image through the lateral compartment of the knee shows bone marrow contusions (arrows) in locations commonly associated with an anterior cruciate ligament tear: the posterolateral tibial plateau and the mid-lateral femoral condyle just above the anterior horn of the lateral meniscus. The bone marrow contusions are identified by the amorphous foci of low-intensity tissue that replace normal high-intensity fatty marrow.

SE 600/20

Question 46

Concerning bone marrow contusions,

    (A) they have no prognostic significance
    (B) medial contusions of the femur and tibia are commonly associated with anterior cruciate ligament tears
    (C) bone scintigraphy is usually normal in areas of bone contusion seen by MRI
    (D) follow-up MR examinations show resolution of abnormal signal intensity by about 3 months after the injury
    (E) the abnormal signal intensity is postulated to be the result of endosteal callus formation

    MRI is capable of demonstrating fractures that are very subtle or not visible at all on conventional radiographs (Figure 11-26). These include osteochondral fractures, occult complete fractures that breach the cortex, stress fractures, and bone marrow contusions (also called occult fractures or bone bruises).

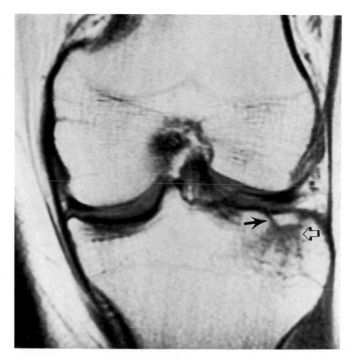

SE 800/20

Figure 11-26. Occult lateral tibial plateau fracture. A T1-weighted coronal MR image shows tibial plateau fracture that could not be detected on conventional radiographs. MR features include demonstration of the fracture line (solid arrow) and the associated bone marrow hemorrhage and edema (open arrow).

Bone marrow contusions are believed to be caused by trauma with trabecular microfractures, hemorrhage, edema, and hyperemia. There is no histologic proof of this hypothesis since there is no logical reason to perform a biopsy of the lesions. The microfracture hypothesis is favored because bone scintigrams show increased tracer activity with the same distribution as the MR abnormality **(Option (C) is false)** and because both tests show a return to normal by about 3 months after the injury (Figure 11-27) **(Option (D) is true).**

Bone marrow contusions are typically located in subcortical cancellous bone, but they may be extensive enough to also involve greater regions of a metaphysis. T1-weighted images of bone marrow contusions show low-intensity reticular, geographic, amorphous, or even discrete linear areas. These transform into high-intensity areas on T2-weighted or T2*-weighted images. Edema of the injured marrow is the primary determinant of these changes in MR signal intensity **(Option (E) is**

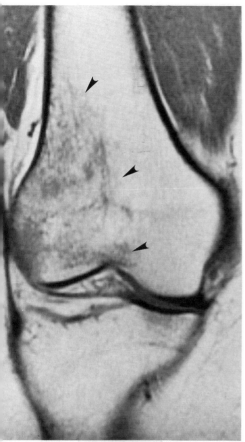 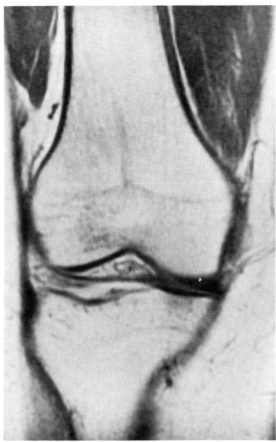

SE 800/20   SE 800/20   **B**

Figure 11-27. Resolution of bone marrow contusion. (A) A T1-weighted coronal MR image shows extensive patchy low-signal-intensity bone marrow contusion (arrowheads) within the femoral metaepiphysis. The conventional radiographs were normal. (B) A T1-weighted coronal MR image of the same patient obtained 4 weeks later shows almost total resolution of the contusion. The femoral marrow signal intensity has reverted to nearly homogeneous fat signal intensity.

false). Articular cartilage overlying the bone marrow contusion is often injured, but the injury is usually too subtle to be detected by MRI. The subcortical location and morphologic appearance allow the diagnosis of bone marrow contusion to be made by MRI.

Accurate diagnosis and detection of bone marrow contusions are important for several reasons. The contusions may be the only abnormalities present and can therefore explain the patient's symptoms and obviate arthroscopy. Second, avoidance or proscription of weight bearing is often required to prevent compression of bone in the areas of trabecular fracture, which could lead to collapse and damage of the overlying articular cartilage and hence to pain or premature degenerative joint disease **(Option (A) is false).** Finally, ligamentous abnormalities are known to occur in association with bone marrow contusions, and these abnormalities are often of greater clinical significance than the occult fractures. Thus, detection of the contusion should cause the interpreter to pay particularly close attention to the ligamentous structures.

Approximately 80% of all bone marrow contusions of the knee occur in the lateral compartment. A certain pattern of lateral compartment contusions is commonly associated with anterior cruciate ligament tears: contusion of the posterolateral tibial plateau alone or in combination with contusion of the mid-lateral femoral condyle directly above the anterior horn of the lateral meniscus **(Option (B) is false).** These specific bone contusions are found in over half of the patients with acute anterior cruciate ligament tears (Figure 11-25).

A common mechanism of injury causes both the anterior cruciate ligament tear and the characteristic associated bone marrow contusions. Anterior cruciate ligament tears are usually acquired with the knee in near full extension, with the foot fixed in position, and from valgus forces causing compression of the lateral side of the knee. When the anterior cruciate ligament ruptures under this stress, the tibia undergoes anterior subluxation relative to the femur. The lateral side of the tibia undergoes more subluxation than does the medial side, causing a relative external rotation of the femur on the fixed tibia. This event is termed pivot shift. If the pivot shift phenomenon occurs with enough force, a unique pattern of occult fracture occurs in the midportion of the lateral femoral condyle and the posterior lateral tibial plateau as the bones are compressed against one another (sometimes termed kissing contusions). The posterior lateral tibial plateau is structurally weaker than the lateral femoral condyle, and therefore it is fractured more often. The pivot shift motion cannot occur if the anterior cruciate ligament is intact; therefore, the fracture patterns described above do not exist if the anterior cruciate ligament is intact.

Phoebe A. Kaplan, M.D.
Robert G. Dussault, M.D.

SUGGESTED READINGS

MENISCAL TEARS

1. Crues JV III, Mink J, Levy TL, Lotysch M, Stoller DW. Meniscal tears of the knee: accuracy of MR imaging. Radiology 1987; 164:445–448
2. Reicher MA, Hartzman S, Bassett LW, Mandelbaum B, Duckwiler G, Gold RH. MR imaging of the knee. Part I. Traumatic disorders. Radiology 1987; 162:547–551
3. Reicher MA, Hartzman S, Duckwiler GR, Bassett LW, Anderson LJ, Gold RH. Meniscal injuries: detection using MR imaging. Radiology 1986; 159:753–757
4. Singson RD, Feldman F, Staron R, Kiernan H. MR imaging of displaced bucket-handle tear of the medial meniscus. AJR 1991; 156:121–124
5. Weiss KL, Morehouse HT, Levy IM. Sagittal MR images of the knee: a low-signal band parallel to the posterior cruciate ligament caused by a displaced bucket-handle tear. AJR 1991; 156:117–119

NORMAL VARIATIONS

6. Herman LJ, Beltran J. Pitfalls in MR imaging of the knee. Radiology 1988; 167:775–781
7. Vahey TN, Bennett HT, Arrington LE, Shelbourne KD, Ng J. MR imaging of the knee: pseudotear of the lateral meniscus caused by the meniscofemoral ligament. AJR 1990; 154:1237–1239
8. Watanabe AT, Carter BC, Teitelbaum GP, Seeger LL, Bradley WG Jr. Normal variations in MR imaging of the knee: appearance and frequency. AJR 1989; 153:341–344

INTRAMENISCAL SIGNAL PATTERNS

9. Dillon EH, Pope CF, Jokl P, Lynch JK. Follow-up of grade 2 meniscal abnormalities in the stable knee. Radiology 1991; 181:849–852
10. Hajek PC, Gylys-Morin VM, Baker LL, Sartoris DJ, Haghighi P, Resnick D. The high signal intensity meniscus of the knee. Magnetic resonance evaluation and in vivo correlation. Invest Radiol 1987; 22:883–890
11. Kornick J, Trefelner E, McCarthy S, Lange R, Lynch K, Jokl P. Meniscal abnormalities in the asymptomatic population at MR imaging. Radiology 1990; 177:463–465
12. Stoller DW, Martin C, Crues JV III, Kaplan L, Mink JH. Meniscal tears: pathologic correlation with MR imaging. Radiology 1987; 163:731–735

LIGAMENTOUS INJURY

13. Grover JS, Bassett LW, Gross ML, Seeger LL, Finerman GA. Posterior cruciate ligament: MR imaging. Radiology 1990; 174:527–530
14. Lee JK, Yao L, Phelps CT, Wirth CR, Czajka J, Lozman J. Anterior cruciate ligament tears: MR imaging compared with arthroscopy and clinical tests. Radiology 1988; 166:861–864

15. Mink JH, Levy T, Crues JV III. Tears of the anterior cruciate ligament and menisci of the knee: MR imaging evaluation. Radiology 1988; 167:769–774

16. Turner DA, Prodromos CC, Petasnick JP, Clark JW. Acute injury of the ligaments of the knee: magnetic resonance evaluation. Radiology 1985; 154:717–722

17. Vahey TN, Broome DR, Kayes KJ, Shelbourne KD. Acute and chronic tears of the anterior cruciate ligament: differential features at MR imaging. Radiology 1991; 181:251–253

18. Zeiss J, Saddemi SR, Ebraheim NA. MR imaging of the quadriceps tendon: normal layered configuration and its importance in cases of tendon rupture. AJR 1992; 159:1031–1034

BONE MARROW CONTUSIONS

19. Kaplan PA, Walker CW, Kilcoyne RF, Brown DE, Tusek D, Dussault RG. Occult fracture patterns of the knee associated with anterior cruciate ligament tears: assessment with MR imaging. Radiology 1992; 183:835–838

20. Lynch TC, Crues JV III, Morgan FW, Sheehan WE, Harter LP, Ryu R. Bone abnormalities of the knee: prevalence and significance at MR imaging. Radiology 1989; 171:761–766

21. Mink JH, Deutsch AL. Occult cartilage and bone injuries of the knee: detection, classification, and assessment with MR imaging. Radiology 1989; 170:823–829

22. Yao L, Lee JK. Occult intraosseous fracture: detection with MR imaging. Radiology 1988; 167:749–751

Notes

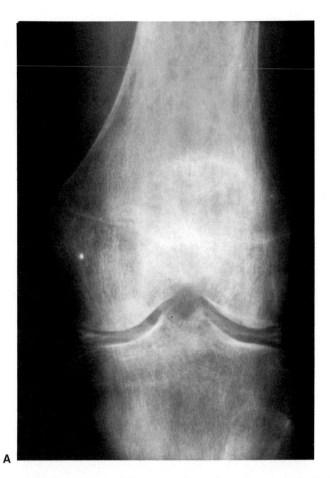

A

Figure 12-1. This 57-year-old woman has chronic musculoskeletal pain and increasingly frequent fractures. You are shown anteroposterior radiographs of her left knee (A) and hip (B).

Case 12: Hypophosphatasia

Question 47

Which *one* of the following is the MOST likely diagnosis?

(A) Postmenopausal osteoporosis
(B) Osteogenesis imperfecta tarda
(C) Mastocytosis
(D) X-linked hypophosphatemia
(E) Hypophosphatasia

The anteroposterior radiograph of the knee (Figure 12-1A) shows osteopenia characterized by cortical thinning, irregular or patchy demineralization of the metaepiphyseal regions of the femur and tibia, and prominence of the longitudinal trabeculae in both epiphyses. The reason why these major trabeculae are conspicuous is that the minor horizontal trabeculae that normally cross between and obscure them have been resorbed, thereby uncovering the presence of the larger longitudinal trabeculae. Also evident in the knee radiograph is chondrocalcinosis of the hyaline articular and meniscal fibrous cartilages (Figure 12-2A).

The anteroposterior radiograph of the hip (Figure 12-1B) shows osteopenia and chondrocalcinosis similar to those found about the knee. In addition, soft tissue mineralization is noted just distal to the femoral head. It is faint and linear and appears to be distributed within muscle. In fact, the mineral crystals are probably within the pectineus muscle. Also evident in the hip radiograph is a short linear lucency, representing an incomplete stress fracture (forming Looser's zone or pseudofracture), in the lateral femoral cortex (Figure 12-2B).

This constellation of findings including osteopenia, coarsened trabeculae, soft tissue mineralization, chondrocalcinosis, and a Looser's zone indicates the presence of osteomalacia. The patient has osteopenia, is in the postmenopausal age group, has experienced fractures, and may well have a degree of osteoporosis, but the diagnosis of postmenopausal osteoporosis (Option (A)) does not account for the other features shown in the test images and is therefore unlikely.

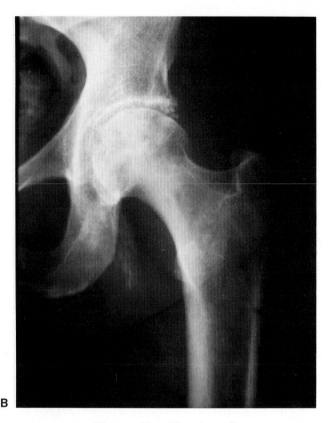

B

Figure 12-1 (Continued)

Osteogenesis imperfecta tarda (Option (B)) can certainly have a clinical presentation in the adult years and can be accompanied by osteopenia and fractures. The degree of osteopenia is highly variable, but in some patients it is moderately severe. In patients with mild forms, the bone can appear radiographically normal. Interestingly, the frequency of fractures increases in affected women following menopause. However, the diagnosis of osteogenesis imperfecta tarda does not account for the chondrocalcinosis or the Looser's zone and is therefore unlikely.

Similarly, mastocytosis (Option (C)) can affect adult women in the postmenopausal age group and can have osteopenia as a prominent manifestation. Again, the other radiographic findings evident in the test images are not features of mastocytosis.

X-linked hypophosphatemia (XLH) (Option (D)), formerly termed vitamin D-resistant rickets, is a chronic condition characterized by features of osteomalacia including coarsened trabeculae, Looser's zones, and even some chondrocalcinosis. However, chondrocalcinosis occurs in

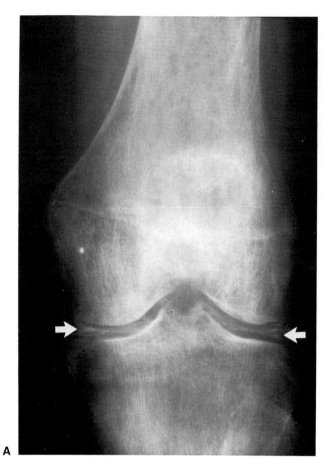

A

Figure 12-2 (Same as Figure 12-1).   Hypophosphatasia. (A) An antero-posterior radiograph of the knee shows generalized osteopenia, thin femoral cortices, thickened trabeculae, and chondrocalcinosis (arrows). (B) An anteroposterior radiograph of the hip shows osteopenia, chondrocalcinosis (solid straight arrow), intramuscular mineralization (curved arrows), and a Looser's zone (an incomplete insufficiency stress fracture) of the lateral femoral cortex (open arrow).

less than 10% of affected individuals and tends to be less severe than that shown in the test images. Moreover, XLH is accompanied by bowing of the femur in at least 75% of affected individuals, a finding not present in the test patient. Also, adults do not experience increasingly frequent fractures as part of their condition. For these reasons, XLH is unlikely.

Hypophosphatasia is the most likely diagnosis **(Option (E) is correct).** The adult form of hypophosphatasia is variable in its clinical expression. However, it is characterized by osteomalacia, and so clinically apparent adult hypophosphatasia is typically accompanied by

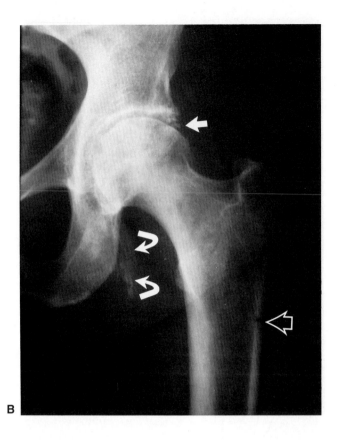

B

radiographically evident osteopenia, coarsened trabeculae, and Looser's zones. These Looser's zones typically occur in the lateral femoral cortex, as in the test patient. Chondrocalcinosis is not an invariable feature of this condition, but it is often present and is a helpful diagnostic feature. Medical attention for increasingly frequent fractures commonly leads to the diagnosis. Hypophosphatasia accounts for all the features detected in the clinical history and images of the test patient.

Question 48

Concerning mastocytosis,

(A) approximately 90% of patients have cutaneous manifestations
(B) systemic symptoms are caused by release of chemical mediators
(C) only 25% of patients with multiorgan involvement have skeletal lesions
(D) its manifestations include both osteopenia and osteosclerosis
(E) bone lesions are symptomatic in about 75% of patients

The mast cell was first described by Ehrlich in 1877 as a "well-fed" ("mast" is the German word for "food") connective tissue cell. We now know that mast cells are of hematopoietic origin and arise from pluripotential bone marrow cells. These cells have a normal distribution throughout the connective tissues. Concentrations of mast cells are found beneath the epithelial surfaces of skin, in the respiratory system, in the gastrointestinal and genitourinary tracts, and in association with blood vessels, lymphatic vessels, and peripheral nerves.

Mast cells contain or elaborate many bioactive compounds including histamine, heparin or chondroitin sulfates, neutral proteases, acid hydrolases, cathepsin G, carboxypeptidase, prostaglandin D_2, leukotriene C_4, and platelet-activating factor. Their locations in connective tissue allow mast cells to receive stimuli from the environment and to affect the response of other tissues by release of mast cell products. These chemical mediators influence adjacent connective tissue cells, as well as nearby nerve and smooth muscle cells.

Mast cells are normal constituents of all connective tissues, but their population can become hyperplastic and result in the group of conditions generally categorized as mastocytosis. The division of mastocytosis into meaningful clinical subgroups has been debated and is confusing. However, a simple scheme is to divide mastocytosis into localized and systemic forms.

By far the most common form of mastocytosis is the localized cutaneous condition, which generally presents in childhood, has a good prognosis, and can resolve spontaneously. The typical manifestation involves scattered pigmented maculopapular lesions (urticaria pigmentosa) that urticate when scratched. Cutaneous mastocytosis can also manifest with diffuse skin involvement or with small papular, nodular, or bullous lesions. In its early stage, cutaneous mastocytosis can have no visible manifestation. Rarely, a localized mastocytoma occurs in a child and can be cured by excision.

Systemic mastocytosis represents 10 to 30% of cases and is characterized by mast cell infiltration of multiple organs other than the skin. Typically, the bone marrow, liver, spleen, gastrointestinal tract, and lymph nodes are involved. Most patients with systemic mastocytosis have cutaneous mast cell infiltration. When all forms of mastocytosis are considered, approximately 90% of affected persons have cutaneous manifestations **(Option (A) is true).**

Mastocytosis can be asymptomatic, or symptoms can be mild and intermittent; these situations delay diagnosis. The condition is often indolent, but patients with systemic mastocytosis generally become sufficiently symptomatic to require medical attention. Their symptoms can be categorized into those caused by organ infiltration and those caused by release of biologically active mediators.

Hepatomegaly occurs in at least 60% of individuals with the systemic condition. These patients may have pain, and some develop fibrosis with associated portal hypertension and varices. Approximately half of affected individuals have splenomegaly, and a few develop associated myelofibrosis. Interestingly, more than 90% of patients with systemic mastocytosis have some fraction of the bone marrow replaced by the hyperplastic mast cell population. This can result in thrombocytopenia and anemia.

Systemic symptoms are caused by release of chemical mediators by the mast cells **(Option (B) is true)** and are characterized by intermittent, generally self-limited attacks. Such attacks often begin with a sensation of flushing or warmth, followed by palpitations, light-headedness, and sometimes syncope. Other symptoms include nausea, abdominal pain, diarrhea, headache, paresthesia, dyspnea, and chest pain. Most attacks begin spontaneously, but the onset can be triggered by heat, stress, and certain medications including intravascular radiographic contrast agents.

With bone marrow involvement so common in patients with systemic mastocytosis, it is not surprising that 50 to 70% of these patients have bone lesions that can be detected by conventional radiography or radionuclide scintigraphy **(Option (C) is false).** It is now well recognized that systemic mastocytosis has a spectrum of radiographic patterns ranging from diffuse osteopenia (Figure 12-3) to diffuse osteosclerosis (Figure 12-4) **(Option (D) is true).** There are many patterns of mixed osteopenia and osteosclerosis. These mixtures include focal lytic or sclerotic lesions ranging from 1 to 2 mm to several centimeters in diameter (Figure 12-5).

In patients who have only osteopenia, mastocytosis is difficult to diagnose. The single most important step in its diagnosis is to remember to include mastocytosis in the differential diagnosis of diffuse osteopenia. The diagnosis may then be supported by measurements of the levels of chemical mediators in the blood or, more definitively, by results of bone biopsy. The diagnosis should always be considered in patients who have

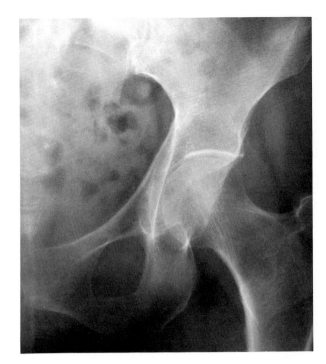

Figure 12-3 (left). Systemic mastocytosis. An anteroposterior radiograph of the left hip shows generalized osteopenia manifested by too few trabeculae and sharply visualized cortices. This 60-year-old woman had a 10-year history of heat-induced urticaria and sequential vertebral-body compression fractures.

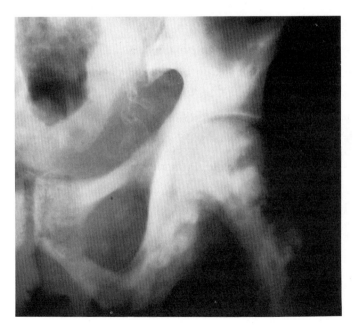

Figure 12-4. Systemic mastocytosis. An anteroposterior radiograph of the left hip shows generalized osteosclerosis. This 71-year-old man had rough skin with multiple macules and papules, lymphadenopathy, and hepatomegaly. He complained of itching and diarrhea but had no bone pain.

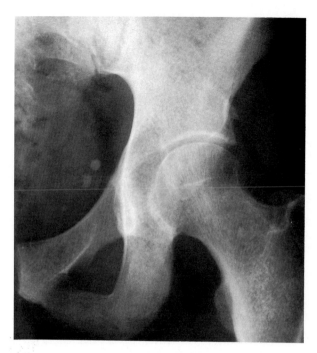

Figure 12-5. Systemic mastocytosis. An anteroposterior radiograph of the left hip shows innumerable tiny discrete trabecular densities. This 39-year-old man was totally asymptomatic and had a normal physical examination at the time his radiologic skeletal abnormalities were discovered.

osteopenia and vertebral compression fractures (Figure 12-6) but in whom there is no reason to suspect postmenopausal osteoporosis, steroid-induced osteopenia, or multiple myeloma.

The precise pathophysiology of the bone changes in systemic mastocytosis remains elusive, but there is evidence from tissue culture research that implicates the mast cell mediators as causative agents in osteopenia and osteosclerosis. It has been demonstrated that prostaglandins increase bone resorption and decrease collagen synthesis, both of which contribute to osteopenia. Heparin is also known to increase bone resorption and decrease bone formation, leading to osteopenia. Conversely, histamine has been shown to increase fibroblast proliferation, and this could result in bone marrow fibrosis with associated osteosclerosis.

Data from histopathologic analysis of bone support these *in vitro* observations. In patients with mastocytosis-induced osteopenia, the rate of bone remodeling is increased but shifted toward resorption as demonstrated by increased osteoclast activity. Osteoblast activity is theorized

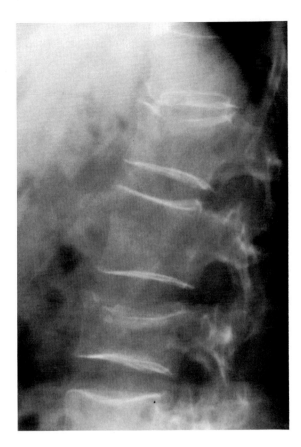

Figure 12-6. Same patient as in Figure 12-3. Systemic mastocytosis. A radiograph of the lateral lumbar spine shows osteopenia and compression fractures of the L1 and L3 vertebral bodies.

to be defective. The number of mast cells in the bone marrow of patients with systemic mastocytosis and osteopenia is absolutely increased and many times normal. Nodules of mast cells are found in all osteopenic patients with mastocytosis.

Patients who have osteosclerosis as the manifestation of systemic mastocytosis have a different histologic pattern. Their bone marrow shows dramatically increased mast cell infiltration, typically several times that found in patients with osteopenia. Patients with the osteosclerotic form also have diffuse bone marrow fibrosis and increased bone remodeling, but the net result is shifted to bone formation.

The differential diagnosis of the radiographic manifestations depends on the mineralization pattern found in a particular patient. For patients with demineralization, the many causes of osteopenia must be considered. In most cases a bone biopsy is required for definitive diagnosis. For patients with osteosclerosis, the pattern of osteosclerosis can resemble metastatic carcinoma, sarcoidosis, and, rarely, Paget's disease of bone. Again, a bone biopsy is usually required for final diagnosis.

Bone pain can certainly result from bone involvement in patients with mastocytosis, particularly if a pathologic fracture (such as a vertebral body compression fracture) is present. However, bone pain is found in less than one-third of patients with systemic mastocytosis. Therefore, despite the sometimes dramatic bone alterations demonstrated radiographically, patients are typically asymptomatic with respect to skeletal anatomy **(Option (E) is false).**

Treatment of systemic mastocytosis is directed toward relief of symptoms. Antihistamines alone have not proven sufficiently effective. The current approach is to identify the symptom complex and direct a specific agent toward the chemical mediator suspected to cause the symptoms. Combinations of agents are used when several mediators appear to be active.

Question 49

Concerning X-linked hypophosphatemia,

(A) proximal renal tubules fail to reabsorb filtered phosphate
(B) it is typically diagnosed before 12 months of age
(C) affected men have more severe deformities than do affected women
(D) most affected adults have measurably diminished bone mass
(E) enthesopathy is a characteristic feature
(F) the principal cause of morbidity in affected adults is lower extremity degenerative joint disease

Historically, rickets resulted from dietary vitamin D deficiency. With the nearly complete disappearance of this deficiency from many nations, it has become apparent that rickets can occur despite normal or supernormal vitamin D intake. Individuals with rickets despite adequate vitamin D intake are considered resistant to the vitamin, and a large number of these persons have persistent hypophosphatemia. The best characterized form of hypophosphatemic rickets is the X-linked dominant type.

XLH is expressed as rickets in children and as osteomalacia in adults. It is inherited as a result of a dominant gene defect at the Xp22 region on the short arm of the X chromosome. The hypophosphatemia is a result of phosphate wasting caused by failure of the renal proximal tubules to reabsorb filtered phosphate **(Option (A) is true).** Renal function is otherwise normal. The intestines also fail to absorb normal amounts of calcium and phosphate, but this is not believed to be a primary cause of this condition. Another characteristic of XLH is that circulating levels of calcium, parathyroid hormone, and the vitamin D metabolites generally remain normal. The gene defect is expressed as growth retardation in children and as short stature with lower extremity bowing and osteomalacia in adolescents and adults.

Infants with XLH are born without clinical, laboratory, or radiographic evidence of rickets. This is true even when their mothers are hypophosphatemic, probably because placental transport of phosphate is not impaired. After the first few months, biochemical changes can be detected in the blood, and after about 6 months, early radiographic alterations can be found. However, unless there is a family history of the condition and because there are no clinically evident features, laboratory studies and radiographs are not obtained. Therefore, the diagnosis of XLH is typically delayed until growth retardation becomes evident or bowing of the lower extremities develops as the child begins to walk. For these reasons, the diagnosis is typically delayed beyond the first year of life **(Option (B) is false)**.

Approximately one-third of all new cases of XLH arise by spontaneous mutation or in persons whose affected mother has no evident manifestation of the disease. The clinical manifestations in children can be quite mild or even nonexistent. These complicating features mean that the definitive diagnosis can be delayed for a long time or never made.

This condition is controlled by an X-linked dominant gene. Therefore, affected men are hemizygotes, because they have only one X chromosome. They transmit the gene to all their daughters but never to their sons. Affected women are typically heterozygous for the defective gene and transmit the defect to 50% of their offspring, either male or female. As is often the case with this genetic pattern, men are more severely affected than women **(Option (C) is true)**. Additionally, men have a more homogeneous expression of the condition, whereas women have more-variable severity of disease. It is possible for an affected woman with demonstrated hypophosphatemia to have no other manifestation. In general, the degree of hypophosphatemia is similar between the sexes but the radiographic features and clinical symptoms are more pronounced in men.

Because XLH is expressed as osteomalacia, osteopenia might be expected and resultant fractures might be anticipated, particularly as these patients become older. A few studies have found diminished bone mass in children, but most studies have found normal or mildly increased bone mass in adults **(Option (D) is false)**. Some studies have found slightly diminished appendicular bone mass in adults, but axial bone mass is not diminished. In fact, some affected patients have dramatically increased axial bone mass. The degree of increased bone mass cannot be predicted on the basis of any measure of disease severity. Concordant with the observation that adults with XLH typically have nor-

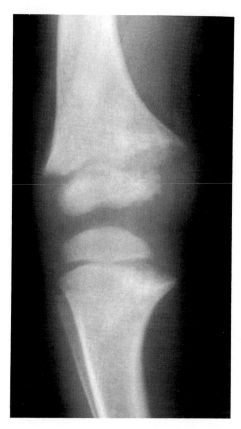

Figure 12-7. Rickets in a 5-year-old boy with XLH. An anteroposterior radiograph of the knee shows lateral bowing of the extremity with typical rachitic changes at the growth plates, particularly on the medial side. The physes are thickened, and the metaphyses are widened and frayed.

mal to increased bone mass is the fact that they have no more fractures than are expected in the general population.

XLH has many radiographic features. Among the features present in children are the typical findings of rickets, with thickening of the physis and fraying, widening, and cupping of the adjacent metaphysis (Figure 12-7). These features are more pronounced in the lower extremities, particularly at the knees, than in the upper extremities. Bowing deformities of the long bones of the lower extremity can be pronounced (Figure 12-8).

Radiographic features of XLH in adults are many and varied. Looser's zones, unhealed insufficiency stress fractures (Figure 12-9), are a typical manifestation of osteomalacia and occur in about half of affected adults. They are most commonly found along the medial aspect of the femoral shaft and are more common in affected men than women. New bone formation is a prominent feature of XLH and occurs at endosteal and periosteal surfaces of long bones. Periosteal hyperostosis develops along adjacent interosseous borders. In some patients the distal femur

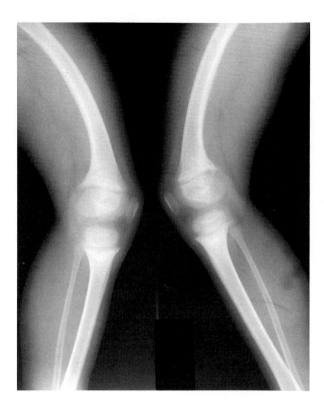

Figure 12-8 (left).
Femoral bowing in
a 7-year-old girl
with XLH. A lateral
radiograph of both
knees shows ante-
rior bowing of both
femora. Note the
rachitic changes of
the growth plates.

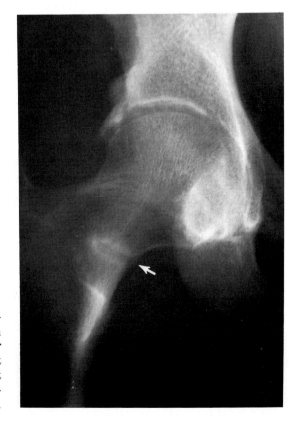

Figure 12-9 (right).
Looser's zone in a 35-
year-old woman with
XLH. An anteroposterior
radiograph of the right
hip shows a distinct
Looser's zone in the femoral neck (arrow).

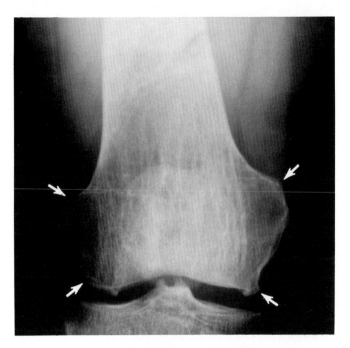

Figure 12-10. Trapezoidal-shaped femoral condyles in a 46-year-old woman with XLH. An anteroposterior radiograph of the knee shows angular deformity of the distal femoral condyles (arrows). The appearance is reminiscent of a trapezoid.

remodels such that the condyles assume a trapezoidal shape (Figure 12-10).

Bowing and shortening of the long bones of the lower extremities is one of the primary manifestations of XLH. Most subjects have this finding, and femoral bowing (Figure 12-11) is slightly more common than tibial bowing. Men and women are affected with equal frequency, but the degree of bowing is greater in men.

Enthesopathy (bone proliferation at sites of ligament, tendon, and joint capsule attachment to bone) is now recognized as a characteristic manifestation of XLH **(Option (E) is true).** About 70% of adults with XLH demonstrate this finding. Men are more likely than women to have this feature and to have more sites of involvement. The ankle is most commonly involved, but various sites in the pelvis are also frequently affected (Figure 12-12). By age 30, enthesopathy is a constant finding.

Extra ossicles occur in about one-third of patients and are found more frequently in older patients. These ossicles are juxta-articular and are encountered primarily in the hands, wrists, feet, and ankles (Figure 12-13).

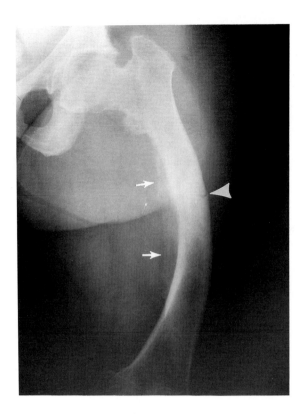

Figure 12-11. Femoral bowing in a 33-year-old woman with XLH. An anteroposterior radiograph of the left femur shows profound lateral bowing of the femur, an incomplete insufficiency stress fracture of the lateral cortex (arrowhead), and extensive periosteal hyperostosis along the medial aspect of the diaphysis (arrows).

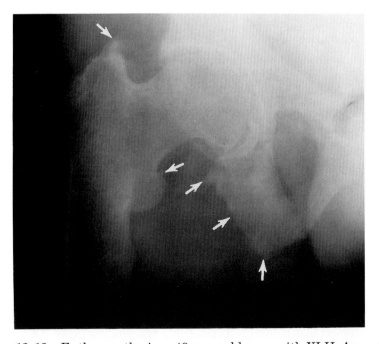

Figure 12-12. Enthesopathy in a 49-year-old man with XLH. An anteroposterior radiograph of the right hip shows mineralization at musculotendinous insertion sites on the surfaces of the greater and lesser trochanters of the femur and along the ischium (arrows).

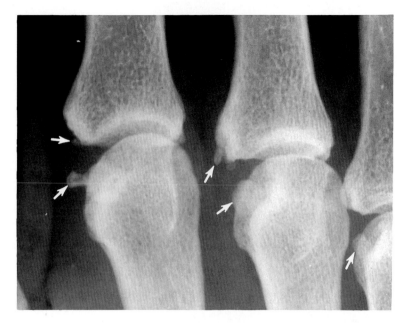

Figure 12-13. Extra ossicles in a 43-year-old woman with XLH. A posteroanterior radiograph of the metacarpophalangeal joints shows multiple juxta-articular ossicles (arrows).

Osteoarthritis of the lower extremity joints is a common finding and occurs in nearly all older patients. It has the cartilage loss, subarticular sclerosis, and spur formation typical of osteoarthritis (Figure 12-14).

Clinically, most patients with XLH present with rickets in childhood and are diagnosed because they are evaluated for growth retardation and for development of lower limb bowing. Most of these children have at least one orthopedic surgical procedure to correct tibial or femoral bowing (Figure 12-15). Adults with XLH are typically symptomatic. They complain of pain, which can be divided into pain of bone origin and pain of joint origin. Joint pain is by far the most common complaint and is the greatest cause of morbidity for these patients. Joint pain is attributed to osteoarthritis **(Option (F) is true).** Bone pain is much less frequent and is commonly attributed to Looser's zones. Enthesopathy does not correlate with pain.

One other cause of morbidity in persons with XLH is dental disease. The underlying problem appears to be defective dentin that permits communication between the pulp space and the enamel layer. This leads to direct bacterial inoculation of the pulp space, with resultant tooth abscesses and dental sepsis. These problems are managed by extraction

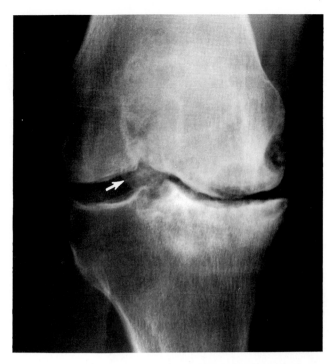

Figure 12-14. Same patient as in Figure 12-13. Osteoarthritis in XLH. An anteroposterior radiograph of the right knee shows classic features of medial compartment osteoarthritis including cartilage loss, subarticular sclerosis, peripheral spurs, and attrition of the tibial plateau. Note the partially hidden osteocartilaginous body that overlies the tibial spines (arrow).

or root canal surgery. Many adults with XLH ultimately undergo complete dental clearance.

Principles of therapy for individuals with XLH are straightforward. When the diagnosis is made early in childhood, the aim is to prevent rickets, growth disturbance, and lower extremity deformity. This is accomplished by use of supraphysiologic doses of 1,25-dihydroxyvitamin D$_3$ and aggressive inorganic phosphate replacement. This simple regimen results in an improved growth rate and healed rickets. Individuals who do not receive treatment until later in childhood may also benefit from the treatment and experience healing of rickets. Their bone deformities may be surgically corrected. In adults, the same medication protocol can be used to relieve the bone pain associated with osteomalacia. Looser's zones require internal stabilization with orthopedic rods, and osteoarthritis is managed by combined medical and orthopedic approaches as indicated for the particular joint.

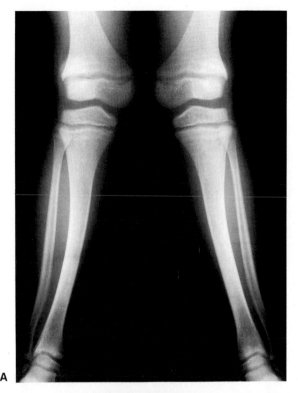

A

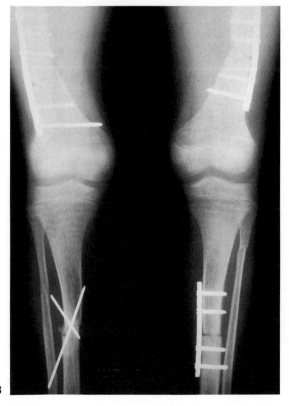

B

Figure 12-15. Surgical correction of bowed lower extremities in a boy with XLH. (A) An anteroposterior radiograph of both distal femora and tibiae shows bilateral genu valgum deformities due to medial bowing of both limbs. Note the rachitic changes of the growth plates. The patient was 10 years 2 months old at the time this radiograph was obtained. (B) An anteroposterior radiograph shows the result of medical and surgical management. The rachitic changes have resolved. Both limbs have been straightened following osteotomies and internal fixation. The patient was 11 years 6 months old at the time this radiograph was obtained.

Question 50

Concerning hypophosphatasia,

(A) the plasma concentration of inorganic phosphate is decreased
(B) half of patients with the infantile form die in infancy
(C) the childhood form is characterized by the combination of rachitic deformities and premature loss of deciduous teeth
(D) nearly 100% of patients with the adult form have a history of symptoms during infancy or childhood
(E) in patients with the adult form, some pseudofractures progress to complete fractures
(F) soft tissue calcification is common

Hypophosphatasia is an inherited metabolic bone disease characterized by subnormal serum alkaline phosphatase activity. Isoenzyme analysis reveals a deficiency of the tissue-nonspecific alkaline phosphatase isoenzyme, a glycoprotein; the gene coding for this protein is localized to the short arm of chromosome 1. There is variability in the relative amounts of the several components of alkaline phosphatase activity (liver, bone, kidneys, and intestines) depending on the individual patient studied and perhaps on the form of hypophosphatasia in a particular patient.

Diminished alkaline phosphatase activity is associated with abnormalities of several phosphorylated biocompounds including inorganic phosphate, phosphoethanolamine, and pyridoxal 5'-phosphate. These three phosphocompounds accumulate in patients with hypophosphatasia and are therefore considered the natural substrates for tissue-nonspecific alkaline phosphatase. Typically, patients with hypophosphatasia have elevated plasma concentrations of inorganic phosphate (**Option (A) is false**).

Defective mineralization of bones and teeth is the characteristic expression of hypophosphatasia. It is believed that the extracellular accumulation of the phosphocompounds, in particular inorganic phosphate, is responsible for this abnormal mineralization. The clinical severity of the mineralization defect is significantly variable, and at least four forms of hypophosphatasia are recognized. These are categorized as perinatal, infantile, childhood, and adult forms. In general, the clinical severity inversely correlates with the age of onset.

Perinatal hypophosphatasia is the most severe form of the condition and is always lethal. Many of these gestations spontaneously abort. Newborns can have normal weight but have a profound mineralization defect (Figure 12-16). The skull can be completely unossified, and the remaining bones can be undermineralized, short, deformed, and fractured. Fetuses that survive birth usually die within a few days, com-

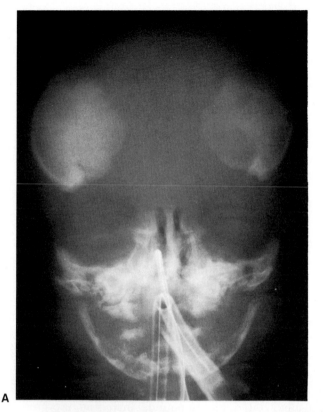

A

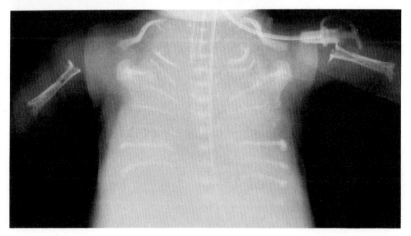

B

Figure 12-16. Perinatal hypophosphatasia in a stillborn infant. (A) An anteroposterior radiograph of the skull shows profound failure of mineralization. Only thin parietal bones are present. (B) An anteroposterior radiograph of the thorax shows short undermineralized bones. The lungs are not aerated. Nasogastric and endotracheal tubes are in place. (Courtesy of Michael P. Whyte, M.D., Washington University School of Medicine, St. Louis, Mo.)

monly of respiratory distress, central nervous system hemorrhage, or renal failure.

Infantile hypophosphatasia is less severe. Pregnancy and delivery are usually normal. There can be episodic respiratory distress postna-

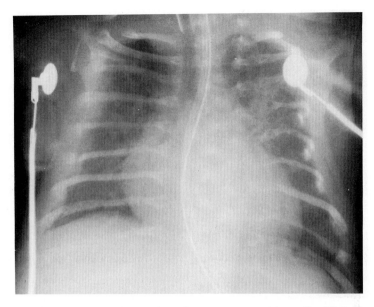

Figure 12-17. Infantile hypophosphatasia in a 23-week-old infant. An anteroposterior chest radiograph shows severe osteopenia, short ribs, many rib fractures, bulbous rib tips, and left upper lobe pneumonia. The infant was experiencing severe respiratory distress. (Courtesy of Michael P. Whyte, M.D.)

tally, and short limbs or wide cranial sutures and fontanels may be detected at birth. Most infants remain symptom free for approximately 6 months. Thereafter they typically develop a failure-to-thrive syndrome characterized by vomiting, hypotonia, convulsions, respiratory difficulty, and irritability. Some show evidence of mental retardation. The course of infantile hypophosphatasia is variable, but about half the affected infants die in infancy, usually of pneumonia (Figure 12-17) **(Option (B) is true).** Some infants show a progressive mineralization defect prior to death. Of those who survive infancy, some improve, although impaired growth and both motor and mental retardation are the expected outcomes of survival.

Generalized osteopenia is the radiographic hallmark of infantile hypophosphatasia. The axial skeleton is severely osteopenic (Figure 12-18). The long bones are typically short and bowed, and they fracture easily. The metaphyses are demineralized and commonly have radiolucent columns of unmineralized tissue projecting from the adjacent growth plates (Figure 12-19). The physes are usually wide, and the zone of provisional calcification is frayed or unsharp. The ribs are often short with bulbous costochondral junctions. The skull is poorly mineralized and soft to the touch.

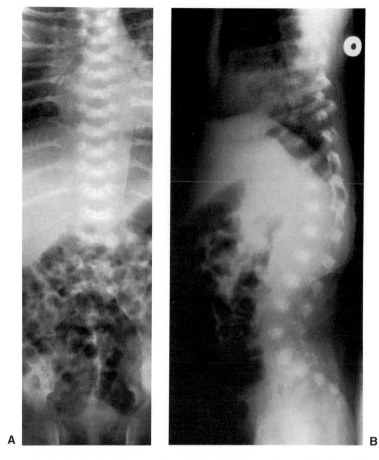

Figure 12-18. Infantile hypophosphatasia in a 14-week-old infant. Anteroposterior (A) and lateral (B) radiographs of the thoracolumbar spine show severe osteopenia. (Courtesy of Michael P. Whyte, M.D.)

Childhood hypophosphatasia is much milder than perinatal or infantile hypophosphatasia. These patients usually present before age 5 because of dental problems, typically unexplained premature loss of deciduous teeth. Some affected children never have any other manifestation of the disease. Most, however, have both dental and skeletal features. Skeletal manifestations of childhood hypophosphatasia include growth retardation and rachitic deformities such as swollen wrists and a rachitic rosary **(Option (C) is true)**. The skeletal manifestations are variable as assessed radiographically. Osteopenia is usually present but can be localized as opposed to generalized. Bone age can be normal or delayed. Metaphyses are usually osteopenic and broad. The growth plate is often wide and poorly mineralized. Large radiolucent zones can extend

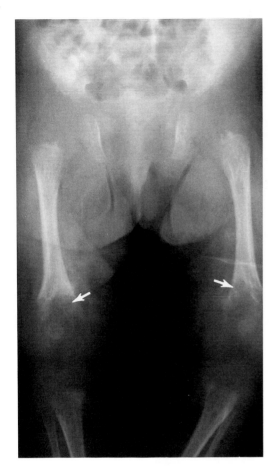

Figure 12-19. Same patient as in Figure 12-18. Infantile hypophosphatasia. An anteroposterior radiograph of the pelvis and lower extremities shows osteopenia and rachitic alterations of the growth plates with large columns of unmineralized tissue extending into the distal femoral metaphyses (arrows). (Courtesy of Michael P. Whyte, M.D.)

from the growth plates deep into the metaphyses (Figure 12-20). These features also account for the clinical manifestation of the rachitic rosary (Figure 12-21).

Long bones can be bowed or otherwise deformed in the childhood form, but fractures are much less common than in patients with the perinatal or infantile form. The skull is also better mineralized but can appear to have persistently open fontanels. However, premature closure of sutures with functional craniostenosis is an important complication of the childhood form.

Over the long term, patients with childhood hypophosphatasia tend to improve spontaneously. Characteristically, the radiographic evidence of rickets resolves, but most individuals have residual osteopenia or deformities. All have persistent evidence of osteomalacia on bone histologic examination when examined as adults.

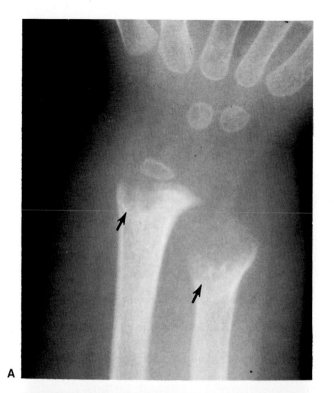

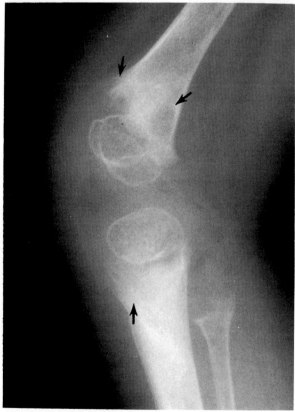

Figure 12-20.
Childhood hypo-
phosphatasia with
rachitic alterations
of growth plates.
(A) An anteroposte-
rior radiograph of
the wrist in a 22-
month-old boy
shows thickened
physes and widened,
frayed metaphyses
(arrows). (B) A lat-
eral radiograph of
the left knee ob-
tained when the boy
was 41 months old
shows similar find-
ings. Note the col-
umns of unmineral-
ized tissue that
extend into the
metaphyses (ar-
rows). (Courtesy of
Michael P. Whyte,
M.D.)

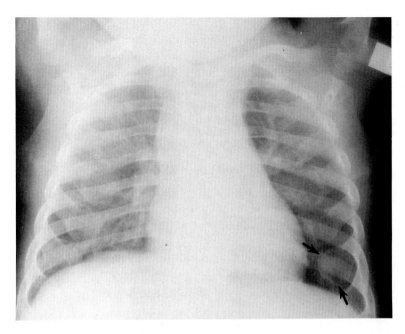

Figure 12-21. Same patient as in Figure 12-20. Childhood hypophosphatasia. The rachitic rosary is manifested on this anteroposterior chest radiograph obtained when the patient was 10 years old as bulbous costochondral junctions of the ribs. Arrows show the extent of process in one rib. All ribs are equally affected. (Courtesy of Michael P. Whyte, M.D.)

Adult hypophosphatasia can develop slowly and can be very difficult to recognize. Less than half of symptomatic adults recall childhood symptoms or give a history of the infantile or childhood condition **(Option (D) is false).** If a careful history is taken, many will have had premature dental problems such as enamel hypoplasia, severe caries, or "loose" teeth. Skeletal manifestations develop long after the dental conditions have been resolved, usually by dental clearance.

Onset of adult hypophosphatasia is usually heralded by bone pain, back pain, arthritis, and recurring pathologic fractures. Physical examination often reveals localized tenderness due to underlying fractures. In severe forms, the fractures heal poorly, bowing of the long bones develops, and kyphosis due to thoracic vertebral body fractures is found.

Radiographs show osteopenia, sometimes of profound degree and greatly out of proportion to the patient's age. However, the spectrum of severity is very broad. Some adults with the enzyme deficiency have normal skeletal mineral mass.

As a result of the underlying osteomalacia, fractures are quite common. These are of various types including typical fractures that occur fol-

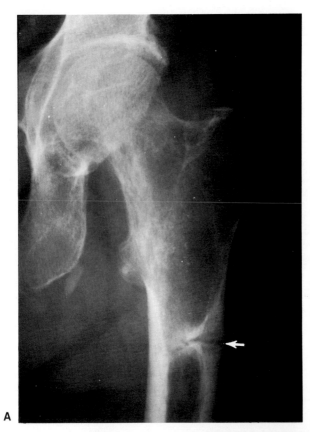

Figure 12-22. Adult hypophosphatasia in a 62-year-old woman. A fracture through the lateral femoral Looser's zone is shown in sequential anteroposterior radiographs of the left femur. (A) At presentation, the Looser's zone (arrow) is accompanied by bone pain. (B) At 5 months after presentation, minor trauma has forced a complete fracture through the preexisting Looser's zone.

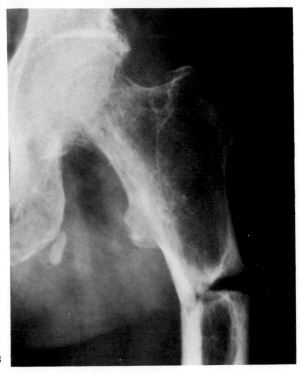

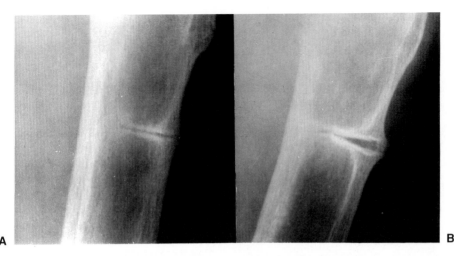

Figure 12-23. Adult hypophosphatasia in a woman aged 53 years at presentation. Persistence and slow progression of a lateral femoral Looser's zone are shown in sequential anteroposterior radiographs of the left femur at presentation (A) and 8 years after presentation (B).

lowing trauma, insufficiency fractures that occur after minor trauma, stress fractures that occur with repetitive normal activity, Looser's zones (pseudofractures) that occur in areas of chronic stress, and completed fractures that occur through preexisting Looser's zones (Figure 12-22).

Looser's zones are typical features of adult hypophosphatasia. They occur in the long bones, commonly involving the femur; most are found in the lateral femoral cortex. Sequential radiographs sometimes demonstrate widening or elongation of Looser's zones, indicating progression or propagation of the pseudofracture (Figure 12-23). When this happens, it is likely that the pseudofracture will progress to a complete fracture **(Option (E) is true),** and internal fixation, usually with an intramedullary rod, is recommended to avoid this complication (Figure 12-24). In general, fractures of any type heal slowly in patients with adult hypophosphatasia.

Soft tissue calcification is a common and important feature of all forms of hypophosphatasia but is particularly important in the adult form **(Option (F) is true).** Mineralization occurs in cartilage, periarticular tissue, muscle, and kidneys. In theory, inorganic phosphate is the controlling factor in the magnitude and type of crystal deposition. *In vivo* experiments indicate that hydroxyapatite formation is inhibited by inorganic phosphate, whereas calcium pyrophosphate dihydrate (CPPD) crystal formation is facilitated. Therefore, the chondrocalcinosis that is often found in adults with hypophosphatasia is presumably formed from CPPD crystals induced by the underlying metabolic condition.

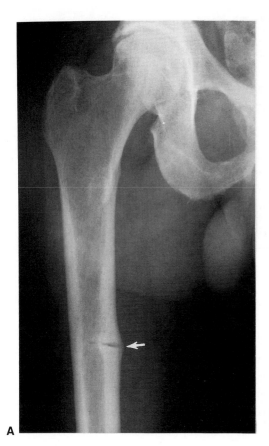

A

Figure 12-24. Adult hypophosphatasia in a man aged 40 years at presentation. Intramedullary rod stabilization of a femoral Looser's zone is shown in sequential anteroposterior radiographs of the right femur. (A) At presentation, the Looser's zone (arrow) is accompanied by bone pain. (B) At 3.5 years after internal fixation, the Looser's zone is partially healed. A complete fracture was avoided by prophylactic surgery.

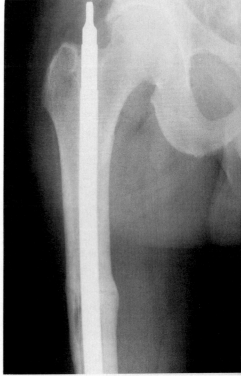

B

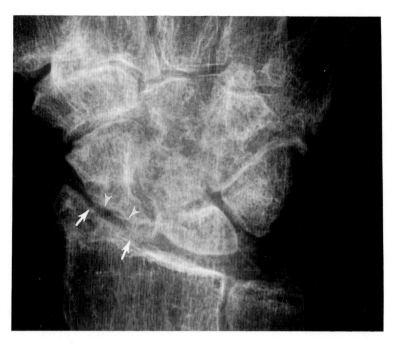

Figure 12-25. Adult hypophosphatasia in a 60-year-old woman. Wrist arthropathy is manifested as diffuse osteopenia, radioscaphoid cartilage loss (arrows), and partial collapse of the articular surface of the scaphoid (arrowheads). Only minor chondrocalcinosis is present in the triangular fibrocartilage region. These features are the same as those encountered in patients with idiopathic CPPD crystal arthropathy.

Of interest, some adults with hypophosphatasia have a CPPD arthropathy indistinguishable from idiopathic CPPD arthropathy. This arthropathy occurs in the usual locations such as the wrist (Figure 12-25) and can develop with or without the presence of chondrocalcinosis. Adult hypophosphatasia has a variable prognosis. However, in general, the condition shows relentless progression with increasing pain, osteopenia, fractures, and resultant deformity. There is no effective medical treatment. Careful orthopedic management is important for fracture prevention and treatment when fractures inevitably occur.

Question 51

Concerning osteomalacia,

    (A) it is characterized by defective mineralization of osteoid matrix

    (B) it is usually caused by excessive hydroxylation of vitamin D in the kidneys

    (C) it is occasionally caused by a mesenchymal tumor

    (D) deficient quantities of osteoid result in a coarsened and unsharp trabecular pattern

    (E) the presence of Looser's zones differentiates it from Paget's disease

    (F) bone pain is infrequent

Historically, the term "osteomalacia" was used to indicate any generalized bone softening disorder that led to crippling deformities. Currently, osteomalacia is histologically defined as the accumulation of osteoid tissue as a result of defective bone mineralization **(Option (A) is true)**. This is differentiated from osteoporosis, in which mineralization of lamellar bone is normal but of subnormal volume, and from osteitis fibrosa, in which normal lamellar bone is replaced by a complex mixture of woven bone and fibrous tissue.

Most types of osteomalacia are caused by a primary disorder of vitamin D metabolism or by a primary defect of renal tubular reabsorption of phosphate. In patients with vitamin D deficiency, hypocalcemia and secondary hyperparathyroidism are typical while hypophosphatemia is mild. In patients with phosphate-wasting conditions, serum calcium levels are usually normal, secondary hyperparathyroidism is absent or mild, and hypophosphatemia is more severe. Other, much less common causes of osteomalacia include the presence of a mineralization inhibitor such as fluoride, a primary abnormality of bone matrix such as fibrogenesis imperfecta ossium, and a defect in alkaline phosphatase such as hypophosphatasia.

The availability of vitamin D can be diminished at any of six levels. The first level is extrinsic depletion. Body stores of vitamin D, calciferol, are maintained by dietary intake and intestinal absorption, as well as by photochemical production in the skin. Decreased dietary intake or skin synthesis can lead to extrinsic depletion. The second level is intrinsic vitamin D depletion, most commonly by intestinal malabsorption associated with gastrointestinal and hepatobiliary diseases. Increased hepatic catabolism of vitamin D to inactive metabolites can augment intrinsic depletion.

The third level is impairment of the first step in vitamin D metabolism. Calciferol undergoes 25-hydroxylation to calcidiol in the liver, and cirrhosis will impair this biochemical reaction. The fourth level is increased hepatic catabolism of calcidiol to inactive metabolites as can occur with hepatic enzyme induction by therapeutic drugs, and increased serum levels of calcitriol or parathormone. This augments depletion of the 25-hydroxylated form of vitamin D.

The fifth level is impairment of the second step in vitamin D metabolism. Calcidiol undergoes 1-α-hydroxylation in the kidneys to become 1,25-dihydroxyvitamin D or calcitriol. This step is impaired by chronic renal failure or by a specific genetic defect in the biochemical pathway within the kidneys.

The sixth and final level of disturbed vitamin D metabolism is ineffective activity of calcitriol as a result of a defective receptor for the vitamin. None of these levels of abnormal vitamin D metabolism involve excessive hydroxylation of vitamin D in the kidneys or in any other organ **(Option (B) is false).**

The plasma phosphate level is essentially under renal control through tubular reabsorption of phosphate. The only exception to this is the profoundly decreased intestinal absorption of phosphate caused by prolonged ingestion of antacids (phosphate-binding aluminum salts). Hypophosphatemia can be secondary to hyperparathyroidism or can be due to a hereditary or nonhereditary intrinsic tubular defect. The classic hereditary form of hypophosphatemia is XLH, as described in the discussion of Question 49. Nonhereditary hypophosphatemia is most commonly caused by a mesenchymal tumor **(Option (C) is true),** and the condition is often termed oncogenous osteomalacia.

Oncogenous osteomalacia must always be considered when osteomalacia first appears during adult years. Although it can begin at any age, most examples of oncogenous osteomalacia have occurred in patients from 20 to 50 years of age. Most of these patients have bone pain, muscle weakness, and difficulty in walking. Some have Looser's zones. Osteopenia tends to be generalized and can be profound, with vertebral body compression features and resultant kyphosis. Biochemically, characteristic features include calcium malabsorption, hypophosphatemia, and low plasma calcitriol levels.

Diagnosis of oncogenous osteomalacia is often delayed for years, sometimes more than 10 years, because physicians may not be aware of the condition or because the responsible tumors cannot be located. Nearly all responsible tumors are of mesenchymal origin, but they are of variable location in soft tissues and bone. All share features of hypervascularity and large numbers of spindle cells and multinucleated giant cells. Many of the tumors appear to be hemangiopericytomas or are of fibrous origin such as fibrous dysplasia or a form of fibro-osseous lesion. Tumor resection leads to dramatic response within days or weeks. Pain disappears, biochemical values return to normal, bone remineralizes, and Looser's zones heal. If the tumor cannot be found, treatment with

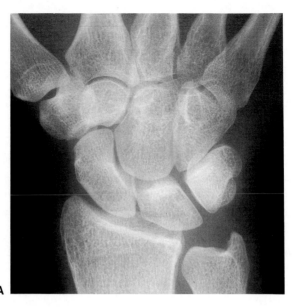

A

Figure 12-26. Normal and abnormal trabecular patterns as shown on posteroanterior radiographs of the wrists. (A) Normal trabeculae-rich bone in a 23-year-old woman. There are so many small trabeculae contributing to the internal cancellous architecture that the larger trabeculae and the carpal bone cortices are obscured. (B) Moderately severe osteopenia in a 66-year-old woman with postmenopausal osteoporosis. The rich small-trabecular architecture is gone, with unmasking of the larger trabeculae and the carpal bone cortices. (C) Severe osteomalacia in a 29-year-old man. The usual innumerable small trabeculae have been replaced by thick, coarse, irregular, and unsharp trabecular plates. (D) Acute osteopenia caused by reflex sympathetic dystrophy in a 50-year-old man. This differs from the osteomalacia shown in panel C because the patchy pattern is due to focal loss of small trabeculae. None of the trabeculae are coarse or thick. The areas that appear dense are actually residual normal trabeculae.

pharmacologic doses of vitamin D generally improves symptoms, biochemical values, and the radiographic appearance.

The radiographic features of osteomalacia are often nonspecific. In general, osteomalacia leads to osteopenia with thin cortices and a diminished number of trabeculae. This pattern can be indistinguishable from osteoporosis; therefore, the neutral term osteopenia is chosen to signify evidence of decreased bone mass. The only form of osteomalacia that regularly leads to osteosclerosis is XLH.

Distinctive qualitative trabecular abnormalities occur in patients with severe osteomalacia. Osteomalacic trabeculae are prominent and replace the usual small structural trabeculae. The remaining trabeculae

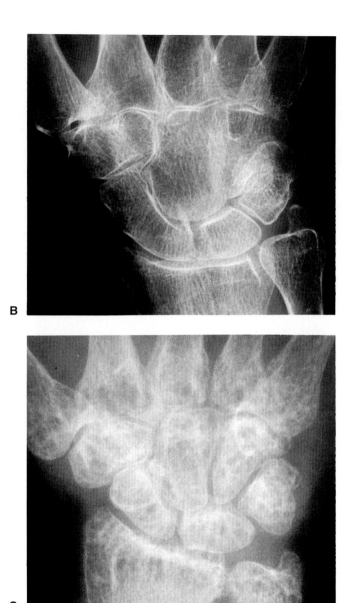

B

C

become thickened, coarse, unsharp, and irregular (Figure 12-26). This requires years of excess osteoid production **(Option (D) is false)** coupled with deficient mineralization.

Looser's zones are lucent bands that are perpendicular to cortices and that extend from the periosteal surface of a bone for a variable distance into the medullary cavity but not the entire distance across the bone. They result from repetitive stress at unique locations and repre-

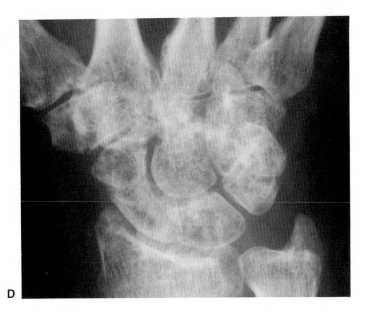

D

sent unhealed insufficiency stress fractures. They are commonly found at sites where daily activities require repeated compression, tension, or bending forces. Typical locations include the shafts of long bones, the femoral neck, metatarsals, scapulae, and pubic rami. Looser's zones occur most frequently in patients with osteomalacia and are a characteristic feature of that condition, but they are not specific for it. Other bone-softening conditions, in particular Paget's disease of bone, can also give rise to Looser's zones (Figure 12-27) **(Option (E) is false).**

The classic clinical features of osteomalacia are bone pain, musculoskeletal tenderness, muscle weakness, and difficulty in walking. Residual deformities from rickets can be present, and deformities such as kyphosis, protrusio acetabuli, and coxa vara can develop in adults. Fractures as described in the preceding discussions are important complications of osteomalacia.

Bone pain is the foremost clinical feature of osteomalacia, and only a few affected individuals are completely free of pain **(Option (F) is false).** The pain is characteristically dull and poorly localized. However, it is clearly bone centered rather than joint related, and it is typically worse with weight bearing. Pain tends to begin in the low back and spreads to the pelvis, hips, thighs, ribs, and dorsal spine. Tenderness is found in a similar distribution and tends to be symmetric. The magnitude of pain ranges from slight to overwhelming. Interestingly, patients with XLH have fewer symptoms of pain than do persons with other causes of osteomalacia, and they have little pain until middle age.

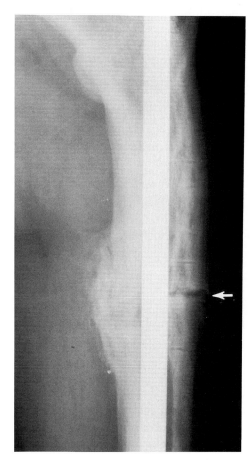

Figure 12-27. Paget's disease with Looser's zones in a 69-year-old man. An anteroposterior radiograph of the proximal left femur shows intramedullary rod fixation of a proximal femoral fracture. The thick, porous femoral cortex is a result of Paget's disease. The fracture occurred through a Looser' zone (arrow) that had formed in the stressed lateral cortex. The traumatic portion of the fracture through the medial cortex has healed with abundant callus. The stress fracture portion (Looser's zone) remains unmineralized. Note the many other lateral cortical Looser's zones.

Muscle weakness is usually of a proximal limb-girdle distribution and varies from barely detectable to near paralysis. These features are termed myopathy, but the pathophysiology of the condition is unknown. Muscle atrophy is disproportionately minor compared with the degree of weakness.

Pain and muscle weakness both contribute to the degree of difficulty in walking. Some patients have pain only when walking. Bowing deformities contribute to the gait disturbance pattern.

Principles of medical management include prevention and treatment. Vitamin D-related osteomalacia can usually be predicted from the family history or the presence of another causative condition and can often be prevented. Unfortunately, phosphate-related osteomalacia is rarely predictable and is therefore not usually preventable. The goals of treatment are relief of symptoms, restoration of bone strength, and preservation of mineral mass. Treatment with vitamin D, calcium, and phosphate supplementation must be tailored for the specific metabolic problem. Orthopedic evaluation and intervention are important for management of the typical complications of skeletal deformity and the various fractures.

William A. Murphy, Jr., M.D.

SUGGESTED READINGS

HYPOPHOSPHATASIA

1. Caswell AM, Whyte MP, Russell RG. Hypophosphatasia and the extracellular metabolism of inorganic pyrophosphate: clinical and laboratory aspects. Crit Rev Clin Lab Sci 1991; 28:175–232
2. Chuck AJ, Pattrick MG, Hamilton E, Wilson R, Doherty M. Crystal deposition in hypophosphatasia: a reappraisal. Ann Rheum Dis 1989; 48:571–576
3. Coe JD, Murphy WA, Whyte MP. Management of femoral fractures and pseudofractures in adult hypophosphatasia. J Bone Joint Surg (Am) 1986; 68:981–990
4. Lassere MN, Jones JG. Recurrent calcific periarthritis, erosive osteoarthritis and hypophosphatasia: a family study. J Rheumatol 1990; 17:1244–1248
5. Whyte MP, Teitelbaum SL, Murphy WA, Bergfeld MA, Avioli LV. Adult hypophosphatasia. Clinical, laboratory, and genetic investigation of a large kindred with review of the literature. Medicine (Baltimore) 1979; 58:329–347

MASTOCYTOSIS

6. Arrington ER, Eisenberg B, Hartshorne MF, Vela S, Dorin RI. Nuclear medicine imaging of systemic mastocytosis. J Nucl Med 1989; 30:2046–2048
7. Bardin T, Lequesne M. The osteoporosis of heparinotherapy and systemic mastocytosis. Clin Rheumatol 1989; 85:119–123
8. Chines A, Pacifici R, Avioli LV, Teitelbaum SL, Korenblat PE. Systemic mastocytosis presenting as osteoporosis: a clinical and histomorphometric study. J Clin Endocrinol Metab 1991; 72:140–144
9. de Gennes C, Kuntz D, de Vernejoul MC. Bone mastocytosis. A report of nine cases with a bone histomorphometric study. Clin Orthop 1992; 279:281–291
10. Galli SJ. New concepts about the mast cell. N Engl J Med 1993; 328:257–265
11. Huang TY, Yam LT, Li CY. Radiological features of systemic mast-cell disease. Br J Radiol 1987; 60:765–770
12. Lidor C, Frisch B, Gazit D, Gepstein R, Hallel T, Mekori YA. Osteoporosis as the sole presentation of bone marrow mastocytosis. J Bone Miner Res 1990; 5:871–876

13. Metcalfe DD. The treatment of mastocytosis: an overview. J Invest Dermatol 1991; 96:55S–59S
14. Travis WD, Li CY, Bergstralh EJ, Yam LT, Swee RG. Systemic mast cell disease. Analysis of 58 cases and literature review. Medicine (Baltimore) 1988; 67:345–368

X-LINKED HYPOPHOSPHATEMIA

15. Burnstein MI, Lawson JP, Kottamasu SR, Ellis BI, Micho J. The enthesopathic changes of hypophosphatemic osteomalacia in adults: radiologic findings. AJR 1989; 153:785–790
16. Chan JC, Alon U. Tubular disorders of acid-base and phosphate metabolism. Nephron 1985; 40:257–279
17. Chan JC, Alon U, Hirschman GM. Renal hypophosphatemic rickets. J Pediatr 1985; 106:533–544
18. Econs MJ, Feussner JR, Samsa GP, et al. X-linked hypophosphatemic rickets without "rickets." Skeletal Radiol 1991; 20:109–114
19. Hardy DC, Murphy WA, Siegel BA, Reid IR, Whyte MP. X-linked hypophosphatemia in adults: prevalence of skeletal radiographic and scintigraphic features. Radiology 1989; 171:403–414
20. Polisson RP, Martinez S, Khoury M, et al. Calcification of entheses associated with X-linked hypophosphatemic osteomalacia. N Engl J Med 1985; 313:1–6
21. Reid IR, Hardy DC, Murphy WA, Teitelbaum SL, Bergfeld MA, Whyte MP. X-linked hypophosphatemia: a clinical, biochemical, and histopathologic assessment of morbidity in adults. Medicine (Baltimore) 1989; 68:336–352
22. Reid IR, Murphy WA, Hardy DC, Teitelbaum SL, Bergfeld MA, Whyte MP. X-linked hypophosphatemia: skeletal mass in adults assessed by histomorphometry, computed tomography, and absorptiometry. Am J Med 1991; 90:63–69
23. Verge CF, Lam A, Simpson JM, Cowell CT, Howard NJ, Silink M. Effects of therapy in X-linked hypophosphatemic rickets. N Engl J Med 1991; 325: 1843–1848

OSTEOMALACIA

24. Parfitt AM. Osteomalacia and related disorders. In: Avioli LV, Krane SM (eds), Metabolic bone disease and clinically related disorders, 2nd ed. Philadelphia: WB Saunders; 1990:329–396
25. Pitt MJ. Rickets and osteomalacia. In: Resnick D, Niwayama G (eds), Diagnosis of bone and joint disorders, 2nd ed. Philadelphia: WB Saunders; 1988:2086–2126
26. Vogler JB, Genant HK. Metabolic and endocrine disease of the skeleton. In: Grainger RG, Allison DJ (eds), Diagnostic radiology. An Anglo-American textbook of imaging, 2nd ed. Edinburgh: Churchill Livingstone; 1992: 1601–1643

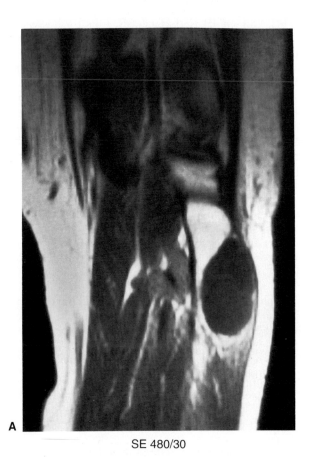

SE 480/30

Figure 13-1. This 39-year-old woman has pain radiating down the lateral aspect of the left leg. You are shown coronal T1-weighted (A) and transaxial T2-weighted (B) MR images of the knee.

Case 13: Ganglion Cyst

Question 52

Which *one* of the following is the MOST likely diagnosis?

(A) Cavernous hemangioma
(B) Ganglion cyst
(C) Meniscal cyst
(D) Baker's cyst
(E) Lipoma

The test MR images show a lobulated soft tissue mass adjacent to the fibula (Figure 13-1). It has low signal intensity on the T1-weighted image (Figure 13-2A) and high signal intensity on the T2-weighted image (Figure 13-2B). Because of its high signal intensity, the mass is more obvious on the T2-weighted image, which also reveals faint septations within the mass. A ganglion cyst can have these MR features, and the tibiofibular joint is one of the typical locations of ganglion cysts. In this location a ganglion cyst sometimes compresses the peroneal nerve as it winds around the neck of the fibula, resulting in pain that radiates down the lateral aspect of the knee. The MR findings, lesion location, and clinical history make ganglion cyst the most likely diagnosis **(Option (B) is correct).** This diagnosis was confirmed at surgery.

Ganglion cysts most commonly present as a palpable mass, but their location is variable. They may arise from the synovium of a joint capsule, but they may not have a definable connection with the adjacent joint at the time of diagnosis. Ganglion cysts may also be attached to tendons and ligaments, or they may be intramuscular. About the knee, they are often found adjacent to the tibiofibular joint. Internally, ganglion cysts are composed of a viscous gelatinous fluid, which may produce an intermediate signal intensity on short-TR/short-TE pulse sequences, a finding not demonstrated in the test images. The main cyst may communicate with adjacent daughter cysts, which are called pseudopods.

On MR images, a cavernous hemangioma (Option (A)) appears as a well-circumscribed soft tissue mass, which may have internal septations.

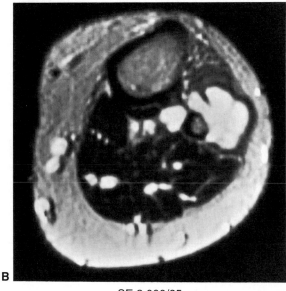

B

SE 2,000/85

Figure 13-1 (Continued)

However, other MR features of cavernous hemangiomas, such as a serpentine pattern, the presence of phleboliths (signal voids), and visualization of feeding and draining vessels, are not present in the test images.

A meniscal cyst (Option (C)), which is always associated with a meniscal tear, is located close to the menisci. In the test patient, however, the mass is located inferior to the tibiofibular joint, quite distant from the menisci. A Baker's cyst (or popliteal cyst) (Option (D)) is a synovial cyst, which occasionally causes peroneal nerve entrapment. However, a typical Baker's cyst would be located in the medial aspect of the popliteal region and would not be immediately lateral to the fibula and hence distal to the knee joint.

A lipoma (Option (E)) is a benign fatty tumor. On MR examination, the intrinsic tissue relaxation parameters are the same for lipomas and subcutaneous fat. Hence, lipomas have the same signal intensity as subcutaneous fat on all pulse sequences (Figure 13-3). The mass in the test images, however, has a lower signal intensity than that of subcutaneous fat on the T1-weighted image and higher signal intensity than subcutaneous fat on the T2-weighted image.

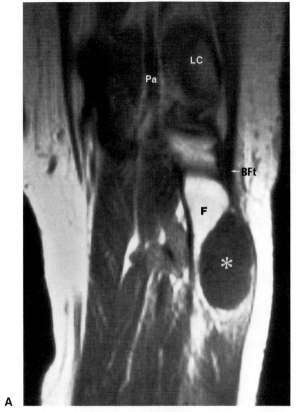

A

SE 480/30

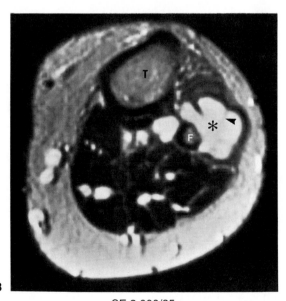

B

SE 2,000/85

Figure 13-2 (Same as Figure 13-1). Coronal T1-weighted (A) and trans-axial T2-weighted (B) MR images show the mass (✻) adjacent to the fib-ula (F), just below the insertion of the biceps femoris tendon (BFt). On the T2-weighted image, low-intensity septa (arrowhead) are faintly visi-ble within the mass. LC = lateral condyle of femur; T = tibia; Pa = popliteal artery.

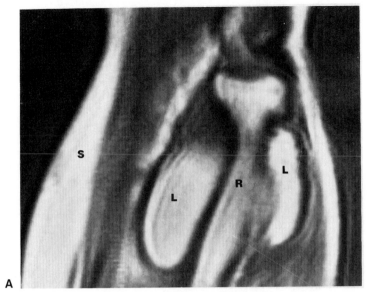

SE 700/30

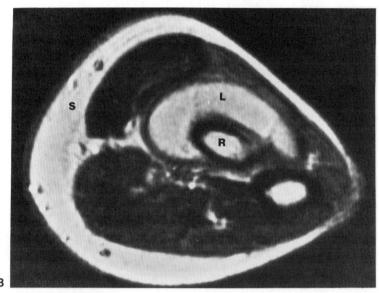

SE 2,000/85

Figure 13-3. Lipoma of the elbow. Coronal T1-weighted (A) and transaxial T2-weighted (B) MR images show that the lipoma (L), which is
wrapped around the proximal radius (R), has the same signal intensity
as the subcutaneous fat (S) on both pulse sequences.

Questions 53 through 58

For each of the descriptions listed below (Questions 53 through 58), indicate whether it is MORE closely associated with meniscal cyst (A) or synovial cyst (B), equally associated with both types of cyst (C), or associated with neither cyst (D). Each lettered option may be used once, more than once, or not at all.

53. Easily diagnosed by arthrography
54. Common on the lateral aspect of the knee
55. Recurs after surgical resection
56. Rupture resembles thrombophlebitis clinically
57. Congenital in origin
58. Gelatinous contents

   (A) Meniscal cyst
   (B) Synovial cyst
   (C) Both
   (D) Neither

Synovial cysts and meniscal cysts of the knee are common clinical entities that may or may not be symptomatic. Both types of cysts are acquired lesions **(Option (D) is the correct answer to Question 57).** Synovial cysts are cavities that have synovial or occasionally fibrous linings and are filled with synovial fluid. These cysts result from the pressure of chronic joint effusion secondary to inflammatory, degenerative, or traumatic conditions. The most common type of synovial cyst is the popliteal cyst (or Baker's cyst), first described in 1840, which forms in the gastrocnemio-semimembranosus bursa in the medial aspect of the popliteal fossa. Popliteal cysts are frequently discovered in patients with joint effusions due to meniscal tears or rheumatoid arthritis. These cysts are usually asymptomatic.

Radiographs of a knee with a synovial cyst may demonstrate a soft tissue mass in the popliteal region associated with a knee joint effusion, and occasionally osteochondral bodies are seen trapped within the popliteal cyst. Baker's cysts can usually be diagnosed easily during arthrography, because the cyst freely communicates with the joint space **(Option (B) is the correct answer to Question 53).** Rarely, if the cyst is filled with fibrinous material or adhesions, it is not depicted on arthrograms. Pressure applied over the suprapatellar bursa during arthrography may aid in visualization of a popliteal cyst by forcing a positive contrast agent, air, or both into the cyst. A lateral view of the knee in 90° of flexion can reveal popliteal cysts that do not appear on routine arthrography.

Sonography is accurate in the diagnosis of popliteal cysts over 1 cm in diameter, and it can usually differentiate a popliteal cyst from other

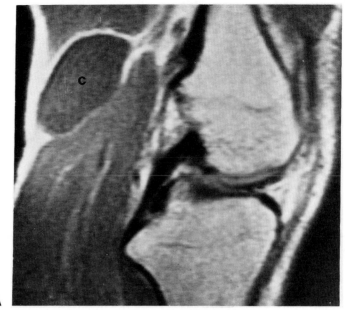

SE 800/30

Figure 13-4. Popliteal cyst. (A) Sagittal T1-weighted MR image. The cyst (C) has the same signal intensity as surrounding muscles. (B) Transaxial T2-weighted MR image. The cyst (c) is easily distinguished from surrounding muscles because of the high signal intensity of the cyst fluid.

masses in the popliteal space, such as a popliteal artery aneurysm, abscess, or tumor. MRI depicts synovial cysts as circumscribed masses, which are best seen on T2-weighted images because of the high signal intensity of their fluid contents (Figure 13-4).

Popliteal cysts usually produce few, if any, symptoms; occasionally they compress the popliteal vein and produce signs and symptoms suggestive of chronic thrombophlebitis. Rupture of a distended popliteal cyst may lead to severe pain, swelling, and tenderness in the leg, a clinical picture mimicking that of acute thrombophlebitis **(Option (B) is the correct answer to Question 56).** Synovectomy is the most effective treatment for popliteal cysts, because cyst recurrence and fistula formation commonly occur after a simple cystectomy.

Meniscal cysts were first reported in 1904. They are characteristically located at the joint line on the medial or lateral side of the knee. Unlike popliteal cysts, meniscal cysts are commonly located on the lateral aspect of the knee joint **(Option (A) is the correct answer to Question 54).** Meniscal cysts are always associated with meniscal tears,

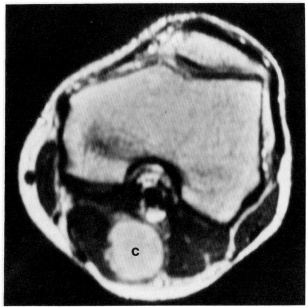

SE 2,000/85

usually horizontal tears or tears with a horizontal component (Figure 13-5). It has been proposed that a pumping mechanism propels synovial fluid through the meniscal tear into the surrounding soft tissues, leading to formation of the meniscal cyst at the meniscocapsular margin. Meniscal cysts are usually filled with a viscous, gelatinous fluid and are therefore often difficult to visualize by arthrography **(Option (A) is the correct answer to Question 58).** As with Baker's cysts, recurrence of meniscal cysts is common following surgical resection of the cyst alone **(Option (C) is the correct answer to Question 55).** Therefore, to avoid recurrence, it is important that the meniscal tear be repaired at the time a meniscal cyst is resected.

Cysts of the knee can be evaluated effectively by MRI. Because of their fluid content, synovial cysts, meniscal cysts, and ganglion cysts all have markedly increased signal intensity on long-TR/long-TE pulse sequences or on images made with fast-scanning techniques that offer some of the imaging advantages of long-TR sequences (i.e., the high signal intensity of fluid and tumors, but with shorter examination times). Each of these cysts is well circumscribed and has smooth walls. Once the diagnosis of a cystic lesion of the knee is made, a combination of location, MR findings (e.g., communication with a meniscal tear, internal septations), and clinical history contributes to the exact diagnosis.

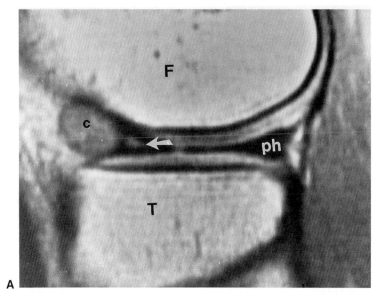

SE 800/30

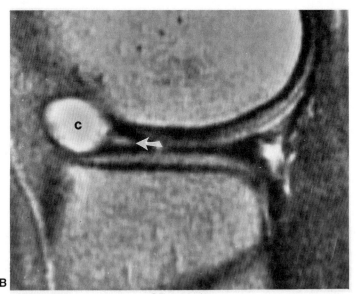

SE 2,000/85

Figure 13-5. Meniscal cyst. Sagittal T1-weighted (A) and T2-weighted (B) MR images depict the cyst (c) near the anterior horn of the lateral meniscus. The cyst communicates with a horizontal tear (arrow) in the meniscus. F = femur; T = tibia; ph = posterior horn of lateral meniscus.

Question 59

Concerning angiovenous dysplasias of the extremities,

    (A) hemangiomas are the most common type
    (B) they are associated with leg length discrepancies
    (C) calcification is uncommon
    (D) periosteal new bone formation is a typical feature
    (E) they are best categorized by the caliber of their vessels
    (F) hemangiomas and venous malformations have a similar appearance on angiography
    (G) MRI commonly shows fat between the vascular channels
    (H) synovial hemangiomas occur most frequently in the hip

The classification of angiovenous dysplasias is somewhat complicated and subject to controversy. However, it is generally agreed that angiovenous dysplasias can be classified into three major groups: hemangiomas, arteriovenous malformations, and venous malformations. The most common of these is the hemangioma **(Option (A) is true).** Hemangiomas can occur in any tissue, but they are found most commonly in the skin and striated muscle. They are divided into capillary and cavernous types, a distinction that can be made on angiography. A hemangioma composed exclusively of normal-sized capillaries is a capillary hemangioma, and a hemangioma that has capacious dilatation of the capillaries is termed a cavernous hemangioma. Histologically, a capillary hemangioma is a mass with newly forming capillaries and a sparse fibrous stroma, whereas a cavernous hemangioma has large blood-filled spaces lined by flat epithelium. Deep soft tissue hemangiomas of the extremities may involve muscle, tendon, connective tissue, fatty tissue, synovium, or bone. Hemangiomas have a predilection for the limbs, and they are more likely to occur distal to the elbows or knees.

Most deep soft tissue angiovenous dysplasias of the extremities are asymptomatic. When they are symptomatic, they may be associated with the following signs and symptoms: pain, swelling, a palpable mass, an audible bruit, cardiac decompensation, osteolysis, and discrepancies in growth of the extremity. Leg length discrepancies are a typical feature of angiovenous dysplasias of the extremities **(Option (B) is true).** Increased blood flow stimulates bone and soft tissue growth so that the involved extremity is usually larger than normal.

Radiographs of angiovenous dysplasias usually show a poorly defined soft tissue mass, which may have tortuous vessels leading to and from it. The tumor may cause smooth pressure erosions of the adjacent bone (Figures 13-6 and 13-7). Calcification is the most commonly encountered radiographic finding **(Option (C) is false).** It is present most frequently in the form of phleboliths (Figure 13-8), but amorphous and curvilinear

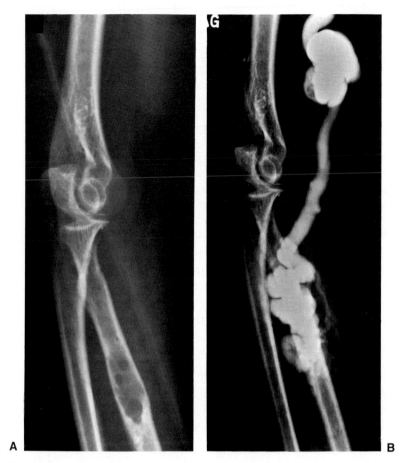

A   B

Figure 13-6. Arteriovenous malformation of the arm in a 40-year-old woman. (A) A radiograph of the proximal forearm and elbow shows a localized, well-circumscribed lytic lesion of the radius associated with expansion of the bone and both cortical thinning and thickening. (B) An arteriogram reveals that the bony changes are caused by the tortuous dilated arteries of a large arteriovenous malformation.

"spongelike" calcifications (Figure 13-9) can also be seen. Localized osteoporosis (Figures 13-7 and 13-10), cortical hyperostosis, and periosteal new bone formation (Figure 13-8) can be seen, but they are rare manifestations **(Option (D) is false).**

 Angiography will depict the different features of the different types of angiovenous dysplasias. The most important feature demonstrated by angiography is the caliber of the vessels in the lesion, which forms the basis for classification of the angiovenous dysplasias **(Option (E) is true).** Therefore, hemangiomas can be distinguished from arteriovenous

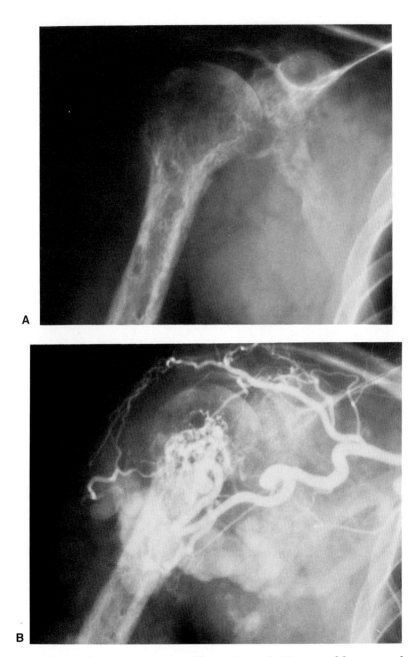

A

B

Figure 13-7. Arteriovenous malformation. A 30-year-old woman had a slowly enlarging soft tissue mass and a loud bruit over her right shoulder. (A) A radiograph shows well-defined erosions and osteoporosis of the scapula and proximal humerus (the ribs are normal). (B) An angiogram shows enlarged arteries with multiple branches supplying an arteriovenous malformation.

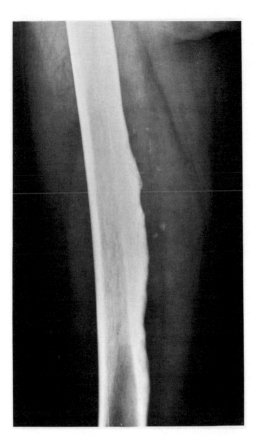

Figure 13-8 (left). Hemangioma in a 26-year-old woman. A radiograph of the thigh shows marked cortical thickening of the femur. Multiple phleboliths adjacent to the cortical thickening indicated the presence of a hemangioma.

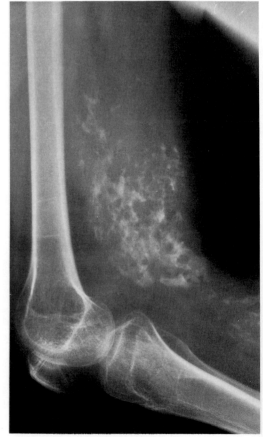

Figure 13-9 (right). Hemangioma in the posterior thigh of a 21-year-old woman. Extensive mineralization in the hemangioma has the appearance of a "calcified sponge."

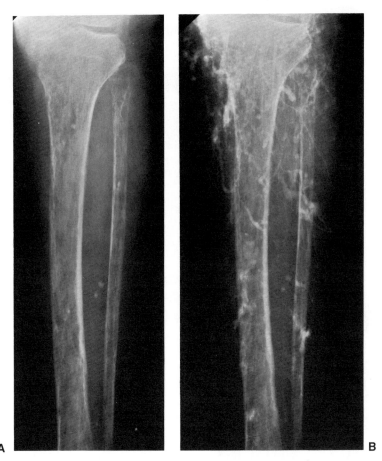

A   B

Figure 13-10. Gradually enlarging cavernous hemangioma of the left lower extremity in a 40-year-old woman. (A) A radiograph shows severe osteoporosis of the tibia and fibula with many discrete lucencies. Phleboliths are identified in the soft tissues. (B) An arteriogram shows enlarged venous structures, many of which correspond to the focal lucencies seen in panel A.

malformations and venous malformations on the basis of their angiographic features **(Option (F) is false).** Hemangiomas are hamartomas of vascular tissues and therefore have contrast opacification of dilated vascular structures. Arteriovenous malformations have large, tortuous arteries and veins and early draining of veins. Venous malformations have large, dilated venous spaces with very slow flow, or their feeding vessels may be thrombosed, so that they are frequently not seen on arteriography.

Largely because of its high soft tissue contrast, MRI is useful in depicting angiovenous dysplasias, particularly in demonstrating the

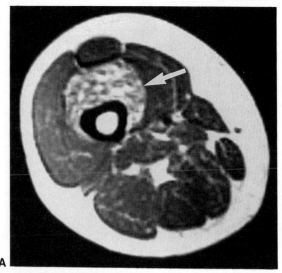

SE 1,083/20

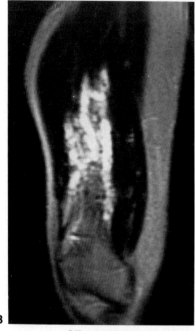

B

SE 2,016/100

Figure 13-11. Hemangioma of vastus intermedius in a 17-year-old boy. (A) A transaxial proton-density MR image shows a heterogeneous high-intensity mass (arrow) involving the right vastus intermedius muscle. There is also focal muscle atrophy. (B) A coronal T2-weighted MR image shows extremely high signal intensity in this serpentine lesion with striated internal septations. (Reprinted with permission from Yuh et al. [16].)

extent of the lesion (Figure 13-11). Reported findings in MR images of angiovenous dysplasias include a serpentine pattern, striated internal septations, lobulations, and characteristic feeding and draining vessels. In addition, fat is commonly seen between the vascular channels of an

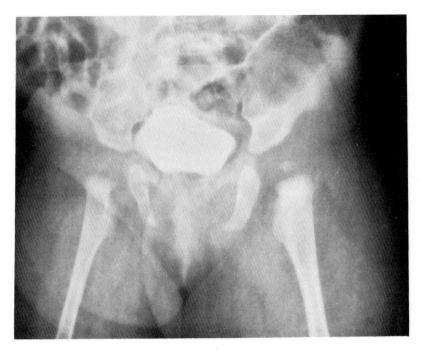

Figure 13-12. Klippel-Trenaunay-Weber syndrome. A 5-month-old girl with cutaneous hemangiomas of the left lower extremity had ipsilateral increase in leg length. An anteroposterior radiograph of her pelvis reveals increased size of the left pubic bone, proximal femur, and soft tissues of the thigh compared with the right side.

arteriovenous malformation **(Option (G) is true).** These MR imaging features will aid in distinguishing angiovenous dysplasias from other soft tissue masses.

The Klippel-Trenaunay-Weber syndrome usually affects infants less than 1 year of age and is characterized by a hemangioma, usually in a lower extemity, which is asymptomatic until it suddenly increases in size (Figure 13-12). The syndrome includes varicose veins, bony and soft tissue hypertrophy, and cutaneous hemangiomas. It can occur in patients of either sex and may be detected at any time from birth to adulthood. Infants with this syndrome are subject to a generalized bleeding tendency with bruising, petechiae, and purpura.

Maffucci's syndrome is a nonhereditary condition consisting of soft tissue hemangiomas and multiple enchondromas. It is seen in male and female patients with equal frequency, most commonly in those younger than 10 years. The clinical findings are usually related to the skeletal deformities caused by the multiple enchondromas. The enchondromas are most commonly found in the metacarpals or phalanges. In addition

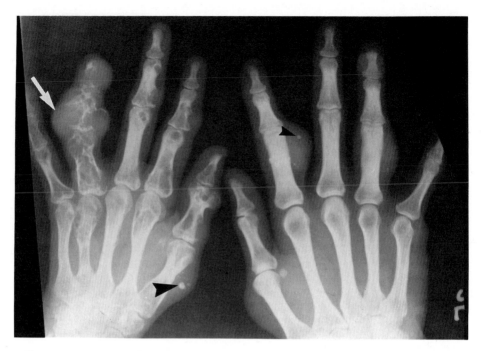

Figure 13-13. Maffuci's syndrome: enchondromatosis with hemangiomas. Multiple bone-deforming enchondromas (arrow) are present in the left hand. The distribution of the hemangiomas, identified as soft tissue masses containing phleboliths (arrowheads), does not correleate with that of the enchondromas. This is a typical radiographic appearance.

to enchondromas, phleboliths may be seen within the overlying soft tissue hemangiomas on radiography (Figure 13-13). Patients may suffer a variety of complications including limb length discrepancies. The most ominous complication of Maffucci's syndrome, however, is malignant transformation of an enchondroma into a chondrosarcoma; this occurs in 20% of patients.

Synovial hemangiomas are uncommon, occurring most frequently in the knee (Figure 13-14) and only rarely in other locations **(Option (H) is false).** They are found in adolescent or young adult women and frequently cause symptoms such as pain, swelling, or locking of the joint. The features of synovial hemangiomas as revealed by various imaging tests are no different from those of hemangiomas found in other anatomic sites. Often, adjacent cutaneous or deep soft tissue hemangiomas are present. Synovial hemangiomas are difficult to treat, and they often recur after surgery.

Vijay P. Chandnani, M.D.
Lawrence W. Bassett, M.D.

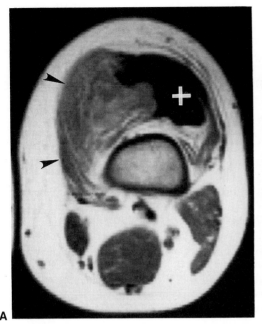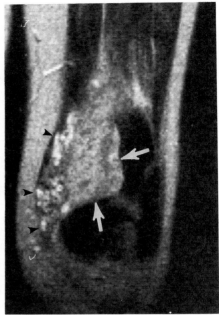

A

SE 1,500/35   SE 1,500/120   B

Figure 13-14. Synovial hemangioma in a 12-year-old boy. (A) A transaxial proton-density MR image shows the suprapatellar region of the distal thigh following instillation of air into the knee joint (+). The mass (arrowheads) is a hemangioma with both intramuscular and synovial components. The mass fills the medial portion of the bursa. (B) A coronal T2-weighted MR image reveals a homogeneous pattern within the synovial portion (arrows) and a serpentine pattern with focal high signal intensity within the intramuscular portion (arrowheads).

SUGGESTED READINGS

CYSTS OF THE KNEE

1. Barrie HJ. The pathogenesis and significance of menisceal cysts. J Bone Joint Surg (Br) 1979; 61:184–189
2. Burgan DW. Arthrographic findings in meniscal cysts. Radiology 1971; 101:579–581
3. Burk DL Jr, Dalinka MK, Kanal E, et al. Meniscal and ganglion cysts of the knee: MR evaluation. AJR 1988; 150:331–336
4. Clark JM. Arthrography diagnosis of synovial cysts of the knee. Radiology 1975; 115:480–481
5. Guerra J Jr, Newell JD, Resnick D, Danzig LA. Pictorial essay: gastrocnemio-semimembranosus bursal region of the knee. AJR 1981; 136:593–596

6. Lapayowker MS, Cliff MM, Tourtellotte CD. Arthrography in the diagnosis of calf pain. Radiology 1970; 95:319–323

7. Lindgren PG, Willen R. Gastrocnemio-semimembranosus bursa and its relation to the knee joint. I. Anatomy and histology. Acta Radiol Diagn 1977; 18:497–512

8. Swett HA, Jaffe RB, McIff EB. Popliteal cysts: presentation as thrombophlebitis. Radiology 1975; 115:613–615

ANGIOVENOUS DYSPLASIAS

9. Allen PW, Enzinger FM. Hemangioma of skeletal muscle. An analysis of 89 cases. Cancer 1972; 29:8–22

10. Bliznak J, Staple TW. Radiology of angiodysplasias of the limb. Radiology 1974; 110:35–44

11. Cohen EK, Kressel HY, Perosio T, et al. MR imaging of soft-tissue hemangiomas: correlation with pathologic findings. AJR 1988; 150:1079–1081

12. Cohen JM, Weinreb JC, Redman HC. Arteriovenous malformations of the extremities: MR imaging. Radiology 1986; 158:475–479

13. Greenspan A, McGatian JP, Vogelsang P, Szabo RM. Imaging strategies in the evaluation of soft-tissue hemangiomas of the extremities: correlation of the findings of plain radiography, angiography, CT, MRI, and ultrasonography in 12 histologically proven cases. Skeletal Radiol 1992; 21:11–18

14. Heitzman ER, Jones JB. Roentgen characteristics of cavernous hemangioma of striated muscle. Radiology 1960; 74:420–427

15. Lenchik L, Poznanski AK, Donaldson JS, Sarwark JF. Case report 681. Synovial hemangioma of the knee. Skeletal Radiol 1991; 20:387–389

16. Yuh WT, Kathol MH, Sein MA, Ehara S, Chiu L. Hemangiomas of skeletal muscle: MR findings in five patients. AJR 1987; 149:765–768

MRI OF SOFT TISSUE TUMORS

17. Dooms GC, Hricak H, Sollitto RA, Higgins CB. Lipomatous tumors and tumors with fatty component: MR imaging potential and comparison of MR and CT results. Radiology 1985; 157:479–483

18. Pettersson H, Gillespy T III, Hamlin DJ, et al. Primary musculoskeletal tumors: examination with MR imaging compared with conventional modalities. Radiology 1987; 164:237–241

19. Pettersson H, Slone RM, Spanier S, Gillespy T III, Fitzsimmons JR, Scott KN. Musculoskeletal tumors: T1 and T2 relaxation times. Radiology 1988; 167:783–785

20. Totty WG, Murphy WA, Lee JK. Soft-tissue tumors: MR imaging. Radiology 1986; 160:135–141

Notes

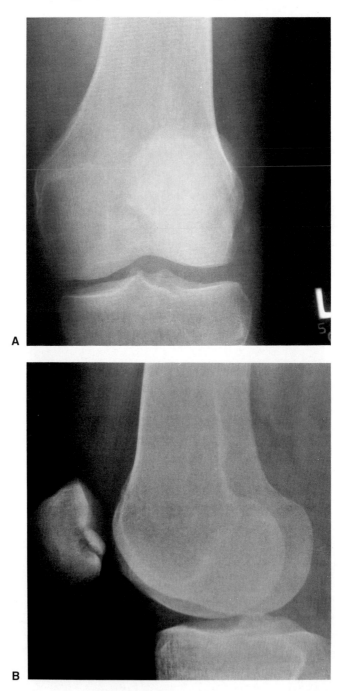

Figure 14-1. This 21-year-old man has pain and swelling of his left knee. You are shown anteroposterior (A) and lateral (B) radiographs of the left knee.

Case 14: Osteochondritis Dissecans of the Patella

Question 60

Which *one* of the following is the MOST likely diagnosis?

(A) Bipartite patella
(B) Osteochondritis dissecans
(C) Chondromalacia patellae
(D) Dorsal defect
(E) Osteoid osteoma

The anteroposterior radiograph of the knee (Figure 14-1A) shows no abnormalities. However, the lateral radiograph (Figure 14-1B) shows subtle evidence of a suprapatellar joint effusion and an ovoid irregular radiolucency in the subchondral area of the inferior pole of the patella (Figure 14-2). A well-defined, dense, osseous fragment rests within the radiolucency. The radiographic features exhibited by the test patient are characteristic of osteochondritis dissecans (OCD), even though the patella is a rare site for this condition **(Option (B) is correct).** When OCD occurs in the patella, the typical site of involvement is the middle or inferior portion of the medial patellar facet, as in the test patient.

A bipartite patella (Option (A)) is a patella with two ossification centers (Figure 14-3). The smaller, accessory ossification center of a bipartite patella is nearly always located in the superolateral aspect of the patella. A bipartite patella is best demonstrated on an anteroposterior radiograph and is identified by the separate well-marginated ossific fragment. The secondary ossification center does not fit perfectly into the patellar defect. Its slight enlargement typically distorts the contour of the patella. In the test images the frontal view is normal and the ossification is inferior and subarticular; bipartite patella is therefore unlikely.

Bipartite patella is found in 2% of the adult population and is bilateral in up to 40% of cases. In some cases the patella may have more than one accessory ossification center (Figure 14-4). The lesion is generally

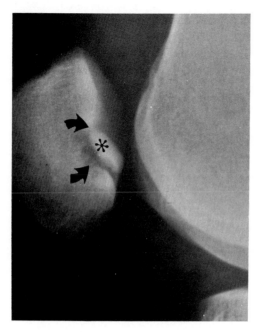

Figure 14-2 (Same as Figure 14-1B). Osteochondritis dissecans of the patella. The coned-down lateral radiograph shows a radiolucent area in the subchondral region of the inferior pole of the patella (arrows) associated with a central osseous fragment (✳).

considered to be congenital, but another proposed theory is that a bipartite patella results from chronic mechanical stress. This type of trauma causes separation of accessory ossification centers during development of the patella. In keeping with this latter theory, a bipartite patella is sometimes associated with clinical complaints. Moreover, bipartite patellae have histologic similarities to other osteochondroses that occur about the knee.

Chondromalacia patellae (Option (C)) typically manifests no conventional radiographic findings, although osteoporosis is seen in some cases. Therefore, this is an unlikely diagnosis in the test patient. Chondromalacia patellae is believed to be a degenerative process. It is seen mainly in adolescents and young adults and is characterized by progressive stages of fibrillation, fissuring, and erosion of articular cartilage with eventual development of patellofemoral joint arthrosis. Either MRI or CT-arthrography is necessary for radiographic demonstration of the early stages of this cartilaginous abnormality. Direct visualization by arthroscopy is the most sensitive diagnostic method.

Dorsal defect of the patella (Option (D)) is a well-defined radiolucency in the patella, most often found in the superior pole and averaging 9 mm in diameter (Figure 14-5). There is no associated loose osseous fragment, and the overlying hyaline cartilage is intact. Therefore, dorsal defect of the patella is an unlikely diagnosis in this case. Its prevalence

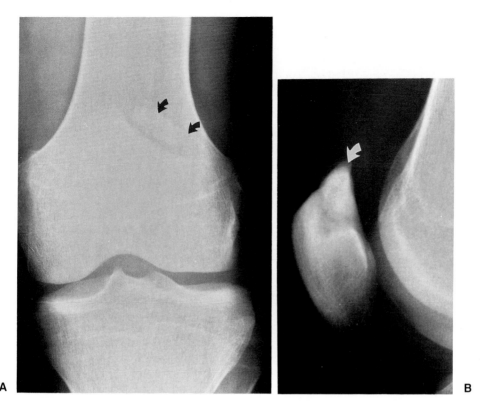

Figure 14-3. Bipartite patella. Anteroposterior (A) and lateral (B) radiographs show an accessory ossification center (arrows) in the superolateral aspect of the patella. The border of the secondary ossification center is continuous with the border of the patella.

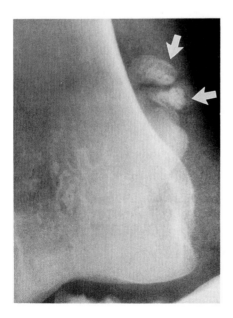

Figure 14-4. Tripartite patella. An anteroposterior radiograph shows two separate accessory ossification centers in the superolateral aspect of the patella (arrows). (Courtesy of Stanley P. Bohrer, M.D., Bowman Gray School of Medicine, Winston-Salem, N.C.)

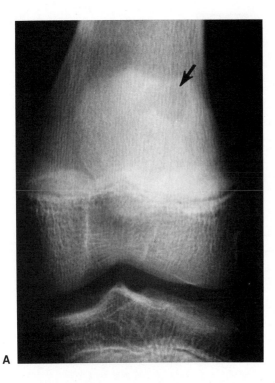

A

Figure 14-5. Dorsal defect of the patella. Anteroposterior (A) and lateral (B) views show a lucency in the superodorsal aspect of the patella (arrows).

in the population is much less than 1%, and it may be bilateral. Dorsal defect of the patella is best demonstrated on lateral or tunnel radiographs and may be difficult to appreciate on frontal radiographs. The exact cause of a dorsal defect of the patella is not known, but stress and normal developmental variation have been proposed as etiologies. A dorsal defect of the patella is an incidental radiographic finding and is of no clinical significance.

Osteoid osteoma (Option (E)) is typically characterized by laminated or solid periosteal reaction surrounding a radiolucent nidus that is usually less than 1 cm in diameter. CT is often required either to confirm the diagnosis by demonstrating the lucent nidus or to establish the exact location of the nidus prior to surgical excision. The lesion may occur in cortical, cancellous, or subperiosteal locations. Osteoid osteoma most commonly affects the tibia, femur, vertebrae, and small bones of the hands and feet. The patella is a distinctly unusual location. Furthermore, even though some patients may have a radiolucency without sclerosis or periosteal reaction and others may have a tiny calcification within the radiolucent nidus, osteoid osteoma should not be associated with an osteocartilaginous fragment.

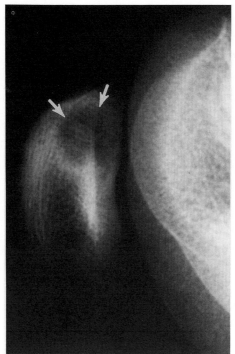

B

Question 61

Concerning osteochondritis dissecans,

    (A) remote or subacute infection is considered the cause
    (B) it usually affects patients under 10 years of age
    (C) the most common site is the medial femoral condyle
    (D) the stability of the osteochondral fragment determines management
    (E) premature osteoarthritis is a sequela

OCD is thought to be a sequela of a transchondral articular injury and might be better designated as an osteochondral defect or osteochondral lesion. Proposed etiologies for the condition include direct or indirect trauma, ischemic necrosis, ossification anomalies, and genetic predisposition. The suffix "-itis" suggests an inflammatory etiology; however, infection is not implicated as a cause of this disorder **(Option (A) is false).** By far the most tenable explanation is that OCD results from shearing, rotatory, or tangentially oriented impaction forces that cause an osteochondral fracture. When OCD is found in the patella, there may be a history of patellar subluxation and ligamentous laxity.

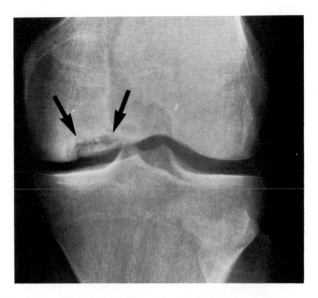

Figure 14-6. Osteochondritis dissecans of the medial femoral condyle. An anteroposterior radiograph of the knee shows a crescentic lucency (arrows) containing an irregular ovoid osteochondral fragment.

Approximately 75% of cases of OCD involve the posterolateral aspect of the medial femoral condyle (Figure 14-6) **(Option (C) is true).** Femoral OCD can be divided into five categories by site and degree of involvement: (1) focal involvement of the lateral aspect of the medial femoral condyle; (2) more extensive involvement of the medial femoral condyle, from its apex to the intracondylar notch; (3) inferocentral involvement of the most medial aspect of the medial femoral condyle; (4) involvement of the inferior and central portion of the lateral femoral condyle; and (5) involvement of the anterolateral aspect of the lateral femoral condyle. OCD also occurs in the patella, talar dome (Figure 14-7), capitellum of the humerus (Figure 14-8), tarsal bones, tibia, humeral head, and wrist.

Men have OCD of the femur more often than women do. Patients with OCD are usually 15 to 20 years of age at the time of onset of symptoms. OCD is rare in patients under 10 years of age **(Option (B) is false)** and is also extremely uncommon in persons over 50 years. Patients usually present with anterior knee pain and "locking," especially when the knee joint is in the flexed position. Although OCD of the femur may be asymptomatic at the time it is incidentally discovered on a radiograph, most patients have a history of recurrent swelling, stiffness, pain aggravated by movement, clicking, locking, or "giving way" of the knee. Physical examination may show a joint effusion, localized tender-

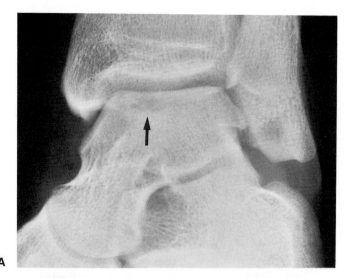

A

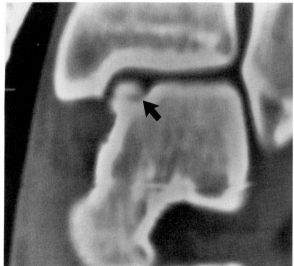

B

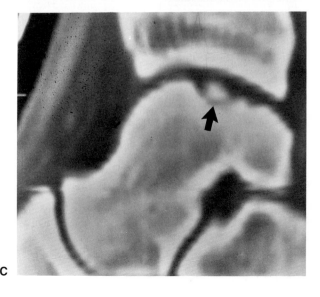

C

Figure 14-7. Osteochondritis dissecans of the talus. (A) An oblique radiograph of the ankle shows an ovoid radiolucency (arrow) in the talar dome. OCD in this location is typically difficult to detect. Reformatted coronal (B) and sagittal (C) CT images confirm the lesion and show its location, extent, and central osteochondral fragment (arrow) more clearly.

377

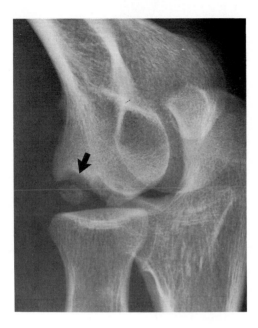

Figure 14-8. Osteochondritis dissecans of the capitellum. An oblique radiograph of the elbow shows OCD (arrow) of the capitellum.

ness, and muscle atrophy or weakness around the involved joint. Femoral OCD is bilateral in about 30% of cases.

The classic conventional radiographic features of OCD are a subchondral juxta-articular crescentic radiolucency with a border of sclerotic trabecular bone of varying thickness surrounding a subchondral ossified density. This "osteochondral fragment" may be attached to the adjacent epiphyseal cancellous bone and hence will be stable, or it may be mobile and unstable or even displaced within the joint. The mobile osteochondral fragment has also been termed a loose body or joint mouse (Figure 14-9).

Management and treatment of OCD are determined by the degree of stability of the osteochondral fragment **(Option (D) is true).** Stable lesions (those with no evidence of separation of the osteochondral fragment from the host bone) are treated nonoperatively by limitation of joint motion and by non-weight bearing for 6 to 12 weeks. If there is evidence that the osteochondral fragment has separated from the subarticular bone, arthroscopic or open surgery is used to debride the area, to remove any fragments that might become loose in the joint, and to stimulate healing. As a general rule, lesions smaller than 0.2 cm^2 are usually stable, whereas lesions larger than 0.8 cm^2 and those having a margin of sclerotic trabecular bone over 3 mm thick usually have a separated osteochondral fragment.

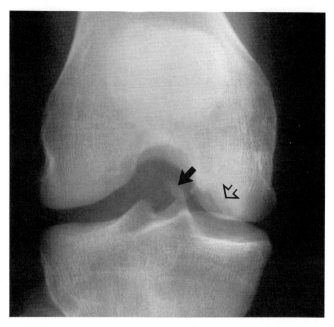

Figure 14-9. Osteochondritis dissecans of the femur with a detached fragment ("loose body"). Intercondylar notch (tunnel) radiograph of the knee shows a radiolucent donor site (open arrow) in the medial femoral condyle and a displaced osteochondral fragment (solid arrow) near the anterior tibial spine.

Conventional radiographs reliably demonstrate a grossly loose fragment. However, the presence of an ossified fragment within the lucent zone is not a foolproof indicator of stability. For example, a significant number of functionally loose *in situ* fragments appear to have an intact overlying articular cartilage. These partially attached fragments require drilling, surgical debridement, resection, or internal fixation. CT, arthrography, bone scintigraphy, and MRI have all been used to evaluate the stability of the osteochondral fragment. Of these, MRI may prove to be the most reliable.

The major advantage of MRI in imaging OCD is that it shows the discrete relationship of the subchondral fragment to the underlying host bone and adjacent hyaline cartilage without the need for intravenous or intra-articular injection of a contrast agent. The MR protocol should include both coronal and sagittal sections to allow for estimation of the three-dimensional size and shape of the lesion. In addition to T1-weighted images that define morphology, T2-weighted spin-echo or gradient-echo images are used to help predict fragment stability. The presence of a continuous high-intensity line or of high-intensity "cystic" areas

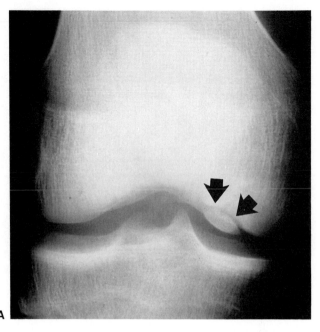

A

Figure 14-10. Osteochondral fragment. (A) An anteroposterior radiograph shows OCD of the medial femoral condyle (arrows). The stability of the fragment cannot be determined. (B) A T1-weighted sagittal MR image shows the low-intensity fragment within the donor site (arrows) but does not predict fragment stability. (C) A gradient-echo sagittal MR image shows a continuous high-intensity line between the osteochondral fragment and the native bone (solid arrows), as well as tiny "cysts" in the adjacent host bone (open arrow), suggesting instability.

between the osteochondral fragment and underlying bone on T2-weighted spin-echo or gradient-echo images correlates with instability. These high-intensity features are believed to represent granulation tissue or synovial fluid interposed between the osteochondral fragment and the donor site (Figure 14-10). The presence of normal-appearing articular cartilage surrounding the osteochondral fragment has not correlated with stability.

Adequate and reliable evaluation of the stability of osteochondral fragments has important prognostic implications. If not treated, partially attached, grossly loose, or fragmented osteochondral bodies may displace into the joint. Small particles may become a nidus for the development of larger loose bodies. The irregular articular cartilage and surface at the host site and the migrating osteochonrdal fragments predispose to premature osteoarthritis **(Option (E) is true).**

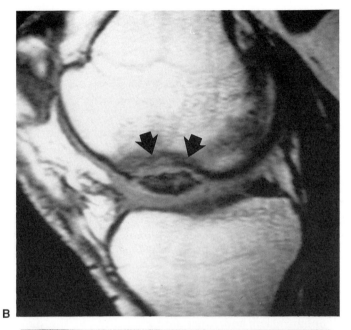

B

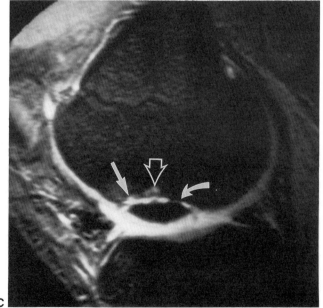

C

Question 62

Concerning lesions of the patella,

(A) chondromalacia patellae is the most common cause of pain
(B) chondromalacia patellae is best evaluated on T2-weighted spin-echo MR images
(C) medial patellar plicae are more likely than other plicae to be symptomatic
(D) acute dislocations are associated with fractures of the lateral patellar facet
(E) enchondroma is the most common primary tumor

The patella, a sesamoid bone arising in the quadriceps tendon, appears in the third month of gestation and is first evident on radiographs at about 3 years of age. The patella articulates with the anterior femoral metaepiphyseal surface. Its articular surface is divided into medial and lateral facets, each covered by hyaline articular cartilage. Generally, the lateral facet is larger than the medial facet. The patella functions as a spacer and pivot for the quadriceps extensor mechanism. As such, it is subject to large compressive forces during flexion and extension.

Chondromalacia patellae is a syndrome of patellofemoral pain caused by damage to the patellar articular cartilage. As a result of the anatomic configuration and functional capacities of the patellofemoral joint, even small aberrations of morphology or alignment can predispose to damage to the articular cartilage and subchondral bone. Chondromalacia patellae is a common cause of patellar pain **(Option (A) is true)**.

Chondromalacia patellae is usually diagnosed in adolescents and young adults. In older adults, the same syndrome is classified as osteoarthritis. The condition may be caused by direct or indirect trauma, patellar subluxation or dislocation, extensor mechanism malalignment, previous knee surgery, or prominence of the medial femoral condylar ridge (Outerbridge's ridge). The most common presenting complaints are anterior knee pain, swelling, retropatellar noise, and "giving way" of the knee. Clinical signs include lateral patellar tenderness, limping, knee joint effusion, crepitus with motion, and patellar malalignment. The gross morphologic changes in this condition are characterized by progressive stages of fibrillation, fissuring, and erosion of the patellar or femoral trochlear articular cartilages and subchondral bone. The diagnosis is suggested by the clinical history and physical findings and can be confirmed by arthroscopy.

Conventional radiographs are usually normal in chondromalacia patellae. As the condition progresses, axial views of the patellofemoral articulation, when obtained with various degrees of knee flexion, may show patellar malalignment and subluxation. However, even when these

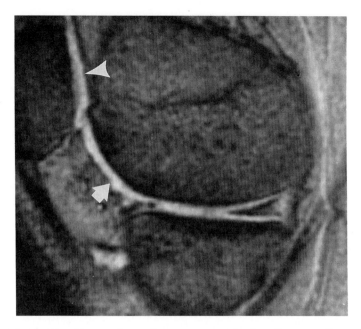

Figure 14-11. Gradient-echo pulse sequence for hyaline cartilage. A sagittal gradient-echo MR image shows high-intensity normal femoral (arrow) and patellar (arrowhead) articular cartilages.

findings are present, the radiographs do not reveal the status of the articular cartilage. Conventional arthrography and CT-arthrography have been used to evaluate the patellar articular cartilage. However, these arthrographic examinations are invasive and typically do not show early hyaline cartilage changes. Bone scintigraphy shows increased radiopharmaceutical uptake in up to 50% of cases, but the changes are nonspecific.

Recently, MRI has been evaluated as a diagnostic tool in patients with patellar pain. Because of its high protein and water content, hyaline cartilage can be depicted without the use of contrast agents. Adequate evaluation of the patellar cartilage requires imaging in both sagittal and coronal planes. Pulse sequences that maximize the differentiation of hyaline cartilage from subchondral bone and synovial fluid must be used. T1-weighted spin-echo, long-TR/short-TE (proton-density) spin-echo, or gradient-echo (Figure 14-11) pulse sequences are most useful. T1-weighted spin-echo sequences with fat suppression (Figure 14-12) have also shown promise. Normal cartilage has an intermediate-intensity pattern on T1-weighted spin-echo sequences and a relatively high-intensity pattern on T2-weighted spin-echo or gradient-echo sequences. In gen-

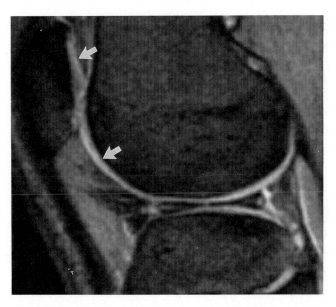

Figure 14-12. Fat-suppression technique for hyaline cartilage. A sagittal T1-weighted fat-suppression MR image shows high-intensity normal femoral and patellar articular cartilages (arrows).

eral, T2-weighted spin-echo imaging is not routinely used, because it does not adequately differentiate hyaline cartilage from joint fluid, and because it has a lower signal-to-noise ratio and requires a longer imaging time than T1-weighted imaging **(Option (B) is false).**

In the sagittal plane, the MR features of normal patellar cartilage include a uniform homogeneous signal pattern within the substance of the cartilage and a smooth, well-defined articular surface (Figure 14-13). On the axial projection, the homogeneous signal pattern within the substance of the cartilage is preserved and there is a well-defined low-intensity line between the apposed patellar and femoral trochlear cartilages (Figure 14-14). This junction line is an important indicator that a normal interface exists between the patellofemoral hyaline cartilages.

The signs of chondromalacia patellae on T1-weighted spin-echo sequences have been categorized according to the stage of the disease. Grade I changes, reflecting softening of hyaline cartilage, are not shown on MR images but are detected by arthroscopy. In grade II disease, the surface of the cartilage appears normal but low-intensity foci ("blisters") exist within the substance of the hyaline cartilage. These foci may extend to the surface of the cartilage (Figure 14-15). In grade III disease, the sharp interface between the patellar and femoral trochlear cartilages is focally lost and there may be decreased signal intensity within the car-

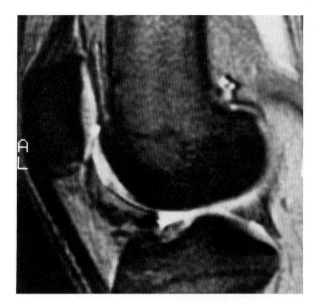

Figure 14-13 (left).
Normal patellar cartilage. A sagittal gradient-echo MR image shows a uniform-signal-pattern patellar cartilage with a smooth articular wall, characteristic features of normal patellar hyaline cartilage.

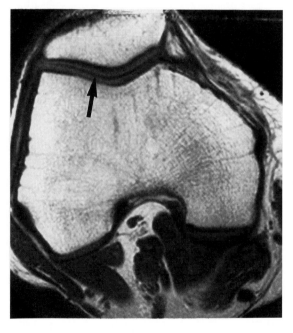

Figure 14-14 (right).
Normal patellar cartilage. An axial T1-weighted spin-echo image at the midpatella shows a smooth uniform low-intensity line (arrow) separating the patellar and femoral articular cartilages. This line represents the normal interface between the two cartilaginous surfaces.

tilage (Figure 14-16). The obliteration of the interface represents articular surface cartilage fibrillation, ulceration, and fragmentation. Grade IV disease is manifested by more numerous decreased-intensity foci, now extending from the cartilage surface to the subchondral bone. The carti-

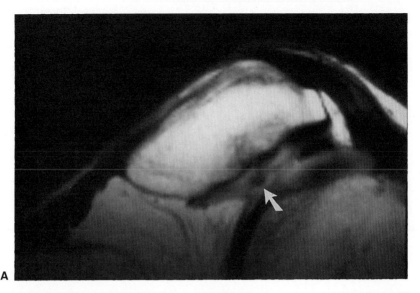

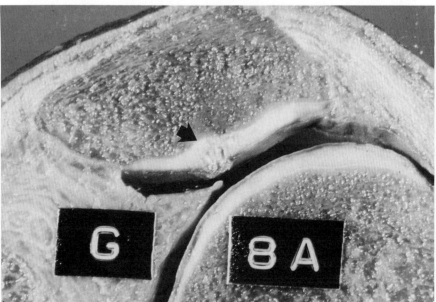

Figure 14-15. Grade II chondromalacia patellae. (A) A sagittal T1-weighted MR image of a cadaver knee shows a small focal area of abnormally decreased intensity within the hyaline cartilage (arrow) with a mild irregularity of the subjacent subchondral bone. (B) A sagittal anatomic section of the patella shown in panel A demonstrates a focal blisterlike lesion (arrow), which was filled with fibrillated vertical cartilage. (Reprinted with permission from Hayes et al. [43].)

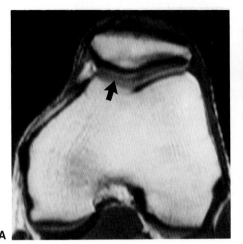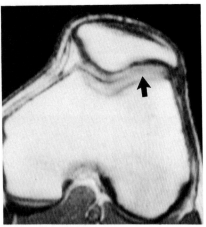

A   B

Figure 14-16. Grade III chondromalacia patellae. Axial T1-weighted spin-echo MR images from two patients with patellar pain show focal obliteration of the black junction lines (arrow) medially (A) in one patient and laterally (B) in the other.

lage is irregular and of nonuniform thickness. Decreased-intensity subchondral bone is found; this represents bony eburnation or sclerosis (Figure 14-17). Later, patellar and femoral osteophytes may be seen.

The therapeutic management of chondromalacia remains an enigma. In general, treatment should be directed toward correcting the underlying problem. However, the etiology is often multifactorial. For early cases, modification or limitation of activity produces the most consistent improvement. Other approaches include physical therapy to strengthen surrounding muscles, anti-inflammatory medications, knee bracing, and foot orthoses. It is generally believed that surgery should not be considered unless conservative methods have failed and results of surgical interventions have been disappointing. Arthroscopic surgery has been directed at shaving or drilling the articular cartilage to improve the motion between the contacting surfaces. Open surgery is aimed at improving biomechanical stability. Surgical procedures for improving biomechanics include tightening or loosening the patellar retinaculum, advancing the quadriceps muscle, pes transfer, tubercle transfer, or a combination of these.

Patellar plicae are another common cause of knee pain and symptoms that may mimic meniscal or chondral lesions, especially in children. Plicae are remnants of embryonic septations within the knee joint, which appear arthroscopically as synovial folds (Figure 14-18). There are three major plicae: (1) the suprapatellar plica; (2) the medial patellar plica, or

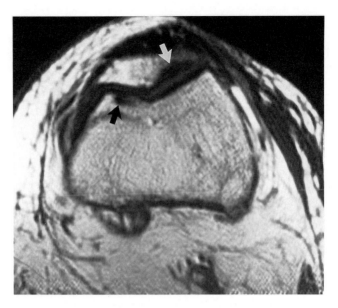

Figure 14-17. Grade IV chondromalacia patellae. An axial T1-weighted spin-echo MR image of a patient with severe osteoarthritis shows diffuse narrowing of the patellofemoral compartment, decreased signal intensity of the femoral and patellar cartilages, and subchondral low signal intensity (sclerosis) in the medial patellar facet (white arrow) and lateral femoral condyle (black arrow).

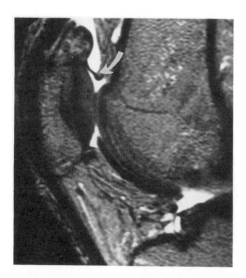

Figure 14-18. Suprapatellar plica. A sagittal T2-weighted MR image shows a low-intensity linear structure (arrow), the suprapatellar plica, outlined by a small suprapatellar joint effusion.

shelf; and (3) the infrapatellar plica, or ligamentum mucosum. The reported prevalence of patellar plicae varies, ranging from 5 to 55% of the population.

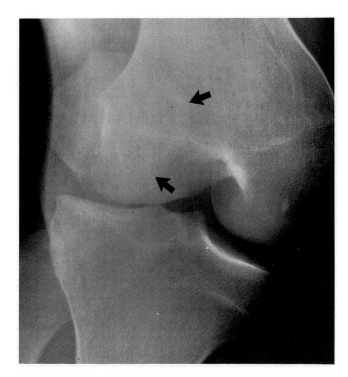

Figure 14-19. Acute dislocation of the patella. An anteroposterior radiograph following trauma shows lateral dislocation of the patella (arrows). The medial facet of the patella has locked against the lateral femoral condyle.

Patellar plicae may become thickened and inflamed. The medial patellar plica is the most likely to cause symptoms **(Option (C) is true).** The plica syndrome, consisting of snapping, "pseudolocking," crepitus, and aching with prolonged sitting or exercise, results from impingement of the medial patellar plica on the medial femoral condyle or from entrapment of the plica within the patellofemoral joint. Chondromalacia patellae and groove formation in the medial femoral condyle or medial patellar facet have also been attributed to thickened plicae. Normal suprapatellar plicae are commonly observed during MRI of the knee; however, most abnormal medial patellar plicae require arthroscopy for diagnosis. Initially, a symptomatic plica is treated conservatively with rest and anti-inflammatory drugs. If pain and disability continue, the plica is resected at arthroscopy.

Acute dislocations of the patella are most likely to occur during forced contraction of the quadriceps muscle when the knee is in a partly flexed and valgus position. Under these circumstances, the patella is pulled laterally so that its medial facet lies adjacent to the margin of the lateral femoral condyle (Figure 14-19). The dislocated patella may reduce spontaneously or lock in this lateral position. The most common sequela of acute patellar dislocation is chondral or osteochondral fracture of the medial patellar facet **(Option (D) is false).** This occurs because the

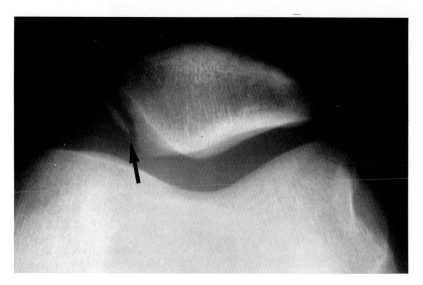

Figure 14-20. Osteochondral patellar fracture following patellar dislocation. A postreduction axial radiograph of the patella shows medial osteochondral fracture (arrow) with a linear fragment.

patella impacts on the lateral femoral condyle at the time of the dislocation (Figure 14-20). Often these injuries spontaneously reduce before
radiographs are acquired. Patellar osteochondral fracture fragments are
best seen on axial or internal oblique projections of the patella, and these
radiographs should be included during the workup of a patient with a
history of patellar dislocation.

Primary tumors of the patella are uncommon. In his review of 8,542
primary bone tumors, Dahlin encountered only 6 (0.07%) primary
tumors of the patella. A circumscribed lytic area with a variably sclerotic
margin is the most common radiographic feature of primary tumors of
the patella, but soft tissue masses, effusions, and patellar sclerosis also
occur. Most primary tumors of the patella are benign, and the most common of these is chondroblastoma (Figure 14-21) **(Option (E) is false).**
Giant cell tumor, aneurysmal bone cyst, solitary bone cyst, hemangioma,
osteochondroma, enchondroma, lipoma, osteoblastoma, lymphoma, hem-
angioendothelioma, angiosarcoma, and osteosarcoma have also been
found in the patella. However, most malignant lesions encountered in
the patella are metastases from extraosseous primary cancers. Because
of the pain and disability associated with any of these lesions, surgical
resection of the patella is usually performed.

Thomas L. Pope, Jr., M.D.
Lawrence W. Bassett, M.D.

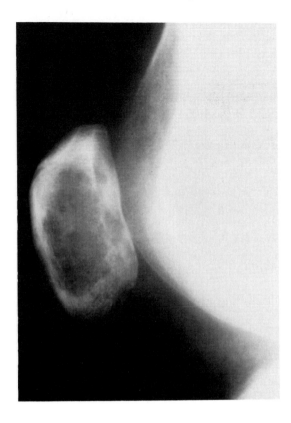

Figure 14-21. Chondro-
blastoma of the patella. A
lateral radiograph of the
knee shows a large radi-
olucent lesion with rela-
tively well marginated
borders occupying most of
the patella.

SUGGESTED READINGS

OSTEOCHONDRITIS DISSECANS

1. Clanton TO, DeLee JC. Osteochondritis dissecans. History, pathophysiology and current treatment concepts. Clin Orthop 1982; 167:50–64
2. Desai SS, Patel MR, Michelli LJ, Silver JW, Lidge RT. Osteochondritis dissecans of the patella. J Bone Joint Surg (Br) 1987; 69:320–325
3. De Smet AA, Fisher DR, Burnstein MI, Graf BK, Lange RH. Value of MR
   imaging in staging osteochondral lesions of the talus (osteochondritis
   dissecans): results in 14 patients. AJR 1990; 154:555–558
4. De Smet AA, Fisher DR, Graf BK, Lange RH. Osteochondritis dissecans of
   the knee: value of MR imaging in determining lesion stability and the
   presence of articular cartilage defects. AJR 1990; 155:549–553
5. Edwards DH, Bentley G. Osteochondritis dissecans patellae. J Bone Joint
   Surg (Br) 1977; 59:58–63
6. Howie JL. Computed tomography in osteochondritis dissecans of the
   patella. J Can Assoc Radiol 1985; 36:197–199
7. Hughston JC, Hergenroeder PT, Courtenay BG. Osteochondritis dissecans
   of the femoral condyles. J Bone Joint Surg (Am) 1984; 66:1340–1348

8. Mesgarzadeh M, Sapega AA, Bonakdarpour A, et al. Osteochondritis disse-cans: analysis of mechanical stability with radiography, scintigraphy, and MR imaging. Radiology 1987; 165:775–780

9. Nelson DW, DiPaola J, Colville M, Schmidgall J. Osteochondritis dissecans of the talus and knee: prospective comparison of MR and arthroscopic classifications. J Comput Assist Tomogr 1990; 14:804–808

10. Pfeiffer WH, Gross ML, Seeger LL. Osteochondritis dissecans of the patella. MRI evaluation and a case report. Clin Orthop 1991; 271:207–211

11. Schwarz C, Blazina ME, Sisto DJ, Hirsh LC. The results of operative treat-ment of osteochondritis dissecans of the patella. Am J Sports Med 1988; 16:522–529

BIPARTITE PATELLA

12. Lawson JP. Symptomatic radiographic variants in extremities. Radiology 1985; 157:625–631

13. Lawson JP. Not-so-normal variants. Orthop Clin North Am 1990; 21:483–495

14. Weaver JK. Bipartite patellae as a cause of disability in the athlete. Am J Sports Med 1977; 5:137–143

CHONDROMALACIA PATELLAE

15. Bentley G. Articular cartilage changes in chondromalacia patellae. J Bone Joint Surg (Br) 1985; 67:769–774

16. Bentley G, Dowd G. Current concepts of etiology and treatment of chondro-malacia patellae. Clin Orthop 1984; 189:209–228

17. Christensen F, Sballe K, Snerum L. Treatment of chondromalacia patellae by lateral retinacular release of the patella. Clin Orthop 1988; 234:145–147

18. Cox JS. Patellofemoral problems in runners. Clin Sports Med 1985; 4:699–715

19. Ficat RP, Philippe J, Hungerford DS. Chondromalacia patellae: a system of classification. Clin Orthop 1979; 144:55–62

20. Hille E, Schulitz KP, Henrichs C, Schneider T. Pressure and contact-surface measurements within the femoropatellar joint and their variations fol-lowing lateral release. Arch Orthop Trauma Surg 1985; 104:275–282

21. Huberti HH, Hayes WC. Contact pressures in chondromalacia and the effects of capsular reconstructive procedures. J Orthop Res 1988; 6:499–508

22. Insall J. Current concepts review: patellar pain. J Bone Joint Surg (Am) 1982; 64:147–152

23. Kohn HS, Guten GN, Collier BD, Veluvolu P, Whalen JP. Chondromalacia of the patella: bone imaging correlated with arthroscopic findings. Clin Nucl Med 1988; 13:96–98

24. Meachim G. Age-related degeneration of patellar articular cartilage. J Anat 1982; 134:365–371

25. Outerbridge RE. The etiology of chondromalacia patellae. J Bone Joint Surg (Br) 1961; 43:752–757

26. Unneberg K, Reikeras O. The effect of lateral retinacular release in idiopathic chondromalacia patellae. Arch Orthop Trauma Surg 1988; 107:226–227

27. Zorman D, Prezerowitz L, Pasteels JL, Burny F. Arthroscopic treatment of posttraumatic chondromalacia patellae. Orthopedics 1990; 13:585–588

DORSAL DEFECT

28. Goergen TG, Resnick D, Greenway G, Saltzstein SL. Dorsal defect of the patella (DDP): a characteristic radiographic lesion. Radiology 1979; 130:333–336

29. Haswell DM, Berne AS, Graham CB. The dorsal defect of the patella. Pediatr Radiol 1976; 4:238–242

OSTEOID OSTEOMA

30. Dahlin DC, Unni KK. Bone tumors: general aspects and data on 8,542 cases, 4th ed. Springfield, Ill: Charles C Thomas; 1986:88–101

31. Kransdorf MJ, Stull MA, Gilkey FW, Moser RP Jr. Osteoid osteoma. RadioGraphics 1991; 11:671–696

PLICAE

32. Lupi L, Bighi S, Cervi PM, Limone GL, Massari L. Arthrography of the plica syndrome and its significance. Eur J Radiol 1990; 11:15–18

33. Ogata S, Uhthoff HK. The development of synovial plicae in human knee joints: an embryologic study. Arthroscopy 1990; 6:315–321

34. Patel D. Plica as a cause of anterior knee pain. Orthop Clin North Am 1986; 17:273–277

TRAUMA

35. Gilley JS, Gelman MI, Edson DM, Metcalf RW. Chondral fractures of the knee. Arthrographic, arthroscopic, and clinical manifestations. Radiology 1981; 138:51–54

36. Kennedy JC, Grainger RW, McGraw RW. Osteochondral fractures of the femoral condyles. J Bone Joint Surg (Br) 1966; 48:436–440

37. Milgram JW, Rogers LF, Miller JW. Osteochondral fractures: mechanisms of injury and fate of fragments. AJR 1978; 130:651–658

38. Rogers LF. Radiology of skeletal trauma, vol 2, 2nd ed. New York: Churchill Livingstone; 1992:1257–1281

PATELLAR TUMORS

39. Ehara S, Khurana JS, Kattapuram SV, Rosenburg AE, el-Khoury GY, Rosenthal DI. Osteolytic lesions of the patella. AJR 1989; 153:103–106

40. Kransdorf MJ, Moser RP Jr, Vinh TN, Aoki J, Callaghan JJ. Primary tumors of the patella. A review of 42 cases. Skeletal Radiol 1989; 18:365–371

41. Moser RP Jr, Brockmole DM, Vinh TN, Kransdorf MJ, Aoki J. Chondroblastoma of the patella. Skeletal Radiol 1988; 17:413–419

MRI

42. Chandnani VP, Ho C, Chu P, Trudell D, Resnick D. Knee hyaline cartilage evaluated with MR imaging: a cadaveric study involving multiple imaging sequences and intraarticular injection of gadolinium and saline solution. Radiology 1991; 178:557–561
43. Hayes CW, Sawyer RW, Conway WF. Patellar cartilage lesions: *in vitro* detection and staging with MR imaging and pathologic correlation. Radiology 1990; 176:479–483
44. König H, Sauter R, Deimling M, Vogt M. Cartilage disorders: comparison of spin-echo, CHESS, and FLASH sequence MR images. Radiology 1987; 164:753–758
45. Lynch TC, Crues JV III, Morgan FW, Sheehan WE, Harter LP, Ryu R. Bone abnormalities of the knee: prevalence and significance at MR imaging. Radiology 1989; 171:761–766
46. Mink JH, Deutsch AL. Occult cartilage and bone injuries of the knee: detection, classification, and assessment with MR imaging. Radiology 1989; 170:823–829
47. Reiser MF, Bongartz G, Erlemann R, et al. Magnetic resonance in cartilaginous lesions of the knee joint with three-dimensional gradient-echo imaging. Skeletal Radiol 1988; 17:465–471
48. Totterman S, Weiss SL, Szumowski J, et al. MR fat suppression technique in the evaluation of normal structures of the knee. J Comput Assist Tomogr 1989; 13:473–479
49. Vellet AD, Marks PH, Fowler PJ, Munro TG. Occult posttraumatic osteochondral lesions of the knee: prevalence, classification, and short-term sequelae evaluated with MR imaging. Radiology 1991; 178:271–276
50. Wojtys E, Wilson M, Buckwalter K, Braunstein E, Martel W. Magnetic resonance imaging of knee hyaline cartilage and intraarticular pathology. Am J Sports Med 1987; 15:455–463
51. Yulish BS, Montanez J, Goodfellow DB, Bryan PJ, Mulopulos GP, Modic MT. Chondromalacia patellae: assessment with MR imaging. Radiology 1987; 164:763–766

Notes

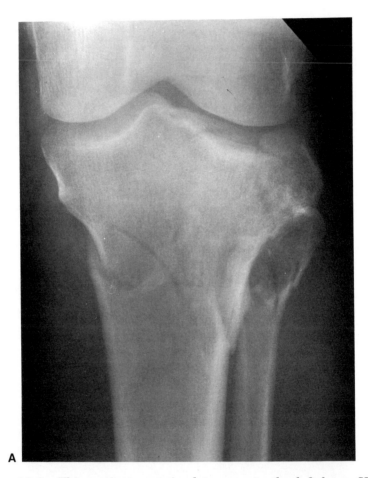

A

Figure 15-1. This patient sustained trauma to the left knee. You are shown anteroposterior (A) and lateral (B) radiographs of the knee.

Case 15: Tibial Plateau Fracture

Question 63

Concerning the injury to the test patient,

   (A) the fracture affects only the lateral tibial plateau and fibula
   (B) the lateral collateral ligament is likely to be ruptured
   (C) closed treatment by traction and early motion should not be used
   (D) an associated distal fibular fracture is likely
   (E) knee instability is a likely long-term complication of inadequate treatment

The test images (Figure 15-1) consist of an anteroposterior radiograph and a slightly oblique lateral radiograph of the left knee. Together, they reveal a fracture of the lateral tibial condyle. This fracture consists of a minimally displaced, vertically cleaved component and a compressed articular segment (Figure 15-2). There is also a mildly comminuted fracture of the fibula. The tibial fracture also has a secondary transverse component that extends across the metaphyseal-diaphyseal junction. The fracture thus involves more than just the lateral tibial plateau and the fibula **(Option (A) is false).**

Tibial plateau fractures account for approximately 1% of all fractures and 8% of fractures in the elderly. The typical mechanism for a tibial plateau fracture is a valgus stress or, less commonly, a varus stress applied with a variable amount of axial loading. Kennedy and Bailey, using cadaver knees, were able to reproduce clinical fracture patterns with controlled axial and varus or valgus stresses. The most frequent result of the application of these forces was either a fracture or a ligamentous tear, but not both. The postulated mechanism of injury requires an intact collateral ligament that initially stabilizes the condyle, which subsequently fractures. The medial collateral ligament, for instance, acts as a hinge, allowing the lateral femoral condyle to be forced into the lateral tibial condyle and hence creating a lateral tibial plateau fracture. If the force persists after the fracture occurs, the medial collateral ligament may then tear. Valgus stress, the most common traumatic force that produces this type of fracture, is more likely to lead to a tear of the medial

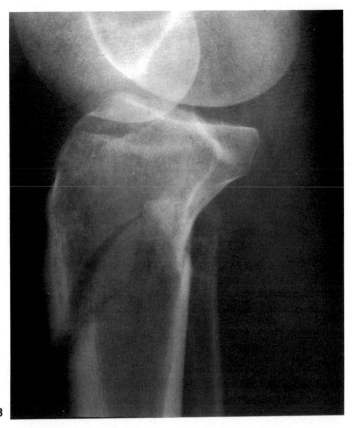

B

collateral ligament than of the lateral collateral ligament. Hence, rupture of the lateral collateral ligament is not likely to be an associated feature of the test patient's injury **(Option (B) is false)**. Lateral tibial plateau fractures typically result from auto-pedestrian or auto accidents. Falls from heights, slipping and twisting injuries, and other accidents may also cause these fractures.

Fractures of the tibial condyles have been organized into several classification schemes by different authors. For the purposes of this discussion they fall into several major groups: the vertical split fracture, the pure compression fracture, the combination of split and compression fractures, and the bicondylar fracture. About 55 to 70% involve the lateral plateau, about 10 to 23% involve the medial plateau, and 11 to 31% involve both plateaus. The various types are represented in the classification of Moore and Hohl (Figure 15-3).

Minimally displaced fractures are those with less than 4 mm of displacement or depression. They comprise about 25% of all tibial plateau fractures and usually do well with nonoperative treatment. The local

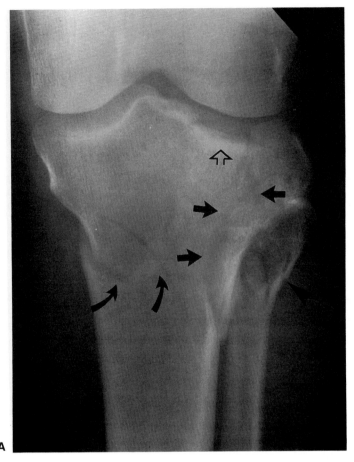

A

Figure 15-2 (Same as Figure 15-1). Tibial and fibular fractures. The tibial fracture has the following components: a minimally displaced vertical component (straight arrows), a compressed articular segment (open arrow), and a transverse metaphyseal component (curved arrows). The proximal fibula is also fractured (arrowhead).

compression (or depression) type of fracture affects the central part of the lateral plateau, usually causing a mosaic-like pattern of comminution. Those in the anterior part of the plateau are usually depressed no more than 6 to 7 mm, whereas those lying more posteriorly may be depressed up to 10 to 30 mm. They comprise about half of all tibial plateau fractures.

Split compression-type fractures affect the lateral plateau, comprise only about 6% of all plateau fractures, and produce a wedge-shaped articular fragment that is displaced laterally and a more central depression fracture of the articular surface. They are occasionally associated

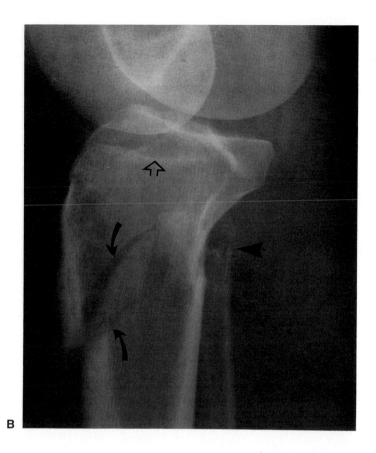

B

with cruciate ligament or medial collateral ligament injuries. Adequate treatment depends on restoring and maintaining support of the lateral tibial condyle, usually requiring open reduction and internal fixation.

The total condylar or total depression-type fracture comprises 6% of all plateau fractures, is usually medial, and usually results in some comminution of the metaphyseal cortex where the fracture line exits inferiorly. Because it affects the medial plateau, little or no articular surface depression can be tolerated, so adequate treatment depends on restoring the surface to near anatomic position either by closed or open treatment.

The bicondylar-type fracture comprises about 15% of plateau fractures and may have a T-, Y-, or V-shaped configuration. It has a higher frequency of meniscal injuries than do other types but rarely causes ligamentous injury. It occasionally results in a shattered comminution of the proximal tibia.

Schatzker's classification (Figure 15-4) is quite similar to that of Moore and Hohl but adds an additional type. The Schatzker Type I is a wedge or split fracture of the lateral condyle that occurs most commonly

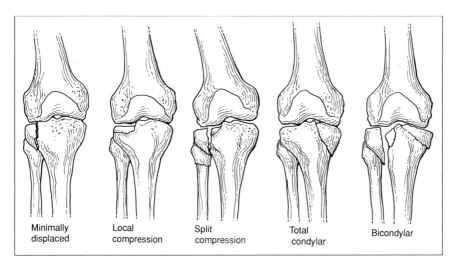

Figure 15-3. Moore and Hohl classification of tibial plateau fractures. The different types are discussed in more detail in the text. (Reprinted with permission from Hohl and Moore [4].)

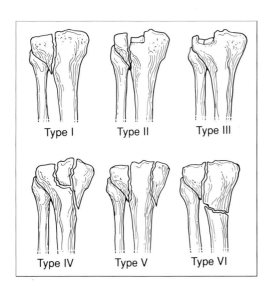

Figure 15-4. Schatzker's classification of tibial plateau fractures. This classification is very similar to the Moore and Hohl classification but adds the Type VI fracture. It is discussed in more detail in the text. (Reprinted with permission from Schatzker et al. [7].)

in young people. Type II is a split depression fracture of the lateral plateau typically occurring in older, osteoporotic patients. Type III is a pure depression fracture of the central part of the lateral plateau. Type IV is a split or a split depression fracture of the medial tibial plateau. This type requires greater force than the typical lateral plateau fractures and often involves rupture of the lateral collateral ligament or damage to cruciate ligaments, the peroneal nerve, or the popliteal artery. Type V is a bicondylar split fracture typically resulting from axial loading.

Schatzker's Type VI is not represented in the Moore and Hohl classification. This type includes a transverse subcondylar fracture that separates the condyles from the diaphysis. Many of these are associated with depression or split depression fractures of one or both articular surfaces. The fracture in the test case is a Schatzker Type VI because of the transverse metaphyseal fracture.

Split-type fractures are more likely to occur in younger patients, who have normally mineralized bone. Compression-type fractures are more likely to occur in older patients with underlying osteoporosis.

Treatment options for tibial plateau fractures fall into three general categories: traction and early motion, reduction and casting, and operative reduction with internal fixation. Many fractures may be treated successfully with traction and early motion; however, this is not an option in the test patient because traction would cause distraction of the associated diaphyseal-metaphyseal fracture line **(Option (C) is true).**

Fibular fractures may be associated with tibial condylar fractures, but they are usually related to the same forces that cause the tibial fracture. Therefore, the companion fracture involves the proximal fibula rather than the distal fibula **(Option (D) is false).** There is no force acting to separate the tibia from the fibula. Hence, no energy is dissipated along the interosseous membrane and the distal fibula is not affected.

Major sequelae of tibial condylar fractures evident in the knee joint include instability, deformity, posttraumatic arthritis, and loss of range of motion. Hohl, in an evaluation of 445 patients, estimated that instability of the knee develops in approximately 30% of patients by 2 years after the fracture **(Option (E) is true).** He further stated that knee instability results when an articular fracture fragment heals below its normal articular level or when torn collateral ligaments heal with excessive length and residual laxity. The frequency of posttraumatic arthritis may be as high as 20% after 2 years and 50% at 15 years. Chronic instability contributes to the development of osteoarthritis.

Question 64

Concerning complications of tibial plateau fractures,

    (A) popliteal artery damage is likely
    (B) peroneal nerve palsy occurs in about 5% of cases
    (C) the medial collateral ligament is the most commonly torn ligament
    (D) tears of the menisci are unlikely
    (E) there is a high frequency of nonunion

Complications of tibial plateau fractures parallel the extent and type of injury. Fractures that involve the medial condyle or both condyles indicate a more severe injury and are more likely to have associated injuries than are those limited to the lateral condyle. Development of an anterior compartment syndrome is one possible complication. Popliteal artery injury is another possible complication, but, fortunately, arterial injuries are extremely uncommon **(Option (A) is false).**

Peroneal nerve palsy occurs in up to 5% of patients with a proximal tibial fracture **(Option (B) is true).** This injury may be due to direct trauma or to stretching of the nerve during the injury. The peroneal nerve runs in close association with the head of the fibula near the proximal tibiofibular joint, and so it is at risk for injury during valgus stress. Such injuries frequently accompany a fibular fracture. The peroneal nerve may also be damaged during treatment. Fortunately, in most cases the nerve injury is self-limited and recovery of neurologic function can be expected.

Tibial condyle fractures are associated with ligament injuries frequently enough to merit evaluation of the several knee ligaments in these patients. The number of documented ligament injuries reported varies with the diligence and skill of the observer. MRI may assist in this determination and make ligament assessment easier in the future. Ligament injuries most commonly involve the medial collateral ligament and less commonly involve the anterior cruciate or lateral collateral ligaments. Medial collateral ligament injury is most commonly associated with a lateral condyle fracture (valgus injury), and lateral collateral ligament injury is most commonly associated with a medial condyle fracture (varus injury). Lateral fractures are more common than medial fractures, making medial collateral ligament injuries more common than lateral collateral ligament injuries **(Option (C) is true).** In fact, medial collateral ligament tears are reported to occur in 10 to 30% of cases.

Anterior cruciate ligament tears are uncommon in isolation. They are usually combined with medial collateral ligament tears, and the combination portends a poor outcome.

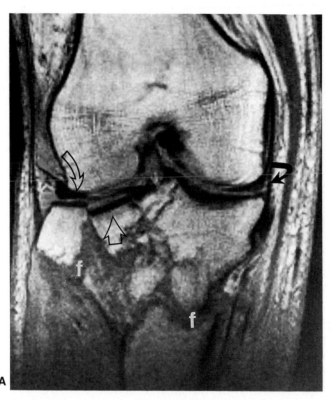

Figure 15-5. MRI of type VI tibial condyle fracture. (A) A coronal T1-weighted MR image of a fractured proximal tibia shows that the lateral meniscus (open curved arrow) has migrated laterally, maintaining its relationship to a displaced tibial condyle articular fragment. The fracture lines (f) are identified as decreased-intensity lines between higher-intensity fragments. The compressed articular segment (open straight arrow) is well demonstrated. The medial collateral ligament (black curved arrow) remains intact. (B) A sagittal T1-weighted MR image shows an increased-intensity dot within the posterior horn of the lateral meniscus (black arrow), which may represent a meniscal substance injury. A fat-fluid level (white arrow) is demonstrated in the joint, consistent with a lipohemarthrosis. The fracture lines (f) and multiple condylar fragments are again clearly visible.

Tears of the menisci have been reported to occur in 10 to 20% of tibial condyle fractures **(Option (D) is false).** There may be separation of the meniscus from the joint capsule or vertical, horizontal, or complex intra-substance tears. Occasionally, the meniscus is driven down into the fracture, and in that location it interferes with fracture reduction. MRI is not yet a fully established technique for evaluating complete plateau frac-

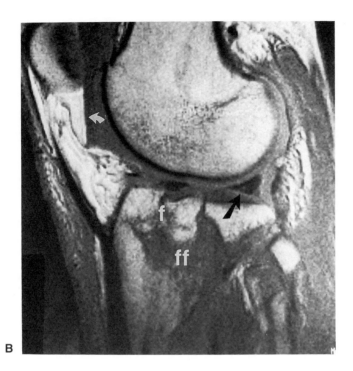

B

tures, but it is known to be effective for demonstration of meniscal tears and displacement (Figure 15-5).

Nonunion of tibial condyle fractures is extremely rare **(Option (E) is false),** but malunion is common. Fractures that split the condyle(s) are more likely to result in malunion secondary to loss of prior reduction. Loss of reduction occurs most commonly in bicondylar fractures. In patients with compression-type fractures, avascular necrosis of individual fracture fragments may develop.

Question 65

Concerning the treatment of tibial plateau fractures,

    (A) nonoperative treatment of uncomplicated fractures with less than 4 mm of displacement yields good results

    (B) residual varus deformity correlates with a poor functional result

    (C) collateral ligament tears usually heal well with nonoperative treatment by immobilization

    (D) cast immobilization of the knee joint for 8 to 12 weeks is required to ensure solid bony union

    (E) open reduction is required in less than 25% of patients

The treatment of tibial plateau fractures is directed toward returning knee alignment, stability, and range of motion to normal or as close to normal as possible. Fractures with less than 4 mm of articular-surface depression or displacement are considered minimally displaced fractures in the classification of Moore and Hohl. By this classification, minimally dispaced fractures can have any fracture configuration; approximately 20% of tibial condyle fractures in their series fell into the minimally displaced category.

The major determinant of whether a minimally displaced fracture requires surgery is the detection of instability. Instability is usually defined as more than 5° of varus or valgus deformity resulting from stress applied through the range of flexion and extension. Stable fractures in this group have an excellent prognosis when treated by closed reduction **(Option (A) is true).**

The surgeon's decision on how to best treat a tibial plateau fracture is based on many features including characteristics of the patient as well as the fracture. The patient's age, general health, occupation, and expectations as to function may affect the decision. In general, the goal is to restore and maintain normal alignment and stability to the knee. How this is achieved depends on the nature of the fracture and the quality of the bone. Local compression (depression) fractures of the lateral plateau commonly are treated surgically to elevate the articular surface when there is 8 to 10 mm of depression. Fractures with less than 6 to 8 mm of articular-surface depression have a good prognosis following either surgery or closed reduction. However, less depression is acceptable when the fracture involves the medial plateau. On the medial side, if there is more than about 5 mm of depression, operative treatment is usually chosen.

Angular deformity of the leg following fracture reduction may result from failure to attain or maintain correct tibial articular levels. Either varus or valgus deformity may result from tibial plateau fractures. Varus deformity is associated with medial condylar or bicondylar fractures, whereas valgus deformity is more likely with the more common lateral condylar fractures. Either of these complications may result in joint instability and eventual osteoarthritis. Genu valgum is somewhat better tolerated than genu varum. Early studies by Rasmussen showed that 56% of knees with greater than 10° of valgus deformity developed osteoarthritis, whereas essentially all knees with greater than 10° of varus deformity developed osteoarthritis. Varus deformity may ultimately require tibial osteotomy to restore alignment or joint replacement to relieve pain and restore function **(Option (B) is true)**.

The knee has a relatively rich blood supply, and ligaments and meniscal injuries usually heal well. Anterior cruciate ligament tears are repaired primarily only if the injury is of the avulsion type, in which case the attached bone fragment may be reaffixed to the host bone. Intrasubstance cruciate ligament tears are not repaired initially since healing requires prolonged immobilization. This interferes with the more important goal of early mobilization of the joint.

Operative treatment is currently recommended for collateral ligament tears if there is demonstrable knee instability. Failure to repair the collateral ligaments properly may result in a lax or abnormally long ligament, which in turn results in chronic knee instability **(Option (C) is false)**. Osteoarthritis subsequently occurs.

Salvage of the menisci is recommended if at all possible. It is theorized that the menisci help mold the injured joint as well as cushion it. Meniscal retention theoretically prevents early osteoarthritis.

The goal of treatment is to obtain a stable knee without osteoarthritis. This may be accomplished by a variety of methods, depending on the type of fracture. These methods include closed reduction and traction, percutaneous fixation, and operative reduction and internal fixation. Some fractures may be treated by arthroscopy as an adjunctive technique.

A cast or cast brace may be used for some fractures, but only as a temporary measure. Current approaches recognize that intra-articular fractures result in exuberant fibrous proliferation within the joint, which can result in extreme joint stiffness. Therefore, early mobilization has become a major treatment goal. The period of immobilization should be as short as possible without jeopardizing reduction. Passive range-of-motion physical therapy is started as soon as possible and is followed by active motion. Schatzker recommends using a passive-motion machine as soon as it can be tolerated. Weight bearing may be begun as early as 8 weeks by patients with uncomplicated fractures but may be deferred to 10 to 12 weeks by those with more complex fractures. Immobilization for so long would be extremely undesirable **(Option (D) is false)**.

Open reduction is recommended when closed reduction cannot be accomplished or maintained, when there is major ligament damage, or when the joint is unstable. Open fractures, which occur 1 to 3% of the time, require irrigation, debridement, and subsequent management based on the fracture type. Vascular injuries or compartment syndromes usually require operative intervention. Currently, approximately 50% of tibial plateau fractures are treated operatively **(Option (E) is false).**

William A. Fajman, M.D.
Terry M. Hudson, M.D.

SUGGESTED READINGS

GENERAL

1. Bowes DN, Hohl M. Tibial condylar fractures. Evaluation of treatment and outcome. Clin Orthop 1982; 171:104–108
2. Burri C, Bartzke G, Coldewey J, Muggler E. Fractures of the tibial plateau. Clin Orthop 1979; 138:84–93
3. Hohl M. Fractures of the proximal tibia and fibula. In: Rockwood CA, Green RP, Buchholz RW (eds), Rockwood and Green's fractures in adults. Philadelphia: JB Lippincott; 1991:1725–1751
4. Hohl M, Moore TM. Articular fractures of the proximal tibia. In: Evarts CM (ed), Surgery of the musculoskeletal system. New York: Churchill Livingstone; 1983:3471–3496
5. Kennedy JC, Bailey WH. Experimental tibial-plateau fractures. Studies of the mechanism and a classification. J Bone Joint Surg (Am) 1968; 50:1522–1534
6. Schatzker J. Tibial plateau fractures. In: Browner BD, Jupiter JB, Levine AM, Trafton PG (eds), Skeletal trauma. Philadelphia: WB Saunders; 1992:1745–1769
7. Schatzker J, McBroom R, Bruce D. The tibial plateau fracture. The Toronto experience 1968–1975. Clin Orthop 1979; 138:94–104

COMPLICATIONS

8. Delamarter RB, Hohl M, Hopp E. Ligament injuries associated with tibial plateau fractures. Clin Orthop 1990; 250:226–233
9. Kettelkamp DB, Hillberry BM, Murrish DE, Heck DA. Degenerative arthritis of the knee secondary to fracture malunion. Clin Orthop 1988; 234:159–169
10. Moore TM, Meyers MH, Harvey JP Jr. Collateral ligament laxity of the knee. Long-term comparison between plateau fractures and normal. J Bone Joint Surg (Am) 1976; 58:594–598
11. Rasmussen PS. Tibial condylar fractures as a cause of degenerative arthritis. Acta Orthop Scand 1972; 43:566–575

TREATMENT

12. Caspari RB, Hutton PM, Whipple TL, Meyers JF. The role of arthroscopy in the management of tibial plateau fractures. Arthroscopy 1985; 1:76–82
13. Delamarter R, Hohl M. The cast brace and tibial plateau fractures. Clin Orthop 1989; 242:26–31
14. Duwelius PJ, Connolly JF. Closed reduction of tibial plateau fractures. Clin Othop 1988; 230:116–126
15. Gausewitz S, Hohl M. The significance of early motion in the treatment of tibial plateau fractures. Clin Orthop 1986; 202:135–138
16. Hohl M. Managing the challenge of tibial plateau fractures. J Musculoskel Med 1991; 8:70–86
17. Jennings JE. Arthroscopic management of tibial plateau fractures. Arthroscopy 1985; 1:160–168
18. Lachiewicz PF, Funcik T. Factors influencing the results of open reduction and internal fixation of tibial plateau fractures. Clin Orthop 1990; 259:210–215
19. Moore TM, Patzakis MJ, Harvey JP. Tibial plateau fractures: definition, demographics, treatment rationale, and long-term results of closed traction management or operative reduction. J Orthop Trauma 1987; 1:97–119

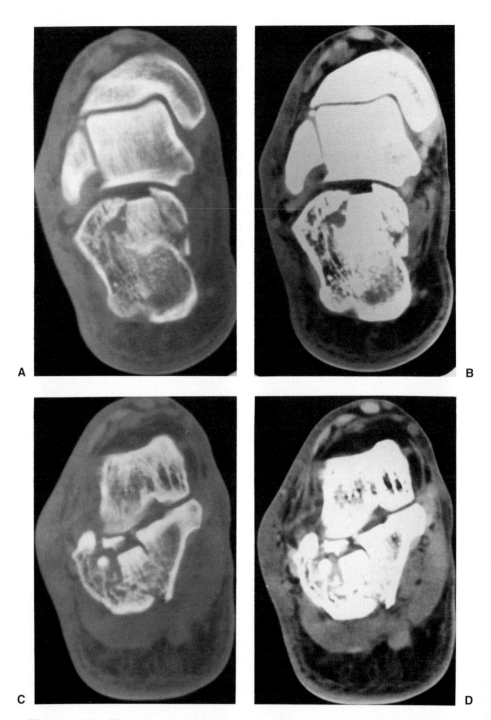

Figure 16-1. This 36-year-old man injured his right foot while under the influence of alcohol. You are shown direct coronal CT scans displayed with bone and soft tissue windows of the ankle (A and B) and hind foot (C and D).

Case 16: Calcaneal Fractures

Question 66

Concerning the injury to the test patient,

    (A) the fracture involves both the posterior and middle calcaneal articular facets
    (B) peroneal tendinitis is likely to develop
    (C) subtalar osteoarthritis is a likely complication
    (D) forced dorsiflexion was the mechanism of injury
    (E) assessment for possible vertebral fracture is appropriate

The CT images of the test patient (Figure 16-1) show a comminuted fracture of the calcaneus. The posterior facet of the calcaneus is fractured and divided into three major fragments (Figure 16-2A). These fragments are impacted into the body of the calcaneus, with resultant spreading of the sides of the calcaneus. There is obvious incongruity of the posterior facet articular surface as a result of the variable displacement of the fragments. The middle calcaneal facet supported by the sustentaculum tali is spared (Figure 16-2C) **(Option (A) is false).**

The peroneal tendons are visible just inferior to the tip of the lateral malleolus. Careful inspection shows that the tendons are pinched between the fibula and the laterally displaced calcaneal fracture fragment (Figure 16-2B and D). Such impingement may lead to peroneal tendinitis. Rosenberg and colleagues reviewed CT examinations of calcaneal fractures and showed that 22 of 24 patients with intra-articular fracture had acute abnormalities of the peroneal tendons. In order of frequency, peroneal tendon abnormalities included lateral displacement (58%), impingement by fragments (33%), subluxation or dislocation (25%), surrounding masses of either scar or hematoma (25%), and entrapment between the calcaneus and fibula (13%). Impingement by bony fragments correlated well with subsequent development of tenosynovitis **(Option (B) is true).** Peroneal tenosynovitis results in pain, swelling, and tenderness along the course of the tendons, as well as weakness, which may result in involuntary inversion of the foot. This may lead to lateral instability, twisting, or repeated sprains.

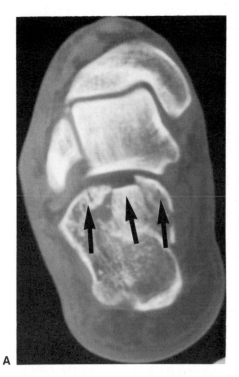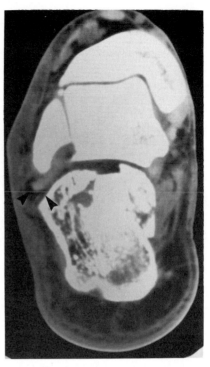

A B

Figure 16-2 (Same as Figure 16-1).   Calcaneal fracture. (A) A bone-windowed direct coronal CT section through the ankle and subtalar joints
shows a comminuted fracture of the calcaneus with three major posterior
calcaneal facet articular fragments (arrows). (B) A soft tissue-windowed
CT section (same as panel A) shows peroneal tendons (arrowheads) entrapped between the tip of the lateral malleolus and the lateral calcaneal
fracture fragment. (C) A bone-windowed direct coronal CT section
through the sustentaculum tali (S), middle subtalar joint (arrow), and
middle calcaneal facet shows a comminuted fracture of the lateral half of
the calcaneus but no fracture of the sustentaculum tali or medial facet.
(D) A soft tissue-windowed CT section (same as panel C) shows displaced
peroneal tendons (arrowheads) surrounded by swollen soft tissues.

Intra-articular fractures of the calcaneus are disabling injuries, and
their treatment remains somewhat controversial. Choices of treatment
include (1) aggressive open reduction and internal fixation and (2) conservative closed reduction and casting. Historically, either subtalar or
triple arthrodesis was the initial treatment, but this surgical approach is
no longer the treatment of choice.

The results of treatment are difficult to evaluate because of the lack
of a uniform classification scheme for these fractures and because of the
different measures of outcome used to assess the effectiveness of treat-

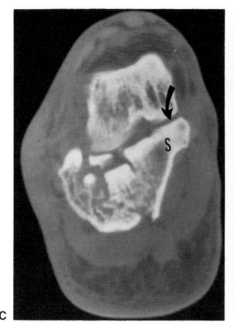
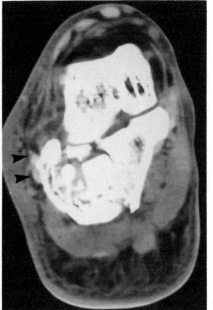

C   D

ment. However, there are several well-accepted causes of long-term disability. One of the major causes is the inability to obtain or the failure to hold adequate reduction, leading to subtalar osteoarthritis. Because of the extensive damage to the subtalar joint, subtalar osteoarthritis is likely to develop in the test patient **(Option (C) is true)**. Posttraumatic osteoarthritis is manifested by pain in the subtalar region referable to the sinus tarsi.

Prolonged disability due to peroneal tenosynovitis has been discussed above. Another complication is formation of bone spurs on the plantar aspect of the calcaneus, which may cause pain. Less common disabilities include pain from abutment of the widened calcaneus against the fibula, entrapment of the medial or lateral plantar branches of the posterior tibial nerve medially, and entrapment of the sural nerve laterally.

The mechanism of injury in the calcaneal fracture in the test patient was through axial and shear forces applied to the calcaneus at the crucial angle of Gissane (see below), with resultant involvement of the posterior facet. This usually results from a high-impact or jumping injury in which the calcaneus is driven upward into the lateral process of the talus **(Option (D) is false)**. In contrast, forced dorsiflexion of the ankle is more likely to fracture the talar neck.

Other musculoskeletal injuries occur in association with calcaneal fractures. Up to 30% of patients with a calcaneal fracture demonstrate other injuries of the ipsilateral limb, and 9% of calcaneal fractures are bilateral. An association is also noted with compression injuries of the spine, typically in the lumbar region. Compression fractures of vertebral bodies are reported in up to 10% of patients with calcaneal fractures **(Option (E) is true).**

Question 67

Concerning the subtalar joint,

    (A) the sinus tarsi separates the anterior and middle calcaneal facets
    (B) the anterior and middle calcaneal facets are in the same joint space
    (C) the facets are best shown by CT images parallel to the long axis of the calcaneus
    (D) Boehler's angle is estimated by drawing lines parallel to the middle and posterior facets

The talocalcaneal articulation (Figure 16-3) consists of two synovial joints, the subtalar or posterior subtalar joint and the talocalcaneonavicular or anterior subtalar joint. The posterior subtalar joint is formed between the convex posterior calcaneal facet and the corresponding concave posterior talar facet. The capsule of this joint contributes to the interosseous talocalcaneal ligament, which is the strongest ligamentous connection between the talus and the calcaneus.

The anterior subtalar joint is the second joint supporting the talus. Part of the floor of this joint is made up of the plantar calcaneonavicular ligament, also termed the "spring" ligament, which aids in supporting the plantar arch. The posterior portion of the articular capsule of the talocalcaneonavicular joint contributes to the interosseous ligament.

The interosseous ligament resides within the sinus tarsi, which separates the anterior and posterior subtalar joints. This ligament carries most of the talar blood supply. The posterior calcaneal facet lies behind the sinus tarsi, and the middle and anterior calcaneal facets are anterior to it **(Option (A) is false).** The anterior and middle calcaneal facets are within the anterior subtalar joint **(Option (B) is true),** and the posterior calcaneal facet is within the posterior subtalar joint. Thus, there are usually three calcaneal facets but only two subtalar joints. Occasionally, the anterior and middle calcaneal facets blend into a single continuous anterior calcaneal facet that covers the same anatomic area as the two individual facets.

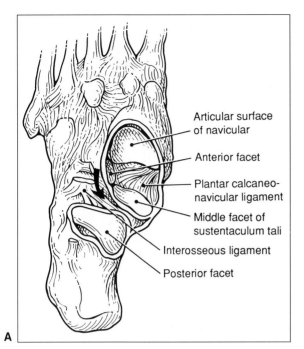

A

Articular surface
of navicular

Anterior facet

Plantar calcaneo-
navicular ligament

Middle facet of
sustentaculum tali

Interosseous ligament

Posterior facet

Figure 16-3. Talocalca-
neal articulation. As
seen from above (A) and
in a sagittal section (B),
the structures of the
subtalar joints are la-
beled as described in the
text. Note the interos-
seous ligament lying in
the sinus tarsi (curved
arrow in panel A) be-
tween the anterior and
posterior subtalar joints.

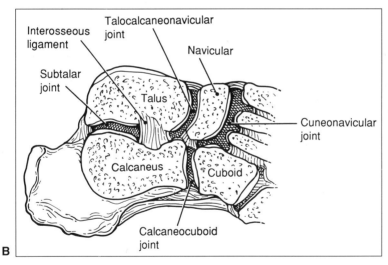

B

When evaluating the fractured calcaneus with CT, the goal is to demonstrate the configuration of each calcaneal facet and in particular the
posterior facet, which is the largest and most important of the three. CT
should be performed such that the plane of the CT scans is perpendicular
to the posterior facet. This is best accomplished when the CT scan plane
is angled approximately 30° craniad from the sole of the foot, thereby
obtaining a direct coronal section. This ideal is not always possible since

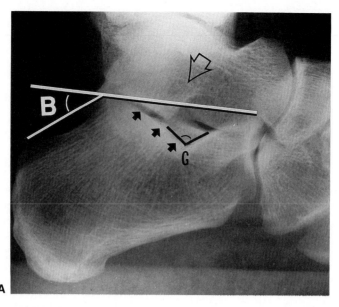

Figure 16-4. Calcaneal angles and measurements. (A) A lateral radiograph of the normal calcaneus shows the angle of Gissane (G) and the lines forming Boehler's angle (B), which in this image measures approximately 40°. The open arrow shows the direction of the desired plane for direct coronal CT sections of the subtalar joints and calcaneus. Small arrows = posterior facet. (B) A lateral radiograph shows an intra-articular fracture (large arrows) of the calcaneus with mild depression of the posterior facet. Boehler's angle is less than 20°. Small arrows = posterior facet. (C) A lateral radiograph shows a more severe calcaneal fracture with a Boehler's angle of 0°. Part of the posterior calcaneal facet (arrowheads) is impacted into the underlying portion of the calcaneus.

the limb may be in a cast or splint and optimal positioning may not be attainable. Alternatively, the fracture itself may result in such distortion of the calcaneal morphology that the otherwise optimal image plane may no longer be perpendicular to the facet. Planes parallel to the long axis of the calcaneus do not show the posterior facet well and are therefore not the best choice **(Option (C) is false).** Thin, overlapped coronal sections permit good sagittal reconstructions. Coronal scans should be acquired far enough distally to include the calcaneocuboid joint in order to evaluate for extension of the fracture into this joint.

A decrease in Boehler's angle indicates depression of the posterior facet. Boehler's angle is measured by drawing a line from the highest point on the tuberosity to the highest point of the posterior facet. A second line is drawn from the highest point of the posterior facet to the highest point on the anterior process (Figure 16-4) **(Option (D) is**

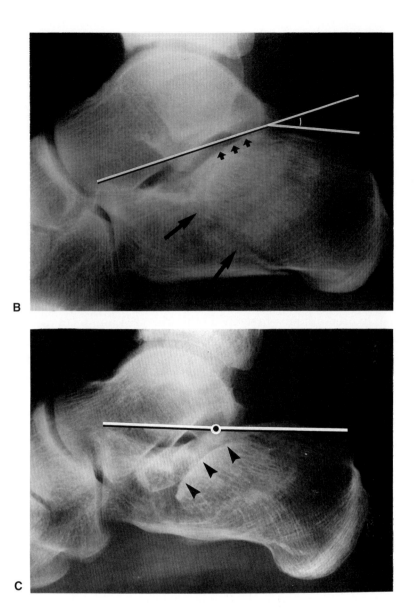

false). The angle typically averages approximately 30° (range, 25 to 40°). In patients with severely depressed fractures, the landmarks may be distorted; measurement of Boehler's angle may then be difficult, and the result may be inaccurate. Using CT sagittal reconstructions for measurement may permit more accurate evaluation of the angle.

Question 68

Concerning calcaneal fractures,

    (A) forces at the angle of Gissane result in either joint depression- or tongue-type fractures
    (B) approximately 75% are extra-articular
    (C) extra-articular fractures have an excellent overall clinical outcome
    (D) restoration of Boehler's angle is predictive of an excellent surgical result
    (E) an abnormal Boehler's angle indicates a requirement for open reduction and internal fixation

The calcaneus is the most commonly fractured tarsal bone. Various systems for classification of types of calcaneal fractures have been devised to facilitate understanding the pathophysiology and anatomy, predicting the outcome, and planning the appropriate treatment. The most commonly used systems first divide the fractures into intra- and extra-articular categories depending on whether or not a fracture involves the superior articular surface of the calcaneus. For extra-articular fractures, a modified Rowe classification system is widely used (Figure 16-5). A popular classification system of intra-articular fractures was devised by Essex-Lopresti. It first divides these fractures into tongue and central depression types (Figure 16-6).

Intra-articular calcaneal fractures usually result from axial and shear forces focused at the crucial angle of Gissane. The angle of Gissane is the angle formed by the posterior facet where it intersects with the thickened cortex of the anterior process of the calcaneus (Figure 16-4A). Force applied at the lateral talar process results in a primary vertical fracture extending through the apex of the angle of Gissane. As force increases or continues, a secondary fracture line may extend under the posterior calcaneal facet. This results in a joint depression-type injury, which is the most common intra-articular fracture. The fragment formed is sometimes referred to as the thalamic fragment. The degree of depression and comminution depends on the magnitude of the force. Less commonly, the secondary fracture line extends back to the tuberosity from the apex of the crucial angle, creating a large fragment containing most of the posterior facet. This is referred to as a tongue-type fracture **(Option (A) is true).**

In the past, the classification of intra-articular calcaneal fractures was based on plain radiographic fractures. Because CT has provided more-detailed assessment of calcaneal fractures, newer classification systems based on CT features have appeared. One recent classification of intra-articular fractures has been proposed by Sanders (Figure 16-7). This particular classification may or may not become generally accepted,

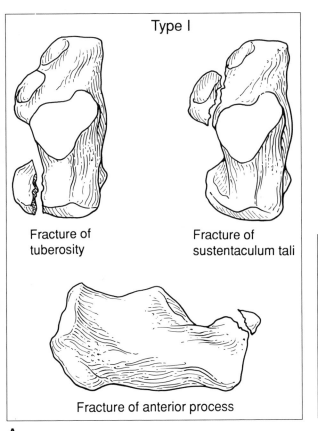

Type I

Fracture of
tuberosity

Fracture of
sustentaculum tali

Fracture of anterior process

A

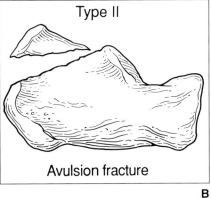

Type II

Avulsion fracture

B

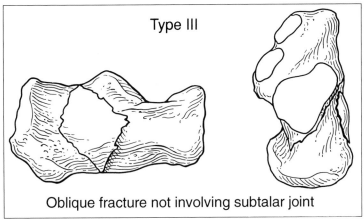

Type III

Oblique fracture not involving subtalar joint

C

Figure 16-5. Extra-articular calcaneal fractures, modified Rowe classification. (A) Type I: avulsion injuries. (B) Type II. Originally, these infrequent fractures were thought to comprise two types, one of which was due to avulsion. Now, however, both are believed to result from avulsion injury by the Achilles tendon. (C) Type III fractures involve the body of the calcaneus. If severely displaced, they may lead to long-term complications. (Reprinted with permission from Rowe CR, Sakellarides HT, Freeman PA, Sorbie C. Fractures of the os calcis. JAMA 1963; 184:920–923.)

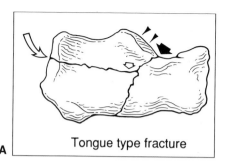
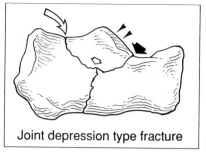

A | Tongue type fracture | | Joint depression type fracture | **B**

Figure 16-6. Intra-articular calcaneal fractures classified into two basic types by Essex-Lopresti. Both types include a primary vertical fracture line extending down from the angle of Gissane (solid arrows). (A) Tongue-type fracture. A secondary fracture line extends horizontally back to the posterior cortex (curved arrow). More severe force drives the anterior end of the superior tuberosity fragment down into the body of the calcaneus (open arrow). (B) Joint depression-type fracture. The secondary fracture line (curved arrow) extends across the body posteroinferior to the posterior facet. More severe force drives the posterior facet fragment down into the body (open arrow). Arrowheads = posterior articular facet. (Adapted with permission from Giannestras NJ. Foot disorders: medical and surgical management. Philadelphia: Lea & Febiger; 1973:536.)

but it provides an example of how CT can be used to refine the classification of calcaneal fractures. The coronal CT images are evaluated at the widest point of the posterior facet. The body of the calcaneus and the posterior facet are divided into lateral, central, and medial columns. These three columns and the sustentaculum result in a potential for four fragments. Type I fractures include all nondisplaced fractures. Type II fractures are two-part fractures and are described as IIA, IIB, or IIC, depending on the position of the fracture line. Type III fractures are three-part fractures that feature a centrally depressed fragment and are categorized as IIIAB, IIIAC, or IIIBC, depending on the fracture lines. Type IV fractures are four-part fractures that are typically badly comminuted. Use of this system by its creator has proven prognostic. The outcome was excellent in all Type I fractures, good to excellent in Type II fractures, and poor or failed in Type III and IV fractures. Operative intervention in Type IV fractures was mainly aimed at restoring calcaneal shape.

About 25% of calcaneal fractures are extra-articular, and the remainder have some intra-articular component **(Option (B) is false)**. Extra-articular fractures may involve the medial process of the tuberosity, the sustentaculum tali, the anterior process, the upper part of the tuberosity, the anterior dorsolateral surface of the calcaneus, and even the body of the calcaneus (Figure 16-5). Many extra-articular calcaneal fractures

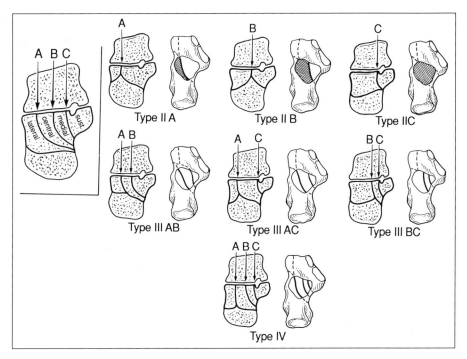

Figure 16-7. Sanders classification of calcaneal fractures, an example of a system based on CT images rather than on plain radiographs. All non-displaced fractures are Type I. Type II fractures divide the articular surface into two parts, Type III into three parts, and Type IV into four parts. (Reprinted with permission from Sanders R. Intra-articular fractures of the calcaneus: present state-of-the-art. J Orthop Trauma 1992; 6:252–262.)

result from twisting of the foot or from avulsive injuries. The fractures generally heal well with good results. The fracture of the medial process of the tuberosity probably results from either a direct shearing force or avulsion by the medial origin of the plantar fascia (Figure 16-5A, top left). Fracture of the sustentaculum tali is an unusual injury and is probably due to landing on the inverted foot (Figure 16-5A, top right). If the sustentaculum is significantly depressed, treatment involves elevating it back to its normal position. A fracture of the anterior process of the calcaneus results from avulsion by the insertion of the bifurcate ligament (Figure 16-5A, bottom, and Figure 16-8). This fracture is easily missed on routine radiographs but is usually best seen on the oblique view of the foot. A fracture of the superior aspect of the tuberosity (Figure 16-5B) apparently results from avulsion by the Achilles tendon due to a fall from a small height and usually occurs among patients in their sixties. The origin of the extensor digitorum brevis sometimes avulses a small fracture fragment from the anterior, dorsolateral surface of the calcaneus

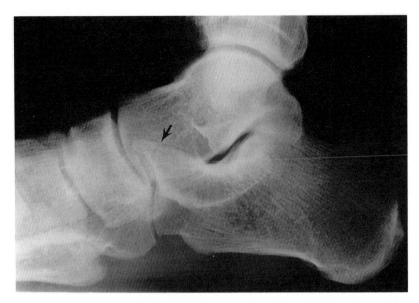

Figure 16-8. Fracture of the anterior process of the calcaneus (arrow). The mechanism is avulsion by the bifurcate ligament. The fracture is usually more clearly visible on an oblique view of the foot, which was not obtained in this case.

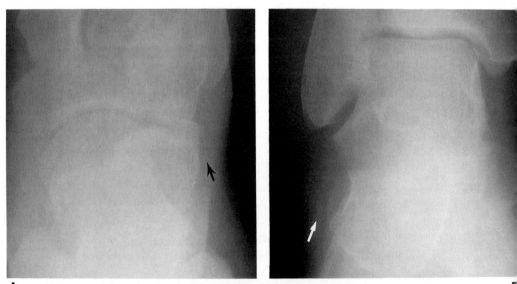

A   *Figure 16-9.*   Avulsion fracture at the origin of the extensor digitorum   B
brevis muscle. The tiny flake of bone (arrow) avulsed from the anterolateral surface of the calcaneus is visible on anteroposterior views of the foot (A) and ankle (B).

(Figure 16-9). Extra-articular fractures of the body of the calcaneus (Figures 16-5C and 16-10) account for up to 20% of calcaneal fractures and vary greatly in their configuration. They can result in widening of the calcaneus and a decrease in Boehler's angle, thus leading to complications such as shoeing problems and peroneal tendon impingement. However, most extra-articular calcaneal fractures may be treated conservatively and have an excellent prognosis **(Option (C) is true)**.

Kathol et al. recently described 14 calcaneal insufficiency avulsion fractures in patients with long-standing diabetes (Figure 16-11). These fractures occurred in the same location as fatigue fractures in nondiabetic patients, i.e., in the posterior calcaneus parallel to the apophyseal growth plate. The fracture line usually extended through the superior cortex and sometimes through the inferior cortex. A secondary horizontal fracture line almost always extended to the posterior cortex just distal to the Achilles tendon insertion. Some fractures were comminuted. Cephalad displacement of the posterior-superior fracture fragment due to the pull of the Achilles tendon was common, in contrast to the usual insufficiency fractures in nondiabetic patients, which are almost always nondisplaced. The authors felt these fractures occurred because of weakened bone due to the diabetes, neuropathy, steroids (eight of the patients had received renal transplants and were on steroids), infection, and probably the stresses of abnormal gait due to the various diabetic foot abnormalities.

The restoration of Boehler's angle is usually used as a gauge of reduction of intra-articular calcaneal fractures. However, as mentioned above, there are so many causes of a poor result that attention to Boehler's angle alone is not sufficient. A persistent severe abnormality of Boehler's angle may result in pain secondary to abnormal weight-bearing pressure on the calcaneus anterior to the tuberosity. Normally, pressure is centered over the tuberosity, which is protected by the heel pad. Some surgeons believe that a severely depressed Boehler's angle, by causing a relative lengthening of the Achilles tendon, can result in weak plantar flexion. However, others believe that muscle contraction can compensate for this abnormality. It appears that a persistent severe decrease in Boehler's angle can lead to a poor result, whereas a persistent minor abnormality is not significant. However, it appears that the most important determinant of a good result is restoration of the congruity of the posterior facet. A minor degree of residual tuber angle depression with a satisfactorily restored joint surface is often a better predictor of acceptable clinical outcome than is restoration of a normal Boehler's angle with an incongruous posterior subtalar joint **(Option (D) is false)**.

There is a difference of opinion about the optimum method of treating intra-articular fractures. Some surgeons avoid open reduction,

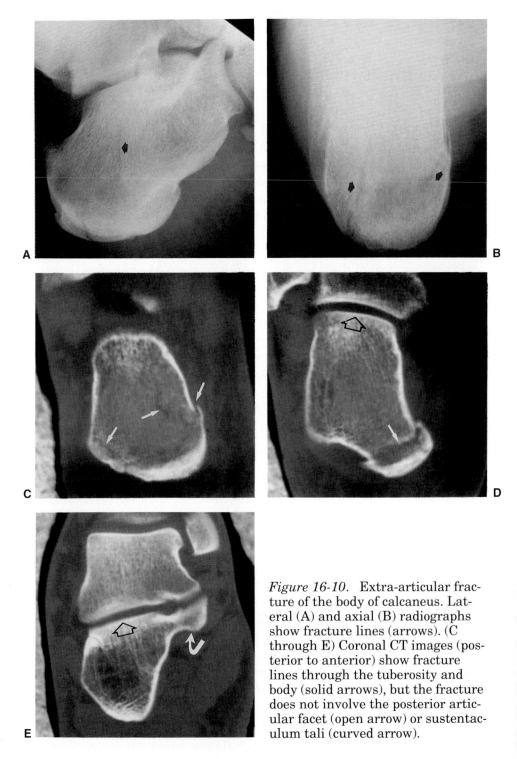

Figure 16-10. Extra-articular fracture of the body of calcaneus. Lateral (A) and axial (B) radiographs show fracture lines (arrows). (C through E) Coronal CT images (posterior to anterior) show fracture lines through the tuberosity and body (solid arrows), but the fracture does not involve the posterior articular facet (open arrow) or sustentaculum tali (curved arrow).

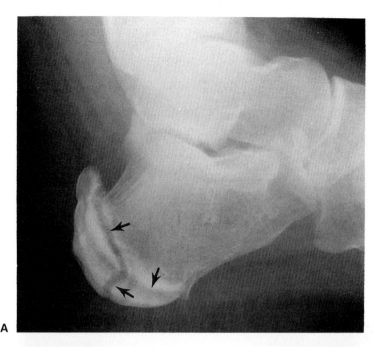

A

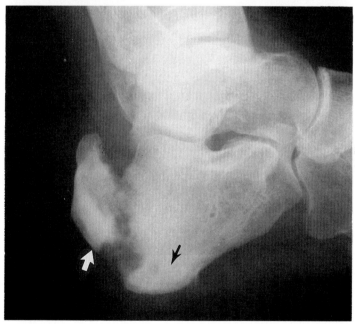

B

Figure 16-11. Calcaneal insufficiency avulsion fracture in a patient with diabetes mellitus. (A) The fracture (arrows) initially was minimally displaced. (B) Five months later, the inferior fracture line has healed (black arrow) but the superior fragment (white arrow) has displaced upward due to the pull of the Achilles tendon. (C) Internal fixation led to complete fracture union, but note the development of neuropathic arthropathy (arrows) due to diabetic neuropathy. (Reprinted with permission from Kathol et al. [6].)

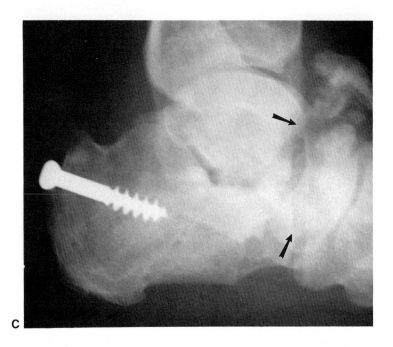

c

whereas others are more aggressive and attempt to achieve surgical restoration of the anatomic congruity of the posterior facet. No single factor determines whether open reduction is indicated **(Option (E) is false).** The treatment depends on the age and overall medical condition of the patient, the degree of comminution of the fracture, the involvement of the peroneal tendons, the widening of the lateral wall, and, of course, the skill of the surgeon.

William A. Fajman, M.D.
Terry M. Hudson, M.D.

SUGGESTED READINGS

CALCANEAL FRACTURES: GENERAL

1. Carr JB, Hamilton JJ, Bear LS. Experimental intra-articular calcaneal fractures: anatomic basis for a new classification. Foot Ankle 1989; 10:81–87
2. Crosby LA, Fitzgibbons T. Computerized tomography scanning of acute intra-articular fractures of the calcaneus. A new classification system. J Bone Joint Surg (Am) 1990; 72:852–859
3. Gilmer PW, Herzenberg J, Frank JL, Silverman P, Martinez S, Goldner JL. Computerized tomographic analysis of acute calcaneal fractures. Foot Ankle 1986; 6:184–193

4. Heckmer JD. Fractures of the foot. In: Rockwood CA, Green R, Buchholz RW (eds), Rockwood and Green's fractures, 3rd ed. Philadelphia: JB Lippincott; 1991:2103–2139
5. Heger L, Wulff K. Computed tomography of the calcaneus: normal anatomy. AJR 1985; 145:123–129
6. Kathol MH, el-Khoury GY, Moore TE, Marsh JL. Calcaneal insufficiency avulsion fractures in patients with diabetes mellitus. Radiology 1991; 180:725–729
7. Resnick D. Radiology of the talocalcaneal articulations. Anatomic considerations and arthrography. Radiology 1974; 111:581–586
8. Sanders R, Hansen ST, McReynolds IS. Fractures of the calcaneus. In: Jahss MH (ed), Disorders of the foot and ankle. Philadelphia: WB Saunders; 1991:2326–2354

CALCANEAL FRACTURES: COMPLICATIONS

9. Isbister JF. Calcaneo-fibular abutment following crush fracture of the calcaneus. J Bone Joint Surg (Br) 1974; 56:274–278
10. Rosenberg ZS, Feldman F, Singson RD, Price GJ. Peroneal tendon injury associated with calcaneal fractures: CT findings. AJR 1987; 149:125–129

CALCANEAL FRACTURES: TREATMENT

11. Hammesfahr JF. Surgical treatment of calcaneal fractures. Orthop Clin North Am 1989; 20:679–689
12. Hammesfahr R, Fleming LL. Calcaneal fractures: a good prognosis. Foot Ankle 1981; 2:161–171
13. Paley D, Hall H. Calcaneal fracture controversies. Can we put Humpty Dumpty together again? Orthop Clin North Am 1989; 20:665–677

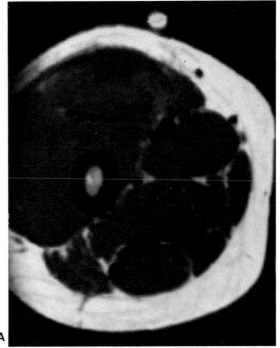

SE 300/15

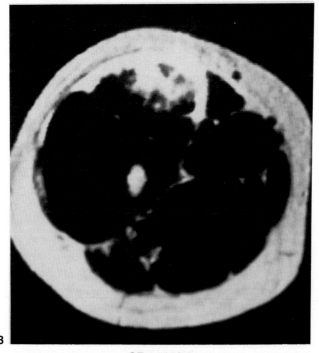

SE 2,500/80

Figure 17-1. This is a 19-year-old man. Additional history is withheld. You are shown T1- and T2-weighted MR images of the right thigh.

428 / *Musculoskeletal Disease*

Case 17: Muscle Tear

Question 69

Which *one* of the following is the MOST likely diagnosis?

(A) Rhabdomyosarcoma
(B) Muscular dystrophy
(C) Muscle tear
(D) Plexiform neurofibroma
(E) Hemangioma

The test images (Figure 17-1) show disruption and edema of the rectus femoris muscle fibers on the T1-weighted image, with a dramatic increase of muscle signal intensity on the T2-weighted image (Figure 17-2). Subtle increased signal of muscle on the T1-weighted image, combined with the increased signal intensity on the T2-weighted image, suggests hemorrhage. The contour of the signal abnormality is irregular, and it does not appear to be a solid mass. Adjacent muscle (vastus intermedius and posterior vastus lateralis) is normal and without evidence of additional increased signal intensity that would indicate edema on the T2-weighted image. A band of intermediate (T1-weighted) and increased (T2-weighted) signal intensity representing fluid can be seen in the lateral aspect of the thigh. The subcutaneous fat and bone marrow appear to be normal. These findings are most consistent with a traumatic injury to the muscle or with muscle tear **(Option (C) is correct).** This 19-year-old athlete had pain immediately following a soccer game, a history totally in keeping with the MR features.

Rhabdomyosarcoma (Option (A)) typically presents in patients younger than the test patient; the median age at presentation is 5 years. Grossly, rhabdomyosarcomas form a solid mass within skeletal muscle and typically exhibit a smooth or lobulated but not an irregular margin, unlike the abnormality seen here. These tumors usually exhibit intermediate signal intensity (equal to that of muscle) on T1-weighted images and high signal intensity on T2-weighted images (Figure 17-3). The tumor mass is frequently associated with edema of the surrounding mus-

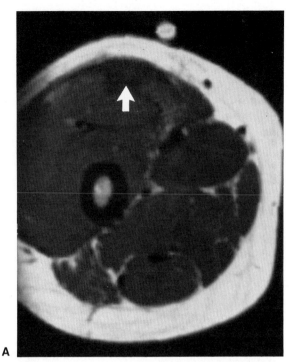

A

SE 300/15

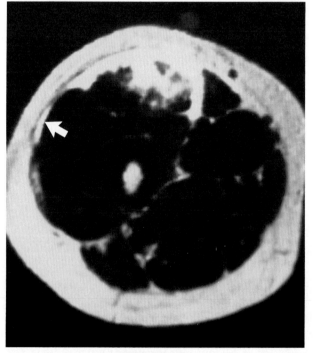

B

SE 2,500/80

Figure 17-2 (Same as Figure 17-1). Muscle tear. Transaxial T1-weighted (A) and T2-weighted (B) MR images show abnormal right thigh muscle. On the T1-weighted image, there is subtle disruption of the muscle fibers of the rectus femoris in the anterior thigh (arrow) with subtle increased signal intensity of the muscle. On the T2-weighted image, the rectus femoris muscle shows fluid with dramatically increased signal intensity, a finding associated with fluid lateral to the vastus lateralis (arrow). The increased signal intensity has a somewhat stellate pattern. These findings are typical for a muscle tear.

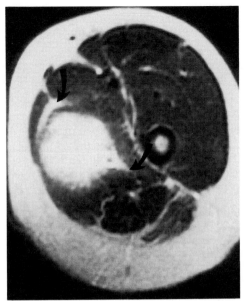

SE 2,500/80

Figure 17-3. Rhabdomyosarcoma. A T2-weighted transaxial MR image through the left
thigh in a 16-year-old boy
shows a tumor mass of high
signal intensity with adjacent
edema (arrows).

culature and violation of adjacent soft tissue planes. Rhabdomyosarcoma
is difficult to diagnose on conventional radiographs, since bone is seldom
involved. On CT examination, the soft tissue mass is usually appreciated
when surrounding muscle and soft tissue planes are distorted. The use of
intravenous contrast agents will result in tumor enhancement and
improved tumor recognition. Scintigraphy is not particularly useful in
diagnosing rhabdomyosarcoma, since there are no agents specific for
rhabdomyosarcoma and there typically is no osseous involvement. The
age of the test patient, the ill-defined lesion margins, the lack of a space-
occupying mass, and the absence of surrounding edema all make rhabdomyosarcoma an unlikely diagnosis for the test patient.

MRI has increasingly been used in the evaluation of muscular dystrophy (Option (B)). In general, transaxial T1- and T2-weighted images
are adequate to evaluate neuromuscular disorders. Short-tau inversion-
recovery (STIR) and fat-suppression images can also be helpful since
water-containing pathologic processes and muscle edema can be more
conspicuous on such images. If needed, coronal or sagittal views can be
obtained to evaluate the entire length of a muscle in a single image. Neuromuscular disorders are characterized clinically by muscle volume
changes (both "pseudohypertrophy" and atrophy) and muscle weakness.
Muscle volume changes can be seen on the MR image, as can the fatty
replacement of muscle fibers commonly seen in such disorders (Figure

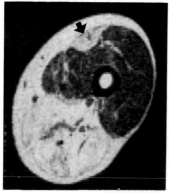

Figure 17-4. Facioscapulohumeral dystrophy. A T1-weighted transaxial MR image of left thigh shows fatty replacement of the rectus femoris (arrow) and hamstring muscles.

SE 300/30

17-4). This fatty replacement is easily recognized on both T1- and T2-weighted images.

"Muscular dystrophy" is a general term used to describe a variety of neuromuscular disorders. In general, muscle signal intensity in patients with muscular dystrophy reflects the fatty replacement of muscle and is therefore increased on both T1- and T2-weighted images. This is the typical appearance in patients with X-linked Duchenne muscular dystrophy. The outlines of individual muscles are clear since the curvilinear fibrous intermuscular septa of low signal intensity persist. These findings can be accompanied by either increased muscle volume (pseudohypertrophy) (Figure 17-5) or decreased muscle volume (atrophy). Relative sparing of the sartorius and gracilis muscles can be seen in Duchenne dystrophy.

Patients with limb-girdle muscular dystrophy uniformally show fatty replacement of thigh muscle. Fatty replacement of calf muscle can also be seen. Fatty changes can be severe or moderate, symmetric or asymmetric. While MRI has not yet proven useful in the evaluation of disease duration, it can be useful in directing biopsies. Patients with mitochondrial myopathy have severe fatty replacement of musculature, whereas those with amyotrophic lateral sclerosis and hereditary sensorimotor neuropathy have only slight fatty replacement. In the test patient, the abnormal muscle signal intensity is not characteristic of fat, nor is there evidence of pseudohypertrophy or atrophy. Therefore, muscular dystrophy is an unlikely diagnosis.

Neurofibromatosis type 1, a hereditary, hamartomatous disorder arising from neuroectoderm, mesoderm, and endoderm, can result in abnormalities in any organ system of the body. Involvement of both the skeleton and soft tissues is frequent. In the soft tissues, neurofibromas can either be singular or form an interdigitating network referred to as a

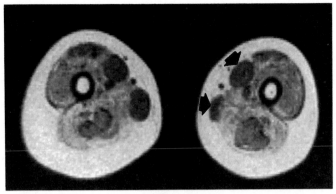

SE 500/30

Figure 17-5. Muscular dystrophy. A T1-weighted transaxial MR image of both thighs shows partial fatty replacement of muscle with asymmetric pseudohypertrophy of the sartorius and gracilis muscles (arrows).

plexiform neurofibroma (Option (D)). These plexiform neurofibromas infiltrate the soft tissues, usually adjacent to osseous defects in the bone. It is uncertain whether the osseous defects are related to the adjacent plexiform neurofibroma or whether the occurrence of these two lesions in adjacent tissues is fortuitous.

On T1-weighted MR examination, a plexiform neurofibroma typically presents as a moderate-sized to large mass of irregular nodules with intermediate signal intensity. On T2-weighted images, these lesions have a heterogeneous "salt and pepper" appearance or they can exhibit fairly uniform increased signal intensity. The appearance may be similar to that of a hemangioma. In the test patient, there is no evidence of a nodular intermediate-signal-intensity mass within the muscle. In addition, the fluid associated with the lesion in this case would not be typical of a plexiform neurofibroma. Thus, plexiform neurofibroma is an unlikely diagnosis.

Hemangioma (Option (E)), a benign, slowly growing neoplasm arising from newly formed blood vessels, can be small and self-limited or large and invasive. Pathologically, hemangiomas are classified as cavernous, capillary, or mixed. Cavernous hemangioma is characterized by large, thin-walled vessels and sinuses lined by a single layer of endothelial cells. Capillary hemangioma consists of fine capillary loops that spread outward in a sunburst pattern. Mixed hemangioma has elements of both of the other two types. Hemangiomas are associated with an underlying stroma of either fatty or fibrous tissue. Soft tissue hemangio-

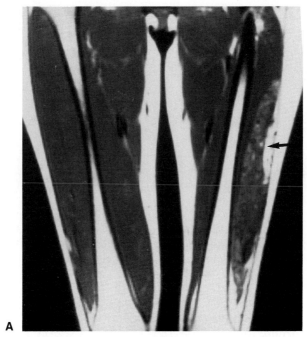

A

SE 800/20

Figure 17-6. Hemangioma of vastus lateralis muscle. T1-weighted coronal (A) and proton-density (B) and T2-weighted transaxial (C) MR images of the thighs in a 16-year-old girl show the "serpentine" appearance and the fatty matrix (arrow in panel A) of the hemangioma. Note the typical increased signal intensity on the T2-weighted image. As compared with the right side, the relative hypoplasia or atrophy of surrounding musculature in the left thigh (vastus intermedius and vastus medialis muscles) is apparent.

mas are characterized radiographically by a soft tissue mass that sometimes contains multiple phleboliths.

The MR appearance of a soft tissue hemangioma generally reflects the underlying histologic composition of the neoplasm, including densely packed, vascular networks separated by stroma, adipose tissue, fibrous tissue, calcium, hemosiderin, thrombosis, and hemorrhage. Hemangiomas are most often heterogeneous and have a typical serpentine intermediate-signal-intensity appearance on T1-weighted images. The signal intensity of a hemangioma is usually increased on T2-weighted images, although intermediate signal intensity can occasionally be seen. High signal intensity on both T1- and T2-weighted images can be seen with hemorrhage, fat deposition, or both. Homogeneous intermediate signal intensity on T1-weighted images with homogeneous high signal intensity

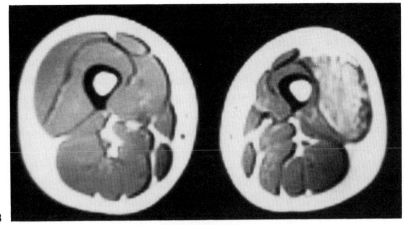

B

SE 2,000/20

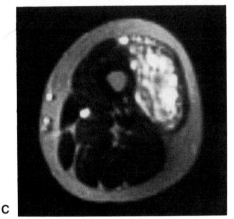

C

SE 2,000/80

on T2-weighted images has been reported in small, cavernous hemangiomas with a maximum diameter of less than 2 cm. However, not all small (<2 cm) hemangiomas have this appearance.

There are several useful MR criteria in the diagnosis of a soft tissue hemangioma. A serpentine pattern of low to intermediate signal intensity intermixed with areas of intermediate to high signal intensity on T1-weighted images that increases in intensity on T2-weighted images is highly suggestive of a hemangioma (Figure 17-6). This is particularly true when there is an underlying fatty stroma. The absence of an identifiable fatty or fibrous stroma does not exclude hemangioma. Infiltration of subcutaneous fat is best seen on T1-weighted images, whereas involvement of muscle is best seen on T2-weighted images. Vessels can be seen in the subcutaneous tissues surrounding the lesion; however, this appearance is variable, and a lack of feeding vessels in the surrounding tissues does not exclude the diagnosis of hemangioma.

Soft tissue edema has not been associated with intramuscular hemangioma, even when the hemangioma crosses fascial planes or invades surrounding structures. The presence of edema suggests an inflammatory or neoplastic process. Finally, uninvolved musculature surrounding deeper muscular hemangiomas can be either normal or decreased in size, although a muscle replaced by hemangioma can be larger than expected. Atrophy or hypoplasia of surrounding musculature is unlikely in acute inflammatory or neoplastic processes and suggests the presence of a slowly growing process such as hemangioma. Phleboliths, a highly specific finding on radiography and CT, are not readily identified on MR images. However, the combination of conventional radiography and MRI will adequately visualize any calcifications or phleboliths.

There are two phases of hemangioma described by Mulliken and Glowacki: (1) a proliferative phase with high cellular content, and (2) an involuting phase with a lower cellular content. To date, no study of hemangiomas has described findings that allow one to distinguish between an involuting and a proliferating hemangioma.

Muscle tear is part of the spectrum of muscular injury that can be evaluated by MRI. Muscle strain or injury can occur anywhere within the muscle, although the origin or insertion of the muscle is the most likely region. The diagnosis of muscle injury is suspected following a history of trauma or in patients with pain following physical activity. Athletes with a specific training regimen that is then modified are also at risk for developing muscular injury. Physical examination frequently elicits tenderness with deep palpation of the muscle or pain with resistive muscle contraction.

Muscular injury can be graded using a system similar to that used for ligamentous injuries. Grade-1 muscle strain results from muscle use or minimal trauma and is usually due to muscle spasm or cramp. Grade-2 strain, the result of true muscle overuse, is characterized by pain during activity and resolution of the pain with adequate rest. In these two strains there is usually muscle fiber injury with or without partial muscle tear. Grade-3 strain represents a true muscle tear that occurs within the belly of the muscle, at the musculotendinous junction, or at the origin or insertion of the muscle.

Muscle injury is associated with both abnormal signal intensity of muscle (particularly on T2-weighted images) and muscle contour abnormality. In general, muscle tears have a varied signal intensity on T1-weighted MR images and increased signal intensity on T2-weighted

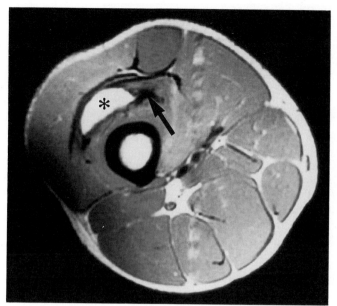

SE 2,000/20

Figure 17-7. Muscle tear with hematoma. A proton-density transaxial MR image through the thigh in a 16-year-old boy with an athletic injury shows a focal high-intensity well-defined mass (✻) within the vastus intermedius muscle. Linear low-intensity fibers of the vastus intermedius muscle (arrow) surrounding the mass represents the muscle tear. The high-intensity well-defined mass is characteristic of an intramuscular hematoma, which was also of high intensity on the T1- and T2-weighted images. (Case courtesy of George S. Bisset III, M.D., Childrens Hospital Medical Center, Cincinnati, Ohio.)

images. This high signal intensity on T2-weighted images likely reflects both edema and hemorrhage at the site of the muscle tear. The transaxial plane allows visualization of the origin or insertion of the muscle, as well as the muscle belly. Coronal or sagittal images are useful for evaluation of the entire muscle on a single image and can be particularly helpful in the evaluation of insertion or origin sites.

MRI of Grade-1 strain shows edema or hemorrhage of the muscle and preservation of muscle morphology. Grade-2 strain, in which up to 50% of the muscle fibers can be injured, is characterized by disruption of fibers, subacute hemorrhage, and edema. When present, subacute hemorrhage in the muscle is characterized by increased signal intensity on both T1- and T2-weighted images (Figure 17-7). MRI of muscle injury or strain often reveals an abnormality that involves more than one muscle group. This distribution to more than one muscle is also characteristic of

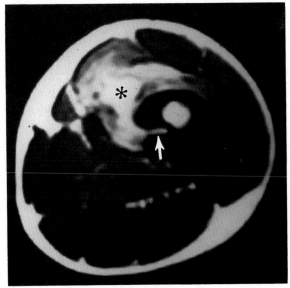

Figure 17-8. Muscle infection. A proton-density transaxial MR image shows osteomy-elitis of femur with a sinus tract (arrow) connecting the bone abscess with an adjacent intramuscular abscess (✻). Note the edema of adjacent muscles. (Case courtesy of George S. Bisset III, M.D.)

SE 2,000/20

soft tissue infection (Figure 17-8), which can have an appearance similar to that of Grade-1 and Grade-2 muscle injuries. However, muscle infection is typically characterized only by edema, with intermediate signal intensity on T1-weighted images and increased signal intensity on T2-weighted images. Muscle infection is infrequently complicated by intramuscular hemorrhage.

Grade-3 injury, i.e., complete muscle tear, can have a variety of appearances. Acute tears are invariably associated with signal abnormality on both T1- and T2-weighted images. The signal-intensity abnormality is variable on T1-weighted images (intermediate or high) and increased on T2-weighted images. Frequently, acute muscle tears will be associated with a fairly linear abnormal signal within the muscle. These findings are all seen in the test images. Alternatively, a focal hematoma can be seen, suggesting a mass rather than a linear tear (Figure 17-7). There can also be a palpable mass in patients with a Grade-3 injury, since torn muscle can either become edematous and swollen or else retract.

Subacute muscle tear is characterized by increased signal intensity on both T1- and T2-weighted images. Again, the abnormal signal can be linear or appear as a focal mass. The high signal intensity can occasionally be surrounded by a rim of low signal intensity, likely representing hemosiderin. Signal abnormality of muscle in patients with chronic tears is more varied than is the muscle signal intensity with acute or subacute tears. The signal abnormalities seen reflect several different processes including resolving hemorrhage and fatty replacement of muscle in the region of the tear. A low-signal-intensity linear abnormality with a high-signal rim is thought to represent both fibrous and fatty healing of torn muscle fibers. The signal intensity of muscle can also return to normal. Alterations in muscle contour can be seen with more-chronic injuries, particularly when there is hypertrophy of adjacent musculature to compensate for the torn muscle or loss of muscle fiber as a result of the injury.

When performing MRI for muscle injury, it is best to image in a transaxial plane, using a body coil and a field-of-view large enough so that the two sides of a patient can be compared and abnormalities of muscle signal intensity or contour can be more easily seen. Comparison of muscle bulk between the affected and nonaffected sides can reveal subtle changes in muscle contour. Contour changes result from either focal mass effect (from acute hemorrhage and edema) or muscle tear and retraction, as well as from muscle atrophy in more chronic injuries. Retraction of muscle bundles during muscle contraction can be evaluated by dynamic MRI. In MR images obtained with the muscle in contraction, retraction of muscle bundles can simulate a mass.

The signal-intensity abnormalities of injured and torn muscle reflect both edema and hemorrhage within the muscle. The predominantly linear morphologic pattern seen in many muscle tears likely represents blood that has dissected between muscle bundles. More-focal or mass-like collections of blood suggest localized hematoma rather than dissecting hemorrhage.

The MR appearance of soft tissue blood has been extensively studied both *in vitro* and *in vivo*. To date, there have been inconsistent signal-intensity patterns reported for intramuscular blood, with some investigators reporting increased signal intensity on T1-weighted images and others reporting intermediate or low signal intensity. The signal intensity of acute hemorrhage increases on T2-weighted images. Both subacute and chronic hemorrhage exhibit intermediate or high signal intensity on T1-weighted images and high signal intensity on T2-weighted images.

These differences in reported signal intensity may reflect extrinsic factors such as acquisition technique or magnetic field strength or may reflect intrinsic factors such as differing rates of blood breakdown in localized hematomas as opposed to dissecting hemorrhage within muscle tear. Following muscle injury, fatty replacement of muscle is frequent. Low-intensity zones on both T1- and T2-weighted images in old muscle injury likely reflect fibrosis that has occurred as a result of healing.

Question 70

Concerning rhabdomyosarcoma,

    (A) the median age at presentation is 5 years
    (B) most arise within the striated muscle of the extremities
    (C) at clinical presentation, skeletal metastases occur in over 50% of patients
    (D) direct cortical bone invasion by the primary tumor is common

Rhabdomyosarcoma accounts for 10 to 15% of all childhood solid tumors. The median age at presentation is 5 years **(Option (A) is true).** It is an aggressive tumor, which occurs in multiple sites. Approximately 35 to 50% of embryonal rhabdomyosarcomas originate in the head and neck, followed in frequency by a tumor origin in the pelvic region (urinary bladder, prostate, vagina, testes and peritesticular tissues, pelvic floor, and perineum). Only one-third of cases arise within striated muscle of the extremities and trunk **(Option (B) is false).** The remainder of these tumors arise at other anatomic sites, including regions where striated muscle is not normally present. Metastatic disease and recurrence are common. Metastases are found in the lung, lymph nodes, brain, liver, mediastinum, and skeleton. Therapy consists of surgical removal of the tumor with adjunctive chemotherapy and radiation therapy in patients with gross or microscopic residual disease.

Grossly, these tumors form either a singly solid mass or an extensively lobulated mass (the so-called "sarcoma botryoides"). The latter is most frequently found in hollow viscera such as the bladder, vagina, and common bile duct. Histologically, these are tumors of embryonic mesenchyme. The small, round rhabdomyoblasts vary in size and maturation and may contain acidophilic cytoplasm. They are considered one of the "small blue round-cell tumors of childhood" along with leukemia, Ewing's sarcoma, and neuroblastoma.

Radiographically, the tumor manifests as a localized or diffuse soft tissue swelling that displaces adjacent structures (Figure 17-9). When the tumor occurs in the abdomen or pelvis, displacement of pelvic or colonic structures on excretory urogram, voiding cystourethrogram, or barium enema examination may provide the only clue to the diagnosis by conventional radiography. CT, sonography, and MRI all reveal a soft tissue mass in the region of origin and are used to diagnose and characterize the tumor.

Approximately 20% of patients develop skeletal metastases during the course of their disease **(Option (C) is false).** Bone metastases appear as ill-defined lytic or permeative lesions in the metaphyses. Metastases are more likely to occur in areas of rapid skeletal growth, such as the distal femoral metaphysis. However, invasion of a primary

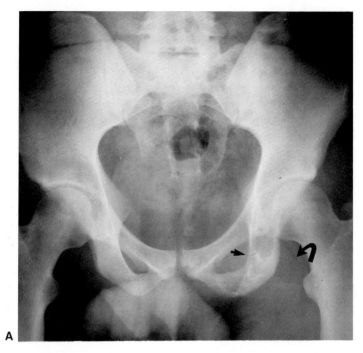

A

Figure 17-9. Rhabdomyosarcoma in a 19-year-old man. (A) An anteroposterior radiograph of the pelvis shows permeative changes in the left
inferior pubic ramus and ischium (straight arrow). The cortical bone is
eroded. Note the soft tissue mass (curved arrow), which displaces the fat
plane delineating the left hip joint laterally. Compare the abnormal contour of the fascial plane on the left with the normal fascial plane on the
right. (B) A T1-weighted coronal MR image through the lower pelvis and
proximal femora shows an intermediate-intensity soft tissue mass
involving the medial aspect of the left thigh and pelvis. The signal intensity of tumor is slightly higher than that of surrounding muscle. Note the
well-defined margins and the overall increase in muscle size as a result
of the tumor. (C) A STIR coronal image at the same level helps to distinguish tumor from surrounding musculature. Minimal edema of surrounding musculature is seen inferiorly (arrow).

soft tissue tumor into bone occurs infrequently (Figure 17-9) **(Option
(D) is false).** Local spread of disease to surrounding soft tissue structures is common. Parenchymal and subpleural nodular metastases are
characteristic of metastatic spread to the lungs.

On MRI, rhabdomyosarcoma has a fairly well defined soft tissue
mass of intermediate signal intensity (equal to muscle) on T1-weighted
images and high signal intensity on T2-weighted images (Figures 17-3
and 17-9). There are no CT or MR criteria that distinguish rhabdomyo-

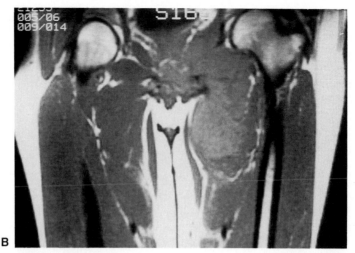

B

SE 600/25

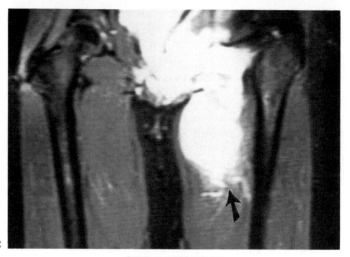

C

STIR 2,500/40/160

sarcoma from other soft tissue tumors of childhood. Therefore, the major role of both CT and MRI is pretherapeutic tumor staging. Transaxial images are the most useful for determining the involvement of surrounding musculature and violation of the soft tissue planes. MRI seems superior to CT for staging these tumors since T2-weighted images provide optimized contrast among the high-signal tumor, the intermediate-signal muscle, and the other surrounding soft tissues. While T2-weighted MR images are best for distinguishing tumor from muscle, involvement of subcutaneous fat, bone, and mediastinal structures is best assessed on T1-weighted images.

Head and neck rhabdomyosarcomas (35 to 50% of all tumors) frequently require both CT and MR examination for full evaluation. MR images are preferable to CT to determine the soft tissue extent of tumor and to evaluate the spread of tumor into the spinal canal and the cranial vault. Thin-section CT examination is currently superior to MRI in the evaluation of subtle bone erosion in the face and the skull base.

Question 71

Concerning the MR evaluation of muscle,

- (A) increased signal intensity on both T1- and T2-weighted images likely represents subacute hemorrhage or fat
- (B) on T2-weighted images, acute muscle tears are accompanied by increased signal intensity
- (C) neuromuscular disorders are characterized by focal muscle atrophy and fatty replacement
- (D) in acute myonecrosis, muscle signal is frequently normal on T1-weighted images
- (E) exercise increases muscle signal intensity on short-tau inversion-recovery (STIR) images

Currently, only a small percentage of the musculoskeletal MR studies performed in the United States are done primarily for the evaluation of muscle diseases. As knowledge regarding the appearance, specificity, sensitivity, and accuracy of MRI for these disorders increases, its use will likely increase. Evaluation of muscle contour, position, homogeneity, and MR signal intensity on both T1- and T2-weighted images provides the basis for image evaluation. In the evaluation of muscle trauma and muscle tears, changes in muscle configuration and abnormal signal intensity within the muscle are readily appreciated.

Abnormal signal intensity within muscle is felt to result predominantly from intramuscular hemorrhage. This signal intensity will vary depending on the age, character, and tissue of origin of the hemorrhage. Acute hemorrhage has an appearance different from that of subacute or chronic hemorrhage, a focal hematoma has an appearance different from that of infiltrating hemorrhage, and the time course for lysis and clearance of blood depends to some degree on the surrounding tissue (i.e., whether fat or muscle, etc.).

In cases of acute or subacute trauma, there will almost always be increased signal intensity on both the T1- and T2-weighted images. Occasionally, a central linear region of low signal intensity with a peripheral zone of high signal intensity is seen on the T1- or T2-weighted image. These findings are typical for subacute hemorrhage, with the central zone likely representing methemoglobin as the blood begins to lyse. Fat within muscle, such as that seen in patients with healed muscle tears, is also seen as increased signal intensity on both T1- and T2-weighted images. However, the signal intensity of the fat is less on the T2-weighted image, whereas the signal intensity of hemorrhage is usually greater on the T2-weighted image **(Option (A) is true).** The signal intensity of acute muscle tears is always increased on T2-weighted images **(Option (B) is true).**

Neuromuscular disorders encompass a wide range of muscle abnormalities. Denervation is the primary histopathologic finding and is characterized by relatively greater atrophy of type 2 muscle fibers than of type 1 muscle fibers. In most cases, neuromuscular disorders are seen on MR examination as muscle atrophy and fatty replacement of muscle bulk **(Option (C) is true),** as characterized by shortening of the T1 relaxation time and correspondingly increased signal intensity on T1-weighted images. While atrophy and fatty replacement are the most readily recognized MR findings, there is evidence that prolonged T1 and T2 relaxation times occur during the early stages of disease and denervation. Although changes in signal intensity may not be evident during these early stages of disease on spin-echo images, STIR images show high signal intensity, indicating the increase in extracellular water content of muscle fibers as denervation occurs.

Myonecrosis results from a variety of insults. The basic histopathologic feature is muscle fiber necrosis, and this is reflected clinically by increased serum levels of creatine kinase and myoglobin. Some of the causes of myonecrosis include exertional rhabdomyolysis, crush injury, thermal injury, chemical injury, and inherited disorders of metabolism (e.g., McArdle's disease, myophosphorylase deficiency). Inflammatory conditions, such as polymyositis, dermatomyositis, and drug reaction polymyositis, can also result in myonecrosis. Myonecrosis also occurs as a complication of diabetes mellitus.

The sonographic examination of muscle in cases of myonecrosis usually shows a hypoechoic region within the muscle, although occasionally an echogenic focus can be seen. Although ultrasonography can be a useful screening modality if it is positive, its sensitivity is only about 40%, and so a negative sonogram does not preclude the diagnosis of myonecrosis. CT is more sensitive for the detection of myonecrosis, particularly when intravenous contrast agents are used. In comparison, MRI is very sensitive for detecting myonecrosis, which exhibits high signal intensity on proton-density, T2-weighted, and STIR sequences, probably reflecting the increased water content of the necrotic muscle. On T1-weighted images, the intermediate signal intensity of myonecrosis is commonly indistinguishable from that of normal muscle **(Option (D) is true).**

After exertion, muscle has an MR appearance similar to that of acute traumatic or thermal injury. However, with both acute traumatic and thermal injury there is frequently swelling of the affected muscle. Exertion does not result in swelling of the affected muscle. Caution must be used in evaluating muscle on MR images since exertional muscle activity just prior to the MR examination can cause transient increased signal intensity of the exercised muscle on both T2-weighted and STIR images **(Option (E) is true).**

Discussion

Skeletal muscle is the primary organ of movement and the major metabolic reservoir for the body. It constitutes up to 40% of body weight, and muscle pain and weakness are among the most common symptoms for which patients seek medical care.

Although soft tissue radiography of muscle was first reported in 1928, little advancement was made in the imaging of muscle until the advent of CT and MRI. Disorders that involve skeletal muscle include primary neurogenic disorders (e.g., amyotrophic lateral sclerosis), muscular dystrophy (e.g., Duchenne muscular dystrophy), metabolic myopathies, inflammatory muscle disease (e.g., polymyositis), trauma (e.g., crush injury, burn, contusion, strains and ruptures, and overuse syndromes), and neoplastic disease. Although conventional radiographs can be used to evaluate muscle, they are relatively insensitive and abnormalities are barely reflected as atrophy, fatty replacement, or alterations of fat planes.

Sonography can detect gross changes in muscle composition and size but is relatively insensitive to many of the changes that occur in muscle. It is useful in distinguishing muscle from hematoma and solid from cystic masses. CT provides high resolution and is sensitive to alteration in tissue density, including fatty infiltration, necrosis, and inflammation. However, since most pathologic processes decrease muscle attenuation, CT is relatively nonspecific in the evaluation of muscle disorders. In addition, evaluation of muscle by CT typically requires intravenous injection of a contrast agent. Finally, the radiation required, as well as the beam-hardening artifact from adjacent bone, can limit muscle evaluation by CT. MRI is the most sensitive modality for imaging muscle abnormalities. MRI can provide quantitative information about muscle size and signal and can distinguish fatty from fibrous, neoplastic, and water (edema) infiltration.

Trauma results in contour abnormalities of muscle, disruption of muscle fibers, and signal-intensity abnormalities on both T1- and T2-weighted images. Linear or stellate regions of low signal intensity are often seen within the muscle in cases of muscle tear. In cases of acute muscle rupture or musculotendinous separation, large gaps between muscle fibers or else a soft tissue mass simulating tumor may be seen. Edema, acute swelling, surrounding hemorrhage, and fluid collections are also apparent.

Myonecrosis can result from a variety of causes, including overexertion, thermal injury (particularly high-voltage injury), drugs, crush injury, and inherited disorders of carbohydrate metabolism. The MR signal-intensity findings of myonecrosis are essentially indistinguishable from those of traumatic injury, with intermediate signal intensity of muscle seen on T1-weighted images and increased signal intensity seen on T2-weighted and STIR images. Myonecrosis secondary to crush injury is interesting in that the pattern of distribution of muscle abnormality does not necessarily conform to that expected on the basis of the crush injury alone; conversely, drug overdose frequently results in a strikingly focal distribution of muscle necrosis. Thermal myonecrosis is characterized by a more contiguous pattern of muscle involvement, with frequent muscle swelling. Postexertion muscle necrosis is similar to that of thermal myonecrosis except that there is little muscle swelling. Postexertion myonecrosis typically occurs in the "weekend athlete" or, less frequently, in the well-trained athlete. The MR features are increased muscle signal intensity on T2-weighted images, limitation of the abnormality to the muscle fibers themselves, no significant distortion of the surrounding soft tissue planes, and frequently the involvement of contiguous muscle groups.

Neuromuscular disorders have a typical appearance on MRI. They are characterized by denervation and atrophy of muscle fiber. Acute muscle atrophy results in edema and an increased extracellular water content, but with time these denervated areas become chronic and are characterized by diminished muscle bulk and fatty replacement of muscle fibers. This gives a "marbled" appearance to the muscle. The pattern of fatty replacement frequently reflects the underlying neuromuscular disorder. Neuromuscular disorders such as X-linked Duchenne muscular dystrophy and limb-girdle muscular dystrophy show fairly marked fatty replacement of involved muscle. Patients with mitochondrial myopathy show severe fatty replacement of musculature, with little musculature remaining in the extremities. In contrast, patients with amyotrophic lateral sclerosis and hereditary sensory motor neuropathy frequently show only slight fatty replacement of muscle. Asymmetry of muscle size is seen in patients with cerebral palsy. Although the musculature of the involved side is smaller than that of the uninvolved side, muscle signal intensity is fairly normal and does not show the fatty replacement seen with other neuromuscular disorders. This is more consistent with hypoplasia of musculature than with atrophy, reflecting the lack of muscle development in disorders such as cerebral palsy as opposed to the atrophy of muscle that follows from denervation in many neuromuscular disorders. Muscle findings in patients with poliomyelitis show asymmetric involvement of musculature, but intensive fatty replacement is common. While at the present time specific diagnosis of a particular neuromuscular disorder is difficult on the basis of the MR examination alone, MRI is potentially useful for guiding muscle biopsy and for documenting progression or improvement of disease following therapeutic intervention.

Sheila G. Moore, M.D.

SUGGESTED READINGS

MUSCLE TRAUMA

1. De Smet AA, Fisher DR, Heiner JP, Keene JS. Magnetic resonance imaging of muscle tears. Skeletal Radiol 1990; 19:283–286
2. Dooms GC, Fisher MR, Hricak H, Higgins CB. MR imaging of intramuscular hemorrhage. J Comput Assist Tomogr 1985; 9:908–913
3. Ehman RL, Berquist TH. Magnetic resonance imaging of musculoskeletal trauma. Radiol Clin North Am 1986; 24:291–319
4. Fleckenstein JL. Magnetic resonance imaging and computed tomography of skeletal muscle pathology. In: Bloem JL, Sartoris DJ (eds), MRI and CT of the musculoskeletal system. A text atlas. Baltimore: Williams & Wilkins; 1992:176–188
5. Stoller DW, Maloney WJ. The hip. In: Stoller DW (ed), Magnetic resonance imaging in orthopedics and sports medicine. Hagerstown, MD: JB Lippincott; 1993:85–98

RHABDOMYOSARCOMA

6. Kransdorf MJ, Jelinek JS, Moser RP Jr, et al. Soft-tissue masses: diagnosis using MR imaging. AJR 1989; 153:541–547
7. Moore SG. Pediatric musculoskeletal imaging. In: Stark DD, Bradley WG Jr (eds), Magnetic resonance imaging. St. Louis: Mosby-Year Book; 1992:2223–2330
8. Murphy WA, Totty WG, Carroll JE. MRI of normal and pathologic skeletal muscle. AJR 1986; 146:565–574
9. Polak JF, Jolesz FA, Adams DF. Magnetic resonance imaging of skeletal muscle. Prolongation of T1 and T2 subsequent to denervation. Invest Radiol 1988; 23:365–369

10. Shabas D, Gerard G, Rossi D. Magnetic resonance imaging examination of denervated muscle. Comput Radiol 1987; 11:9–13
11. Wilner D. Other malignant disorders of childhood. In: Wilner D (ed), Radiology of bone tumors and allied disorders. Philadelphia: WB Saunders; 1982:3393–3440

PLEXIFORM NEUROFIBROMA

12. Armstrong DC, Harwood-Nash DC. Pediatric spine. In: Stark DD, Bradley WG Jr (eds), Magnetic resonance imaging. St. Louis: Mosby-Year Book; 1992:1370–1398
13. Gundry CR, Patel MM, Kursunoglu-Brahme S. Magnetic resonance imaging of the wrist and hand. In: Bloem JL, Sartoris DJ (eds), MRI and CT of the musculoskeletal system. A text atlas. Baltimore: Williams & Wilkins; 1992:302–312
14. Hall TR. Central nervous system: ear, nose, throat and skull. In: Cohen MD, Edwards MK (eds), Magnetic resonance imaging of children. Philadelphia: BC Decker; 1990:387–419

HEMANGIOMA

15. Cohen EK, Kressel HY, Perosio T, et al. MR imaging of soft-tissue hemangiomas: correlation with pathologic findings. AJR 1988; 150:1079–1081
16. Hawnaur JM, Whitehouse RW, Jenkins JP, Isherwood I. Musculoskeletal hemangiomas: comparison of MRI with CT. Skeletal Radiol 1990; 19:251–258
17. Mulliken JB, Glowacki J. Hemangiomas and vascular malformations in infants and children: a classification based on endothelial characteristics. Plast Reconstr Surg 1982; 69:412–422
18. Wilner D. Benign vascular tumors and allied disorders of bone. In: Wilner D (ed), Radiology of bone tumors and allied disorders. Philadelphia: WB Saunders; 1982:660–782

MYONECROSIS

19. Fleckenstein JL, Weatherall PT, Parkey RW, Payne JA, Peshock RM. Sports-related muscle injuries: evaluation with MR imaging. Radiology 1989; 172:793–798
20. Lamminen AE, Hekali PE, Tiula E, Suramo I, Korhola OA. Acute rhabdomyolysis: evaluation with magnetic resonance imaging compared with computed tomography and ultrasonography. Br J Radiol 1989; 62:326–330

Notes

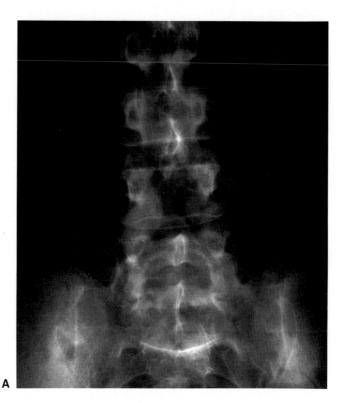

Figure 18-1

Figures 18-1 and 18-2. This patient presented with progressive low back and leg pain 3 years after back surgery. You are shown radiographs of the lumbar spine obtained 1 month apart.

Case 18: Spinal Fusion

Question 72

Which *one* of the following was the MOST likely clinical diagnosis leading to the surgical procedure shown in Figure 18-2?

    (A) Degenerative disk disease
    (B) Failed back syndrome
    (C) Postoperative infection
    (D) Segmental spine instability
    (E) Diskogenic pain

The initial radiographs demonstrate evidence of previous lumbar spine surgery, as manifested by an L4 laminectomy defect in the anteroposterior radiograph (Figure 18-1A). Bone graft donor sites in both posterior iliac crests can be identified in this radiograph (Figures 18-1A and 18-3). This is evidence of an attempted posterior fusion associated with the laminectomy. The lateral radiograph is within normal limits (Figure 18-1B). The second pair of radiographs (Figure 18-2) shows the results of reoperation with insertion of a dorsal spinal fixation system accompanied by additional intertransverse bone graft at the L4-L5 level (Figures 18-2A and 18-4).

The laminectomy was performed 3 years ago, and the patient now has slowly progressive low back and leg pain. This case is illustrative of long-term failure of spine surgery. In patients presenting with a long-term surgical failure and low back pain as the predominant symptom, the differential diagnosis includes the list of possibilities offered in the test question. There is no evidence of postoperative infection (Option (C)) in the initial radiographs (Figure 18-1). Disk space height is maintained, and there are no secondary signs of degenerative disk disease such as end-plate sclerosis or marginal spur formation (Option (A)). Following these relatively easy exclusions, there are three possible choices for the most likely clinical diagnosis: failed back syndrome, segmental spine instability, and diskogenic pain.

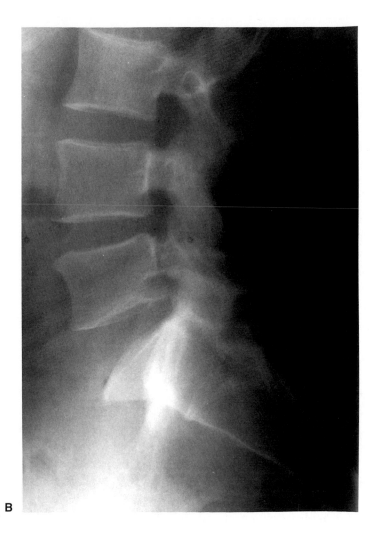

B

Segmental spine instability (Option (D)) is a relatively common cause of persistent low back pain following lumbar disk excision without fusion and has been reported to account for up to 18% of surgical failures in these patients. Generally, patients with segmental instability have a gradual onset of low back pain following resolution of the sciatica for which they underwent the original operation. However, segmental instability is difficult to document clinically and radiographically. It must be kept in mind that segmental instability can be present in patients who have had no operation and in those who have had operations such as disk excisions without fusion. Also, there may be residual or recurrent instability in patients who have had operations that included fusions. This discussion essentially lumps all these patients together in the

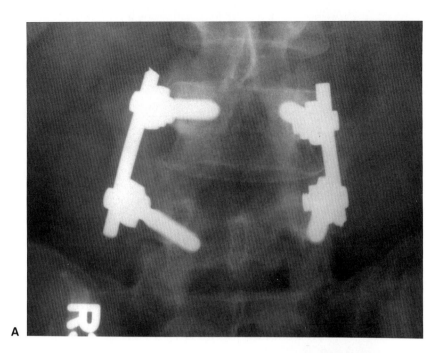

A

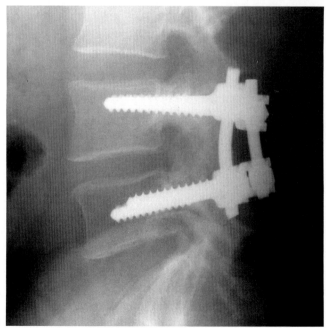

B

Figure 18-2

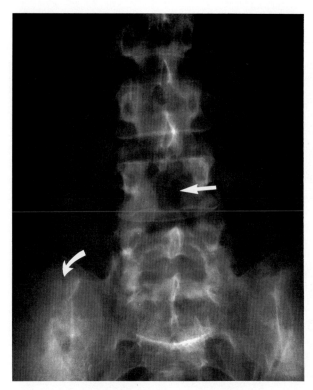

Figure 18-3
(Same as Figure
18-1A). An an-
teroposterior ra-
diograph of the
lumbar spine
demonstrates an
L4 laminectomy
(straight arrow)
with absence of
the spinous pro-
cess and portions
of the laminae.
Note also the
bone graft donor
site in the right
ilium (curved ar-
row). This radio-
graph was ob-
tained because of
progressive low
back pain 3 years
after the surgery.

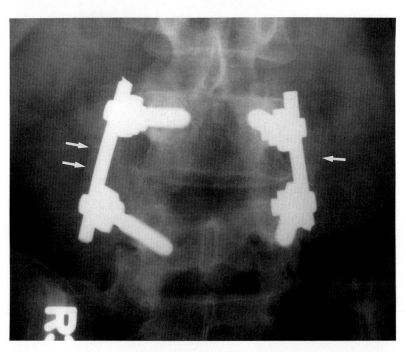

Figure 18-4 (Same as Figure 18-2A). An anteroposterior radiograph
shows a transpedicular screw posterior fixation system with posterolateral (intertransverse) bone graft (arrows) at the L4-L5 spinal segment
level.

description of instability. Patients who have had previous surgery but no fusion procedure can have hypermobility at the operated segment. These patients can be asymptomatic. Therefore, documenting that the identified instability is, in fact, causing the symptoms is very difficult. In patients who have had a fusion procedure, one would expect that the fused segments would be relatively immobile. One can search for instability on flexion and extension radiographs in patients with previous fusions by superimposing the fused segments to see if they stay the same on flexion and extension views. Also, of course, one should look for visually identifiable subluxation.

However, radiographic evidence varies in patients thought to have pain secondary to unstable segments whether they have had previous fusions or not. Some secondary signs include disk space narrowing, excessive vertebral body translation in the sagittal plane on flexion and extension lateral radiographs, development of pseudarthrosis in a bone graft fusion mass (Figure 18-5), and development of traction spurs. (However, it has not been clearly established that traction spurs do indicate spinal instability.) The presence of these findings in asymptomatic patients who have had spinal surgery confuses matters further. The presence of motion in an operated segment is less common in patients who have had fusion procedures than in those who have had only disk excision procedures, but this finding can still occur in patients with fusions but no significant symptoms.

In general, most authors believe that subluxation of 3 to 5 mm between vertebral bodies is abnormal. Some authors believe that the inter- and intra-observer errors require the use of the high number (5 mm), whereas others believe that the estimate of 3 mm is adequate to define abnormal. If there are radiographic signs of instability in a patient with consistent symptoms, the treatment of choice is a spinal fusion. However, if there are no radiographic signs of instability and the clinical symptoms support the diagnosis of instability, it has been our experience that the surgeon will still tend to make the diagnosis of instability and do a fusion procedure. Whether these patients truly have instability or internal disk derangement is not clear.

In spite of the fact that the test patient radiographs show a prior laminectomy followed by a spinal fusion, there is no direct evidence of spinal instability. Support for this diagnosis requires flexion and extension radiographs. Therefore, segmental spine instability is not the best diagnosis for this case.

Diskogenic pain (also known as internal disk derangement or internal disk disruption) (Option (E)) arises from mechanical overload on a disk. This overload results in alterations in the internal structure and metabolic functions of the disk. This concept includes the theory that the

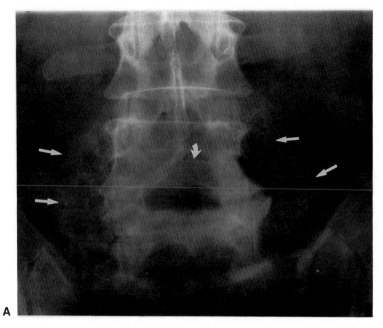

A

Figure 18-5. Failed back syndrome due to segmental instability with pseudarthrosis. (A) Coned-down anteroposterior radiograph of the lower lumbar spine soon after spinal surgery shows a left L4 hemilaminectomy (curved arrow) and L4-S1 intertransverse bone graft bilaterally (straight arrows). The immature bone graft has a mottled, heterogeneous appearance. More graft is visible on the right than on the left. (B) Anteroposterior radiograph of the lumbosacral spine 1 year later shows denser, more mature bone graft, but the patient complained of low back pain. Subtle resorption of the bone graft at L5-S1 on the left is evident (curved arrow). The associated vague radiolucency in the L5-S1 bone graft on the right (straight arrows) is suspicious for the development of a pseudarthrosis. (C) Anteroposterior radiograph the following year shows interval insertion of posterior instrumentation, which was placed to enhance fusion and provide stability. The bilateral radiolucency at L5-S1 (arrows highlight the right side) persists and is consistent with a pseudarthrosis in the bone graft fusion mass.

patient develops symptoms due to catabolites, which pass out of the affected disks via the vascular system, cause adverse reactions in the regional nerves in and around the disks, and produce constitutional disturbances mediated through the body's immune system. One of the more difficult problems in spine imaging and diagnosis is identification of the offending segment. Diskogenic pain is thought to be the type of pain that is exacerbated by provocative diskography. Some workers therefore believe that provocative diskography is a very important method of choice for identifying the symptomatic segments. Others believe that the find-

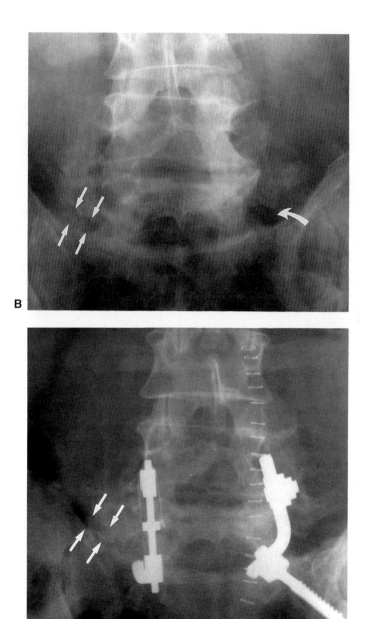

B

C

ing of changes of disk degeneration on MRI is adequate to confirm the diagnosis. The test images do not provide direct evidence of disk degeneration and are insufficient to confirm this diagnosis. Diskogenic pain is therefore not the best clinical diagnosis.

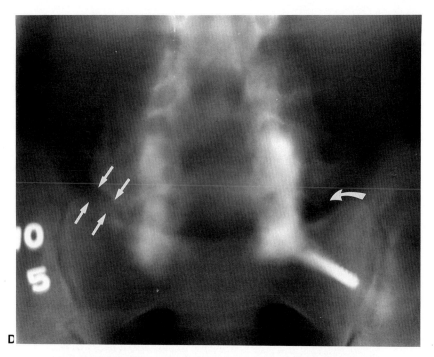

Figure 18-5 (Continued). Failed back syndrome due to segmental instability with pseudarthrosis. (D) The patient's symptoms persist 3 years after the first surgery. An anteroposterior tomogram clearly shows the L5-S1 pseudarthrosis (straight arrows on the right, curved arrow on the left).

"Failed back syndrome" is a general term describing residual or recurrent low back pain or radicular symptoms after spinal surgery. Segmental instability and diskogenic pain are only two of the possible problems that may contribute to failed back syndrome in a patient presenting with a long-term clinical failure (months to years following the original operation). There are several other possible causes of failed back syndrome, including recurrent herniated disk and recurrent radicular pain. Many patients with serious low back pain months to years after surgery have no specific radiographic findings. Failed back syndrome is therefore the best clinical diagnosis **(Option (B) is correct).**

Failed back syndrome due to diskogenic pain or segmental instability is commonly treated with a fusion procedure of the spine by bone grafting alone or combined with instrumentation. The goal is to fuse what is considered to be a painful spinal motion segment. A spinal motion segment is made up of two vertebrae with the intervening disk, two facet joints, and supporting ligamentous structures. In the test patient, both transpedicular screw instrumentation and bone grafting were used to accomplish fusion of L4-L5 (Figure 18-4).

It is important to remember that segmental instability and diskogenic pain can be diagnosed in patients who have had previous spine operations, as well as in those who have not. In patients who have not had surgery, both diskogenic pain and segmental instability are treated with primary spinal fusion. Patients who develop diskogenic pain or instability after a simple disk excision may be treated with secondary spinal fusion. This latter group represents a subgroup of patients with failed back syndrome.

Fusions for low back pain, whether performed as primary or secondary procedures, are done on the premise that some form of instability gives rise to the pain. A basic principle of orthopedic surgery is that fused joints are not painful. Therefore, spine surgeons fuse what they determine to be painful spinal motion segments. Hence, a very important exercise is the determination of the symptomatic level or levels. Unfortunately, the diagnostic means to this end are not well defined or thoroughly understood.

Standard, flexion and extension lateral radiographs and lateral-bending anteroposterior radiographs are poor predictors of symptomatic disease because they can be normal in patients with significant symptoms or abnormal in asymptomatic patients. Diskography is a very controversial procedure. Many physicians believe that it is the method of choice for diagnosing either segmental instability or internal disk disruption, while many others believe that it is an unreliable and unproven procedure. Facet joint injections have also been used to localize painful segments, but their efficacy has been questioned. CT and MRI are nearly always used in the search for reasonable anatomic evidence of contributory disk or osteoarticular abnormalities. However, CT and MRI do not always supply a satisfactory explanation for the patient's low back symptoms. This discussion of diskogenic pain and segmental instability is meant to emphasize the difficulty in making these diagnoses.

It is believed that identification of a painful segment is very important to prediction of successful outcome, and therefore it is common practice to use as many diagnostic tests as necessary to identify the specific spinal motion segments that give rise to the pain. Even with all available studies, however, it is often not possible to be certain which segment to fuse or to predict whether an arthrodesis will relieve the pain and disability. There is considerable controversy about whether spinal fusion procedures are even therapeutically useful. Recently, Esses et al. suggested the use of external spinal fixation as a temporary test to help determine whether permanent internal fixation would be successful. Results of this technique are preliminary.

In the final analysis, the test case demonstrates a patient with recurrent low back pain following a simple laminectomy and disk excision. Among several possibilities, the patient's pain could be due to segmental instability of the operated segment or to internal disk disruption (diskogenic pain). Since these two entities are very difficult to diagnose radiographically and their pathophysiology and treatment remain controversial among orthopedists, the best approach is to use the general diagnosis of failed back syndrome.

Question 73

The fixation system shown in Figure 18-2 (page 453) is:

(A) Harrington
(B) Cotrel-Dubousset
(C) Transpedicular screw
(D) Anterior interbody
(E) Luque

In making a choice of the type of instrumentation to use in spinal fusion procedures, the surgeon generally evaluates the following: (1) ability to provide three-dimensional correction (especially in patients with scoliosis); (2) rigidity of fixation; (3) safety; (4) ability to preserve spinal mobility; (5) technical complexity; (6) overall cost; and (7) ease of postoperative care.

The Harrington fixation system (Option (A)) (Figure 18-6) consists of long rods that are usually ratcheted at their ends and employs attached laminar hooks to hold spinal segments in compression or distraction. This is not the configuration of the instrument shown in Figure 18-2 (page 453). The Cotrel-Dubousset system (Option (B)) (Figure 18-7) involves long dorsal rods to which pedicle screws and laminar hooks can be attached. Transverse traction devices (transverse crosslinks), which connect the dorsal rods, are added to improve stabilization. This system is most commonly used in the treatment of adolescent scoliosis but can be used in other fusion situations as well. The instrument shown in Figure 18-2 has a different configuration.

The system shown in Figure 18-2 is obviously a posterior system; therefore, it cannot be the anterior interbody system (Option (D)). The Luque segmental wiring system (Option (E)) involves long L-shaped rods fixed with sublaminar wires (Figure 18-8). These devices are not present in Figure 18-2.

The device shown in Figure 18-2 is a transpedicular screw system **(Option (C) is correct).** These systems, of which there are several

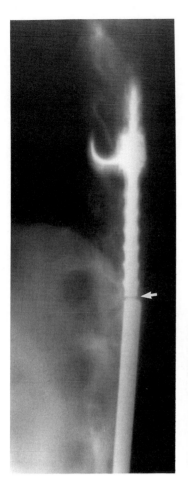

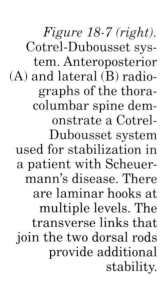

Figure 18-6 (left). Harrington rod with fracture. A lateral tomogram shows a fracture (arrow) through a Harrington distraction rod at the junction of the smooth and ratcheted portions of the rod. The rod had been placed for treatment of scoliosis.

A

B

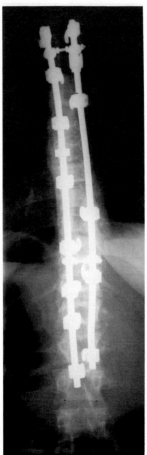

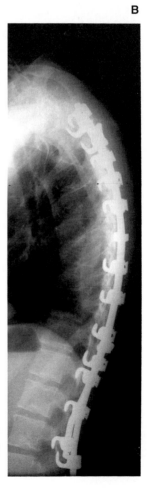

Figure 18-7 (right). Cotrel-Dubousset system. Anteroposterior (A) and lateral (B) radiographs of the thoracolumbar spine demonstrate a Cotrel-Dubousset system used for stabilization in a patient with Scheuermann's disease. There are laminar hooks at multiple levels. The transverse links that join the two dorsal rods provide additional stability.

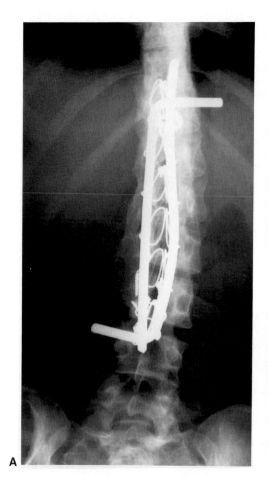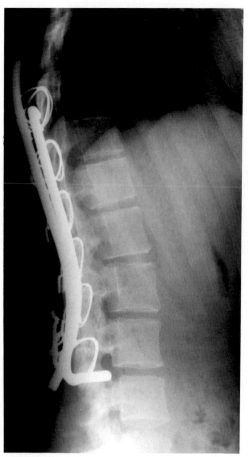

A

B

Figure 18-8. Luque system. Anteroposterior (A) and lateral (B) radiographs demonstrate the use of the Luque fixation system with sublaminar wiring in the treatment of scoliosis.

types, are considered among the major recent advances in spinal instrumentation. Transpedicular screws provide a three-dimensionally controlled grip on the vertebra, unlike hooks, which do not produce as stable a grip. This three-dimensionally controlling grip allows pedicle screw instrumentation to be stable with short-segment instrumentation, as is illustrated in the test images.

Question 74

Concerning the Harrington system of spinal fusion,

  (A) it has been used to treat both vertebral fractures and scoliosis
  (B) postoperative braces are required
  (C) stabilization is inadequate
  (D) short-segment fixation cannot be achieved
  (E) postoperative mobility is facilitated

Harrington instrumentation systems (Figure 18-6) have been used for many years, and the experience with these systems for treatment of vertebral fractures and scoliosis is extensive **(Option (A) is true).** Postoperative bracing is required for up to 6 months **(Option (B) is true),** unlike in some of the other systems, particularly the Cotrel-Dubousset and transpedicular screw systems, which do not require postoperative bracing. Use of the Harrington system is quite successful provided that postoperative care is adequate and fusion occurs. Harrington systems, used properly, certainly provide adequate stabilization **(Option (C) is false).**

Figure 18-6 also demonstrates a complication that can occur in any spinal instrumentation system: fracture of the metallic devices. Harrington rods are particularly susceptible to fracture at the interface between the ratcheted and smooth portions of the rods. This junction produces a stress riser, which increases the risk of metal failure. The occurrence of fracture in a metal fixation device should lead to a high suspicion for the presence of a pseudarthrosis in the fusion with resulting instability in the fused segments.

The original Harrington instrumentation was a major advance introduced in the early 1960s. In 1973, Harrington published an evaluation of 578 patients treated for adolescent scoliosis with an 11-year follow-up. In that series, the average frontal curve correction was 54%. There was only a 4% pseudarthrosis rate in this large series, which was much better than previous results obtained by fusion and casting. However, there is little, if any, rotational correction with the Harrington system. In addition to fracture of a rod, other complications of the Harrington instrumentation reported in the series included 12 hook dislocations and 87 changes in instrument position. Also, the distraction applied across the lumbar spine to correct the scoliosis sometimes caused loss of the normal lumbar lordosis, producing "flat-back syndrome." This syndrome can cause delayed low back pain over time and sometimes requires additional surgery in patients many years after Harrington instrumentation.

Posterior fixation rods with laminar hooks alone require multiple-segment instrumentation. Therefore, unlike the pedicle screw and anterior interbody fusion systems, the Harrington system cannot achieve short-segment (two or three vertebral levels) fixation **(Option (D) is true)**. Because of their less secure "grip" on the spine, the Harrington spinal fusion systems require long periods of postoperative immobilization **(Option (E) is false)**.

Question 75

Which *one* of the following is a characteristic of BOTH transpedicular screw and anterior interbody fixation systems?

    (A) Simple surgical procedure
    (B) Low complication rate
    (C) Usefulness in treating scoliosis
    (D) Stable short-segment fixation
    (E) Few vascular complications

Stable short-segment fixation is a characteristic feature of both transpedicular screw and anterior interbody fixation systems **(Option (D) is correct)**. Both of these systems provide sufficient "grip" across vertebral motion segments that short-segment fixation is adequate.

The increased grip and control of pedicle screw systems are based on the following anatomic observations. Steffee has described a "force nucleus" of the vertebral body pedicle, which is the point on the vertebra where the transverse process, lamina, inferior facet, pars inter-articularis, superior facet, and pedicle all converge. Furthermore, just posterior to the pedicles are the mammillary and accessory processes. These are important posterior sites of muscular attachment for the paraspinal muscles. Considering these anatomic facts, all forces transmitted from the posterior elements to the vertebral body must pass through the force nucleus. Also, the nearby origins and insertions of paraspinal muscles are responsible to some degree for the segmental rotation, side bending, and extension of the spine. Therefore, as the center of convergence of these forces, the anatomic position of the pedicle is extremely important for controlling motion and transmitting force to the anterior vertebral body. As such, placing screws through the pedicle into the vertebral body bilaterally should provide significant control of the entire vertebral complex.

Therefore, in a patient with a single unstable spinal motion segment, the pedicle screw system can be used at the two levels that cross the unstable region. A Harrington system would require that five to seven vertebral levels be crossed by the posterior instrumentation to adequately immobilize the same region of instability. Anterior interbody fusion can be used in short-segment fixation as well. However, since the advent of the pedicle screw system for posterior fixation, the anterior interbody fusion option has been chosen less often.

A benefit of systems that allow short-segment fusion is that adjacent uninvolved segments maintain their mobility. This is a distinct advantage of pedicle screw and anterior interbody systems as opposed to the Harrington system. Traditional Harrington systems required more-extensive surgery to fuse multiple spinal segments, even ones that were not involved with the disease process and did not cause pain.

There are three major categories of pedicle screw systems: screw-plate devices, fixateurs, and screw-malleable rod devices. The screw-plate devices include screws connected to slotted plates (Steffee system) and to plates with holes rather than slots (Roy-Camille). These systems provide rigidity for a motion segment but do not allow for compression or distraction forces. Therefore, pedicle screw systems alone usually are not used for the treatment of scoliosis, because the compression and distraction forces are needed to treat long-segment scoliosis effectively with instrumentation. However, some of the newer systems used to treat scoliosis, such as the Cotrel-Dubousset system (Figure 18-5C), employ pedicle screws in addition to lamina hooks. Also, pedicle screw systems alone can be used to treat adult short-segment scoliosis.

Pedicle screw systems can involve simple surgical procedures relative to other spinal fixation systems, but anterior interbody systems cannot be considered simple. The pedicle screw instrumentation systems do have a relatively low complication rate, but anterior instrumentation systems have a higher risk of operative complications due to the location of the devices and the required approach. Although retroperitoneal approaches can decrease these complications, this approach still has a greater risk of damage to visceral, vascular, and neural structures. Also, the proximity of these devices to the great vessels can result in vascular erosion. The Dunn device is an anterior interbody fusion system that uses curved plates and staples. This system resulted in significant rates of vascular erosion with severe complications. These complications were sufficiently frequent that the Dunn device is no longer used.

Anterior interbody fusion systems have been used to treat patients with scoliosis. These devices, usually applied in the thoracolumbar spine, were developed in an attempt to produce compression on the convex side of the scoliotic curve and therefore help curve correction. One of the first of these devices was developed by Dwyer (and thus called the Dwyer device); vertebral body screws were connected by cables with the cable tightened to apply tension to the convex side, thus correcting the curve. The cable was later modified to a threaded rod by Zielke. Although these anterior instrumentation devices allow greater correction of the frontal curve than does the Harrington system (up to 70% correction), they do have some disadvantages, including more-complicated surgical approaches and increased risk of complications.

Question 76

Advantages of the Cotrel-Dubousset spine fixation system include:

    (A) derotation of the scoliotic curve
    (B) correction of the rib-hump deformity
    (C) no postoperative brace
    (D) use in a variety of spinal problems
    (E) short operative time

The Cotrel-Dubousset system was introduced in 1984. It uses knurled rods to which laminar and pedicle hooks and pedicle screws can be attached at any point along the rods. Figure 18-7 shows a Cotrel-Dubousset system in place for treatment of an S-shaped thoracolumbar scoliosis in an adolescent. The system depends on multiple hooks at multiple levels throughout the spine. Some of the hooks are in distraction, and others are in compression. This configuration induces derotation of the spinal curvature. The rods can be bent and contoured along a scoliotic deformity and then rotated appropriately to correct the deformity. The bars that join the posterior rods in a transverse plane, transverse traction devices, add to the overall stability of the spinal fixation and improve the mechanical performance of this system. Similar transverse traction devices can be used in other systems, including short-segment pedicle screw systems, with the same biomechanical effect.

The Cotrel-Dubousset system has several advantages. It permits derotation of the scoliotic curve **(Option (A) is true)** while correcting the sagittal-contour deformity, thus producing three-dimensional spinal correction in the coronal, sagittal, and axial planes. This derotation helps correct the rib-hump deformity of scoliosis **(Option (B) is true),** which is one of the major goals in management of adolescent idiopathic scoliosis. The Harrington system can produce some correction of rib-hump deformity, but the Cotrel-Dubousset system does a better job. The Cotrel-Dubousset system has sufficient intrinsic stability that postoperative external bracing is not required **(Option (C) is true).** This is an improvement over the Harrington system, which requires postoperative bracing for rather long periods.

The Cotrel-Dubousset system has been used for treatment of adolescent scoliosis, unstable vertebral fractures, and degenerative diseases of the spine **(Option (D) is true)**. However, it is relatively new, and so its long-term efficacy is not clear for all clinical settings in which it is used.

The larger number of hook sites required and the complexity of the Cotrel-Dubousset system have lengthened the operating time for application of this device over the time for other techniques **(Option (E) is false)**.

Question 77

Fracture of a posterior fixation rod is frequently associated with:

(A) pseudarthrosis
(B) postoperative infection
(C) neurologic injury
(D) severe preoperative deformity

The goal of a spinal fusion procedure is to eliminate motion in the spinal motion segments. This is achieved by bone graft material, either anteriorly, posteriorly, or both. Often, metallic instrumentation devices are also placed to provide rigidity while the bone graft material consolidates and heals solidly to the native bone. The later development of a pseudarthrosis is a major potential complication of spinal fusion. Pseudarthrosis is defined as a defect in the otherwise solid fusion mass (comprising bone graft healed to native bone). This is analogous to the development of a pseudarthrosis with chronic non-union of a fracture. In essence, the pseudarthrosis allows motion, thus interrupting the solid fusion. Once a pseudarthrosis develops, the fusion can be a therapeutic failure. On the other hand, it is probable that some patients who develop pseudarthrosis nevertheless have a clinically successful result. If a patient who has had a spinal fusion procedure develops recurrent back pain and has a radiographically identifiable pseudarthrosis, the pseudarthrosis is usually assumed to be the cause of the recurrent symptoms. However, it is important to note that radiographically apparent pseudarthroses can be present in patients with no symptoms.

Other causes of pain following spinal fusion include spinal stenosis, nerve root pain due to scarring, degenerative alterations at adjacent unfused motion segments including disk and facet joints, and pain arising from the graft donor site.

The radiographic diagnosis of a pseudarthrosis requires the identification of an abnormal radiolucency crossing and interrupting the bone graft fusion mass. Sclerotic borders along the lucency make the diagnosis of pseudarthrosis more likely. While pseudarthroses can be visible on standard radiographs, they are sometimes difficult or impossible to see

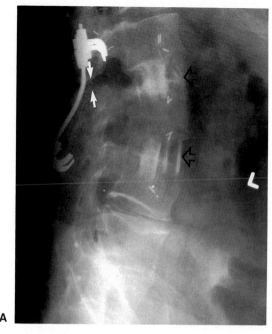

A

Figure 18-9. Pseudarthrosis. (A) Lateral radiograph of the lumbar spine demonstrates a pseudarthrosis (solid arrows) in the posterior fusion mass at the L2-L3 level in a patient who had undergone both anterior interbody (open arrows) and posterior fusions with bone grafts. The posterior compression rods were placed after the development of the pseudarthrosis in an attempt to stabilize the area and to induce fusion at the pseudarthrosis. Anteroposterior (B) and lateral (C) radiographs obtained 6 months after placement of the compression rods show a fracture of the left rod and persistence of the pseudarthrosis.

without use of tomography. Bending or flexion and extension films, angled and oblique views, CT, and bone scintigraphy are also used to try to identify pseudarthroses following spinal fusion.

Pseudarthrosis in a fused spinal segment increases the risk of metal failure and instrument fracture. In fact, detection of an instrument fracture strongly suggests the presence of an underlying pseudarthrosis in the fusion mass **(Option (A) is true).** Figures 18-6 and 18-9 demonstrate fractures in posterior fixation devices in patients with pseudarthroses in posterior fusion masses. Postoperative infection usually occurs earlier in the postoperative period and is not frequently associated with instrument fracture **(Option (B) is false).** However, loosening of the instrumentation from the bone can be seen in patients with infection. Neurologic injury is not frequently associated with instrument failure **(Option (C) is false).** The severity of the preoperative deformity is not

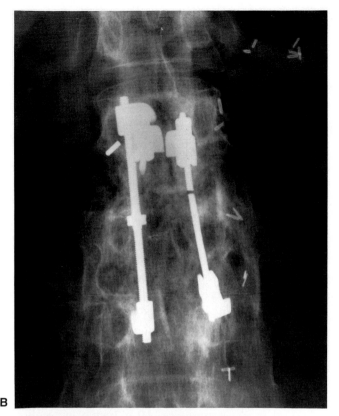

B

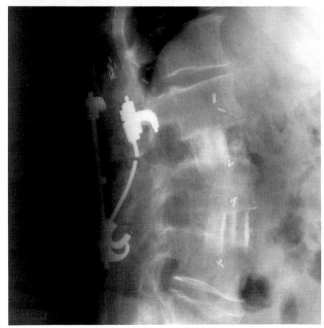

C

necessarily associated with subsequent fracture of instrumentation **(Option (D) is false).**

Question 78

Manifestations of pseudarthrosis developing after spinal fusion for scoliosis include:

(A) loss of correction of the scoliotic curve
(B) pain
(C) fracture of fixation hardware
(D) loss of lumbar lordosis
(E) no symptoms

Development of pseudarthrosis in a fused spine can lead to loss of correction of a scoliotic curve **(Option (A) is true).** However, the loss of correction may not be detected while the patient remains in a cast but may become evident only after the cast is removed. Radiographically, the "fat disk" sign can be seen at the level of the pseudarthrosis. Apparently, this is due to preservation of normal disk height as growth allows spreading apart of the vertebrae at the unfused level while the disks at the fused levels become narrower as vertebral growth continues and compresses them. In patients with scoliosis, pseudarthroses are more likely following fusion for paralytic curves, neurofibromatosis, and kyphoscoliosis and in adult patients. After fusion for scoliosis or other abnormalities, pseudarthrosis can lead to pain **(Option (B) is true)** or fracture of fixation hardware (Figure 18-10) **(Option (C) is true)** or can be asymptomatic **(Option (E) is true).** Loss of lumbar lordosis is not related to pseudarthrosis **(Option (D) is false),** but it is related to place-ment of Harrington fixation systems low in the spine, particularly below L5 or S1. This iatrogenic condition, known as flat-back syndrome, can produce pain and require additional surgery years after fusion of an ado-lescent scoliosis.

Richard G. Stiles, M.D.
Terry M. Hudson, M.D.

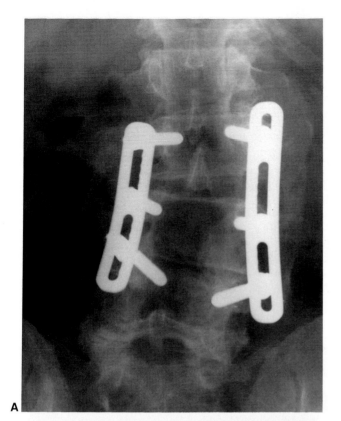

A

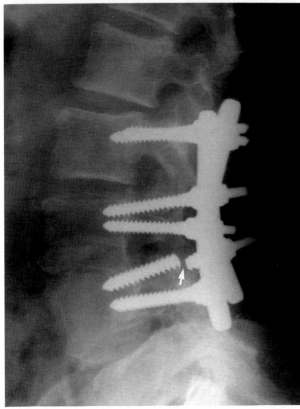

B

Figure 18-10.
Hardware failure.
Anteroposterior (A)
and lateral (B) ra-
diographs of the
lumbar spine dem-
onstrate a broken
pedicle screw (ar-
row in panel B) in a
Steffee plate poste-
rior fixation system.

SUGGESTED READINGS

1. Akbarnia BA. Selection of methodology in surgical treatment of adolescent idiopathic scoliosis. Orthop Clin North Am 1988; 19:319–329
2. Birch JG, Herring JA, Roach JW, Johnston CE. Cotrel-Dubousset instrumentation in idiopathic scoliosis. A preliminary report. Clin Orthop 1988; 227:24–29
3. Cundy PJ, Paterson DC, Hillier TM, Sutherland AD, Stephen JP, Foster BK. Cotrel-Dubousset instrumentation and vertebral rotation in adolescent idiopathic scoliosis. J Bone Joint Surg (Br) 1990; 72:670–674
4. Esses SI, Botsford DJ, Kostuik JP. The role of external spinal skeletal fixation in the assessment of low-back disorders. Spine 1989; 14:594–601
5. Frymoyer JW (ed). The adult spine. Principles and practice. New York: Raven Press; 1991
6. Harrington PR. The history and development of Harrington instrumentation. Clin Orthop 1988; 227:3–5
7. Hu SS, Pashman RS. Spinal instrumentation. Evolution and state of the art. Invest Radiol 1992; 27:632–647
8. Shufflebarger HL. Cotrel-Dubousset instrumentation in neurofibromatosis spinal problems. Clin Orthop 1989; 245:24–28
9. Slone RM, MacMillan M, Montgomery WJ. Spinal fixation. Part 1. Principles, basic hardware, and fixation techniques for the cervical spine. RadioGraphics 1993; 13:341–356
10. Slone RM, MacMillan M, Montgomery WJ, Heare M. Spinal fixation. Part 2. Fixation techniques and hardware for the thoracic and lumbosacral spine. RadioGraphics 1993; 13:521–543
11. Slone RM, MacMillan M, Montgomery WJ. Spinal fixation. Part 3. Complications of spinal instrumentation. RadioGraphics 1993; 13:797–816
12. Steffee AD, Biscup RS, Sitkowski DJ. Segmental spine plates with pedicle screw fixation. A new internal fixation device for disorders of the lumbar and thoracolumbar spine. Clin Orthop 1986; 203:45–53

Notes

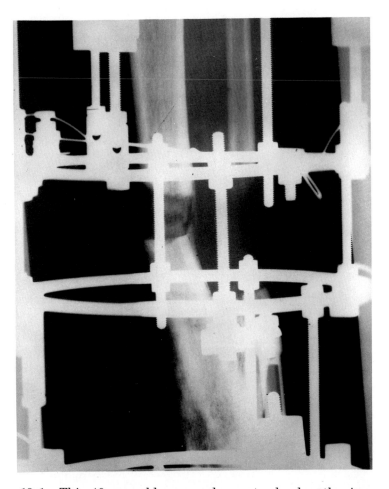

Figure 19-1. This 40-year-old man underwent a leg-lengthening procedure to correct a deformity due to a malunited fracture. You are shown an anteroposterior radiograph of the leg within the lengthening device.

Case 19: Ilizarov Procedure*

Question 79

Which *one* of the following BEST describes this method of bone lengthening?

    (A) Chondrodiatasis
    (B) Callotasis
    (C) Tension-stress
    (D) Epiphysiolysis
    (E) Hemichondrodiatasis

The test image (Figure 19-1) shows a 3-cm segmental defect in the tibial diaphysis, which is partially filled in by longitudinally oriented trabeculae of regenerate bone. The proximal and distal bone segments are secured by an external fixator composed of wires, rings, and interconnecting longitudinal threaded rods. This technique and device make up the Ilizarov method, and regenerate bone forms through the process known as the "tension-stress" effect of Ilizarov **(Option (C) is correct).**

Limb-lengthening procedures are not new. In 1905, Codivilla described a method for forcibly lengthening a bone following oblique osteotomy. The bone segments were held in place by pins and plaster until the osteotomy healed. In 1934, Putti designed a traction device that allowed lengthening and stabilization following a Z-type osteotomy.

It was not until 1956 that the process of induced bone regeneration was described by Gavriil Ilizarov. In 1951, he developed a modular external fixation system consisting of circular components with interconnecting threaded rods. The bone segments are secured by tensioned transfixion wires. Plates, hinges, supports, and other components can be added to allow reduction of fractures and correction of angular and rotational deformity (Figure 19-2). While using his system following open

---

*Orthopedic surgeons George C. Cierny III, M.D., Center for Specialty Medicine, St. Joseph's Hospital, Atlanta, Georgia, and John C. Eldridge, M.D., Emory University College of Medicine, Atlanta, Georgia, provided indispensable help in the preparation of this case by providing patient data, related information, and personal discussions.

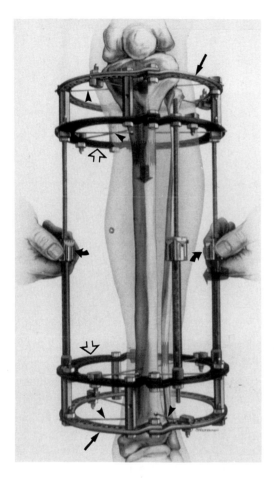

Figure 19-2. Ilizarov device. A drawing of a leg with the device shows the basic Ilizarov configuration with proximal and distal metal (straight black arrows) and graphite (lower weight and lesser radiodensity) (open arrows) rings attached to longitudinal rods. Crossed wires (arrowheads) passed through the bone segments, attached to the rings, and placed under tension provide stability of the proximal and distal bone segments. The patient can adjust the frame in 0.25-mm increments by using the devices connected to the longitudinal rods (curved black arrows). In addition to distraction as shown in the figure, compression can also be performed. (Courtesy of Smith & Nephew Richards, Inc., Memphis, Tenn.)

osteotomy, distraction, and bone grafting to correct a flexion deformity in an ankylosed knee, he noticed new bone formation at the distraction site. Since that time, this phenomenon has been studied in detail and the principle of tension-stress has been developed.

Chondrodiatasis (Option (A)) was described by De Bastiani et al. It is a technique of limb lengthening performed by distracting the growth plate while it is still open. In this procedure, a dynamic fixator is secured to the epiphysis and shaft of the bone to be lengthened. The growth plate is distracted in a symmetric, slow, and controlled manner. Distraction of the growth plate begins at a maximum rate of 0.5 mm per day starting on the first postoperative day. When the desired length is obtained, the distractor can be removed and residual deformities can be corrected. Once the area of distraction shows evidence of mineralization, axial loading can begin. The growth plate may return to a normal appearance once distraction ends; however, abrupt closure of the growth plate often occurs.

Callotasis (Option (B)) is a variation of the Ilizarov procedure. It involves delaying distraction for 10 to 14 days after surgery instead of the 5 to 7 days used in the Ilizarov technique. Callotasis was described by De Bastiani et al., who used a half-pin unilateral fixator instead of a circular external fixator. The half-pin fixators are more rigid with regard to axial loading. The distribution and configuration of the regenerate bone are different from those in the Ilizarov procedure, but there is no significant difference in the overall quality of the regenerate bone produced. The original descriptions involved different types of hardware, but the basic principles of the tension-stress concept and callotasis are the same. Orthopedists are currently combining the use of half-pin fixators with the circular-frame construct of the Ilizarov procedure. The result is a system that is still highly configurable but has the added stability of the larger half-pins (Figure 19-3).

Epiphysiolysis (Option (D)) is another form of epiphyseal or growth plate distraction. Instead of slow distraction as in chondrodiatasis, during which the growth plate is "stretched," epiphysiolysis involves rapid distraction, which actually fractures the plate at the hypertrophic cartilage zone. A hematoma fills the resulting area of distraction, membranous osteogenesis occurs within the hematoma, and the growth plate is eventually replaced by trabecular bone.

Hemichondrodiatasis (Option (E)) is a variation of chondrodiatasis (slow growth plate distraction) in which angular deformities are corrected. Instead of symmetric distraction of the growth plate as in chondrodiatasis, an asymmetric load is applied to correct the initial angular deformity. The ideal time to perform this procedure is near the time of growth plate closure, unless the angular deformity is developing rapidly or exceeds 15 to 20°, in which case hemichondrodiatasis can be done earlier.

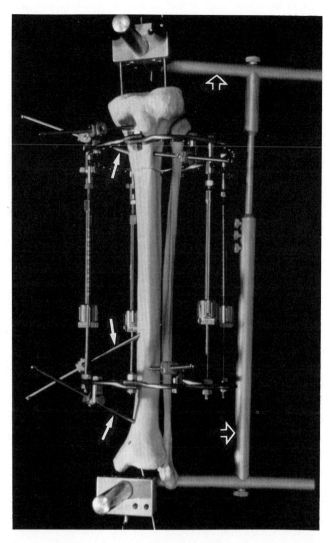

Figure 19-3. De Bastiani modification of the Ilizarov frame by using half-pins. The metal rings and longitudinal rods are the same as those in Figure 19-2. However, instead of the tensioned wires, half pins (solid arrows) have been inserted into the bone segments and are held fixed in the frame. This provides a frame of increased stability while maintaining the highly configurable construct. The metal frame in this model (open arrows) is for display purposes. (Courtesy of Smith & Nephew Richards.)

Question 80

The regenerate bone in the test image is BEST designated as:

(A) normal
(B) atrophic
(C) hypertrophic
(D) fractured
(E) infected

In the test image (Figure 19-1), the distal tibial segment is angulated and there is a fracture line through the regenerate bone (Figure 19-4A and B) **(Option (D) is correct).** Fractures of the regenerate bone occur occasionally but usually heal without compromising the outcome of the lengthening procedure (Figure 19-4C).

The radiographic appearance of normal regenerate bone (Option (A)) that forms as a result of the Ilizarov tension-stress effect is variable and depends on the patient's age and the rate and duration of bone distraction (Figure 19-5). During the first week of distraction, the new bone formation can impart a generalized amorphous increased density to the distraction gap. Ultrasonography has detected new bone formation in the distraction gap as early as 1 to 2 weeks after surgery. Between 6 and 10 weeks, longitudinally oriented trabeculae become visible radiographically. The trabeculae appear more mature nearest the cut bone surfaces and less mature toward the center of the defect. The center of the defect takes on the appearance of a central transverse lucent band. This central transverse lucent band is histologically a region of undifferentiated mesenchymal spindle-shaped cells and has sometimes been referred to as a pseudo-growth plate. The central lucent band in normal immature regenerate bone is characterized by a continuous linear alignment from one bone segment to the other. This appearance differs from that of the test image, in which there is a lateral displacement of the regenerate trabeculae at the lucent fracture site.

Eventually the regenerate bone matures into longitudinally oriented trabeculae extending across the bony defect or distraction site. With time and resumed loading of the bone, the regenerate bone gradually remodels into cortical and medullary bone. Callus and periosteal new bone can be seen if a segment of bone is fractured during the initial corticotomy or osteotomy, but this is associated with the fractured bone and not with normal regenerate bone formation.

Atrophic regenerate bone (Option (B)) is best described as either the absence of regenerate bone formation or a disproportionate lag between the degree of distraction of the bone segments and the degree of bone production. Radiographically this can appear as a spectrum of findings

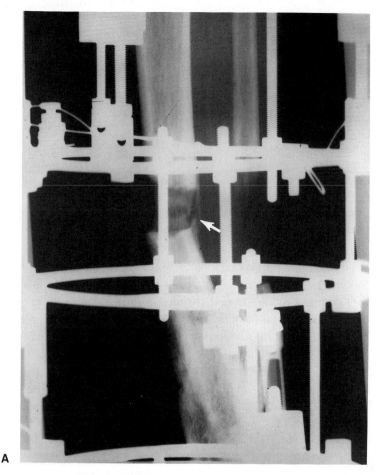

A

Figure 19-4. Same patient as in Figure 19-1. Fracture through regenerate bone during the Ilizarov leg-lengthening procedure. (A) (Same as Figure 19-1) An anteroposterior radiograph shows that the distal tibial segment is posteriorly angulated and the regenerate bone is fractured (arrow). (B) A close-up of the area of regenerate bone visible in panel A shows angulation between the proximal and distal tibial shaft segments, an irregular fracture line through the posterolateral aspect of the regenerate bone (arrow), and longitudinal splitting of the regenerate bone (arrowheads). (C) A radiograph 2 months later shows that the fractured regenerate bone has healed and is maturing. Also, there is solid periosteal bone along the posterolateral aspect of the tibial shaft (arrows).

ranging from complete absence of visible bone formation to tapered regenerate bone with central waisting. The latter form has been termed the "pulled-taffy" appearance (Figure 19-6). In other instances, some regenerate bone is visible but the central transverse lucent zone is dis-

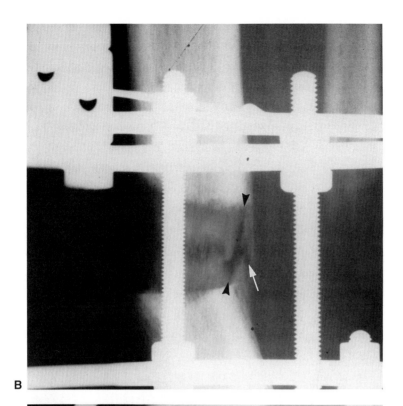

B

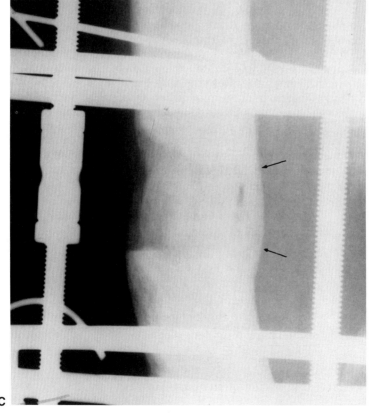

C

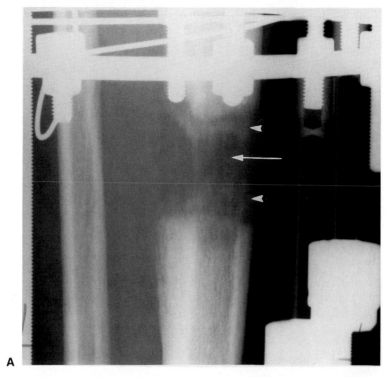

A

Figure 19-5. Normal regenerate bone formation. This patient underwent lengthening of the tibia by the Ilizarov procedure. (A) An anteroposterior radiograph at 32 weeks shows early formation of regenerate bone with longitudinally oriented trabeculae, which are denser and more mature near the cut surfaces of the bone (arrowheads). Note the wide, serrated central lucent band (arrow) and the fact that the trabeculae all have continuous linearity across the osteotomy gaps. (B) At 38 weeks, there are well-formed longitudinal trabeculae and zoning into bands of mature and immature regenerate bone. There is very little periosteal new bone formation, the normal situation. (C) At 17 months, the mature regenerate bone has remodeled into compact cortical bone and a medullary cavity.

proportionately wide. When there are signs of atrophic regenerate bone, the surgeon may decrease the rate of distraction in an attempt to compensate for the slow bone formation. In some patients, cyclic compression and distraction can be performed to stimulate bone production.

Conversely, hypertrophic regenerate bone (Option (C)) forms faster than desired for the degree or rate of distraction. This situation may require an accelerated rate of distraction to compensate for the rapid bone formation. Hypertrophic regenerate bone can lead to early fusion and incomplete distraction of the bone segments. In severe cases, with

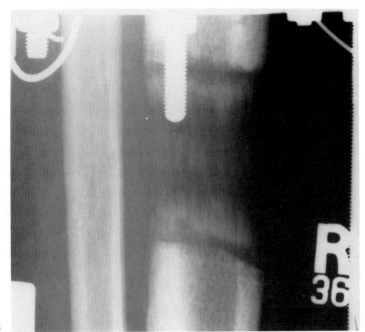

B

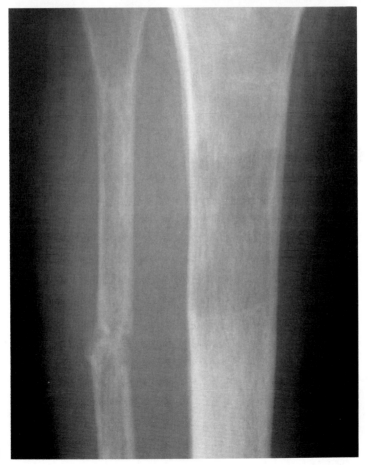

C

483

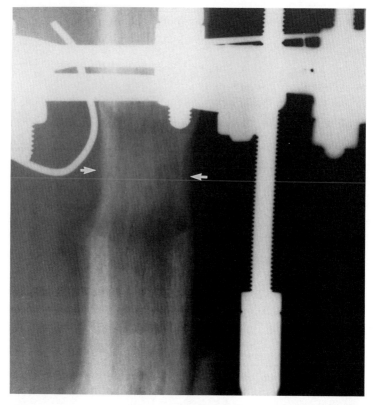

Figure 19-6. Atrophic regenerate bone. Initially, the regenerate bone may form normally but with a delay in maturation. An anteroposterior radiograph of the tibia at 38 weeks shows "waisting" or narrowing (arrows) of the regenerate bone developing as distraction continues. The "pulled-taffy" appearance in this case is mild.

premature fusion, a repeat osteotomy or corticotomy may be necessary to achieve the desired degree of lengthening. In the test patient, however, the regenerate bone is neither atrophic nor hypertrophic but has followed the expected degree of maturation.

Bone infection (Option (E)) can follow any orthopedic surgical procedure, but osteomyelitis rarely follows an Ilizarov procedure. If infection does occur, the pattern of bone destruction can appear as in any long bone. Soft tissue swelling, resorption of bone at the surgical site, subperiosteal-bone resorption, and atrophic regenerate bone can be seen. Chronic osteomyelitis would produce the typical radiographic features, including sclerotic bone, thick periosteal new bone, sequestration, and possibly nonunion. The test image demonstrates none of the expected radiographic features of osteomyelitis.

Question 81

Concerning bone lengthening by the Ilizarov procedure,

    (A) distraction begins immediately after surgery
    (B) osteotomies and corticotomies are equally effective in the production of regenerate bone
    (C) the average distraction rate is 0.25 mm every 6 hours
    (D) distraction is limited to a total of 10 mm per surgical site
    (E) purulent pin tract drainage indicates osteomyelitis

Ilizarov proposed the following seven factors as essential to the proper formation of regenerate bone: (1) maximum preservation of medullary and periosseous blood supply; (2) stable external fixation capable of incremental adjustment; (3) a delay in distraction of 5 to 7 days; (4) a distraction rate of 1 mm/day; (5) distraction in frequent small steps; (6) a period of neutral fixation after distraction; and (7) normal physiologic use of the limb while it undergoes distraction.

Distraction is delayed for 5 to 7 days after surgery **(Option (A) is false).** It is believed that this interval allows for some vascular repair following corticotomy or osteotomy. With bone-lengthening procedures that rely on regenerate bone, every attempt is made to preserve vascular supply, so a corticotomy is often chosen instead of an osteotomy.

Ilizarov showed that the regenerative potential depends on preservation of the vascular supply. In his experiments, three types of osteotomies were performed: (1) open osteotomy with transection of the marrow and nutrient artery; (2) open osteotomy with transection of one-third of the marrow; and (3) closed osteotomy with preservation of the marrow. Regenerate bone formation was best in the third group. However, other studies have shown that although the nutrient artery is compromised with osteotomy, there is no appreciable difference in the pattern of regenerate bone formation or the quality of regenerate bone. In one animal series, osteotomies were compared with corticotomies. The osteotomies were separated into three groups. In the first group only an osteotomy was performed. In the second group the ends of the bone were plugged with bone wax. In the third group the bone ends were plugged with methylmethacrylate. Only the osteotomies that were plugged with methylmethacrylate failed to produce bone. In the other two groups, bone production was similar to that seen with corticotomy **(Option (B) is true).**

Ilizarov noted that the quality of regenerate bone depends on the frequency and rate of distraction. In animal studies, different rates and frequencies of distraction were evaluated. An overall distraction rate of 1 mm/day was found to give the best results. Distraction of 0.5 mm/day often resulted in premature osseous bridging of the distraction site. Distraction of 2 mm/day resulted in damage to the periosteum and suboptimal regenerate bone formation. When the distraction was fractionated into 60 increments per day (16.6 μm per step), the histologic characteristics of the tissues under stress approached that of embyronic and neonatal tissue. The rate of 60 steps per day is not practical with a manual distraction and would require an automatic distractor. (Indeed, automatic distraction devices are now coming into use.) A reduction to a minimum of four times a day (0.25 mm per step) allows the patient to perform the distraction manually and still gives acceptable results. Ilizarov recommended a distraction in frequent small steps of at least four times a day or 0.25 mm every 6 hours **(Option (C) is true).**

There is no accepted limit on the maximum degree of distraction **(Option (D) is false).** Studies of upper-extremity lengthening have indicated that 3 to 10 cm of lengthening can be achieved. In some cases two corticotomies or osteotomies were required. In another study dealing with treatment of bone loss, distraction or transport of bone ranged from 1 to 16 cm. Corticotomies at two levels were necessary in some but not all instances. Some surgeons believe that the limiting factor is not so much the magnitude of bone transport as the amount of soft tissue stress. Complications increase if the degree of distraction or lengthening exceeds 15% of the total limb length. For example, a 50-cm femur will tolerate a 7.5-cm lengthening before the risks of complication increase significantly.

The long-term maintenance of percutaneous pins is not without complications. The motion between the skin and the pin results in local inflammation of the skin. This can lead to local infection, which can spread from the skin to the deeper tissues. Without proper pin tract care, a superficial infection can lead to osteomyelitis. Drainage of purulent material from the pin tract does not necessarily indicate an underlying bone infection **(Option (E) is false).** If pin site care is stressed and pin tract infections are treated appropriately, bone infection can be avoided in most cases.

Question 82

Concerning regenerate bone formed by the Ilizarov procedure,

(A) it is primarily the result of membranous repair
(B) bone marrow is the largest source of interfragment callus
(C) radiographically it appears as longitudinally oriented trabeculae
(D) its formation is compromised by smoking

The process of regenerate bone formation has been studied in both animal models and human patients. These studies have shown that there is very little cartilage formation at the distraction site and that under optimal conditions, the regenerate bone arises from fibrous tissue. Histologically, the area of new bone formation resembles membranous bone formation **(Option (A) is true)**.

In one study comparing corticotomy (marrow and periosteum preserved) with osteotomy (marrow and periosteum transected), the latent period prior to distraction allowed sufficient healing of the medullary vasculature so that there was little difference in regenerate bone formation. With the preservation of a medullary and periosteal blood supply, fibroblasts can invade the distraction gap and produce regenerate bone. However, when the medullary vasculature was completely disrupted, very little regenerate bone formed. It was shown that marrow with an intact blood supply was the principal source of new bone formation **(Option (B) is true)**. However, the importance of periosteal bone production should not be minimized. In patients with absent periosteum, regenerate bone can still form, but its load-bearing capability and stability may be compromised.

Smoking has been shown to diminish the rate of regenerate bone production **(Option (D) is true)**. Apparently it affects not only oxygen transport but also the vascular system. As mentioned above, preservation of a good medullary vascular supply is essential to satisfactory regenerate bone formation.

As discussed in Question 81, the regenerate bone is arrayed as longitudinally oriented trabeculae **(Option (C) is true)**. These first appear near the cut bone ends and later become separate, serrated, dense bands. This appearance is termed "zoning."

Question 83

Complications of the Ilizarov procedure include:

(A) nerve damage
(B) muscle contracture
(C) joint subluxation
(D) vascular damage
(E) premature consolidation of bone across the surgical site
(F) refracture

High complication rates have plagued bone-lengthening procedures since their introduction. The more physiologic standardized and controlled method of lengthening introduced by Ilizarov has reduced but not eliminated complications. As discussed above, the lengthening procedure can be complicated by pin tract infections and osteomyelitis. Other complications include neurologic injury, muscle contracture, joint malalignments, vascular injury, premature consolidation, and refracture **(Options (A) through (F) are all true).**

During initial pin or wire placement, if care is not taken, a pin can pierce a nerve. Although this may result in little damage, the rapidly spinning pin can produce significant thermal injury and, by twisting the nerve around the pin, can produce mechanical injury. There is also potential for nerve injury at the time of corticotomy. This may be the result of direct injury from the saw or osteotome, or it may be a stretch injury as a result of the osteoclasis maneuver required to complete the corticotomy. The nerve can also be injured by the distraction itself. This is less common, but if it is not recognized quickly, it can result in permanent nerve injury. Slowing or stopping the distraction may permit reversal of the neurologic symptoms. In addition to direct distraction of the nerve, the nerve can become tented or entrapped by an initially unoffending wire during the distraction process. This can necessitate removal of the wire.

Muscle contracture is a well-recognized complication of bone-lengthening procedures. The larger and stronger the muscle group, the more resistant it is to distraction. If unopposed, a differential degree of distraction can occur between muscle groups of different size and strength during the distraction process. This can cause joint flexion, which can lead to deformity. An excellent example is the equinus deformity that can occur during tibial distraction. The gastrocnemius muscles are much larger and stronger than the dorsiflexor muscles and are therefore lengthened to a lesser degree, resulting in the equinus deformity. This can be controlled to some degree by fixation of both sides of the joint (Figure 19-7). Contractures can also result from pin transfixion of either

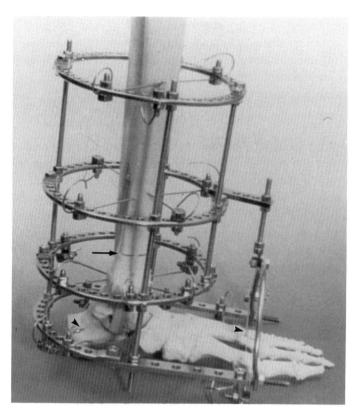

Figure 19-7. The Ilizarov frame applied across the ankle joint. In this example, lengthening of the tibia would be performed through the distal tibial corticotomy (arrow). The frame has been carried across the ankle joint and fixed to the foot by wires through the calcaneus and metatarsals (arrowheads). In this way, the position of the ankle joint can be controlled either to correct preexisting deformity or to prevent the onset of joint deformity. (Courtesy of Smith & Nephew Richards.)

muscle or tendon. Transfixion of tendon or fascia by the pin can also result in restricted joint movement and, potentially, a contracture.

Joint malalignments can result from asymmetric loading of the joint either by the frame or by muscle contracture. This imbalance can result in subluxation, dislocation, or axial deviation of the joint. In many instances, an adjustment of the frame is all that is required to correct the problem. When a large amount of distraction is necessary, both sides of a joint may require fixation. If there is compression across a joint, there is the potential for articular injury as a consequence of immobilization and chronic compression.

As with neurologic injury, vascular damage can occur during surgery or during distraction. There is potential for direct vascular injury at the time of pin placement and at the time of corticotomy. This may be related to direct injury by the osteotome or by stretching at the time of osteoclasis. Deep venous thrombosis is a recognized complication of any surgery and has been reported during bone-lengthening procedures.

Consolidation across the surgical site can be considered a complication if it is delayed or premature. Premature consolidation may be the result of incomplete osteoclasis following corticotomy, and it can also be seen in younger patients in whom the distraction is not rapid enough to match the rate of bone production. Delayed consolidation can be seen in cigarette smokers and patients with malnutrition. Metabolic disorders such as rickets or osteomalacia can also cause delayed consolidation.

Premature removal of the frame can result in fracture of the regenerate bone. Generally, this can be avoided by careful radiologic inspection of the regenerate bone. Prior to removal of the frame, there should be a well-formed cortex bridging the distraction gap, and the overall density of the regenerate bone should equal that of the surrounding bone. Since the affected bone may have been subjected to a long period without weight bearing, significant disuse osteoporosis may result. With resumption of activity and weight bearing, stress fractures can occur in the osteoporotic normal bone.

Discussion

The tension-stress effect of Ilizarov involves the response of tissue to stretching. When slow, steady traction is applied, the tissues at the site of an osteotomy can be induced to produce regenerate bone. The process depends on preservation of the local vascular supply, stresses applied to the bone, and the rate of distraction. In a series of investigations, Ilizarov found that after corticotomy there is an inflammatory response like that seen in fracture healing. On distraction, biologically active fibroblasts appear in the distraction gap and produce collagen. Electron microscopy has shown that these cells are similar to fetal collagenoblasts. The collagen produced by these cells aligns longitudinally in the region of distraction, starting adjacent to the cut surfaces of the bone and extending toward the center of the distraction gap. Capillaries form among these collagen bundles, and osteoblasts line up with the collagen fibers. The osteoblasts produce lamellar bone. All of these elements (fibroblasts, collagen, osteoblasts, and lamellar bone) are aligned in the direction of mechanical stress, hence the term "tension-stress effect."

The Ilizarov procedure includes the use of a stable external fixation frame that permits full weight bearing, normal joint motion, and limb function during treatment. Secure fixation of the bone segments during treatment is essential, because this prevents translational micromotion, which can damage bone circulation, inhibit bone union, and lead to formation of callus rather than of desired regenerate bone alone.

The Ilizarov method has several advantages over other techniques. It is less invasive and permits immediate weight bearing. It involves operating on healthy rather than pathologic bone, and it leads to few failures and complications. The Ilizarov technique can be used to lengthen abnormally short bones caused by dysplasia, congenital defects, metabolic disease, or trauma (Figure 19-8). It can also be used to treat fracture nonunions and bone deformities and to fill in bone defects due to trauma or infection by transporting a segment of bone (Figure 19-9).

The Ilizarov frame is modular; it is built of numerous separate parts like a sophisticated erector set. It permits precise and detailed adjustments of bone angulation, rotation, and translation (transverse motion). Transfixion wires 1.5 to 1.8 mm in diameter are inserted through skin and soft tissues, drilled through bone, and passed on through the skin on the other side. The wires are placed above and below the planned surgical site. It is very important to stretch muscles as the wires are passed through them, because this appears to prevent complications due to traction on muscles during the subsequent bone distraction process. The wires are then bolted to the frame and tightened to a tension of 500 to 1,300 Newtons to functionally stiffen the wires. Wires with attached heads (either "olive" or "stopper" wires) are used to pull on bone fragments. For example, longitudinally placed olive wires could be used to pull a bone segment longitudinally in transporting it to fill a defect. Likewise, olive wires are used to align both proximal and distal fracture sites in segmental fractures.

Ilizarov's original technique emphasized careful corticotomy via a small skin incision to prevent trauma to soft tissues and blood vessels around the bone and within the medullary cavity. After the rings and wires of the Ilizarov frame are applied proximal and distal to the planned site of corticotomy, the skin is incised to expose the bone. To perform corticotomy, a vertical incision is made in the periosteum. The periosteum is carefully elevated, and the anterior two-thirds of the cortex is cut with an osteotome. The posterior portion of the cortex is then fractured by rotating the osteotome 90°. To complete the corticotomy, the proximal and distal rings are rotated in opposite directions. This maneuver is referred to as a rotational osteoclasis.

It is now known that the medullary cavity can reestablish its blood supply even if interrupted by osteotomy. Therefore, corticotomy is not always required and osteotomy is often done. However, it is crucial to avoid early distraction and to maintain rigid immobilization to permit

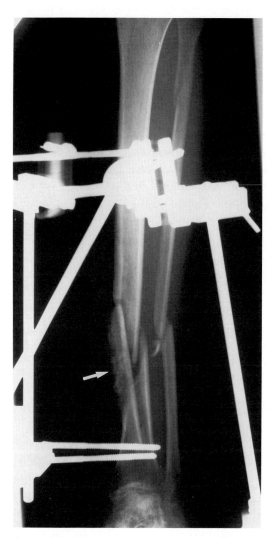
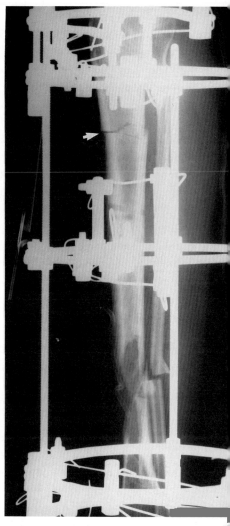

A
B

Figure 19-8. Correction of shortening due to debridement of infected fracture. (A) An anteroposterior radiograph of the left leg shows an open fracture of the distal tibia immobilized by an external fixator. The fracture became infected (arrow). (B) Infected bone has been debrided, the Ilizarov frame has been applied, the tibia has been shortened to provide good contact between the fracture fragments, and a corticotomy has been performed in the proximal tibial shaft (arrow). (C) After several weeks of distraction, abundant maturing regenerate bone is forming at the tibial corticotomy site (arrow), restoring the limb to its normal length. (D) A close-up view of the regenerate bone some weeks later shows continued maturation. The "bumps" on the surface of the regenerate bone (arrowheads) and the irregular lucency across the regenerate bone (arrows) are due to a recent fracture of the regenerate bone sustained when the patient loosened the frame. The final outcome was good, however.

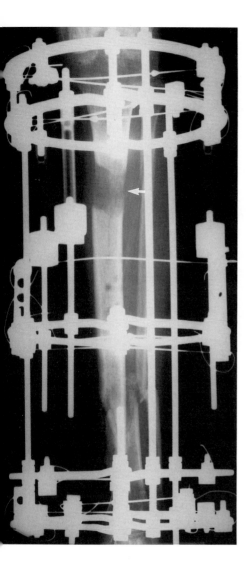 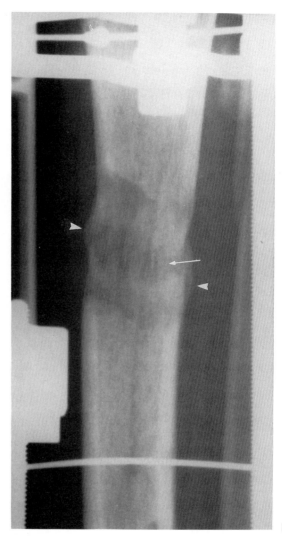

D

this repair to take place. In some instances two distraction sites are needed to obtain the desired lengthening of the bone. In such cases it may be necessary to complete the corticotomy at one level and then perform an osteotomy at the second level because of the inherent instability of the corticotomy. Following corticotomy (or osteotomy), the remainder of the frame is attached and the construct is completed.

After a 5- to 7-day delay, distraction begins. The patient turns the distraction device one click four times a day (0.25 mm per click, 1 mm per day). The surgeon monitors the progress closely, making sure that the patient is performing the distraction correctly and that the frame

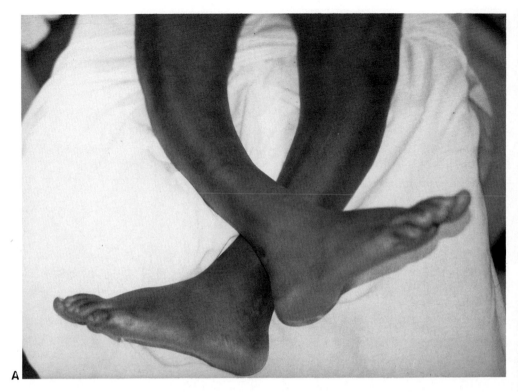

A

Figure 19-9. Correction of marked bowing deformities of the lower extremities due to healed rickets. (A) Initial appearance of the legs. The ankles were actually crossed over because of the severe bowing deformities of the femur (B) and tibia (C). Only the right lower extremity is shown, but the left side was similar.

remains rigid. Malalignment can ensue if undesired angulation or translational motion of one of the bone segments occurs. On the other hand, the surgeon can intentionally adjust the frame to produce angular or translational forces for correction of deformities. The frame can be applied across a joint to better control joint position and prevent malalignment, to correct joint contractures, or to apply compression following surgical joint fusion.

Walter A. Carpenter, Ph.D., M.D.
Terry M. Hudson, M.D.

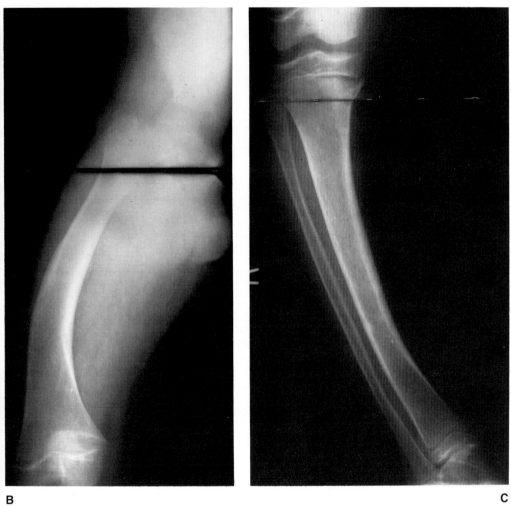

B

C

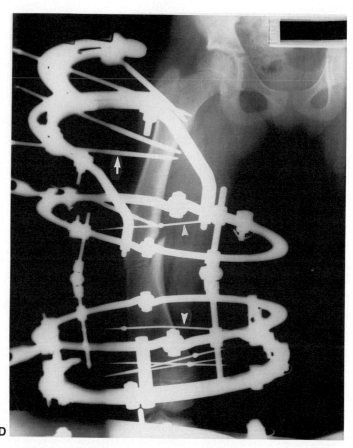

D

Figure 19-9 (Continued). Correction of marked bowing deformities of the lower extremities due to healed rickets. Ilizarov frames were applied to the femur (D) and tibia (E). Corticotomies were performed, and the deformities were gradually corrected. Note the use of half-pins (arrow) in the proximal femur and tensioned wires elsewhere (arrowheads). Because distraction was delayed longer after corticotomy and half-pins were used, the technique here is more correctly called "callotasis."

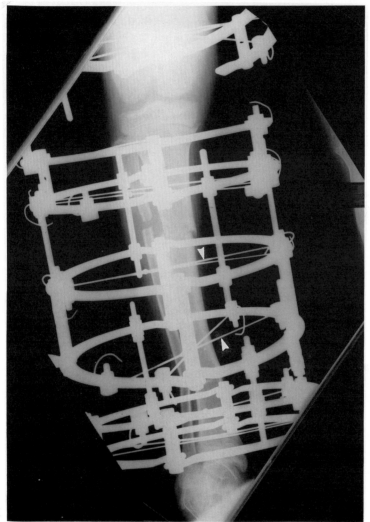

E

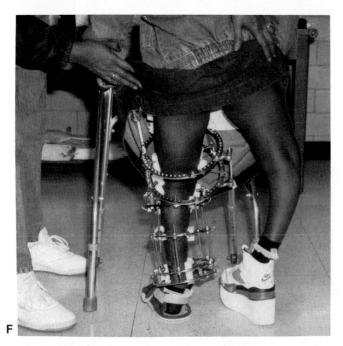

Figure 19-9 (Continued). Correction of marked bowing deformities of the lower extremities due to healed rickets. (F) Posterior view of Ilizarov frames in place around the left lower extremity. Following therapy, the femur (G) and tibia (H) are nearly straight and the corticotomy sites have healed well. (I) Final appearance of the extremities.

F

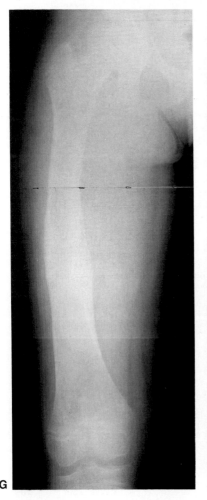

G

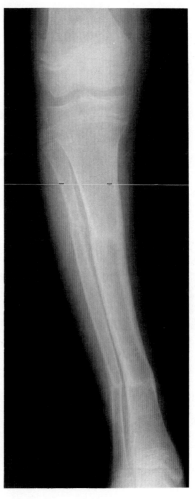

H

498

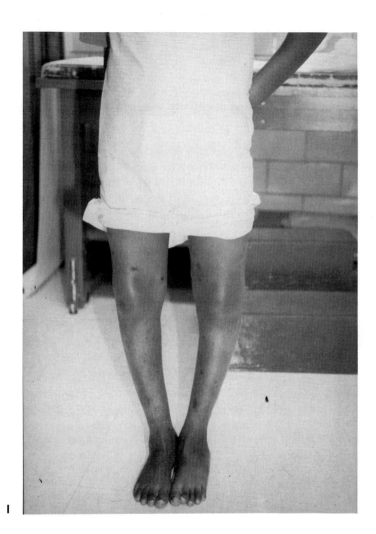

I

SUGGESTED READINGS

METHODS OF LIMB LENGTHENING

1. Aldegheri R, Renzi-Brivio L, Agostini S. The callotasis method of limb lengthening. Clin Orthop 1989; 241:137–145
2. Aldegheri R, Trivella G, Lavini F. Epiphyseal distraction. Chondrodiatasis. Clin Orthop 1989; 241:117–127
3. Aldegheri R, Trivella G, Lavini F. Epiphyseal distraction. Hemichondrodiatasis. Clin Orthop 1989; 241:128–136
4. Behrens F. General theory and principles of external fixation. Clin Orthop 1989; 241:15–23

5. De Bastiani G, Aldegheri R, Renzi-Brivio L, Trivella G. Limb lengthening by callus distraction (callotasis). J Pediatr Orthop 1987; 7:129–134
6. Dahl MT, Fischer DA. Lower extremity lengthening by Wagner's method and by callus distraction. Orthop Clin North Am 1991; 22:643–649
7. Delloye C, Delefortrie G, Coutelier L, Vincent A. Bone regenerate formation in cortical bone during distraction lengthening. An experimental study. Clin Orthop 1990; 250:34–42
8. Guarniero R, Barros TE Jr. Femoral lengthening by the Wagner method. Clin Orthop 1990; 250:154–159
9. Paley D, Fleming B, Catagni M, Kristiansen T, Pope M. Mechanical evaluation of external fixators used in limb lengthening. Clin Orthop 1990; 250:50–57
10. Paterson D. Leg-lengthening procedures. A historical review. Clin Orthop 1990; 250:27–33
11. Price CT, Cole JD. Limb lengthening by callotasis for children and adolescents. Early experience. Clin Orthop 1990; 250:105–111
12. Putti V. The operative lengthening of the femur. 1921 (classical article). Clin Orthop 1990; 250:4–7
13. Yasui N, Kojimoto H, Shimizu H, Shimomura Y. The effect of distraction upon bone, muscle, and periosteum. Orthop Clin North Am 1991; 22: 563–567

ILIZAROV METHOD OF LIMB LENGTHENING

14. Aronson J, Good B, Stewart C, Harrison B, Harp J. Preliminary studies of mineralization during distraction osteogenesis. Clin Orthop 1990; 250: 43–49
15. Aronson J, Harp JH Jr. Mechanical considerations in using tensioned wires in a transosseous external fixation system. Clin Orthop 1992; 280:23–29
16. Aronson J, Johnson E, Harp JH. Local bone transportation for treatment of intercalary defects by the Ilizarov technique. Biomechanical and clinical considerations. Clin Orthop 1989; 243:71–79
17. Calhoun JH, Li F, Ledbetter BR, Gill CA. Biomechanics of the Ilizarov fixator for fracture fixation. Clin Orthop 1992; 280:15–22
18. Cattaneo R, Catagni M, Johnson EE. The treatment of infected nonunions and segmental defects of the tibia by the methods of Ilizarov. Clin Orthop 1992; 280:143–152
19. Cattaneo R, Villa A, Catagni MA, Bell D. Lengthening of the humerus using the Ilizarov technique. Description of the method and report of 43 cases. Clin Orthop 1990; 250:117–124
20. Fleming B, Paley D, Kristiansen T, Pope M. A biomechanical analysis of the Ilizarov external fixator. Clin Orthop 1989; 241:95–105
21. Ilizarov GA. Clinical application of the tension-stress effect for limb lengthening. Clin Orthop 1990; 250:8–26
22. Johnson EE, Weltmar J, Lian GJ, Cracchiolo A III. Ilizarov ankle arthrodesis. Clin Orthop 1992; 280:160–169
23. Kummer FJ. Biomechanics of the Ilizarov external fixator. Clin Orthop 1992; 280:11–14
24. Schwartsman V, Schwartsman R. Corticotomy. Clin Orthop 1992; 280:37–47

25. Tajana GF, Morandi V, Zembo MM. The structure and development of osteogenic repair tissue according to Ilizarov technique in man. Characterization of extracellular matrix. Orthopedics 1989; 12:515–523
26. Tetsworth K, Krome J, Paley D. Lengthening and deformity correction of the upper extremity by the Ilizarov technique. Orthop Clin North Am 1991; 22:689–713
27. Tucker HL, Kendra JC, Kinnebrew TE. Management of unstable open and closed tibial fractures using the Ilizarov method. Clin Orthop 1992; 280: 125–135
28. White SH, Kenwright J. The importance of delay in distraction of osteotomies. Orthop Clin North Am 1991; 22:569–579

COMPLICATIONS OF LIMB LENGTHENING

29. Eldrige JC, Bell DF. Problems with substantial limb lengthening. Orthop Clin North Am 1991; 22:625–631
30. Paley D. Problems, obstacles, and complications of limb lengthening by the Ilizarov technique. Clin Orthop 1990; 250:81–104

RADIOLOGY OF LIMB LENGTHENING

31. Vade A, Eissenstat R. Radiographic features of bone lengthening procedures. Radiology 1990; 174:531–537
32. Walker CW, Aronson J, Kaplan PA, Molpus WM, Seibert JJ. Radiologic evaluation of limb-lengthening procedures. AJR 1991; 156:353–358
33. Young JW, Kostrubiak IS, Resnik CS, Paley D. Sonographic evaluation of bone production at the distraction site in Ilizarov limb-lengthening procedures. AJR 1990; 154:125–128
34. Young JW, Kovelman H, Resnik CS, Paley D. Radiologic assessment of bones after Ilizarov procedures. Radiology 1990; 177:89–93

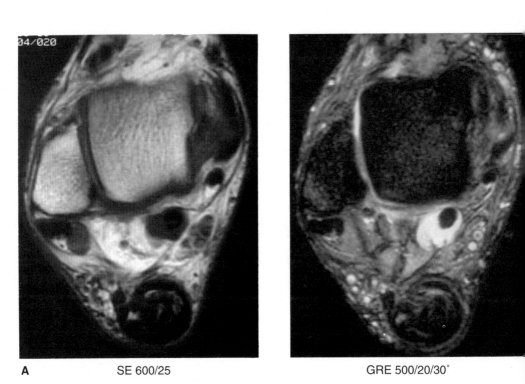

A   SE 600/25   GRE 500/20/30°

Figure 20-1. This ballet dancer presented with ankle pain. You are shown transaxial T1-weighted (A) and gradient-echo (B) MR images of the ankle.

Case 20: Ankle Tendons

Question 84

Concerning the test images,

    (A) there is diffuse soft tissue edema
    (B) there is a partial tear or tendinitis of the flexor hallucis longus tendon
    (C) the posterior tibial tendon is normal
    (D) there is a partial tear or tendinitis of the Achilles tendon
    (E) there is an ankle joint effusion

The test images (Figure 20-1) demonstrate abnormal size, configuration, and signal intensity of the Achilles tendon. It is enlarged, is round rather than oval, and has a convex ventral surface rather than the normal concave configuration. Many areas of abnormal high signal intensity are present within the substance of the Achilles tendon (Figure 20-2A). The flexor hallucis longus tendon is also enlarged; it should normally be about the same size as the adjacent flexor digitorum longus tendon. There is also a subtle area of abnormal signal intensity in the center of the tendon, which should be a homogeneous low-intensity structure. In addition, high-intensity fluid surrounds the tendon and distends the tendon sheath, as is evident on the gradient-echo image (Figure 20-2B). The MR findings of tendon enlargement and signal intensity alteration are characteristic of partial tears and tendinitis **(Options (B) and (D) are true).** Fluid within the flexor hallucis longus tendon sheath indicates tenosynovitis.

All other tendons shown in the test images have normal homogeneous low signal intensity. The peroneal longus and brevis tendons are located posterior to the lateral malleolus. They are very close to one another and are therefore difficult to detect individually. Their combined size and internal signal intensity are normal. Posterior to the medial malleolus, the posterior tibial tendon is seen as an oval structure twice as large as the adjacent and more posterolateral flexor digitorum longus tendon, which is round. These structures are normal in appearance **(Option (C) is true).**

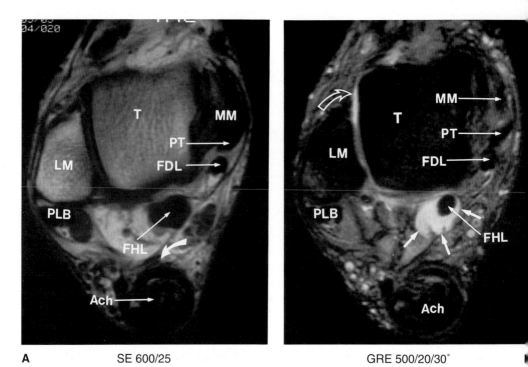

A SE 600/25 GRE 500/20/30°

Figure 20-2 (Same as Figure 20-1). Ankle tendon abnormalities. (A) A T1-weighted MR image shows partial tears of the Achilles and flexor hallucis longus tendons diagnosed by areas of abnormal high signal intensity within the tendons and by enlargement and abnormal configuration of both tendons. The Achilles tendon should be much smaller and more ovoid with the anterior surface flat or concave, rather than convex as it is here (curved arrow). The flexor hallucis longus tendon should be the same size as the adjacent flexor digitorum longus tendon, but it is larger in this case. (B) A gradient-echo MR image shows fluid surrounding the flexor hallucis longus tendon (solid arrows), indicating tenosynovitis, and a small amount of normal ankle joint fluid (open arrow). Ach = Achilles tendon; FDL = flexor digitorum longus tendon; FHL = flexor hallucis longus tendon; MM = medial malleolus; LM = lateral malleolus; PLB = peroneus longus brevis tendon; PT = posterior tibialis tendon; T = talus.

The signal intensity of subcutaneous fat about the ankle is normal, and the skin is of normal thickness. Therefore, soft tissue edema is not present **(Option (A) is false).** Edema infiltrates these tissues and appears as diffuse, indistinct, reticular areas of low signal intensity on T1-weighted images. These wispy streaks of extracellular fluid have increased signal intensity on T2-weighted images.

Fluid in joints also has high signal intensity in T2 (or T2*)-weighted images; this allows the diagnosis of a joint effusion. A very small amount of ankle joint synovial fluid is seen in the test image (Figure 20-1B). This amount of joint fluid is normal **(Option (E) is false).**

Question 85

Concerning MR findings of tendon abnormalities,

(A) ankle joint effusion is a cause of fluid in the sheath of the flexor hallucis longus tendon
(B) the presence of fluid surrounding the peroneus longus tendon is considered abnormal only if there is concomitant abnormal signal intensity within the tendon
(C) tendon enlargement is required to diagnose a partial tear
(D) high signal intensity within the tendon is required to diagnose a partial tear
(E) fluid in the Achilles tendon sheath is a sign of partial tear

Careful attention to proper technique is crucial for obtaining high-quality MR images of tendons. Tailored use of surface coils, thin sections (3 to 5 mm), small fields of view, and both T1- and T2-weighted sequences are required. T1-weighted images effectively demonstrate anatomic detail and the natural contrast between the low-intensity tendons and the surrounding high-intensity fat. Some form of T2-weighted image must be used to demonstrate the presence within a tendon or tendon sheath of subtle high-intensity abnormalities that result from pathologic processes.

The best imaging plane for assessment of tendons is determined by the anatomic location and spatial orientation of the particular tendon. In general, tendon abnormalities are best observed when the plane of imaging is perpendicular to the tendon. A true cross-section of a tendon shows its contour and signal intensity, its relationship to surrounding structures, and the presence of any fluid in the tendon sheath. Determination of the longitudinal anatomy or the extent of a tendon abnormality is facilitated by sagittal or coronal images.

The morphologic and signal intensity patterns of tendons can be explained by their physical and biochemical structure. Tendons are relatively avascular structures composed predominantly of collagen. They also contain some elastin, reticulin fibers, and tenocytes embedded in an amorphous ground substance. The tensile strength of tendons derives mainly from the collagen fibers, which are arranged in a parallel pattern. Collagen fibers are formed from smaller fibrils, which in turn are made of even smaller microfibrils. Collagen microfibrils are composed of a pro-

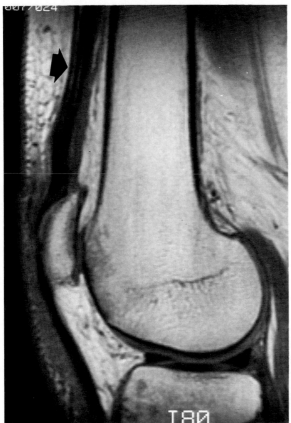

SE 600/25

Figure 20-3. Normal tendon. A T1-weighted sagittal MR image shows linear striations (arrow) within a normal quadriceps tendon, a morphologic pattern caused by slight separation of coarse fascicles of longitudinally arranged collagen.

tein, tropocollagen, which consists of three polypeptide chains arranged in a triple-helix configuration that tightly binds water molecules. Thus, even though tendons are composed largely of water, the lack of rotational motion of the water molecules bound within the triple helix of tropocollagen results in an extremely low signal intensity of tendons on all MR pulse sequences.

As a general rule, normal tendons exhibit low signal intensity throughout; however, there are important exceptions that must not be mistaken for indications of abnormalities. Some large tendons normally have a striated appearance with alternating linear low- and intermediate- intensity layers running longitudinally in the tendon. The quadriceps and triceps tendons routinely demonstrate such striations, which are caused by the longitudinal arrangement of coarse fascicles of collagen separated by zones of "amorphous matrix" (Figure 20-3).

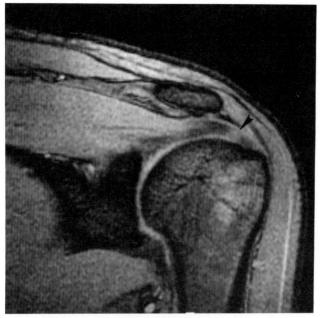

GRE 500/20/30°

Figure 20-4. Normal tendon. A coronal oblique gradient-echo MR image of a normal shoulder shows a focal intermediate-intensity area (isointense with muscle) within the critical zone (arrowhead) of the supraspinatus tendon. This signal intensity pattern is caused by the orientation of collagen fibers with respect to the static magnetic field, the "magic angle" phenomenon, and does not represent abnormalities.

The orientation of a tendon relative to the constant magnetic induction field can also induce intermediate signal intensity within a normal tendon, the so-called "magic angle" phenomenon. This is apparently secondary to the anisotropic biochemical structure of collagen. Isotropic structures have uniform physical properties that behave independently of the direction in which they are measured. Anisotropic structures, such as collagen, have physical properties that vary with the direction of measurement. Structural anisotropy is responsible for the dependence of T2 relaxation times on the orientation of collagen fibers with respect to the magnetic field. When collagen fibers are oriented at about 55°, the "magic angle," with respect to the constant magnetic induction field, intermediate signal intensity becomes evident within the tendon (Figure 20-4). The fiber-to-field orientation angle can be changed by repositioning the patient if necessary to resolve an equivocal MR finding. In a tendon, intermediate signal intensity that is isointense with muscle on both T1-

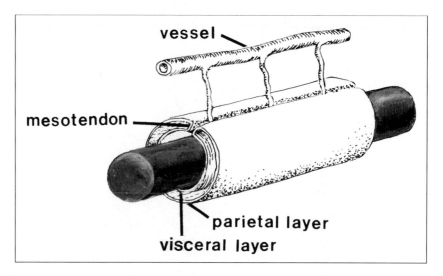

Figure 20-5. Normal tendon anatomy. Where tendons must move in close apposition to adjacent structures, they are invested with a synovial tendon sheath. The tendon invaginates the tendon sheath to form inner (visceral) and outer (parietal) layers and a mesotendon that transmits vascular structures.

and T2-weighted images should not be considered abnormal unless the tendon is also thickened, thinned, or irregular in contour.

Some tendons are partially or completely covered by a sheath. The sheath is invaginated by the tendon such that visceral and parietal layers and a mesotendon are produced (Figure 20-5). The mesotendon is on the nonfrictional surface of the tendon, and blood vessels course within it. The sheath is similar to a synovial membrane. It generates a thin layer of synovial fluid, which acts as a lubricant and allows smooth gliding of the tendon. Tendon sheaths are present in areas where tendons are subjected to high friction, such as in the wrist, hand, foot, and ankle; where closely juxtaposed structures move relative to one another and tendons pass over fascial slings; through fibro-osseous tunnels; or under ligamentous bands. In regions of little friction, there are no tendon sheaths; only loose connective tissue surrounds these tendons.

Under normal conditions, there is an insufficient amount of fluid within the sheaths of normal tendons to be detectable by MRI. The thin sheaths of normal tendons are also not seen by MRI. However, when tendon sheaths communicate with an adjacent joint, fluid from the joint can freely distend the tendon sheath while the underlying tendon remains normal. The two classic examples of this phenomenon are the sheath surrounding the long head of the biceps tendon, which is in communica-

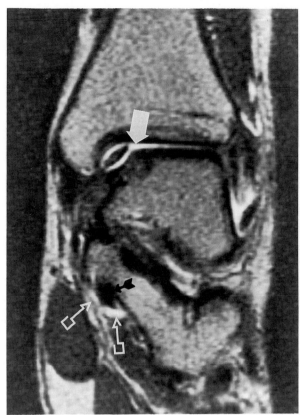

Figure 20-6.
Pseudo-flexor hallucis longus tenosynovitis. A T2-weighted coronal MR image shows a high-signal-intensity ankle joint effusion (solid white arrow) related to the osteochondral fracture of the talar dome. Fluid (open arrows) surrounds the normal flexor hallucis longus tendon (black arrow) because the sheath of this tendon communicates with the ankle joint. In the face of an ankle joint effusion and a flexor hallucis longus tendon of normal size and signal, the diagnosis of tenosynovitis must not be made.

SE 2,000/80

tion with the shoulder joint, and the sheath of the flexor hallucis longus tendon (Figure 20-6), which can normally communicate with the ankle joint **(Option (A) is true).**

Tendon abnormalities result from traumatic, degenerative, and inflammatory processes. A general term applied to any tendon abnormality is tendinopathy, but many other terms are commonly used to describe the abnormalities more specifically.

Tenosynovitis refers to accumulation of abnormal amounts of fluid within a tendon sheath. The underlying tendon may remain of normal signal intensity and size, it may become enlarged, or high-intensity areas may develop within it. These alterations may result from infection, inflammatory arthritides, or traumatic injuries. The diagnosis of tenosynovitis is made by MRI when high-intensity fluid surrounding the tendon is seen on T2-weighted images regardless of the appearance of the underlying tendon or the etiology of the process (Figure 20-7), unless the

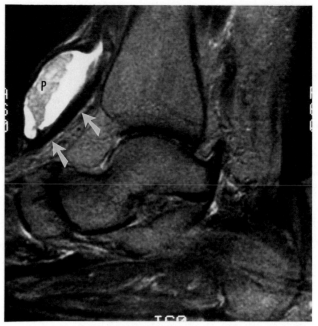

SE 2,000/80

Figure 20-7. Tenosynovitis. A sagittal T2-weighted MR image of the ankle in a patient with rheumatoid arthritis shows severe tenosynovitis involving the anterior tibial tendon sheath. The sheath is distended with high-intensity inflammatory synovial fluid. The low-intensity tendon (arrows) is visible along the deep wall of the tendon sheath. The intermediate-intensity zone within the fluid is hypertrophic pannus (P).

fluid is derived from a joint with which the tendon sheath communicates, as discussed above. Since the peroneus longus tendon sheath does not communicate with the ankle joint, fluid around this tendon is sufficient evidence to diagnose an abnormality of the tendon **(Option (B) is false).**

Inflamed tendons that do not have a synovial tendon sheath will not have a discrete collection of fluid, but they may show amorphous edema in the tissues surrounding the tendon. This is termed peritendinitis. The Achilles tendon is a classic example of a tendon that is not encased by a synovial sheath and does not show MR changes of tenosynovitis in the presence of significant abnormalities (Figure 20-8) **(Option (E) is false).**

Tendinitis is inflammation affecting the substance of a tendon; it is sometimes accompanied by tenosynovitis or peritendinitis. Acute tendinitis may occur from chronic repeated stresses to the tendon (usually

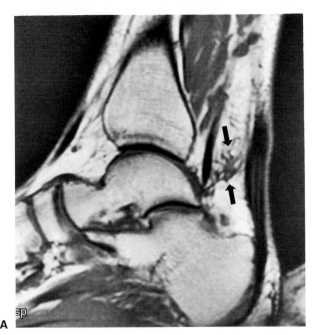

A

SE 600/20

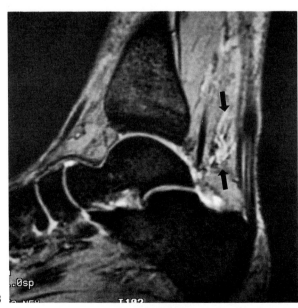

B

GRE 500/20/20°

Figure 20-8. Peritendinitis. T1-weighted (A) and gradient-echo (B) sagittal MR images depict a partial tear or tendinitis of the Achilles tendon, which is thickened and has layered high signal within it. There is edema in the subcutaneous fat dorsal to the tendon and in the pre-Achilles fat (Kager's triangle), creating a reticular pattern (arrows). Edema is evident as low signal intensity on T1-weighted images and high signal intensity on gradient-echo images.

athletic or occupational); from degeneration of the tendon with secondary inflammation; or from inflammatory arthritides, systemic lupus erythematosus, gout, or diabetes mellitus. Tendinitis is considered chronic if symptoms have been present for longer than 6 weeks. MR findings are indistinguishable from those of partial tears or degeneration of tendons.

Tendon degeneration shows increasing frequency with increasing age and affects different tendons to different extents. Biochemical changes that occur within tendons as they age include an increase in collagen, a decrease in elastin, and a decrease in water content. Degenerative tendinopathy affects both tenocytes and collagen fibers. Histologically, tendon degeneration is characterized by variable replacement of a tendon with mucoid material, lipid, calcium, or necrotic debris. Collagen fibers split longitudinally, disintegrate, and become angulated. Available evidence suggests that the key factor in degeneration is decreased arterial blood flow, which leads to local hypoxia, decreased nutrition, and impaired metabolic activity. Tendon degeneration is asymptomatic unless a secondary inflammatory process is superimposed or the tendon spontaneously ruptures because it has been weakened.

Partial or full-thickness tendon tears may occur from acute trauma or repetitive stress. Spontaneous, complete tears following minimal trauma are believed to occur through an area of preexisting tendon degeneration. Impingement on tendons by adjacent osseous or soft tissue structures also contributes to the development of complete and partial tendon tears as a result of mechanical stress.

A complete tendon rupture is manifested as discontinuity of the affected tendon on MR images. In the acute phase, hemorrhage and edema surrounding the torn tendon are seen as intermediate- or low-intensity areas on T1-weighted images and high-intensity zones on T2-weighted images. In chronic complete tendon tears, the hemorrhage and edema may be replaced by low-intensity fibrotic scar or high-intensity fat. The exact site of the tendon tear can be determined by MRI, as can the amount of retraction of the tendon fragments and the presence of any associated soft tissue or bone injuries. This information is helpful to the surgeon in planning therapy.

Partial or incomplete tendon tears have an identical MR appearance to tendinitis and tendon degeneration. The MR features of all three conditions include increased signal intensity within the substance of the tendon, abnormal configuration of the tendon, or both (Figure 20-9) **(Options (C) and (D) are false).** That MRI cannot differentiate among these entities is of little practical significance since, in general, the treatment for all three is conservative and consists of decreased physical activity. Nonsteroidal anti-inflammatory agents are given if the patients are symptomatic.

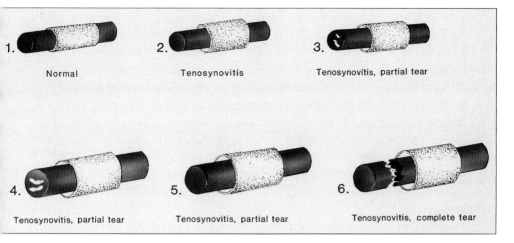

Figure 20-9. Spectrum of tendon abnormalities. (1) Normal tendon and sheath. The tendon has homogeneous low signal intensity and normal size and configuration; there is no fluid in the tendon sheath. (2) Tenosynovitis. The tendon sheath is distended with fluid, but the tendon maintains normal configuration and signal intensity. (3) Tenosynovitis with partial tendon tears. There is fluid in the tendon sheath and increased signal intensity in the tendon, but the tendon has normal configuration and size. (4) Tenosynovitis with partial tendon tear. There is fluid in the tendon sheath and increased signal intensity in the enlarged tendon. (5) Tenosynovitis with partial tendon tear. There is fluid in the tendon sheath and an enlarged tendon with normal low-intensity substance. (6) Tenosynovitis with complete tendon tear. There is fluid in the tendon sheath and discontinuity of the tendon. Tendon fragments may be enlarged and may have abnormal signal intensity. Patterns 3 and 4 could result from tendon degeneration only.

Increased signal intensity in the substance of abnormal tendons on T1-weighted images becomes even higher, similar to that of water, on T2-weighted images. This appearance occurs because collagen fibers have become disrupted, with the result that water molecules in the tendon are less tightly bound. These more mobile protons lengthen the T2 relaxation time within the tendon so that the abnormal areas have an increased signal intensity relative to the very low intensity of the adjacent intact tendon fibers. With even greater disruption of the collagen fascicles, open defects in the tendon develop and can fill with fluid from an adjacent tendon sheath or can be infiltrated by inflammatory transudate.

Tendon degeneration causes abnormal high signal intensity within a tendon; this may persist indefinitely. Acute partial tendon tears or tendinitis also cause high signal intensity within the tendon. However, if the tear or tendinitis heals, the intratendinous signal abnormality often resolves. The time required for resolution of high-intensity regions in different tendons is not known, but these zones may persist for months or longer after the patient has become asymptomatic.

The other major MR finding indicative of a partial tendon tear or tendinitis is an abnormal tendon configuration. A tendon may be focally or diffusely enlarged either with or without abnormal intratendinous signal intensity. Partial tendon tears are occasionally manifested as thinned or irregular tendons rather than abnormally thick tendons. Familiarity with the size and configuration of normal tendons is essential for accurate diagnosis. Tenosynovitis often accompanies tendinitis, degeneration, and tears.

Trauma can cause some tendons to undergo subluxation or to dislocate rather than tear, degenerate, or become inflamed. The tendons that most commonly undergo subluxation or dislocation are the long head of the biceps, the extensor carpi ulnaris, and the peroneus tendons.

Question 86

Concerning the anatomy of the foot and ankle,

    (A) the Achilles tendon uses the anterior tuberosity of the calcaneus as a pulley
    (B) the flexor hallucis longus tendon uses the sustentaculum tali as a pulley
    (C) the peroneus longus tendon attaches to the base of the first metatarsal
    (D) the flexor digitorum longus tendon uses the lateral malleolus as a pulley
    (E) the tibialis posterior tendon uses the medial malleolus as a pulley

The tendons that cross the ankle to act on the foot are depicted well on transaxial MR images of the ankle. These tendons can be divided into groups on the basis of their location and function, and each tendon should be identified and examined in meticulous detail on each section from an MR examination (Figures 20-10 and 20-11).

Posterior ankle. The Achilles tendon is the most posterior tendon of the ankle and can be followed to its attachment on the posterior tuberosity of the calcaneus **(Option (A) is false).** It is the largest and strongest tendon in the body and is formed by the confluence of the gastrocnemius and soleus muscles, which originate from the femoral condyles and posterior tibia and fibula, respectively. It is not invested with a synovial tendon sheath since it is not subjected to high friction forces; therefore, tenosynovitis is not a manifestation of an abnormality in this tendon. The Achilles tendon has a flat or slightly concave anterior margin when imaged in the axial plane (Figure 20-10A). It is also well evaluated in the sagittal plane, where it has a straight anterior margin and is of uniform

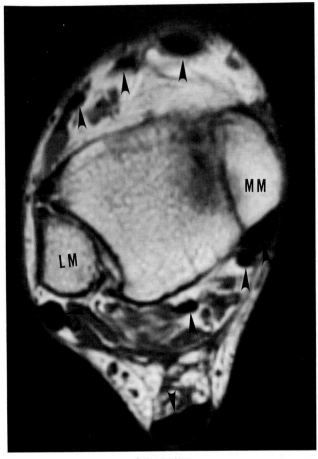

A

SE 600/25

Figure 20-10. Normal ankle tendons. (A) A transaxial T1-weighted MR image through the ankle demonstrates the normal location and configuration of the tendons (arrowheads). (B) A diagram depicts the same ankle anatomy as in panel A. All tendons are labeled. The three tendons on the medial side of the ankle can be remembered by the mnemonic Tom, Dick, And Harry, which is the arrangement of the tendons from medial to lateral. The posterior tibial tendon is oval and twice as big as the round flexor hallucis and flexor digitorum tendons, which are equal in size. The anterior tibial tendon is the largest of the extensors and the most oval. LM = lateral malleolus; MM = medial malleolus.

thickness, never exceeding 1 cm in the anteroposterior dimension (Figure 20-11A). A high-intensity fat pad, the pre-Achilles fat pad, is normally seen anterior to the homogeneously low-intensity Achilles tendon.

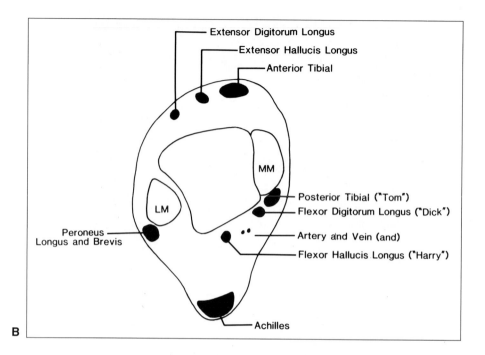

Extensor Digitorum Longus
Extensor Hallucis Longus
Anterior Tibial

MM

Posterior Tibial ("Tom")
Flexor Digitorum Longus ("Dick")

LM

Peroneus
Longus and Brevis

Artery and Vein (and)
Flexor Hallucis Longus ("Harry")

Achilles

B

Medial ankle. The flexor tendons are located on the posteromedial aspect of the ankle and pass through the tarsal tunnel as a group. They are the posterior tibial (or tibialis posterior), flexor digitorum longus, and flexor hallucis longus tendons.

The posterior tibial muscle arises from the proximal and middle portions of the tibia and fibula. The musculotendinous junction is located several centimeters proximal to the medial malleolus, which serves as a pulley for the posterior tibial tendon **(Option (E) is true).** After passing posterior to the medial malleolus, the tendon turns anteriorly underneath the malleolus to insert broadly on the navicular, medial, and intermediate cuneiforms and the bases of the second through fourth metatarsals. The normal posterior tibial tendon on an axial image of the ankle is located just anterior and medial to the flexor digitorum longus and flexor hallucis longus tendons (Figure 20-10). The posterior tibial tendon is oval and about twice as large as the circular flexor hallucis longus and flexor digitorum longus tendons. It is usually very close to the posterior aspect of the medial malleolus, where it blends with the adjacent low-intensity cortex of the bone.

The flexor digitorum longus and flexor hallucis longus tendons are situated more posterior and lateral to the posterior tibial tendon. The flexor digitorum longus tendon uses the medial malleolus as a pulley

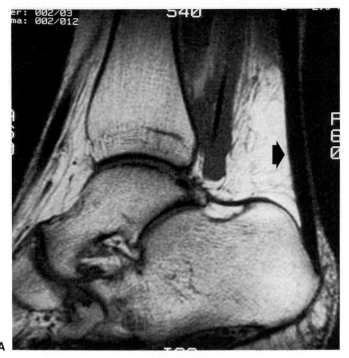

A

SE 600/25

Figure 20-11. Normal ankle tendons. (A) A sagittal T1-weighted MR image shows that the Achilles tendon (arrow) is straight, has uniform thickness, and, as with all ankle tendons, has homogeneous low signal intensity. The high-signal-intensity pre-Achilles fat pad is interposed between the tendon and the deeper structures. (B) A sagittal T1-weighted MR image shows the sustentaculum tali (ST) and the pulley for the flexor hallucis longus (arrows). (C) A sagittal T1-weighted MR image shows the lateral malleolus (LM) with the peroneus longus (PL) and peroneus brevis (PB) tendons running immediately behind it.

(Option (D) is false). The flexor hallucis longus tendon uses the sustentaculum tali of the calcaneus as a pulley **(Option (B) is true).** All tendons of the ankle can be readily recognized in any imaging plane by identifying the more familiar osseous structures to which they relate. Another method of remembering the names and order of the flexor tendons on the medial ankle is by the mnemonic "Tom, Dick, And Harry" (the tendons are arrayed from medial to lateral as follows: posterior Tibial, flexor Digitorum, Artery and vein, flexor Hallucis longus) (Figure 20-10B).

The flexor hallucis longus muscle arises from the proximal tibia and fibula posteriorly. Its tendon descends vertically through a fibro-osseous

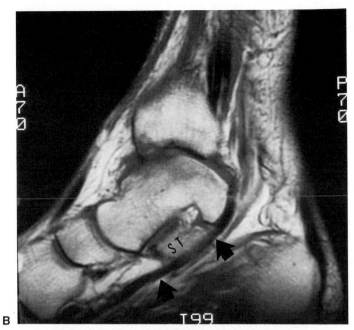

SE 600/25

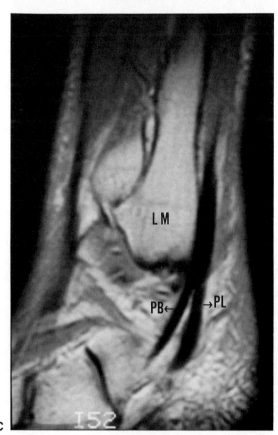

SE 600/25

tunnel posterior to the talus and then turns to run horizontally. It continues beneath the sustentaculum tali of the calcaneus (Figure 20-11B), between the sesamoids on the plantar surface of the first metatarsal, to insert on the great toe.

Lateral ankle. The peroneal muscles originate from the posterior and lateral aspects of the fibula. The peroneal tendons pass posterior to and beneath the lateral malleolus, which they use as a pulley. The peroneus brevis tendon is just anterior and superior to the peroneus longus tendon (Figure 20-11C). The brevis inserts on the base of the fifth metatarsal; the longus passes beneath the calcaneus to insert on the base of the first metatarsal and the medial cuneiform **(Option (C) is true).** In most people, there is a shallow groove in the posterior fibula, the retrofibular sulcus, that partially accommodates the peroneus brevis. Both peroneal tendons are contained within a common tendon sheath and are held in place relative to the lateral malleolus by peroneal retinacula.

Transaxial MR images of the peroneal tendons show that they are round and of nearly equal size (Figure 20-10). The brevis is just anterior and slightly medial to the longus. The tendons are situated so close to one another at the level of the malleolus that it is difficult to distinguish them from one another or at times from the cortex of the adjacent bone.

Anterior ankle. The extensor tendons of the foot are located anterior to the ankle joint. Arranged from medial to lateral, these are the tibialis anterior, extensor hallucis longus, and extensor digitorum longus tendons (Figure 20-10). The tendons are held in place by several retinacula and are surrounded by synovial tendon sheaths. All three anterior tendons are round to oval structures, with the tibialis anterior tendon usually being the largest.

Question 87

Concerning tendons of the foot and ankle,

- (A) posterior tibial tendon abnormalities are most common in ballet dancers
- (B) the flexor hallucis longus tendon is the principal everter of the foot
- (C) peroneal tendon abnormalities are a common cause of pain in patients with a history of calcaneal fractures
- (D) an abnormal flexor digitorum longus tendon is a common cause of a painful flat foot in patients with rheumatoid arthritis
- (E) downhill hiking is a common cause of Achilles tendon injuries

The purpose of a tendon is to transmit force from a contracting muscle to a bone. Tendons can withstand tensile loads far greater than the

Table 20-1: Common athletic activities resulting in ankle tendon injuries

Tendon	Function	Athletic activity
Achilles	Plantar flexion of foot	Running Unconditioned, "weekend" athletes
Tibialis posterior	Inversion of foot Maintains plantar arch Stabilizer of hindfoot	Sudden changes in direction: soccer, ice hockey, tennis
Flexor hallucis longus	Flexion of great toe	Repeated push-off from forefoot: ballet, soccer (affects portion of tendon beneath calcaneus) Running (affected tendon is between sesamoids under first metatarsal head)
Peroneus	Eversion of foot	Mechanical stress against lateral malleolus: running Forced plantar flexion associated with ruptured retinacula: skiing, ice skating, soccer, basketball
Anterior tibial	Dorsiflexion of foot	Downhill hiking and running

corresponding muscle can. Individuals most likely to sustain a tendon abnormality are athletes or others engaged in activities that subject tendons to chronic repetitive stress (Table 20-1). Unconditioned, "weekend" athletes can sustain identical injuries with minimal stress. A prior injury, inadequate warm-up, immobilization, and poor conditioning can all cause weakening of a tendon.

Tendons that are mechanically weakened by underlying degeneration or inflammation can easily sustain partial or complete tendon tears, and this process is accelerated if soft tissue or osseous structures impinge on the tendon. A weakened tendon can tear even when subjected to only routine physiologic stress; patients with rheumatoid arthritis, gout, and diabetes mellitus, whose conditions particularly weaken their tendons, are especially vulnerable. Patients receiving steroid injections also have weakened tendons that are predisposed to tear.

The physical diagnosis of tendon inflammation or tear is often not obvious. Partial tears, in particular, can be misdiagnosed as other disease processes, and without proper treatment the tendon injury can progress to become a complete tear, which requires more lengthy or aggressive therapy.

Achilles tendinitis is a painful inflammatory condition that begins around the Achilles tendon in individuals who suddenly increase their level or frequency of activity, particularly running. In fact, 20% of all injuries caused by running involve the Achilles tendon. The inflammatory process does not cause a focal collection of fluid (tenosynovitis) around the tendon, because the Achilles tendon, unlike most other tendons in the body, does not have a tendon sheath. Thus, the primary inflammatory process occurs in the peritendon. Edema may be seen in the fat pad anterior to the tendon. Chronic tendinitis can lead to longitudinal splitting of the tendon.

MRI of Achilles tendinitis shows focal thickening of the tendon either with or without abnormal high signal intensity within the tendon (Figure 20-12). Sometimes the tendon is thickened diffusely. Subtle amounts of tendon thickening may be recognized on the transaxial view if one recalls that the anterior aspect of the tendon is normally flat or concave; any degree of convexity indicates an abnormality (Figure 20-12C). Partial tears often appear as diffuse tendon thickening with foci of increased signal intensity within the substance of the tendon (Figure 20-13).

Complete ruptures (Figure 20-14) of the Achilles tendon generally occur in unconditioned middle-aged athletes who suddenly increase their level of activity. The rupture probably progresses through an existing region of tendon degeneration. The portion of the Achilles tendon initially or usually involved with tendinitis, partial tears, or complete ruptures is located approximately 4 to 6 cm proximal to the attachment of the tendon on the calcaneus. This is the most hypovascular segment of the tendon.

MRI is helpful in diagnosing complete Achilles tendon rupture even when the diagnosis is evident clinically. Complete rupture is treated surgically if the fragments are widely separated, whereas less severe injuries are treated by immobilization with casting. MRI can help determine which therapy would be more advantageous. If casting is selected, the position of the fragments can be shown post-casting so that the efficacy of the treatment is immediately known.

Achilles tendinitis can be mimicked clinically by retrocalcaneal bursitis in patients with an inflammatory arthritis or mechanical irritation from overuse (as occurs in athletes) (Figure 20-15). MRI can easily differentiate the two conditions because, unlike tendinitis (see above), retrocalcaneal bursitis appears as a teardrop-shaped fluid collection inter-

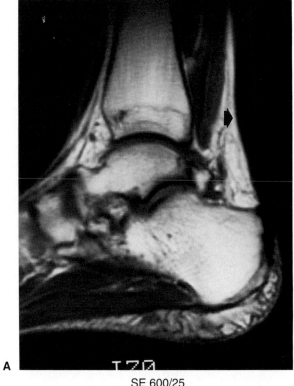

A

SE 600/25

Figure 20-12. Achilles tendinitis and partial tears in a 45-year-old runner. Sagittal T1-weighted (A), sagittal gradient-echo (B), and transaxial gradient-echo (C) MR images demonstrate focal thickening of the Achilles tendon in its most hypovascular region, about 5 cm proximal to its insertion on the calcaneus (arrow in panels A and B). The tendon is recognized as abnormal on the transaxial image (panel C) only by the slight convexity of its anterior surface. The abnormal region has homogeneous low signal intensity on both pulse sequences, suggesting that the condition is probably chronic.

posed between the posterosuperior calcaneus and the overlying normal Achilles tendon.

The posterior tibial tendon is the major invertor of the foot, is one of the main stabilizers of the hindfoot, and maintains the longitudinal arch of the foot. Complete or partial ruptures are most common in middle-aged and older women and are particularly common in patients with rheumatoid arthritis. Posterior tibial tendon injuries are not a major problem in ballet dancers (see below) **(Option (A) is false).** Posterior tibial tendon tears present with a painful flat-foot deformity, and the

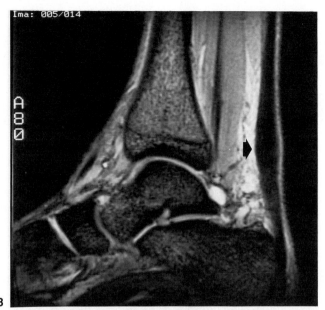

B

GRE 500/20/30°

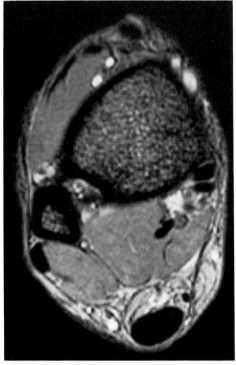

C

GRE 500/20/30°

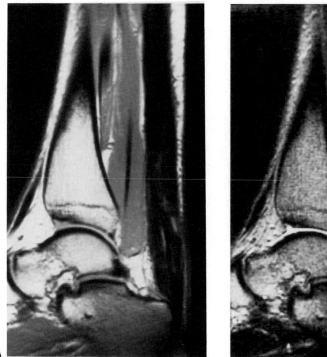

A   B

SE 600/25   SE 2,000/80

Figure 20-13. Partial Achilles tendon tear in a 25-year-old man who experienced severe pain in the posterior ankle while spiking a volleyball several weeks before the MR examination. Sagittal T1-weighted (A) and T2-weighted (B) images through the Achilles tendon show diffuse tendon thickening with several linear areas of intrasubstance high signal intensity representing partial tears.

patient is unable to raise up on the toes; painful flat foot is not a common consequence of flexor digitorum longus tendon injuries **(Option (D) is false).** Other people who sustain this injury include athletes who must change directions quickly, such as soccer, ice hockey, and tennis players. In patients who sustain posterior tibial tendon ruptures that are not related to inflammatory changes of an arthritis, chronic mechanical abrasion of the tendon against the malleolus is believed to be the mechanism of injury.

MRI shows complete or partial ruptures of the posterior tibial tendon or fluid surrounding the tendon. These findings are most frequent at the level of the medial malleolus or distal to it (Figures 20-16 through 20-18). Partial tears may benefit from synovectomy and debridement to prevent

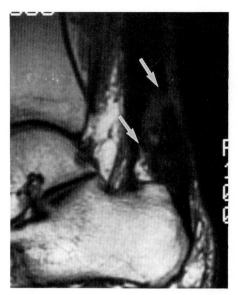

SE 600/25

Figure 20-14 (left). Complete Achilles tendon rupture in a 40-year-old jogger with chronic ankle pain that acutely worsened 2 weeks before the MR examination. Sagittal T1-weighted image shows an oblique complete tendon rupture (arrows) just above the calcaneus. The tendon is very thick, indicating that the tear probably occurred through an area already weakened by chronic tendinitis, partial tear, or degeneration. The tendon fragments are closely apposed; therefore, casting rather than surgery was elected for treatment.

Figure 20-15 (right). Retrocalcaneal bursitis in a 19-year-old college football player suspected clinically of having an Achilles tendinopathy. T2-weighted sagittal MR image of the Achilles tendon shows fluid (arrow) in the retrocalcaneal bursa, which is interposed between the calcaneus and the normal tendon.

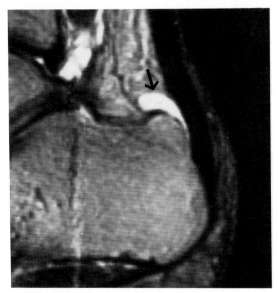

SE 2,000/80

progression to a complete tear. Complete tears are treated surgically, often by transfer of the flexor digitorum longus tendon. If complete posterior tibial tendon tears are not recognized or treated, they may lead to a painful chronic arthritis requiring an arthrodesis.

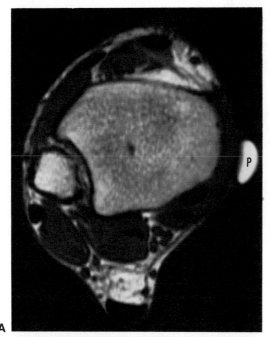

A

SE 600/25

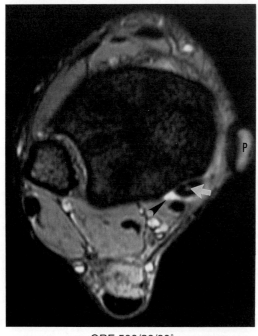

B

GRE 500/20/30°

Figure 20-16. Posterior tibial tendon partial tear and tendinitis, as well as tenosynovitis, in a 44-year-old recreational jogger with chronic medial ankle pain. Transaxial T1-weighted (A) and gradient-echo (B) MR images show abnormal fluid in the tendon sheath surrounding the posterior tibial tendon, indicating tenosynovitis (arrowhead in panel B). The normal size and configuration of the tendon are maintained, but the central high signal intensity (arrow in panel B) is compatible with a partial tear or tendinitis. P = vitamin E pill taped to the ankle to indicate the area of pain.

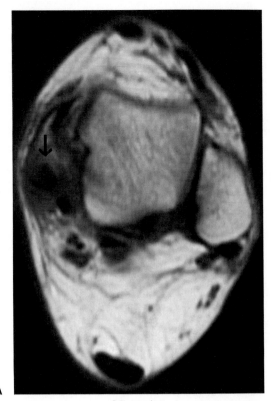

A

SE 600/25

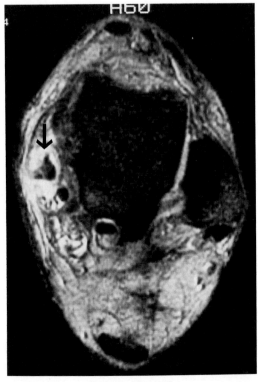

B

GRE 500/20/30°

Figure 20-17. Posterior tibial tendon tears in a 54-year-old woman with pain and flat foot deformity. Transaxial T1-weighted (A) and gradient-echo (B) MR images show that the posterior tibial tendon (arrow) is irregular in shape, contains large areas of high signal intensity, is surrounded by fluid, and has lost its normal oval configuration. These are findings of partial tears and tendinitis, as well as tenosynovitis. Two cuts more distally, the tendon was not visualized because of a complete tendon rupture at the insertion on the navicular bone.

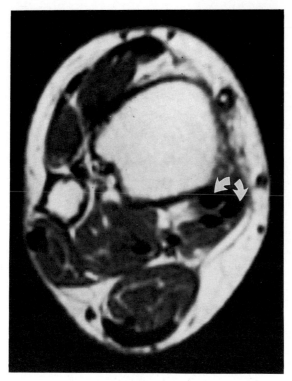

Figure 20-18. Vertical split of posterior tibial tendon in a 50-year-old woman with rheumatoid arthritis and debilitating ankle pain. A T1-weighted axial MR image shows too many tendon structures medially. There appear to be two posterior tibial tendons (arrows), i.e., two Toms, a Dick, and a Harry. This was proven at surgery to be a vertical tear of the tendon. (Courtesy of Joseph Stavas, M.D., Lincoln, Neb.)

SE 600/25

The flexor hallucis longus tendon, which flexes the great toe, rarely undergoes complete rupture. Partial tears and inflammatory changes are most common in individuals who must perform repetitive push-off maneuvers from their forefeet, such as ballet dancers and soccer players (Figure 20-2). The flexor hallucis longus tendon has been called the Achilles tendon of ballet dancers because of the frequency of injury in this population. The usual location for abnormalities in this tendon is the site where the tendon changes direction from its vertical course dorsal to the talus to a horizontal course beneath the calcaneus. Therefore, MR abnormalities are most likely to be identified in that location. Runners may also have flexor hallucis longus tenosynovitis more distally, where the tendon passes between the sesamoids on the plantar aspect of the distal first metatarsal. This causes a painful inability to flex the great toe. MRI may show an abnormal enlargement or signal intensity within the tendon, but fluid distending the tendon sheath from tenosynovitis is the most common finding.

The tendon sheath of the flexor hallucis longus tendon communicates with the ankle joint in 20% of normal individuals. Therefore, in the presence of an ankle joint effusion, fluid around the tendon cannot be interpreted as tenosynovitis unless the tendon has an enlarged girth or contains abnormal signal intensity. Conversely, if no ankle joint effusion is present, MR evidence of fluid surrounding the tendon should always be diagnosed as tenosynovitis. Symptomatic treatment with anti-inflammatory medications and decreased activity is routine for inflammation or partial tears of the flexor hallucis longus tendon.

The peroneus longus and brevis tendons function to evert and pronate the foot **(Option (B) is false).** They are the main stabilizers of the lateral ankle during motion. Peroneal tendons may become inflamed, partially or completely torn, entrapped by bone fragments following calcaneal fractures, or subjected to subluxation or dislocation. Inflammatory changes can result from the inflammatory arthritides or from running. Running may also lead to tears in the peroneus brevis, where there is mechanical stress against the adjacent lateral malleolus. More commonly, the peroneal retinacula rupture during forced plantar flexion of the foot, which permits the tendons to become taut and straight (to "bow-string") with resultant lateral and sometimes anterior subluxation of the tendons relative to the lateral malleolus. This injury occurs in downhill skiers, ice skaters, soccer players, and basketball players, who are often misdiagnosed as having a lateral ankle sprain. The abnormal position of the tendons relative to the malleolus can be demonstrated by MRI.

Entrapment or impingement of the peroneal tendons by bone fragments from a calcaneal fracture commonly causes scarring, fibrosis, and stenosing tenosynovitis with symptoms of lateral ankle pain and difficulty in resisting inversion when walking on uneven surfaces **(Option (C) is true).** The pain is clinically similar to that associated with degenerative subtalar osteoarthritis, another complication of calcaneal fractures. Common peroneal tendon sheath fluid may also follow traumatic rupture of the calcaneofibular ligament. Regardless of etiology, the presence of fluid in this tendon sheath is always abnormal.

The anterior tibial tendon is the main dorsiflexor of the foot. Complete rupture of this tendon generally occurs only in the elderly (Figure 20-19). This may be due in part to mechanical stress on the tendon by the retinacula that hold it in place. The tendon occasionally ruptures from forced plantar flexion in younger individuals. Much more common than a ruptured tendon is tenosynovitis that results from chronic overuse and irritation, usually in downhill hikers and runners **(Option (E) is false).** Treatment is symptomatic for partial tears and surgical for complete tears. The MR signs of anterior tibial tenosynovitis, tendinitis, and partial or complete tears are the same as for all other tendons, i.e., fluid dis-

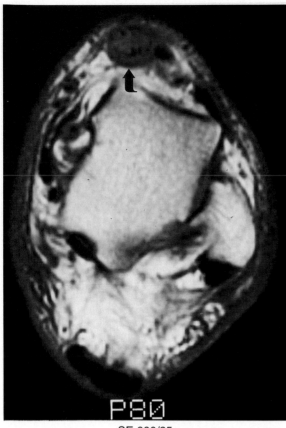

SE 600/25

Figure 20-19. Spontaneous anterior tibial tendon rupture in a 68-year-old man. A T1-weighted transaxial MR image shows absence of the low-intensity anterior tibial tendon (arrow), a manifestation of a chronic complete tear at this level. The ovoid zone of residual intermediate signal intensity in place of the tendon probably represents scarring since the area did not become a high-intensity zone as would be expected for fluid on T2-weighted images. Note the generalized thickening of skin and subcutaneous fat, indicating chronic inflammation about the ankle.

tending the tendon sheath, abnormal size of the tendon, abnormal signal intensity within the tendon, or tendon discontinuity.

Phoebe A. Kaplan, M.D.
Robert G. Dussault, M.D.

SUGGESTED READINGS

NORMAL AND ABNORMAL TENDONS

1. Beltran J, Noto AM, Herman LJ, Lubbers LM. Tendons: high-field-strength, surface coil MR imaging. Radiology 1987; 162:735–740
2. Erickson SJ, Cox IH, Hyde JS, Carrera GF, Strandt JA, Estkowski LD. Effect of tendon orientation on MR imaging signal intensity: a manifestation of the "magic angle" phenomenon. Radiology 1991; 181:389–392

3. Kannus P, Jozsa L. Histopathological changes preceding spontaneous rupture of a tendon. A controlled study of 891 patients. J Bone Joint Surg (Am) 1991; 73:1507–1525

TENDONS OF FOOT AND ANKLE

4. Evarts CM (ed). Surgery of the musculoskeletal system. Edinburgh: Churchill Livingstone; 1983:28–30
5. Fritz RC, Steinbach LS. MRI of the ankle and foot. In: Helms CA (ed), Perspectives in radiology. St. Louis: Quality Medical Publishing; 1990; 3:1–24
6. Netter FH. Ankle and foot. In: Dingle RV (ed), The CIBA collection of medical illustrations. Musculoskeletal system. Part 1. Anatomy, physiology, and metabolic disorders. New Jersey: CIBA-Geigy Summit; 1987; 8:109–120
7. Quinn SF, Murray WT, Clark RA, Cochran CF. Achilles tendon: imaging at 1.5 T. Radiology 1987; 164:767–770

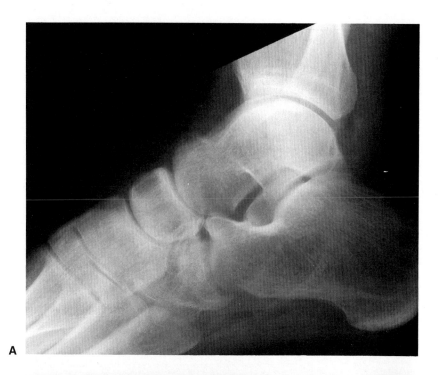

A

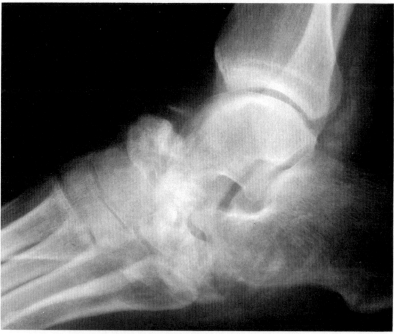

B

Figure 21-1. This 32-year-old man presented with swelling of the left ankle. You are shown lateral radiographs of the ankle obtained at presentation (A) and 1 month later (B).

Case 21: Neuropathic Arthropathy

Question 88

Which *one* of the following is the MOST likely diagnosis?

(A) Septic arthropathy
(B) Calcium pyrophosphate arthropathy
(C) Neuropathic arthropathy
(D) Reiter's arthropathy
(E) Hemophilic arthropathy

The lateral radiograph of the ankle at presentation (Figure 21-1A) shows increased density of the cuboid bone adjacent to the calcaneocuboid joint as a result of an impaction fracture (Figure 21-2A). This has resulted in irregular width of the calcaneocuboid joint and slight narrowing of the talonavicular joint. Vascular calcification of the posterior tibial artery is also present.

A follow-up radiograph obtained 1 month later (Figure 21-1B) shows rapid progression of a destructive process in the midfoot. Apparent "increased density" in this region is due to impaction and fragmentation of fractures of the cuboid, navicular, and distal talus (Figure 21-2B). An important associated finding is absence of demineralization of the neighboring bones. The plantar arch has collapsed.

In summary, the important findings in this case are maintenance of bone mineral content, fracture of several bones with fragmentation, disorganization of local anatomic relationships with malalignment, and rapid progression of the disease process. These features indicate a neuropathic arthropathy **(Option (C) is correct),** and the associated arterial calcification in a 32-year-old patient suggests diabetes mellitus as the etiology.

The other diagnostic choices offered for this case are all less likely because each is more truly a joint-centered process, whereas the process depicted in the test images is bone centered, with fracture and fragmentation being the predominant findings.

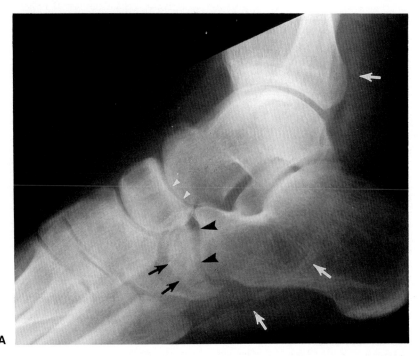

A

Figure 21-2 (Same as Figure 21-1). Diabetic neuropathic arthropathy. (A) The increased density (black arrows) of the cuboid bone adjacent to the calcaneocuboid joint is due to impaction fracture. The width of the calcaneocuboid joint is nonuniform (black arrowheads), and the talonavicular joint is slightly narrowed (white arrowheads). Vascular calcification of the posterior tibial artery (white arrows) suggests that the patient is diabetic. (B) At 1-month follow-up, progressive destruction, fracture impaction, and fragmentation of the cuboid, navicular, and distal talus are evident (arrows). Note the absence of demineralization and the interval collapse of the plantar arch.

Septic arthropathy (Option (A)) is unlikely because demineralization did not occur and, although the bones are fragmented, the osseous and articular margins remain sharply delineated. While the process is destructive, it is important to note the type of destruction present. The test images show destruction due to fragmentation. However, infection typically causes destruction by osteolysis and chondrolysis (Figure 21-3). Infection is a concern in diabetic patients; however, the midfoot is a less common location for septic arthritis than are the metatarsophalangeal joints, which are frequently infected secondary to the spread of bacteria from adjacent soft tissue ulceration. A white blood cell count and a culture of a joint aspirate are appropriate diagnostic measures in cases when the possibility of infection is raised.

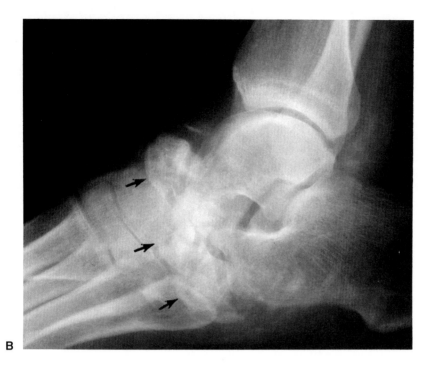

B

Calcium pyrophosphate arthropathy (Option (B)) is unlikely because none of the characteristic joint changes of the crystalline arthropathy, such as cartilage calcification, cartilage loss, articular cortical erosion, subchondral cyst formation, sclerosis, and osteophyte formation, are present. The young age of the patient, absence of generalized osteopenia, rapid progression of the condition, and presence of vascular calcification all favor neuropathic arthropathy. Examination of joint fluid for typical calcium pyrophosphate dihydrate crystals and radiographic examination of the hands and knees to search for other evidence of crystal deposition are useful diagnostic tests in questionable cases.

Reiter's arthropathy (Option (D)) is unlikely for the reasons listed above but particularly because of the absence of periarticular osteopenia, which is usually seen in the early phase of inflammatory synovitis. Other relevant negative findings are the absence of superficial bone erosions at the joints and the absence of enthesitis or calcaneal plantar erosions from adjacent bursitis. The midfoot is also a less common target site for Reiter's arthropathy than are other locations in the foot such as the metatarsophalangeal, interphalangeal, and ankle joints. A young male patient is a good candidate for Reiter's arthropathy. However, a history

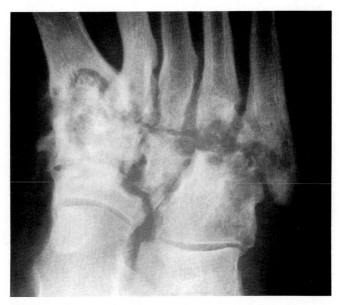

Figure 21-3. Septic (tuberculous) arthropathy. An oblique anteroposterior radiograph of the midfoot shows destruction of the tarsometatarsal and intercuneiform joints, as well as the joints between the cuneiform bones and the navicular and cuboid. Chondrolysis and osteolysis are present with poorly defined articular margins, typical of infection. There is no fragmentation of adjacent bones and no demineralization.

of associated genitourinary, gastrointestinal, or ocular symptoms might be expected.

Hemophilic arthropathy (Option (E)) is unlikely for many of the reasons mentioned above. Osteopenia is an anticipated finding during the acute and subacute phases of hemophilic arthropathy as a result of local hyperemia. Moreover, the talonavicular and calcaneocuboid joints are uncommon sites of hemophilic arthropathy. In this region, the tibiotalar joint is most commonly involved. A young male patient is a good candidate for the diagnosis of hemophilia, but the rapidity and severity of the destructive process seen in the test images would be an atypical clinical course.

Question 89

Concerning calcium pyrophosphate dihydrate crystal deposition,

    (A) pseudogout and pyrophosphate arthropathy are synonyms
    (B) it is associated with diabetes mellitus
    (C) it is associated with scapholunate collapse
    (D) it is associated with scalloped erosion of the anterior cortex of the distal femur
    (E) tophaceous deposits are a rare manifestation

It is useful to clarify the terminology associated with calcium pyrophosphate dihydrate (CPPD) crystal deposition disease.

Chondrocalcinosis is the term used to describe radiographically or pathologically evident cartilage calcification (Figure 21-4). Such calcification may involve articular hyaline cartilage or the fibrocartilage of the menisci and labra. Chondrocalcinosis is not a disease, nor is it a specific feature of any one condition. Instead, it may be found in association with a variety of disorders.

Pseudogout is the term applied to the clinical syndrome characterized by intermittent acute attacks of inflammatory arthritis (usually monoarticular) in association with CPPD crystals; these crystals may be recovered from samples of aspirated synovial fluid. Clinically, these attacks are similar to acute gouty arthritis, except that monosodium urate crystals are not found—hence the term pseudogout.

Pyrophosphate arthropathy is the term used to describe a characteristic arthropathy occurring in CPPD crystal deposition disease. The typical radiographic features of pyrophosphate arthropathy are cartilage loss, erosion of articular cortex, osteosclerosis, subchondral cyst formation, and cartilage calcification. Therefore, pseudogout describes a clinical syndrome consisting of an acutely swollen and painful joint whereas pyrophosphate arthropathy refers to a chronic crystal-induced arthropathy that may not be painful. Pseudogout and pyrophosphate arthropathy are not synonyms **(Option (A) is false).**

Diagnostic criteria for CPPD crystal deposition disease are based on the premise that CPPD crystals are specific for the disease. The criteria include clinical and radiographic features. A definite diagnosis is made if CPPD crystals are demonstrated in tissues or synovial fluid by definitive means (e.g., chemical analysis or X-ray diffraction pattern). A definite diagnosis is also made if crystals compatible with CPPD are demonstrated by compensated polarized light microscopy (e.g., weakly positive or no birefringence) and typical calcification is seen on radiographs. A probable diagnosis is made if only one of the latter two findings is pres-

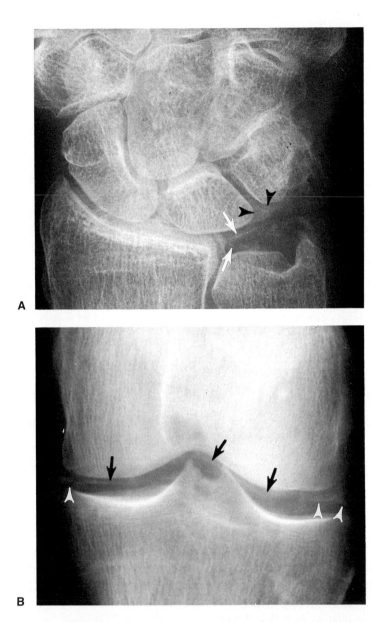

Figure 21-4. Chondrocalcinosis. (A) A posteroanterior radiograph of the
wrist shows calcification in the lunotriquetral ligament (arrowheads),
hyaline articular cartilage, and triangular fibrocartilage (arrows). (B) An
anteroposterior radiograph of the knee shows calcification in the hyaline
articular cartilage (arrows) and meniscal fibrocartilage (arrowheads).

ent. A possible diagnosis can be made in the absence of these criteria if
clinical or radiologic findings are compatible with the diagnosis.

Many metabolic diseases appear to be associated with CPPD crystal deposition disease and may have chondrocalcinosis demonstrated radiographically. The strongest associations are with hyperparathyroidism, hemochromatosis, hypomagnesemia, and hypophosphatasia. In hyperparathyroidism, the mechanism of articular cartilage crystal deposition is thought to be sustained hypercalcemia coupled with nonspecific age-related cartilage changes. In hemochromatosis, the chondrocalcinosis may be caused by a predisposition to precipitation of insoluble pyrophosphate crystals induced by ferrous ions or may somehow be secondary to cartilage degeneration caused by iron. In hypomagnesemia, chondrocalcinosis is hypothesized to occur because of decreased enzyme activity (magnesium acts as a cofactor for alkaline phosphatase), and in hypophosphatasia it may be related to elevated tissue levels of pyrophosphate.

Diabetes mellitus does not have a strong association with CPPD crystal deposition disease; when CPPD crystals are found in a patient with diabetes, the combination represents the coincidence of two common disorders **(Option (B) is false)**.

Hereditary and sporadic forms of CPPD crystal deposition disease exist. Hereditary forms tend to have autosomal dominant inheritance, a younger age of onset, and a more severe arthropathy. Familial CPPD crystal deposition diseases have been described in many countries including Czechoslovakia, Canada, Chile, The Netherlands, Spain, and France. In the sporadic form there is no sex predilection and the condition tends to occur in middle-aged and elderly people.

Several clinical patterns of CPPD crystal deposition have been described by McCarty. He has emphasized that CPPD deposition is a great mimic, often superficially resembling other forms of arthritis. In addition to pseudogout, pseudo-osteoarthritic, pseudorheumatoid, and pseudo-neuropathic forms exist. A large asymptomatic group also exists.

Pyrophosphate arthropathy is commonly encountered without radiographic evidence of articular calcification, and it is usually bilateral but not necessarily symmetric. Joint narrowing, bone sclerosis, and cyst formation simulate osteoarthritis. However, pyrophosphate arthropathy differs from osteoarthritis in at least five respects. First, it tends to have an unusual articular distribution (e.g., radiocarpal, elbow, and glenohumeral joints) as compared with typical osteoarthritis, which involves the interphalangeal joints and the three knee compartments. Second, within a joint, there are unique target sites (e.g., radioscaphoid and patellofemoral). Third, subchondral cyst formation is prominent, and these cysts tend to be clustered and small and to have sclerotic, smudged, and indistinct margins. Fourth, destructive bone changes

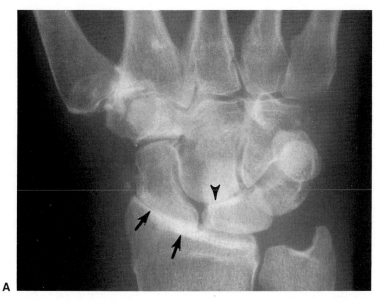

A

Figure 21-5. Scapholunate collapse. (A) A posteroanterior radiograph of the wrist shows CPPD crystal deposition arthropathy with cartilage loss from the radioscaphoid joint, flattening of the subchondral cortical bone of the radius and scaphoid, and subarticular sclerosis (arrows). The scapholunate joint is slightly widened, and there is cartilage loss from the capitolunate joint (arrowhead). The cartilage width of the radiolunate joint is preserved. (B) A posteroanterior radiograph of the wrist shows more advanced scapholunate collapse with small osteophytes at the radial margin of the radioscaphoid joint, erosion of the juxtaposed scaphoid and radius, and increased dissociation of the scaphoid, lunate, and capitate relationships.

include collapse, fragmentation, and the formation of small intra-articular osseous bodies. Fifth, osteophyte formation is often minimal. The variability of these features leads to occasions when individual arthropathies may resemble osteoarthritic or neuropathic conditions.

The joints most commonly affected by pyrophosphate arthropathy are the wrist and knee. Within the wrist, the radioscaphoid joint is characteristically involved and there may be secondary widening of the scapholunate joint due to ligamentous laxity. The scapholunate collapse pattern is characteristic (Figure 21-5) **(Option (C) is true).**

Scapholunate collapse begins in the most radial portion of the radioscaphoid joint. It progressively involves the remainder of the radioscaphoid joint and then the capitolunate joint. Usually the scapholunate joint is abnormally widened, yet there is preservation of the radiolunate joint.

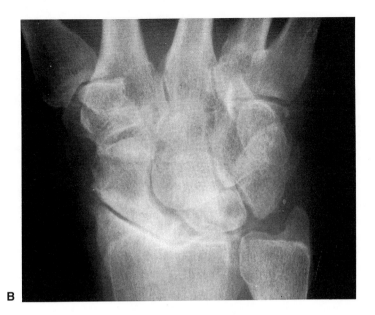

B

Incongruity between the radial and scaphoid articular surfaces caused by ligamentous instability and malalignment leads to cartilage loss and secondary osteoarthritis. The articular surfaces at the radiolunate joint remain congruous even in cases of marked scapholunate ligamentous instability; this probably explains why the radiolunate cartilage is usually preserved.

In the knee joint, the patellofemoral articulation is a target site for CPPD arthropathy. The usual pattern is diffuse cartilage loss of both medial and lateral patellar articular facets and of the adjacent femoral condyles with radiographically demonstrable surface erosion of the subchondral bone. The erosive process may become severe and can even cause scalloped erosion and eburnation of the anterior distal femoral cortex (Figure 21-6) **(Option (D) is true).** When such cortical pressure erosion is encountered, the bone is typically osteopenic. Similar anterior femoral pressure erosions may occur with hyperparathyroidism, renal osteodystrophy, osteoarthritis, and rheumatoid arthritis.

Although CPPD arthropathy is uncommon in the foot, the talonavicular joint is a target site for this disorder.

Tophaceous CPPD crystal deposits are a recognized but rare manifestation of CPPD crystal deposition (Figure 21-7) **(Option (E) is true).** These deposits are probably initiated by chondroid metaplasia, which is subsequently accompanied by massive CPPD crystal deposition. Episodic

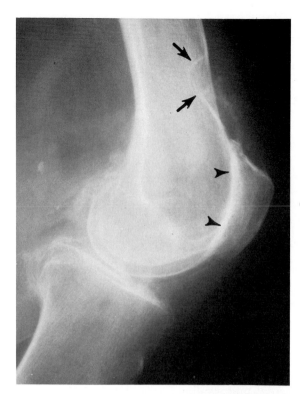

Figure 21-6 (left). Scalloped erosion of the femur. A lateral radiograph of the knee shows chondrocalcinosis and CPPD crystal deposition arthropathy of a patellofemoral joint; this condition is characterized by total loss of cartilage with eburnation of the apposing articular surfaces (arrowheads). Mechanical pressure and repetitive friction between the patella and the anterior femoral cortex have resulted in a superficial scalloped anterior femoral erosion (arrows).

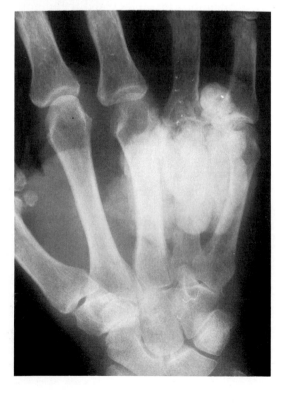

Figure 21-7 (right). Tophaceous CPPD crystal deposit. An oblique radiograph of the hand shows an amorphous lobulated calcified mass on the dorsum of the hand. The opaque sutures are from a recent biopsy. This is the only evidence of CPPD crystal deposition in this patient.

release of crystals from a tophaceous CPPD deposit may precipitate acute episodes of inflammation surrounding the tophus, accompanied by pain (pseudogout). The tophaceous mass enlarges slowly and may cause pressure erosion of adjacent bone. Tophaceous CPPD crystal deposition is a localized soft tissue process rather than a systemic condition.

Question 90

Concerning Reiter's syndrome,

   (A) it is a reactive arthritis
   (B) it typically subsides within 6 months
   (C) upper extremity involvement is more common in men than in women
   (D) periarticular osteopenia accompanies the acute phase
   (E) unilateral sacroiliitis is more common than bilateral sacroiliitis

The American Rheumatism Association (now the American College of Rheumatology) Diagnostic and Therapeutic Criteria Committee proposed in 1981 that Reiter's syndrome be defined as an episode of peripheral arthritis of more than 1 month's duration occurring in association with urethritis or cervicitis.

Reiter's syndrome is considered a form of reactive arthritis **(Option (A) is true).** A reactive arthritis is defined as a joint inflammation initiated by an infectious agent that is either not detected in the joint or not viable when detected in the joint. Reiter's syndrome is frequently subdivided into sexually acquired reactive arthritis and enteric reactive arthritis. The classic triad observed in patients with Reiter's syndrome is the combination of arthritis, urethritis, and conjunctivitis.

The occasional (fortunate) individual with Reiter's syndrome may have a self-limiting disease, but the syndrome is typically a chronic rheumatic disease. The majority of patients with the condition can expect relentless progressive deterioration **(Option (B) is false).** The peak age at diagnosis is 15 to 35 years, and there is a male predominance. There is no significant difference in the course of the disease between patients positive or negative for the HLA-B27 histocompatibility antigen or between men and women.

Prostatitis, cystitis, and circinate balanitis are the most common inflammatory disorders of the genitourinary system in patients with the syndrome. Ocular manifestations include episcleritis, keratitis, uveitis, and iritis. Keratoderma blennorrhagica of the skin is seen, as are oral mucosal and tongue ulcers.

The associated arthropathy typically involves lower extremity joints and is asymmetric in distribution. Men and women are similarly af-

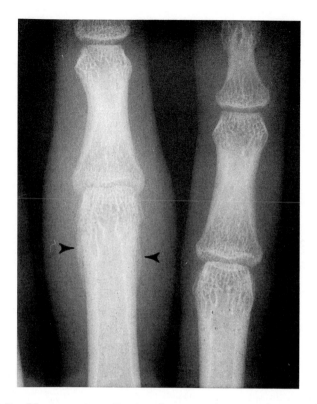

Figure 21-8. Upper extremity involvement in a patient with Reiter's syndrome. A posteroanterior radiograph of the long finger shows fusiform soft tissue swelling around the proximal interphalangeal joint and linear periostitis (arrowheads) along the distal shaft of the proximal phalanx. Compare with the normal adjacent ring finger.

fected. A monoarticular presentation predominates. Although upper extremity involvement is distinctly uncommon, it does occur (Figure 21-8). Neuwelt et al., in a study of 25 patients (12 men and 13 women) with Reiter's syndrome, found that women had more hand and wrist involvement than men; however, this has not been substantiated by other authors. Upper extremity involvement occurs with approximately the same frequency in men and women **(Option (C) is false).**

Reiter's syndrome involves synovial joints, symphyses, and entheses. Target sites are the small articulations of the foot, the calcaneus, and the ankle, knee, and sacroiliac joints. At onset, radiographs are normal in 60 to 80% of patients. Soon, soft tissue swelling is evident clinically and radiographically as a result of joint effusion, periarticular edema, and inflammation of bursal and tendinous structures. Periarticular or regional osteopenia accompanies the inflammation characteristic of acute epi-

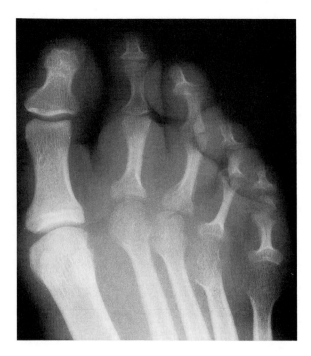

Figure 21-9. Periarticular osteopenia in a patient with early Reiter's syndrome. Anteroposterior radiograph of the forefoot shows periarticular osteopenia of the second, third, and fourth metatarsophalangeal joints.

sodes of the arthritis (Figure 21-9) **(Option (D) is true).** Remineralization generally occurs with prolonged or recurrent bouts of arthritis. Late in the course of the disease, severe cartilage loss and bone erosions are common but without osteopenia.

Diffuse joint space narrowing is a feature of Reiter's syndrome and is more easily detected in small joints. Initially, bone erosions have ill-defined margins and are found at joint margins. Later the erosions involve the more central portions of the articulation. Osseous erosions also occur adjacent to inflamed bursae and tendons.

Bone proliferation is a characteristic finding of Reiter's syndrome and may develop along the periosteum or at tendon and ligament attachments. Periosteal bone proliferation is usually linear and is most commonly encountered along the shafts of metatarsal, metacarpal, and phalangeal bones (Figure 21-10). Periosteal reaction is occasionally found in the malleolar region about the ankle and the metaphyses of the knee. Interestingly, it may occur in the absence of any adjacent articular abnormality. Bone proliferation at tendon and ligament attachments (entheses) produces poorly defined and frayed osseous margins.

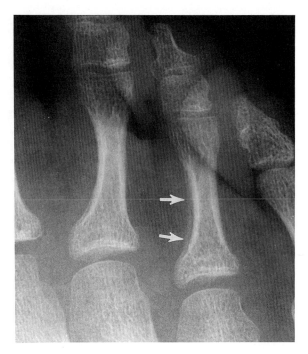

Figure 21-10. Periostitis in a patient with Reiter's syndrome. An antero-posterior radiograph of the third and fourth toes shows linear periosteal new bone formation along the shaft of the fourth proximal phalanx (arrows).

Intraosseous bone production occurs at sites of erosion and may enlarge the articular bone. This process produces subchondral sclerosis and may eventually lead to ankylosis.

In the lower extremity, Reiter's syndrome most frequently involves the forefoot and calcaneus. Asymmetric metatarsophalangeal and inter-phalangeal joint involvement is typical (Figure 21-11). Calcaneal inflammation may be the sole or predominant feature of the syndrome and is frequently bilateral. Involvement of the calcaneus occurs along posterior and plantar aspects with ill-defined erosion (Figure 21-12). Sometimes an irregular fluffy erosion occurs at the attachment of the plantar fascia. Hyperostosis and spur formation follow the initial inflammatory condition, with the osseous margins becoming better defined (Figure 21-13).

Sacroiliac joint involvement is common, with bilateral sacroiliitis (about 80%) being more common than unilateral sacroiliitis **(Option (E) is false).** On radiographs, sacroiliitis is seen initially in 5 to 10% of patients, with changes being recognized in 40 to 60% of patients after several years. Sacroiliitis may be asymmetric or symmetric (Figure 21-14). Reiter's syndrome is often thought to have unilateral or asym-

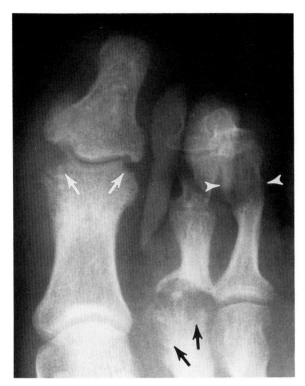

Figure 21-11. Erosions and ankylosis in a patient with Reiter's syndrome. An antero-posterior radiograph of the toes shows marginal erosions (white arrows) and soft tissue swelling involving the great toe interphalangeal joint, marginal and central erosions (black arrows) of the second metatarsophalangeal joint, and ankylosis of the third proximal interphalangeal joint (arrowheads).

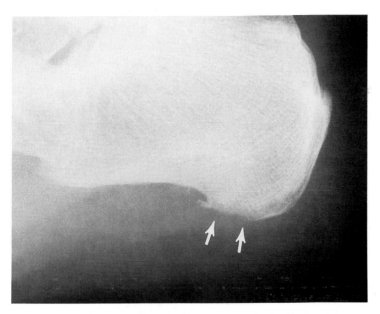

Figure 21-12. Calcaneal erosions in a patient with Reiter's syndrome. A lateral radiograph of the calcaneus shows ill-defined erosion (arrows) involving the cortex of the plantar aspect of the calcaneus at the attachment of the plantar fascia.

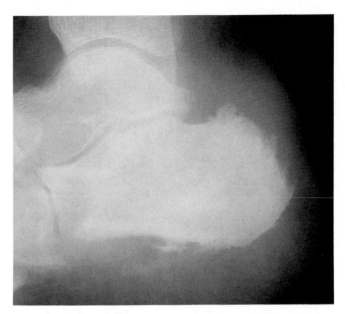

Figure 21-13. Calcaneal bone proliferation in a patient with Reiter's syndrome. A lateral radiograph of the calcaneus shows irregular fluffy bone formation along the cortical surfaces. Overall, the calcaneus is sclerotic.

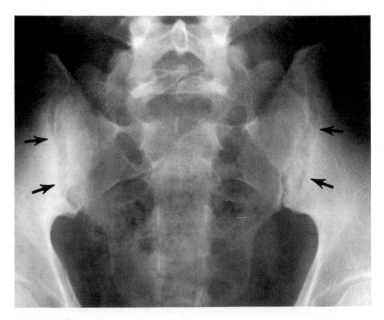

Figure 21-14. Sacroiliitis in a patient with Reiter's syndrome. An anteroposterior radiograph of the sacroiliac joints shows asymmetric sacroiliitis (arrows) with irregular widening of the joint spaces, cortical erosions, and sclerosis.

metric sacroiliac joint involvement, but long duration of the disease results in an increased frequency of bilateral symmetric sacroiliitis.

Question 91

Concerning fractures of the midfoot,

    (A) they are typically isolated to one tarsal bone
    (B) lateral stress injury typically results in cuboid dislocation
    (C) dorsal cortical avulsion fractures of the navicular are most frequent
    (D) medial tuberosity fractures of the navicular are typically displaced
    (E) about 80% of navicular stress fractures occur in the lateral third

The midfoot consists of the navicular, cuboid, and cuneiform bones with their respective joints. The midtarsal joint consists of the talonavicular and calcaneocuboid joints and is also known as Chopart's joint or the transverse tarsal joint. The midfoot is relatively rigid, with the lateral side more stable than the medial side.

Injuries involving the midtarsal joint are rare, found predominantly in young people, and frequently overlooked. When injury occurs, it is typical for more than one bone to be involved; many fracture-dislocation patterns have been reported **(Option (A) is false).** The classification scheme of Main and Jowett describes five patterns of injury, based on the presumed mechanism of injury, the extent of injury, and the direction of displacement of the forefoot. These patterns are categorized as longitudinal, medial, lateral, plantar, and crush.

Longitudinal stress is the most common injury pattern, accounting for approximately 40% of midfoot injuries. It occurs with the foot plantar flexed, the force being transmitted along the metatarsals to disrupt the midtarsal joint and fracture the cuboid or navicular. Navicular fracture tends to occur in line with an intercuneiform joint (Figure 21-15). Damage is usually severe, with a high prevalence of associated fractures and significant residual displacement of fracture fragments.

Medial stress injuries account for approximately 30% of midfoot injuries. These are caused by an inversion force on the forefoot with respect to the midfoot and can result in sprains, fractures, subluxations, and dislocations. A medial swivel dislocation consists of a talonavicular dislocation, with the calcaneocuboid joint remaining intact. Subluxation occurs at the subtalar joint without tearing the talocalcaneal ligament.

Lateral stress injury is characterized by a crush of the cuboid or the anterior calcaneus. This is frequently associated with an avulsion fracture of the navicular tuberosity or a subluxation of the navicular but not with a cuboid dislocation **(Option (B) is false).** A crush of the cuboid

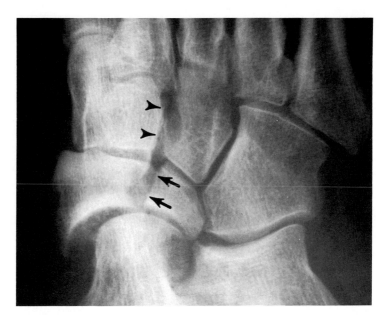

Figure 21-15. Longitudinal navicular fracture. An oblique radiograph of the midfoot shows sagittal fracture of the navicular (arrows) aligned with the intercuneiform joint (arrowheads). The medial portion of the navicular bone is subluxed.

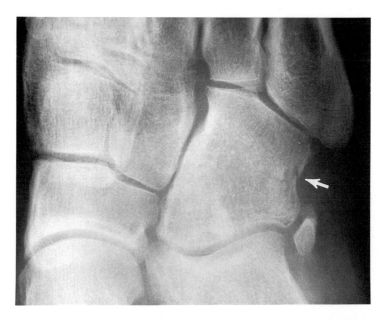

Figure 21-16. Nutcracker fracture. An oblique anteroposterior radiograph of the midfoot shows a crush fracture (arrow) involving the lateral aspect of the cuboid.

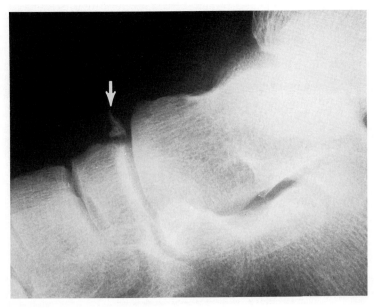

Figure 21-17. Navicular avulsion fracture. A lateral radiograph of the midfoot shows a dorsal avulsion fracture (arrow) that involves only a small portion of the cortex.

between the calcaneus and the bases of the fourth and fifth metatarsals is termed a nutcracker fracture (Figure 21-16).

Plantar stress injury can result in avulsion fractures of the dorsal lip of the navicular, the talus, or the anterior process of calcaneus.

Isolated fractures of the midtarsal bones do occur. The three basic types of navicular fracture are cortical avulsion, tuberosity, and body fractures. Stress fractures constitute a fourth category but result from a different set of mechanical forces.

The cortical avulsion fracture is the most frequent isolated navicular fracture (Figure 21-17) and the most frequent midtarsal fracture overall **(Option (C) is true).** It occurs more frequently in women than in men. The joint capsule or the anteriormost fibers of the deltoid ligament avulse a small region of cortex. Most fragments do not represent a significant portion of the articular surface of the navicular.

Medial tuberosity fractures of the navicular (Figure 21-18) occur from acute eversion of the foot with sudden tension of the posterior tibial tendon or anterior fibers of the deltoid ligament. The avulsed navicular fragment is rarely significantly displaced since other structures hold it in position **(Option (D) is false).** Navicular tuberosity fractures may be found in conjunction with a compression fracture of the cuboid.

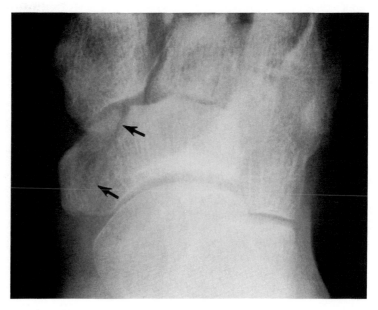

Figure 21-18. Navicular medial tuberosity fracture. An anteroposterior radiograph of the midfoot shows a minimally displaced fracture (arrows).

Navicular stress fractures are usually seen in young athletes, particularly runners and basketball players. Typically the fracture is linear, occurs in the sagittal plane, and involves the midportion of the navicular (Figure 21-19) **(Option (E) is false).** The fracture may be complete or incomplete. A complete fracture can be easily overlooked because the separate lateral fragment is mistaken for a normal tarsal bone. A partial stress fracture is usually confined to the dorsal portion of the navicular and may not be evident on routine foot radiographs. When a stress fracture is suspected, bone scintigraphy or sectional imaging is frequently required to make the diagnosis. Sectional imaging in an axial or coronal plane will best demonstrate the fracture.

Cuneiform fractures are rarely isolated and are usually associated with severe midtarsal or tarsometatarsal joint injuries.

Discussion

Neuropathic arthropathy is a progressive destructive condition that involves articulations and has characteristic clinical and radiologic fea-

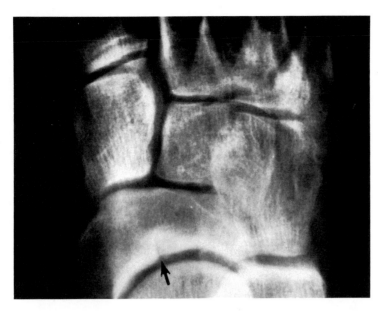

Figure 21-19. Navicular stress fracture. An anteroposterior radiograph of the midfoot shows a subtle partial-thickness stress fracture of the navicular involving the proximal aspect of the navicular at the midline (arrow). (Courtesy of Helene Pavlov, M.D., Hospital for Special Surgery, New York, N.Y.)

tures. The current consensus is that neuropathic arthropathy develops secondary to articular sensory loss and continued weight bearing. The entity was eloquently described by Jean Martin Charcot in 1868 in a patient with tabes dorsalis and has come to bear his name. It is now most commonly encountered as a complication of diabetes mellitus.

Controversy still exists regarding the exact etiology of neuropathic arthropathy. Mitchell and Charcot emphasized a neurotrophic cause wherein joint changes resulted from damage to central nervous system trophic centers that controlled bone and joint nutrition. This has become known as the "French theory." Volkmann and Virchow supported the "German theory," which stated that mechanical stress is the primary abnormality, with joint changes due entirely to repetitive trauma sustained by a joint unable to sense pain. Brower and associates more recently proposed a "vascular theory" wherein a neurally initiated vascular reflex leads to very active osteoclastic bone resorption in an area supplied by a particular vascular bed.

Even though the precise pathophysiology of neuropathic arthropathy remains unknown, a clinically useful theory is generally accepted. Ac-

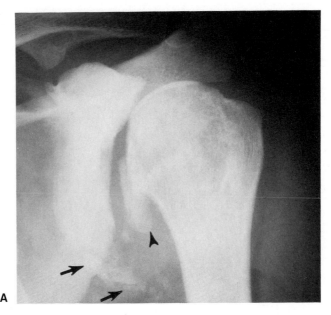

A

Figure 21-20. Neuropathic shoulders in patients with syringomyelia.
(A) An anteroposterior radiograph of the glenohumeral joint shows
hypertrophic neuropathic arthropathy with bone destruction, periarticular sclerosis, fracture fragments (arrowhead), and osseous debris
(arrows). (B) An anteroposterior radiograph of the glenohumeral joint
shows atrophic neuropathic arthropathy. Destruction of the glenoid and
humeral head is profound, with absence of bone repair. The residual joint
is disorganized, and much osseous debris is present.

cording to this summated hypothesis, loss of the protective sensations of
pain and proprioception leads to relaxation of the supporting structures
and chronic instability of the joint. In this setting the daily stresses of
normal movement produce injury, malalignment, and abnormal joint
loading. Cumulative injury leads to progressive degeneration and disorganization. Reactive hypervascularity contributes to the bone resorption.

Several disorders may be complicated by development of a neuropathic joint. These include diabetes mellitus, syphilis, syringomyelia,
meningomyelocele, and congenital insensitivity to pain. The clinical features associated with the abnormal joint vary depending on the underlying disease and the location of the joint. Pain associated with the
involved joint may be present; however, the pain is characteristically
mild relative to the clinical and radiographic findings and is generated
from the adjacent nonarticular soft tissues. Deep joint pain is usually
absent. In diabetic patients, a swollen, warm, mildly painful region of

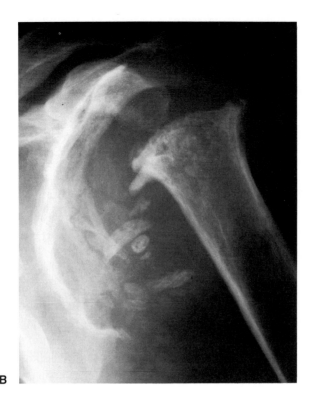

B

the foot or ankle is common. Perforating ulceration associated with infection is a serious complication. In patients with tertiary syphilis, a painless or nearly painless lower extremity monoarthritis is typical, and the joints frequently affected are the knee, hip, ankle, and lumbar spine. In patients with syringomyelia, the upper extremity is frequently involved. In general, the underlying disease can be predicted from the joint involved.

On histopathologic examination, shards of bone and cartilage are found trapped in the synovium, and these constitute an important microscopic feature of neuropathic arthropathy. Other features include cartilage erosion, eburnation of exposed bone, periosteal new bone formation, and extra-articular bone fragments. Coincidence of bone resorption and formation is a major feature.

Radiologically, two classic forms of neuropathic arthropathy exist: hypertrophic and atrophic. The hypertrophic form (Figure 21-20A) is characterized by joint effusion, dissolution and disorganization of the normal joint, abundant juxta-articular new bone formation, massive osteophytes, osseous fragmentation, and intra-articular osseous debris. The atrophic form (Figure 21-20B) is characterized by joint effusion, bone resorption with sharp bone margins, maintenance of bone mineralization, general absence of bone repair, and presence of osseous debris. In any affected joint, the spectrum of changes may range from atrophic to hypertrophic. Mixed patterns are typical.

Early in the process, the radiologic findings may simulate osteoarthritis, with joint space narrowing, sclerosis, and osteophyte formation. An enlarging and persistent joint effusion with subluxation and articular fractures commonly follows. Progression of the destructive process may be very rapid: only days or a few weeks.

In patients with diabetic neuropathic arthropathy, ischemia secondary to small blood vessel disease may act synergistically with sensory loss and repetitive microtrauma to produce a complex osteoarthropathy. Infection may complicate the osteoarthropathy and dramatically accelerate joint destruction. Diabetic osteoarthropathy is encountered in approximately 1 in 680 diabetic patients. Two-thirds of the cases occur in the fifth and sixth decades of life. There is no sex preference. The osteoarthropathy tends to occur with long-standing insulin-dependent diabetes, but no particular subtype of insulin-dependent diabetes is selectively associated with it. There is controversy about whether precise control of diabetes is important in reducing the risk of development of osteoarthropathy.

In diabetic patients, the joints of the forefoot and midfoot are most frequently affected, followed in decreasing order by the ankle, knee, hip, spine, and upper extremities. Involvement may be mono- or polyarticular. At the intertarsal and tarsometatarsal joints, osseous fragmentation, bone sclerosis, and joint subluxation or dislocation are the major features. Characteristic patterns of arthropathy include an appearance that resembles Lisfranc fracture dislocation (Figure 21-21). Another common pattern is involvement of Chopart's joint, with destruction of the talar head and neck, shortening of the foot, and development of a rocker-bottom deformity. At the metatarsophalangeal joints, osseous resorption, flattening, and fragmentation of the metatarsal heads are the predominant features. Pressure erosion of the soft tissue caused by subluxation of the metatarsal heads leads to soft tissue infection with subsequent septic arthritis and osteomyelitis (Figure 21-22).

From 5 to 10% of patients with tertiary syphilis develop neuropathic arthropathy; up to 75% of these have lower extremity involvement. The knee is involved in about 50% of patients, followed in decreasing order by hip, ankle, shoulder, and elbow joints. Approximately 50% of patients have single-joint involvement. When a polyarticular pattern is encountered, up to seven joints may be involved and distribution tends to be

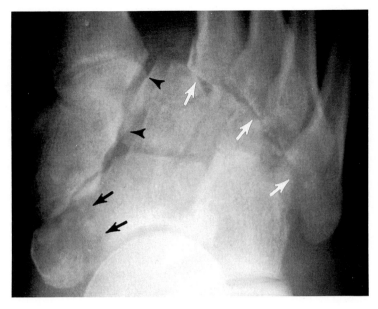

Figure 21-21. Neuropathic midfoot with Lisfranc pattern. An anteroposterior radiograph of the midfoot in a patient with diabetes shows fracture and fragmentation of the navicular (black arrows), subluxation at the joint between the first and second cuneiform bones (arrowheads), and dislocation of the second to fifth metatarsal bones (white arrows). Subtle fragmentation and impaction between the metatarsal bases and adjacent tarsal bones is present.

symmetric. The affected joint is typically painless, swollen, deformed, weak, and unstable. Fractures can occur in neighboring bones with little or no trauma. Fracture tends to heal with abundant callus and may eventually produce a pseudarthrosis.

Spinal involvement develops in up to 20% of individuals with syphilitic neuropathic arthropathy. The prevalence of spinal arthropathy is greater in men than in women and is encountered most frequently in the sixth and seventh decades of life. Involvement is predominantly lumbar, and one or more vertebral segments may be affected. Spinal arthropathy is often symptomatic as a result of preservation of some nerve fibers and compression of adjacent nerve roots. Kyphosis and scoliosis are frequent, and there may be motor and sensory disturbances. Paraplegia is rare. In patients with syphilitic neuropathic spinal arthropathy, productive bone changes are more common than destructive changes. Osteoarticular alterations include disk and apophyseal joint narrowing and bone sclerosis and osteophytosis. Destructive changes can appear acutely, progress rapidly, and mimic infection or metastatic disease.

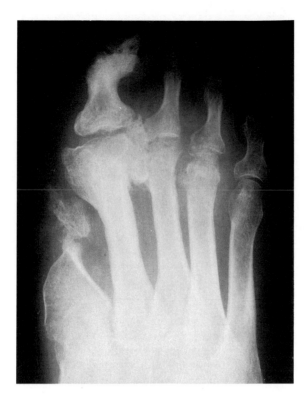

Figure 21-22. Diabetic osteoarthropathy. An anteroposterior radiograph of the forefoot shows transmetatarsal amputation of the great toe, hypertrophy of the second metatarsal head, deformities of the second-toe phalanges, chronic neuropathic arthropathy of the second metatarsophalangeal joint, and subacute inflammation of the third and fourth metatarsophalangeal joints. These features result from the combined effect of neuropathy, vascular insufficiency, and recurrent infection.

Approximately 25% of patients with syringomyelia develop a neuropathic arthropathy, and approximately 80% of affected joints are in the upper extremity. The glenohumeral joint is the usual target; however, involvement of the elbow, wrist, and finger also occurs. Occasionally, spine, hip, knee, or ankle involvement is found. Joint involvement may be bilateral and symmetric. Neuropathic changes generally become evident in the later phases of syringomyelia, but occasionally the arthropathy is the initial or predominant manifestation. Clinical features include rapid and painless swelling of the joint with radiographically apparent fragmentation, sclerosis, and subluxation of the humeral head. Spontaneous fracture of the neighboring glenoid, scapula, ribs, and clavicle can also develop.

Congenital indifference to pain is a feature of several distinct hereditary sensory neuropathies. Most of the these conditions are recognized in infancy or childhood. The skeletal alterations associated with this group of disorders include neuropathic arthropathy, fractures of long bones, epiphyseal separations, and soft tissue ulcerations. These injuries are more frequent in the lower extremity than the upper extremity. Neuropathic arthropathy is especially common in the ankle and tarsal areas, although multiple sites can be affected. Metaphyseal and diaphyseal long bone fractures are thought to result from the combination of osteoporosis and neurologic deficit. Epiphyseal separations similarly result from chronic trauma or stress. Soft tissue ulcerations appear at pressure areas on weight-bearing surfaces or over bony prominences. These may deepen and lead to infection of adjacent bones and joints. Many of the skeletal lesions heal with proper supervision and treatment. Recurrent osteomyelitis, fracture, dislocation, and progressive deformity are common.

An aggressive approach to diagnosis and treatment of neuropathic joints may help the patient. A search for treatable conditions such as syphilis, yaws, or leprosy is indicated.

For the diabetic patient, molded footwear, appropriate immobilization or bracing of joints, and patient education may all be useful in preventing or reducing disability. Elevation of the leg to reduce edema, avoidance of weight bearing, and treatment of infection are fundamental therapeutic concepts. Sprains and fractures are usually immobilized in non-weight-bearing casts until radiographic evidence of improvement is seen. A walking cast is then used until osseous repair and stabilization are radiographically complete. Use of crutches for walking is required when hip and knee involvement is present. Excision of prominent exostoses or subluxed bone surfaces may be required to heal soft tissue ulceration.

Arthrodesis may be necessary to stabilize some joints. Total-joint replacement is generally contraindicated. However, with special care to correct alignment and ligamentous instability, some surgeons have achieved good results from insertion of certain joint replacement devices. Although the various therapeutic approaches are designed to preserve limb function, amputation is occasionally required.

Neal R. Stewart, M.B., Ch.B.
William A. Murphy, Jr., M.D.

SUGGESTED READINGS

NEUROPATHIC ARTHROPATHY

1. Allman RM, Brower AC, Kotlyarov EB. Neuropathic bone and joint disease. Radiol Clin North Am 1988; 26:1373–1381
2. Brower AC. The acute neuropathic joint. Arthritis Rheum 1988; 31:1571–1573

3. Cofield RH, Morrison MJ, Beabout JW. Diabetic neuroarthropathy in the foot: patient characteristics and patterns of radiographic change. Foot Ankle 1983; 4:15–22

4. Ellman MH. Neuropathic joint disease (Charcot joints). In: McCarty DJ (ed), Arthritis and allied conditions, 11th ed. Philadelphia: Lea & Febiger; 1989:1255–1272

5. Jaffe HL. Neuropathic arthropathies and neuropathic fractures of bone shafts. In: Jaffe HL (ed), Metabolic, degenerative and inflammatory diseases of bones and joint. Philadelphia: Lea & Febiger; 1972:847–874

6. Pogonowska MJ, Collins LC, Dobson HL. Diabetic osteopathy. Radiology 1967; 89:265–271

7. Reiner M, Scurran BL, Karlin JM, Silvani SH. The neuropathic joint in diabetes mellitus. Clin Podiatr Med Surg 1988; 5:421–437

8. Resnick D. Neuroarthropathy. In: Resnick D, Niwayama G (eds), Diagnosis of bone and joint disorders, 2nd ed. Philadelphia: WB Saunders; 1988:3154– 3185

9. Scartozzi G, Kanat IO. Diabetic neuroarthropathy of the foot and ankle. J Am Podiatr Med Assoc 1990; 80:298–303

10. Sinha S, Munichoodappa CS, Kozak GP. Neuro-arthropathy (Charcot joints) in diabetes mellitus: clinical study of 101 cases. Medicine 1972; 51:191–210

11. Soudry M, Binazzi R, Johanson NA, Bullough PG, Insall JN. Total knee arthroplasty in Charcot and Charcot-like joints. Clin Orthop 1986; 208:199–204

12. Zlatkin MB, Pathria M, Sartoris DJ, Resnick D. The diabetic foot. Radiol Clin North Am 1987; 25:1095–1105

CPPD CRYSTAL DEPOSITION DISEASE

13. Chen C, Chandnani VP, Kang HS, Resnick D, Sartoris DJ, Haller J. Scapholunate advanced collapse: a common wrist abnormality in calcium pyrophosphate dihydrate crystal deposition disease. Radiology 1990; 177:459–461

14. Komatsu T, Ohira N, Oshida M, Sasaki K. Massive deposition of calcium pyrophosphate dihydrate crystals in the knee. A case report. J Bone Joint Surg (Am) 1990; 72:931–935

15. Ling D, Murphy WA, Kyriakos M. Tophaceous pseudogout. AJR 1982; 138:162–165

16. Moskowitz RW. Diseases associated with the deposition of calcium pyrophosphate or hydroxyapatite. In: Kelley WN, Harris ED (eds), Texbook of rheumatology, 3rd ed. Philadelphia: WB Saunders; 1989:1449–1467

17. Resnick D, Niwayama G. Calcium pyrophosphate dihydrate (CPPD) crystal deposition disease. In: Resnick D, Niwayama G (eds), Diagnosis of bone and joint disorders, 2nd ed. Philadelphia: WB Saunders; 1988:1672–1732

18. Ryan LM, McCarty DJ. Calcium pyrophosphate crystal deposition disease; pseudogout; articular chondrocalcinosis. In: McCarty DJ (ed), Arthritis and allied conditions, 11th ed. Philadelphia: Lea & Febiger; 1989:1711–1736

19. Sissons HA, Steiner GC, Bonar F, et al. Tumoral calcium pyrophosphate deposition disease. Skeletal Radiol 1989; 18:79–87

20. Watson HK, Ballet FL. The SLAC wrist: scapholunate advanced collapse pattern of degenerative arthritis. J Hand Surg (Am) 1984; 9:358–365

REITER'S ARTHROPATHY

21. Calin A. Reiter's syndrome. In: Kelley WN, Harris ED (eds), Textbook of rheumatology, 3rd ed. Philadelphia: WB Saunders; 1989:1038–1052
22. Ford DK. One syndrome—many infectious agents. J Rheumatol 1987; 14:650–652
23. Ford DK. Reiter's syndrome: reactive arthritis. In: McCarty DJ (ed), Arthritis and allied conditions, 11th ed. Philadelphia: Lea & Febiger; 1989:944–953
24. Leirisalo M, Skylv G, Kousa M, et al. Followup study on patients with Reiter's disease and reactive arthritis, with special reference to HLA-B27. Arthritis Rheum 1982; 25:249–259
25. Lipsky PE, Taurog JD. The second International Simmons Center Conference on HLA-B27-related disorders. Arthritis Rheum 1991; 34:1476–1482
26. Martel W, Braunstein EM, Borlaza G, Good AE, Griffin PE Jr. Radiologic features of Reiter disease. Radiology 1979; 132:1–10
27. Michet CJ, Machado EB, Ballard DJ, McKenna CH. Epidemiology of Reiter's syndrome in Rochester, Minnesota: 1950–1980. Arthritis Rheum 1988; 31:428–431
28. Mielants H, Veys EM. Clinical and radiographic features of Reiter's syndrome and inflammatory bowel disease related to arthritis. Curr Opin Rheumatol 1990; 2:570–576
29. Neuwelt CM, Borenstein DG, Jacobs RP. Reiter's syndrome: a male and female disease. J Rheumatol 1982; 9:268–272
30. Resnick D. Reiter's syndrome. In: Resnick D, Niwayama G (eds), Diagnosis of bone and joint disorders, 2nd ed. Philadelphia: WB Saunders; 1988:1199– 1217

MIDFOOT FRACTURES

31. Berquist TH, Morrey BF, Cass JR, Johnson KA. The foot and ankle. In: Berquist TH (ed), Imaging of orthopedic trauma, 2nd ed. Philadelphia: WB Saunders; 1992:453–577
32. Heckman JD. Fractures and dislocations of the foot. In: Rockwood CA Jr, Green DP, Bucholz RW (eds), Rockwood and Green's fractures in adults, 3rd ed. Philadelphia: JB Lippincott; 1991:2041–2182
33. Hermel MB, Gershon-Cohen J. The nutcracker fracture of the cuboid by indirect violence. Radiology 1953; 60:850–854
34. Main BJ, Jowett RL. Injuries of the midtarsal joint. J Bone Joint Surg (Br) 1975; 57:89–97
35. Pavlov H, Torg JS, Freiberger RH. Tarsal navicular stress fractures: radiographic evaluation. Radiology 1983; 148:641–645
36. Rogers LF. The foot. In: Rogers LF (ed), Radiology of skeletal trauma. New York: Churchill Livingstone; 1982:861–920

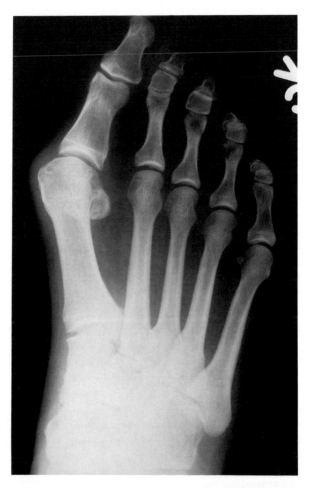

Figure 22-1. This 45-year-old woman complained of foot pain. You are shown an anteroposterior weight-bearing radiograph of the forefoot.

Case 22: Hallux Valgus Deformity

Question 92

Which *one* of the following is the MOST likely diagnosis?

    (A) Hammertoes
    (B) Hallux valgus deformity
    (C) Hallux rigidus deformity
    (D) Systemic lupus erythematosus
    (E) Traumatic dislocation

The conventional anteroposterior radiograph of the forefoot (Figure 22-1) demonstrates lateral deviation of the great-toe-proximal phalanx with respect to the first metatarsal head. The entire first metatarsal is deviated medially. These features are typical of hallux valgus deformity (Figures 22-2 through 22-4) **(Option (B) is correct)**. Also, the sesamoids are no longer centered under the metatarsal head, and a prominent eminence (enlargement) of the medial aspect of the head has developed.

Hammertoes (Option (A)) are a common adult toe deformity. This deformity is frequently related to improper footwear, which accentuates muscle imbalance. However, hammertoes involve the second through fifth digits and are characterized by an extended metatarsal-phalangeal joint, a flexed proximal interphalangeal joint, and a hyperextended distal interphalangeal joint.

Hallux rigidus deformity (Option (C)) is a form of degenerative arthritis (osteoarthritis) involving the first metatarsal-phalangeal joint (Figure 22-5). It is usually idiopathic, but it can result from intra-articular fracture, traumatic compression of the joint surfaces (turf toe), or joint damage due to rheumatoid or septic arthritis. From the initial presentation of pain and synovitis, the degenerative process progresses to osteophyte formation on the metatarsal head, especially dorsally and laterally. Medial and plantar osteophyte formation is rare. The lateral radiograph typically shows a large dorsal osteophyte along with a narrowed joint space dorsally. Bone production enlarges the metatarsal head, and this contributes to loss of great-toe dorsiflexion and increasing

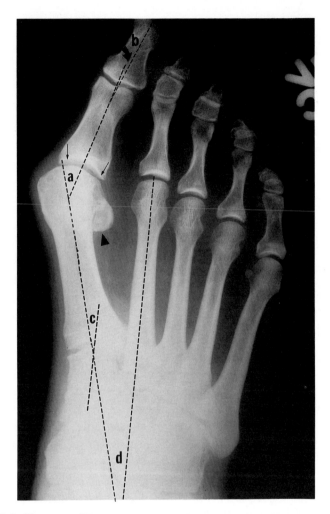

Figure 22-2 (Same as Figure 22-1). Hallux valgus deformity. An antero-posterior weight-bearing radiograph of the right foot shows the funda-mental abnormality, lateral deviation of the great toe at the first metatarsal-phalangeal joint. The joint is still congruent; that is, the articular surfaces are still aligned (small straight arrows). The sesa-moids (arrowhead) are not centered under the metatarsal head, as they would be normally. Important orthopedic measurements include the hal-lux valgus angle (a), the hallux valgus interphalangeal angle (curved arrow, b), the metatarsus primus varus angle (c), and the intermetatar-sal angle (d).

rigidity of the first metatarsal-phalangeal joint. Enlargement of the metatarsal head can also produce neurologic symptoms as a result of pressure on the dorsal medial cutaneous nerve to the great toe. Soft tis-sue callus formation and ulceration caused by pressure of footwear on bone prominences are further complications.

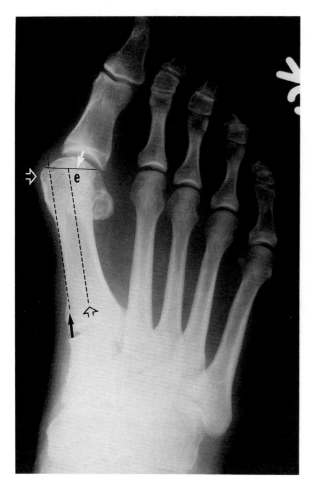

Figure 22-3 (Same as Figure 22-1). Hallux valgus deformity. The size of the median eminence (open white arrow) is determined by a line drawn along the medial aspect of the metatarsal shaft (solid black arrow). The distal metatarsal articular angle (e) is measured between a transverse line across the articular surface (solid white arrow) and a line along the long axis of the metatarsal (open black arrow).

If the pain and other symptoms of hallux rigidus are not relieved with conservative management, such as nonsteroidal anti-inflammatory medications, appropriate footwear, and shoe inserts, surgical intervention may be necessary. Removal of the dorsal 20 to 30% of the metatarsal head, known as cheilectomy, is the initial surgical treatment for hallux rigidus (Figure 22-5C). This procedure decreases the joint bulk by resection of the dorsal osteophytes, which allows increased dorsiflexion and reduces pain. As long as there is some preservation of the metatarsal-phalangeal joint, cheilectomy is the procedure of choice.

If the joint space has been completely obliterated by the degenerative process, arthrodesis can be performed. Other procedures, including resection arthroplasty (Keller procedure) and proximal phalangeal osteotomy, are alternatives depending on the patient's activity level.

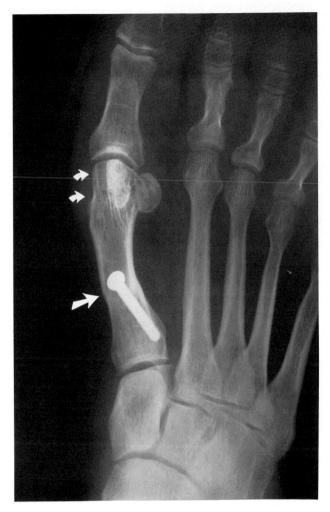

Figure 22-4. Same patient as in Figures 22-1 through 22-3. Appearance of hallux valgus deformity after typical corrective surgery. The alignment between the first metatarsal and the first proximal phalanx has been corrected by soft tissue procedures. The medial eminence has been resected (curved arrows). An osteotomy of the metatarsal shaft (note the bone screw) was performed to correct metatarsus primus varus and restore the intermetatarsal angle. The metatarsal osteotomy is now solidly healed (straight arrow).

Polyarthritis is one of the common manifestations of systemic lupus erythematosus (Option (D)). Typically there is a deforming, nonerosive arthropathy with soft tissue swelling, periarticular osteoporosis, and spontaneous tendon weakening and rupture. Tendinous involvement predisposes these patients to the development of hallux valgus. As in patients with other inflammatory arthropathies, however, such tendon involvement usually causes more severe and widespread alignment abnormalities of the lesser toes than are seen in patients with simple hallux valgus.

Traumatic dislocation (Option (E)) rarely occurs at the first metatarsal-phalangeal joint. Furthermore, the test image shows a subluxation, not a complete dislocation. Finally, the prominent medial eminence and

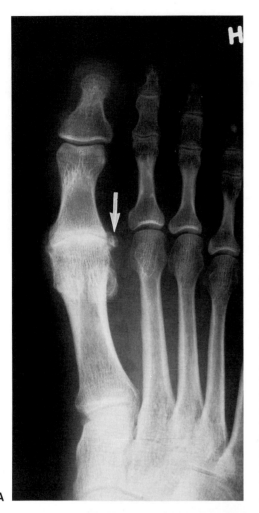

A

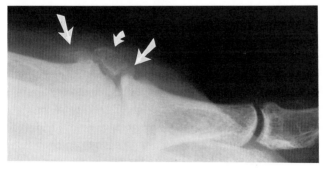

B

Figure 22-5. Hallux rigidus deformity. (A) An anteroposterior radiograph shows severe narrowing of the first metatarsal-phalangeal joint space and osteophyte formation, particularly along the lateral margin (arrow). (B) A lateral radiograph shows prominent dorsal osteophytes (straight arrows) and a large intra-articular osteochondral body (curved arrow). (C) A lateral radiograph shows the result of cheilectomy with removal of the dorsal aspect of the metatarsal head (arrows). The proximal phalangeal osteophyte and the osteochondral fragment were also removed.

the medial angulation of the first metatarsal are typical of a chronic hallux valgus deformity, not an acute traumatic dislocation.

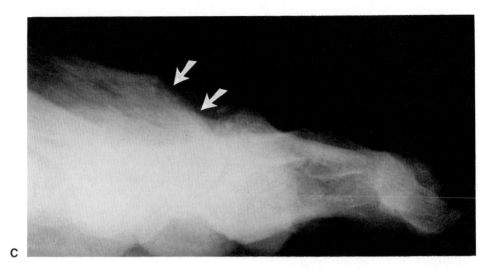

c

Radiographic analysis of hallux valgus deformity requires evaluation of several angles involving the great toe. All measurements are made on the anteroposterior weight-bearing radiograph of the foot. The hallux valgus angle is the angle between the long axes of the proximal phalanx and the first metatarsal shaft (Figure 22-2, angle a). The hallux valgus angle measures the lateral deviation of the proximal phalanx on the metatarsal head. Normally, this angle should be less than 20°. A severe hallux valgus deformity has an angle that measures more than 35°.

The hallux valgus interphalangeal angle measures the lateral deviation of the distal phalanx in relation to the proximal phalanx (Figure 22-2, angle b). This angle ranges from 6 to 24° in normal individuals, but it is usually less than 15°.

The metatarsus primus varus angle (Figure 22-2, angle c) measures the axial relationship between the medial cuneiform and the first metatarsal shaft; it is normally less than 25°. Larger angles indicate medial deviation of the first metatarsal shaft (metatarsus primus varus).

Another important angle is the intermetatarsus angle (Figure 22-2, angle d), which measures the alignment between the first and second metatarsal shafts and is normally less than 10°. Deforming pressures of the first proximal phalanx on the first metatarsal head can displace the first metatarsal medially, thereby widening this angle; however, the intermetatarsus angle can also be affected by intrinsic anatomy. During surgical correction of hallux valgus, the mobility of the first metatarsal-cuneiform joint can be sufficient to reduce this angle to normal once the deforming pressure more distally in the great toe is corrected. However, some surgeons believe that the presence of a lateral facet at the base of

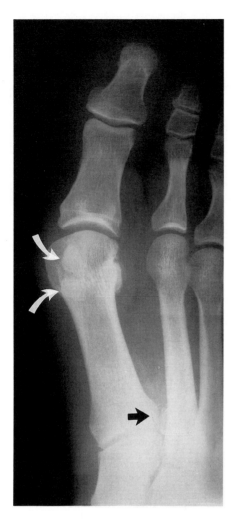

Figure 22-6. Lateral facet of the first metatarsal base and bipartite sesamoid. An anteroposterior radiograph shows a lateral facet at the first metatarsal base (black arrow). Some surgeons think that such a facet prevents adequate reduction of an abnormal intermetatarsal angle unless a first metatarsal osteotomy is performed. A typical bipartite medial sesamoid with rounded edges and relatively equal size of the two components (white arrows) is an incidental feature.

the first metatarsal is an important anatomic variant that can preclude successful reduction of the intermetatarsal angle at surgery unless some form of osteotomy is performed. The implication of this facet is controversial, but its presence or absence can be determined from the radiograph (Figure 22-6).

At least two more useful radiographic observations can be made about the first metatarsal-phalangeal joint. First, the size of the medial eminence can be determined by drawing a line along the medial aspect of the metatarsal shaft (Figure 22-3). Second, the distal metatarsal articular angle (DMAA) is the angle between a line that transversely connects the proximal edges of the articular surface of the first metatarsal head and a line that bisects the long axis of the first metatarsal (Figure 22-3, angle e). In some patients, the hallux valgus deformity is secondary to an abnormal lateral sloping of the distal metatarsal articular surface, indicated by an increased DMAA. The DMAA is normally less than 10°. (The DMAA is not measured directly but is 90° minus angle e in Figure 22-3. That is, the DMAA measures the deviation of the distal articular surface from a 90° alignment.)

The etiology of hallux valgus deformity is multifactorial, involving extrinsic or environmental factors as well as predisposing intrinsic anatomy. A major contributor is tight footwear that produces a laterally directed force against the distal great toe. Intrinsic factors include incompetent or deficient tendon slings, which can result from idiopathic weak ligaments and joint hypermobility or from an underlying disease such as rheumatoid arthritis. Other potentially contributing intrinsic factors include congenital metatarsus primus varus, splay foot, and metatarsus adductus.

Hallux valgus is caused by disruption of the dynamic balance of the soft tissue around the first metatarsal-phalangeal joint. The first metatarsal head and joint capsule rest in a sling of tendons and muscles, which pass by the joint to insert on the proximal and distal phalanges (Figure 22-7). Laterally, the adductor hallucis tendon, inserting into the lateral aspect of the proximal phalanx, provides stability. Medially, the abductor hallucis tendon inserts onto the plantar medial base of the proximal phalanx. Both of these tendons give extensions inferiorly to the sesamoid complex, which gives rise to the sesamoid ligaments and the metatarsal-phalangeal collateral ligaments both medially and laterally. The sesamoids themselves are intratendinous, lying in the flexor hallucis brevis tendon. This sesamoid complex provides stability inferiorly as well as in the transverse plane. Centered on the metatarsal shaft are the tendons of the extensor hallucis longus superiorly and the flexor hallucis longus inferiorly.

For hallux valgus to develop, the balanced interplay of these tendon slings must be disrupted. The tendons can then become destabilizing forces. Pressured by the laterally drifting first proximal phalanx, the first metatarsal head deviates medially. This stretches and attenuates the medial joint capsule. It also stretches the abductor hallucis tendon, which becomes mechanically weakened and migrates both plantarward and laterally and moves under the metatarsal head (Figure 22-8). Consequently, the adductor tendon is no longer balanced by the abductor. Because these two tendons contribute to the sesamoid complex, the tendon sling and sesamoid complex also shift their orientation with respect to the joint (Figure 22-9). The change in position of the sesamoid complex produces an extrinsic force during walking, which promotes further valgus deviation of the toe (Figure 22-10). The flexor hallucis longus

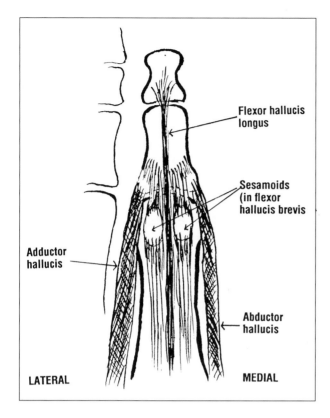

Figure 22-7. Soft tissue sling of normal first metatarsal. The drawing shows a plantar view of the relationships between soft tissue and bone in the normally balanced great toe.

and extensor hallucis longus tendons become bowstrung laterally, further increasing the lateral deviation of the proximal phalanx. The eccentric location of these muscles and tendons continues to magnify the medially directed force on the metatarsal head. The metatarsal head is pushed off the sesamoid sling by pressure from the proximal phalanx, and with a hallux valgus angle greater than 35°, the first metatarsal shaft rotates into pronation, further altering its relationship to the sesamoids.

The articular cartilage of the metatarsal head becomes uncovered medially, and this results in cartilage atrophy. With time, there is bony overgrowth of the medial metatarsal head, producing the so-called medial eminence. Typically, bursal hypertrophy and soft tissue thickening, combined with the medial eminence, result in a prominent bump along the medial side of the great toe. This bump is commonly called a bunion. The term "bunion" is sometimes also used to refer to the entire hallux valgus deformity complex. Because this term is imprecise, it should be avoided.

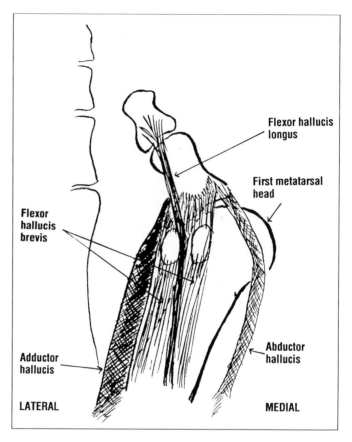

Figure 22-8. Imbalanced soft tissue sling in hallux valgus deformity. The adductor hallucis, flexor hallucis longus, and flexor hallucis brevis muscles and tendons become displaced and contracted laterally, and the abductor hallucis is attenuated medially.

As the first metatarsal is shifted medially by the first proximal phalanx, the metatarsal-phalangeal joint itself can shift, producing an incongruent joint. In the incongruent joint, there is subluxation of the proximal phalangeal base in relation to the metatarsal articulation, so that the two articular surfaces are not parallel (Figure 22-11). Some surgeons think that this increases the risk of progression of the deformity and an unfavorable prognosis. In a congruent joint, there is parallel alignment of the articular surfaces of the metatarsal head and the proximal phalanx and concentric alignment of the articular surface. This is thought to be a more stable configuration (Figure 22-2). The surgical importance of joint congruity is controversial. Some surgeons believe that if the DMAA is more than 20° and the joint is incongruent, a compensating proximal phalangeal osteotomy should be performed.

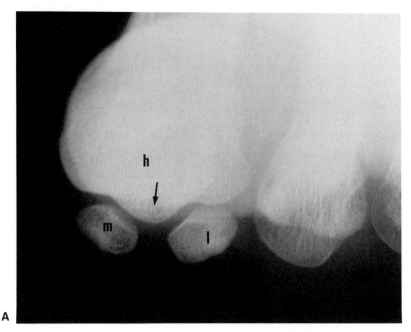

A

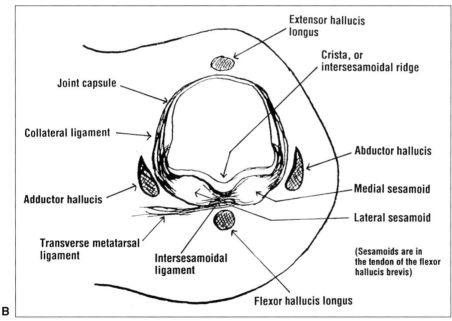

B

Figure 22-9. Cross-sectional anatomy of the normal and abnormal sesamoid complex. (A) An axial radiograph shows the metatarsal-sesamoid joint. h = first metatarsal head; m = medial (tibial) sesamoid; l = lateral (fibular) sesamoid. The prominent crista or intersesamoidal ridge (arrow) separates the two sesamoid articulations. (B) Normal anatomy of the soft tissue sling around the first metatarsal head. (C) Alteration of the normal soft tissue and osseous structures as a result of severe hallux valgus deformity. Note also the atrophy of the crista from valgus pressure and the rotation of the metatarsal head off the sesamoid complex.

573

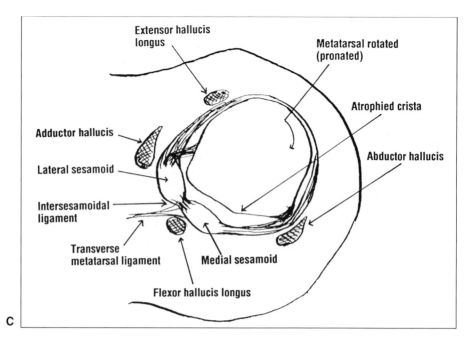

Figure 22-9 (Continued)

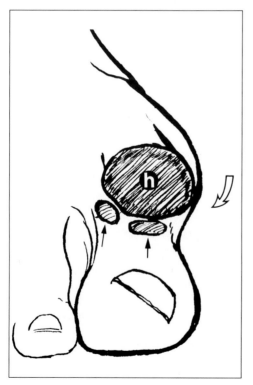

Figure 22-10 (left). Pronation of the first metatarsal. In hallux valgus, weight bearing shifts medially as the first metatarsal head (h) rotates into pronation (open arrow). Small arrows indicate the sesamoids.

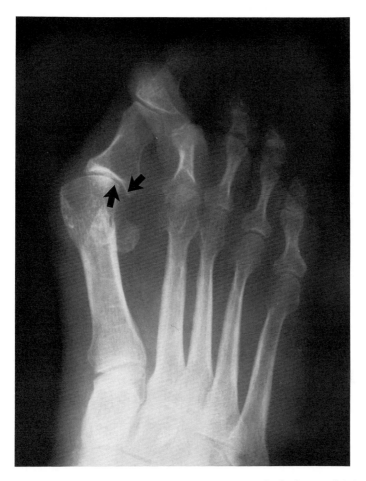

Figure 22-11. Incongruence of the first metatarsal-phalangeal joint. The first metatarsal-phalangeal joint is incongruent, since there is lateral subluxation of the proximal phalangeal base (arrows). Note also the crossover between the great and second toes as a result of the combination of a hallux valgus deformity and disrupted ligamentous and tendinous balance. This patient has rheumatoid arthritis.

Question 93

Components of surgical correction of hallux valgus deformity include:

(A) soft tissue release of lateral contracture
(B) plication of medial capsular structures
(C) removal of the medial eminence
(D) osteotomy to correct metatarsus primus varus
(E) removal of the sesamoid complex

Conservative management consisting of wearing low-heeled shoes with a sufficient toe box area is adequate therapy for most patients with hallux valgus deformity. However, surgical correction of hallux valgus deformity is indicated if conservative management fails to relieve discomfort. The basic goal of hallux valgus surgery is to relieve pain, correct the deformity, and maintain a biomechanically functional foot. However, surgical correction does not necessarily permit unrestricted shoe selection or achieve improved foot function. Recent advances in the understanding of the pathophysiology of this disorder have led most surgeons to believe that both soft tissue correction and bone correction are required for a successful surgical outcome.

The distal soft tissue procedure at the first metatarsal-phalangeal joint involves releasing the lateral contracture **(Option (A) is true)** and plicating the medial joint capsule **(Option (B) is true).** Release of the lateral contracture consists of detaching the adductor hallucis tendon from its insertion into the base of the proximal phalanx. The transverse metatarsal ligament between the lateral sesamoid and the second metatarsal is cut. The lateral joint capsule is then widely torn or cut. These steps reduce the pressure of the proximal phalanx against the first metatarsal and allow the sesamoids to be mobilized and realigned beneath the first metatarsal head. The stretched medial capsular tissue is plicated by excising a 3- to 8-mm wedge of joint capsule tissue (the size depends on the degree of deformity) and resuturing the capsule. The medial eminence can now be excised from the first metatarsal head in line with the medial aspect of the metatarsal shaft **(Option (C) is true).** The surgeon must be careful not to remove too much of the median eminence, because this can result in a hallux varus deformity.

After the soft tissue procedure, the surgeon might be able to realign the first metatarsal with the second metatarsal. If this is not possible, a first metatarsal osteotomy is required; in fact, 80% of patients need such an osteotomy to correct residual metatarsus primus varus **(Option (D) is true).** A crescent-shaped osteotomy at the base of the first metatarsal (Mann osteotomy) maintains stability of the joint and preserves the length of the bone.

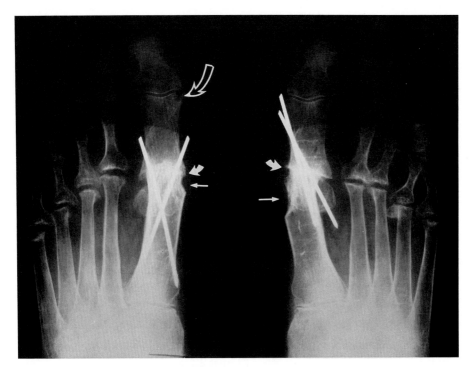

Figure 22-12. Bilateral hallux valgus repair. This patient with rheumatoid arthritis has had bilateral resections of the medial eminences (straight arrows) and arthrodeses of the first metatarsal-phalangeal joints (curved solid arrows). Resection arthroplasties were done at the second through fifth metatarsal-phalangeal joints bilaterally. Typical rheumatoid erosions are present at the interphalangeal joint of the right first toe (open arrow).

Other types of osteotomy can be used to individualize the hallux valgus correction. These include the Akin procedure (medial closing-wedge osteotomy at the proximal phalangeal base) to correct a laterally deviated proximal phalanx, the distal metatarsal chevron procedure (V-shaped intracapsular osteotomy through the metatarsal head) to correct milder forms of hallux valgus, and the Mitchell procedure (osteotomy through the distal metatarsal shaft) to correct the varus position of the first metatarsal.

Patients with associated advanced degenerative arthritis, rheumatoid arthritis, or significant hallux rigidus respond best to an arthrodesis of the first metatarsal-phalangeal joint (Figure 22-12). Historically, surgical procedures involved removal of the lateral sesamoid, but the sesamoid is now left in place to provide greater stability to the sesamoid sling and to help prevent postoperative hallux varus deformity **(Option (E) is false).**

Question 94

Concerning the sesamoid bones of the great toe,

    (A) during walking they absorb most of the weight-bearing stresses on the medial forefoot

    (B) in patients with hallux rigidus deformity, the joints between the sesamoids and the metatarsal head are usually involved by degenerative arthritis

    (C) in patients with hallux valgus deformity, they are tethered to the second metatarsal head by the transverse metatarsal ligament

    (D) bipartite sesamoids and fractured sesamoids can usually be differentiated on standard radiographs

    (E) the anteroposterior radiograph provides adequate evaluation of most sesamoid disorders

The two sesamoids of the first metatarsal-phalangeal joint are located in the tendon of the flexor hallucis brevis muscle and are connected by the intersesamoidal ligament (Figure 22-9). During walking, they absorb most of the weight-bearing stresses on the medial forefoot **(Option (A) is true).** They also protect the tendon of the flexor hallucis longus and increase the mechanical advantage of the flexor hallucis brevis. The stabilizing effect of the sesamoids on the first metatarsal-phalangeal joint can be lost if the angle of weight bearing is shifted anteriorly by elevating the heel several inches, as occurs by wearing shoes with very high heels. Force is then transferred from the sesamoid complex onto the unprotected metatarsal head and articular cartilage.

Most diseases that involve the first metatarsal-phalangeal joint, such as arthritis, trauma, infection, and hallux valgus deformity, can severely affect the sesamoids, because the sesamoids are an integral part of the dynamics of the joint. However, in patients with hallux rigidus deformity, the joints between the metatarsal head and sesamoids are not usually involved in the degenerative process **(Option (B) is false).** The cause of hallux rigidus is unknown, and the relative sparing of the metatarsal sesamoid joints is unexplained.

The sesamoids are connected to the proximal phalanx through the extension of the flexor hallucis brevis tendon and are suspended under the metatarsal head by the metatarsal-phalangeal collateral ligaments and the sesamoid ligaments (Figure 22-9). In patients with hallux valgus deformity, the sesamoids are tethered to the second metatarsal head by the transverse metatarsal ligament and conjoined adductor hallucis tendon **(Option (C) is true).** The sesamoids are intratendinous, except for their dorsal articular surfaces, which articulate with the plantar facets of the first metatarsal head. A crista or intersesamoidal ridge separates the metatarsal facets of the metatarsal head and stabilizes the sesamoid complex (Figure 22-9). In patients with advanced hallux valgus, the intersesamoidal ridge atrophies under the valgus pressure and the metatarsal head migrates medially over the fixed sesamoidal complex (Figure 22-9C). This produces the appearance of laterally drifting sesamoids. In fact, the sesamoids maintain their relationship to the second metatarsal head but do shift in the coronal plane in relation to each other. As the lateral (fibular) sesamoid is displaced into the intermetatarsal space, it migrates dorsally. The medial sesamoid, having traversed the crista, is now held in the lateral sesamoidal groove, which is in a more plantar position. The medial sesamoid alone thus comes to bear all the weight transmitted through the first metatarsal head. The weight-bearing surface of the first metatarsal head is rotated and is now oriented more laterally, i.e., there is eversion or pronation of the metatarsal head (Figure 22-9C).

It can be difficult to distinguish a symptomatic bipartite sesamoid from a fractured sesamoid radiographically **(Option (D) is false).** Typically, the normal bipartite sesamoid (Figure 22-6) is larger than an undivided sesamoid and has a smoothly corticated central lucent cleft, rounded edges, and components of nearly equal size. Fractured sesamoids are usually associated with localized pain and often occur with severe trauma and dislocation of the metatarsal-phalangeal joint. On standard radiographs, it is difficult to see the relatively sharp radiolucent line and subsequent callus formation typical of a fracture.

The anteroposterior radiograph does not provide adequate evaluation of most sesamoidal disorders, because the metatarsal head overlies both sesamoids **(Option (E) is false).** On the lateral view, the sesamoids are also difficult to evaluate because they overlap each other. For fractures (and most sesamoidal disorders), special radiographic projections including the axial sesamoid view (Figure 22-13) and lateral oblique views are helpful. Bone scintigraphy, CT, or MRI can also be useful in the evaluation of symptomatic patients with normal radiographs.

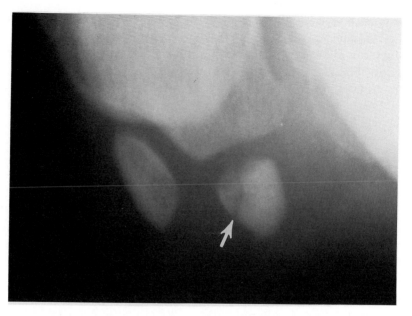

Figure 22-13. Fracture of lateral sesamoid. An axial radiograph of the metatarsal-sesamoid joints shows fracture (arrow) of the lateral sesamoid.

Question 95

Concerning deformities of the second through fifth toes,

    (A) a hammertoe results from a fixed flexion contracture at the proximal interphalangeal joint

    (B) a claw toe results from a fixed extension contracture at the distal interphalangeal joint

    (C) a second-digit crossover toe is the result of a hallux valgus deformity

    (D) a bunionette is characterized by a prominence of the lateral condyle of the fifth metatarsal head

    (E) constricting footwear is a major contributor to their formation and progression

Hammertoes and claw toes are similar in that both are accompanied by extended metatarsal-phalangeal joints and fixed flexion contracture of the proximal interphalangeal joints **(Option (A) is true).** In patients with hammertoe there is hyperextension of the distal interphalangeal joint (Figure 22-14), but in patients with claw toe there is flexion of the distal interphalangeal joint **(Option (B) is false).** These deformities occur because the strong extrinsic muscles of the toe, the extensor digi-

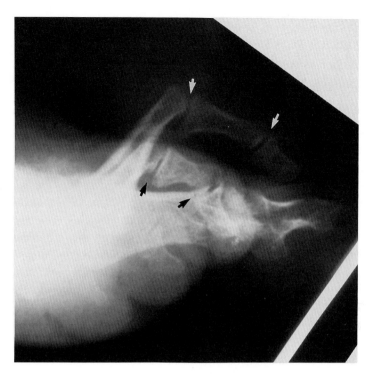

Figure 22-14. Claw toe and hammertoe deformities. A lateral radiograph of the forefoot shows flexion deformities of the proximal and distal interphalangeal joints (black arrows) in a third-digit claw toe. There is flexion of the proximal interphalangeal joint and extension at the distal interphalangeal joint (white arrows) in a second-digit hammertoe. (In a more extreme hammertoe deformity, there would be greater distal interphalangeal joint extension than is shown here.)

torum longus and flexor digitorum longus, overpower the weaker intrinsic muscles, the interossei and lumbricals. In both deformities, the hyperextended metatarsal-phalangeal joint results when the extensor tendons contract dorsally and produce a bowstring effect, which prevents the metatarsal-phalangeal joint from achieving the neutral position necessary to enable the extensor digitorum longus to extend the proximal interphalangeal joint.

Hammertoe and claw toe deformities can be painful and can cause soft tissue callus formation as a result of friction of the shoe over the flexed interphalangeal joints and at the tip of the flexed claw toe deformity. Both deformities can produce dorsal subluxation of the phalanx at the metatarsal-phalangeal joint, and in patients with the most severe deformities there is complete dislocation at the metatarsal-phalangeal joint. Radiographs are useful for evaluation of metatarsal-phalangeal malalignments to determine if an underlying arthropathy exists and to estimate the magnitude of the deformities. Surgical correction, when required, consists of release of the abnormal soft tissues that are the underlying cause of the deformity and sometimes resection of bone and, if needed, internal fixation.

A second-digit crossover toe is a complication of hallux valgus deformity **(Option (C) is true).** As with the great toe, the metatarsal-phalangeal joint of the second toe is held in neutral position by a balance of soft tissue structures. The intrinsic muscles of the second toe differ from those of the other lesser toes in that there are two dorsal interosseous muscles and no opposing plantar interosseous muscles. The lumbricals, which arise from the long flexor tendons and insert onto the medial extensor hood, produce an unopposed adduction force. These intrinsic muscles of the second digit are more susceptible to disruption than those of the other toes because of their potentially unbalanced configuration, and they depend on the plantar aponeurosis and joint capsule to provide stability.

The laterally directed pressure of a hallux valgus deformity pushing on the second toe can be great enough to chronically disrupt the ligamentous and tendinous balance of the second toe, producing subluxation and medial deviation and resulting in crossover between the great and second toes (Figure 22-11). In this circumstance, the great toe displaces the second toe dorsally as the great toe crosses under the second toe. However, in most patients with hallux valgus deformity, the medial deforming pressure is balanced by the pressure of the abutting second toe combined with the intact plantar aponeurosis and joint capsule, and no crossover develops.

A crossover toe can also result when acute trauma causes extensive ligamentous disruption or when there is ligamentous laxity and capsular distension as a result of rheumatoid arthritis or other causes of chronic synovitis. Shoe configuration, especially elevated heels and a small toe box, has also been implicated as a cause of toe crossover, by disrupting the stabilizing ligaments. An unusually long second metatarsal can also be a predisposing factor. If conservative measures are not successful, surgical correction with tendon and capsule releases may be necessary. In patients with severe deformities, resection arthroplasty of the proximal phalangeal head may be required, although this often results in limitation of weight-bearing function. If there is an associated hallux valgus deformity, it must be corrected to ensure stability.

A bunionette (or tailor's bunion) is characterized by a prominence of the lateral condyle of the fifth metatarsal head, analogous to the median eminence of hallux valgus **(Option (D) is true).** A bunionette deformity is associated with a wide range of anatomic variations. It can be limited to the fifth metatarsal head region, but there can also be an increased angle between the fourth and fifth metatarsal shafts or lateral deviation or bowing of the distal fifth metatarsal shaft. In two-thirds of patients, pes planus is an associated deformity. The symptomatic deformity of bunionette results from a thickened bursa and hypertrophic keratosis, and it responds well to conservative care (i.e., proper shoes). The location and extent of the deformity influence the choice of surgical treatment when it is needed. Surgical correction includes lateral condylectomy, distal soft tissue release, and various osteotomies.

Constricting footwear is a major contributor to the formation and progression of abnormalities in the adult forefoot **(Option (E) is true).** Hallux valgus and bunionette deformities are seen most often in women, especially those who favor high-heeled shoes with pointed, constricting toe boxes. Soft tissue instability produced by poor positioning of the foot and toes in tight shoes can either cause or exacerbate any intrinsic conditions that predispose to hallux valgus deformity. Increased heel height has also been blamed for the hyperextension and flexion deformities of claw toe and hammertoe, which position the toes so that the intrinsic muscles provide little resistance to further deformity.

Catherine Brandon, M.D.
Terry M. Hudson, M.D.

SUGGESTED READINGS

1. Coughlin MJ. Subluxation and dislocation of the second metatarsophalangeal joint. Orthop Clin North Am 1989; 20:535–551
2. Coughlin MJ. Sesamoid pain: causes and surgical treatment. Instr Course Lect 1990; 39:23–35
3. Coughlin MJ. Etiology and treatment of the bunionette deformity. Instr Course Lect 1990; 39:37–48
4. Karasick D, Wapner KL. Hallux valgus deformity: preoperative radiologic assessment. AJR 1990; 155:119–123
5. Karasick D, Wapner KL. Hallux rigidus deformity: radiologic assessment. AJR 1991; 157:1029–1033
6. Mann RA. Hallux valgus. Instr Course Lect 1986; 35:339–353
7. Mann RA. Treatment of the bunion deformity. Orthopedics 1987; 10:49–55
8. Mann RA. The great toe. Orthop Clin North Am 1989; 20:519–533
9. Mann RA. Decision-making in bunion surgery. Instr Course Lect 1990; 39:3–13
10. Mann RA. Hallux rigidus. Instr Course Lect 1990; 39:15–21
11. Mann RA, Coughlin MJ, DuVries HL. Hallux rigidus: a review of the literature and a method of treatment. Clin Orthop 1979; 142:57–63

12. Myerson MS, Shereff MJ. The pathological anatomy of claw and hammer-toes. J Bone Joint Surg (Am) 1989; 71:45–49
13. Turan I, Lindgren U, Lundberg I. Surgical treatment of forefoot deformity with special reference to polyarthritis. Clin Orthop 1991; 267:148–151

Notes

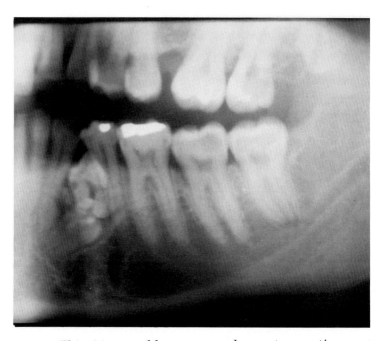

Figure 23-1. This 22-year-old woman underwent a routine pre-orthodontic evaluation. You are shown a panoramic radiograph.

Case 23: Compound Odontoma

Question 96

Which *one* of the following is the MOST likely diagnosis?

(A) Cemental dysplasia
(B) Compound odontoma
(C) Condensing osteitis
(D) Ossifying fibroma
(E) Osteosarcoma

The coned-down portion of the panoramic radiograph (Figure 23-1) shows a cluster of toothlike structures in the region of the mandibular premolars. These structures have a dense outer layer bordering a less dense inner layer (see Figure 23-2), recapitulating the appearance of normal enamel and dentin, respectively. The individual elements have crown and root morphology, and one has partially erupted. The aggregate is surrounded by a radiolucent sac resembling a normal dental sac. These characteristic findings are diagnostic of a compound odontoma **(Option (B) is correct).**

Cemental dysplasia (Option (A)) typically presents as a focal sclerotic lesion with a characteristic crescent shape adjacent to the roots of teeth. However, it does not produce the toothlike structures seen in the test image.

Condensing osteitis, also known as chronic focal sclerosing osteomyelitis (Option (C)), is a response of bone to adjacent infection. It appears as bone sclerosis adjacent to a carious tooth. Condensing osteitis is centered around a tooth rather than between teeth and does not form toothlike structures.

Ossifying fibroma (Option (D)) matures into a solid radiopaque neoplasm that characteristically expands bone through spherical growth. It is always well circumscribed and well demarcated from the surrounding bone. Toothlike structures do not occur.

Osteosarcoma (Option (E)) can arise between teeth, but this malignant neoplasm causes bone destruction. In the osteosclerotic type, exces-

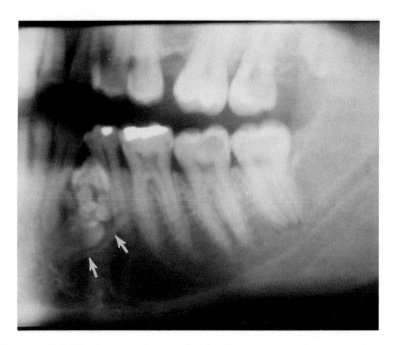

Figure 23-2 (Same as Figure 23-1). Compound odontoma. A cluster of toothlike structures is evident between the canine and the second mandibular premolar. The individual elements have crown and root morphology, and one, probably the original first premolar, has partially erupted. A radiolucent sac is best appreciated at the inferior margin of the mass (arrows).

sive mineral is deposited in a sclerotic mass, sometimes in irregular spicules that form a "sunburst pattern." Toothlike structures do not occur in osteosarcoma.

Questions 97 through 101

For each of the lesions of the osseous portion of the jaw listed below (Questions 97 through 101), select the *one* clinical feature (A, B, C, D, or E) that is MOST closely associated with it. Each clinical feature may be used once, more than once, or not at all.

97. Giant cell reparative granuloma
98. Fibrous dysplasia
99. Osteoma
100. Osteosarcoma
101. Langerhans cell histiocytosis

(A) It is limited to the jaws, hands, and feet.
(B) Its enlargement parallels skeletal growth.
(C) It readily responds to small doses of radiation therapy.
(D) A widened periodontal ligament space is an early finding.
(E) It is associated with intestinal polyposis.

The giant cell reparative granuloma, a benign lesion of uncertain etiology that consists of numerous multinucleated giant cells in a loose fibrillar connective tissue stroma, is a destructive lesion with either smooth or ragged borders (Figure 23-3). Most of these lesions are unilocular, but some have fine trabeculae that confer a multilocular appearance. The granuloma typically expands and thins, and it may perforate the bone cortex. Resorption of tooth root tips is a consistent feature. These tumors occur in children and young adults, with a 2:1 female predominance. They occur in the jaws, hands, and feet but not in other skeletal sites **(Option (A) is the correct answer to Question 97).**

The radiologic and pathologic features of the giant cell reparative granuloma are essentially identical to those of the brown tumor of hyperparathyroidism (Figure 23-4), but the two lesions occur in different clinical settings. In the jaw, osseous changes of hyperparathyroidism are typically accompanied by a diffuse loss of the lamina dura, the dense cortical bone adjacent to the tooth roots. This feature helps differentiate the two lesions but is better demonstrated on individual dental images than on panoramic radiographs. Both the giant cell reparative granuloma and the brown tumor are often locally aggressive and may become large; however, the preferred treatment of these benign conditions is simple curettage or local excision. Local recurrence of granulomas following surgical therapy is much less common than recurrence of the brown tumor of hyperparathyroidism.

Fibrous dysplasia is an important cause of facial asymmetry. It is usually detected between the ages of 10 and 30 years and manifests as painless facial swelling. The lesion enlarges slowly during normal skele-

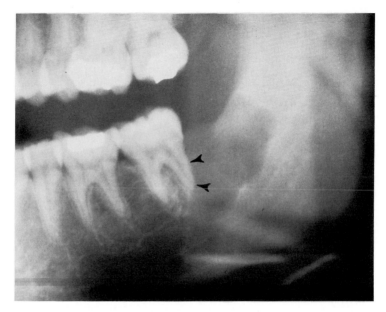

Figure 23-3. Giant cell reparative granuloma. Posterior to the second mandibular molar there is a unilocular lytic lesion with well-defined, scalloped borders. No matrix trabeculation is present in this example. Early resorption of the margin and apex of the adjacent second molar root is noted (arrowheads).

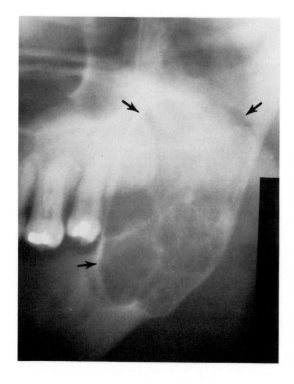

Figure 23-4. Brown tumor of hyperparathyroidism. This large multilocular lytic lesion (arrows) causes bone expansion and cortical thinning of the mandibular angle and ramus. A fine trabecular pattern is present throughout the matrix. Very similar appearances may be encountered with giant cell reparative granuloma and ameloblastoma.

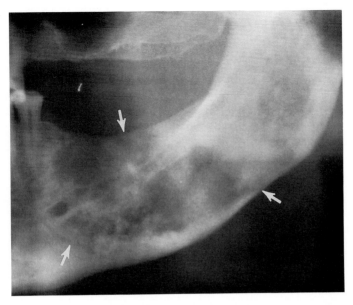

Figure 23-5. Fibrous dysplasia. This mature lesion (arrows) blends into the adjacent normal bone and shows mixed density with mottled areas of sclerosis combined with more-lucent areas containing fine trabeculae. Only mild bone enlargement is present.

tal growth and becomes static with skeletal maturity **(Option (B) is the correct answer to Question 98).** The maxilla is affected more frequently than the mandible. Like other fibro-osseous lesions, the radiographic appearance of fibrous dysplasia varies with the maturity and size of the lesion. In its immature form, fibrous dysplasia presents as a small unilocular or somewhat larger multilocular radiolucency with well-defined borders and a matrix of fine bone trabeculae. As the condition matures, it develops increased trabeculation and a more radiopaque, mottled appearance. Mature fibrous dysplasia is opaque with numerous fine trabeculae giving a "ground-glass" appearance. At this stage, the lesion blends into the surrounding bone (Figure 23-5). In all its forms, fibrous dysplasia enlarges the host bone and causes cortical thinning. Adjacent teeth may be displaced, but actual tooth resorption is uncommon.

Disfigurement caused by fibrous dysplasia may be difficult to manage, and definitive treatment is often withheld until the skeleton is mature. Cosmetic recontouring of affected bone is the treatment of choice; radical excision for this benign condition is not warranted. Radiation therapy has been abandoned due to lack of efficacy and to several instances of presumptive radiation-induced osteosarcoma.

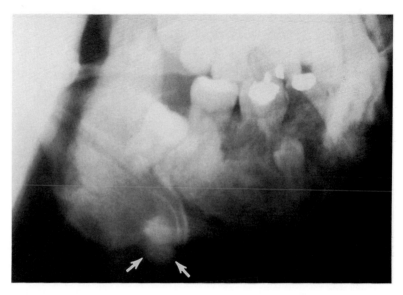

Figure 23-6. Osteomas in a patient with Gardner's syndrome. An oblique radiograph of the mandible shows a well-defined oval radiopaque mass projecting from the cortex (arrows). The areas of amorphous sclerosis throughout the mandibular body are endosteal osteomas.

Osteoma is a benign neoplasm of compact or cancellous bone that arises in either periosteal or endosteal locations. Periosteal osteoma presents as a well-defined, round or oval radiopaque mass that projects away from the normal adjacent bone (Figure 23-6). Endosteal osteoma appears as a radiopaque mass within the confines of the affected bone, at times causing bone expansion. Osteomas of the jaw may be multiple, and when jaw osteomas are accompanied by osteomas of the skull and long bones and by intestinal polyposis, Gardner's syndrome must be considered **(Option (E) is the correct answer to Question 99).** The features of this syndrome include polyposis of the large intestine; multiple osteomas of the long bones, skull, and jaws; multiple epidermoid or sebaceous cysts of the skin; occasional desmoid tumors; impacted supernumary or permanent teeth; and odontomas. On occasion, the presence of multiple osteomas of the jaw is the first evidence of Gardner's syndrome.

About 7% of osteosarcomas arise in the jaws. These malignant tumors commonly present as painful facial swelling, but symptoms may include loosened teeth, paresthesia, bleeding, and nasal obstruction. The mean age at diagnosis is 27 years, a decade later than with primary osteosarcoma found elsewhere in the body. Two appearances of jaw osteosarcoma are described: osteoblastic (sclerotic) and osteolytic. With osteoblastic osteosarcoma, mineral is laid down in amorphous masses. In 25%

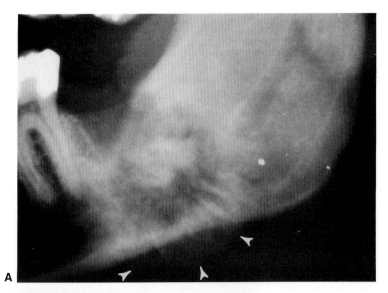

A

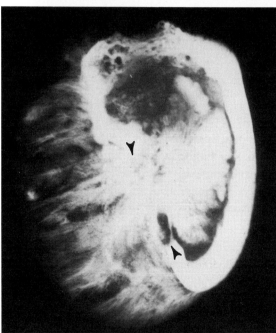

B

Figure 23-7. Osteosarcoma. (A) The mixed osteolytic and osteoblastic mass has characteristic mineralized tumor (arrowheads) projecting beyond the inferior margin of the mandible posterior to the second molar. Note the central sclerotic zone with a more lytic periphery. (B) A specimen radiograph of transverse tumor section demonstrates the central sclerotic mass, the lucent periphery, the cortical destruction (arrowheads), and the "sun-ray" spicules that extend beyond the normal bone.

of such cases, tumor mineralization develops as irregular spicules in a characteristic "sun-ray" or "sunburst" pattern (Figure 23-7). The tumor is initially confined within the jawbone, but the cortex is destroyed as the tumor enlarges. Osteolytic osteosarcoma is a poorly differentiated, very

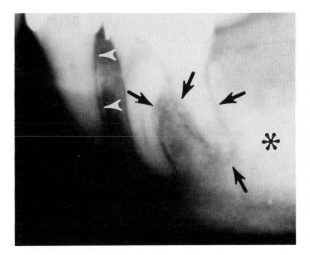

Figure 23-8. Osteosarcoma. The osteoblastic tumor (✳) in the body of the mandible has infiltrated the periodontal ligament and widened the periodontal ligament space around the first molar (arrows). Note the normal periodontal ligament space around the adjacent premolar (arrowheads).

aggressive, destructive lesion with little or no bone formation. A combination of osteoblastic and osteolytic areas is often seen in jaw osteosarcoma.

An early sign of osteosarcoma within the jaw is symmetric widening of the periodontal ligament space around one or more teeth (Figure 23-8) **(Option (D) is the correct answer to Question 100).** A few reported cases of asymmetric widening of the periodontal ligament space have been shown to result from infiltration of the periodontal ligament by osteosarcoma. The widened periodontal ligament space may be the first sign of tumor. Symmetric widening of the periodontal ligament space has been considered relatively specific for osteosarcoma; however, both periodontal disease and scleroderma also cause symmetric periodontal ligament space widening and should be excluded. Another early sign of jaw osteosarcoma is extension of mineralized tissue beyond the normal crest of the alveolar ridge.

Osteosarcoma of the mandible tends to be less anaplastic and has a better prognosis than does osteosarcoma of the maxilla or the remainder of the skeleton. Therapy consists of radical excision of the tumor plus adjuvant chemotherapy.

Langerhans cell histiocytosis, in its localized form (eosinophilic granuloma) and chronic recurring form (Hand-Schüller-Christian disease), may involve the jaw. Lesions manifest as single or multiple radiolucencies in the superficial alveolar bone. Bone destruction may be extensive

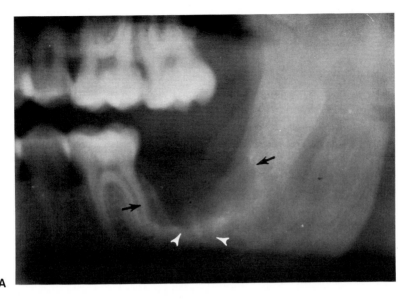

A

Figure 23-9. Langerhans cell histiocytosis (localized form). (A) This purely lytic lesion (arrows) has destroyed the alveolar bone, leaving behind the ghost of a socket (arrowheads) from a recently lost second molar. (B) One year later, following a course of radiation therapy, the lesion has healed completely.

and result in tooth loosening and loss (Figure 23-9A). The area of destruction is sometimes well demarcated and may therefore mimic jaw cysts. Treatment by either curettage or low-dose (6 to 10 Gy) radiation therapy is rapidly curative **(Option (C) is the correct answer to Question 101)** (Figure 23-9B). Currently curettage is the primary form of treatment instead of radiation therapy because there is a small risk of osteosarcoma following radiation therapy. A combination of radiation therapy and chemotherapy is used in recurrent disease or advanced primary disease such as may be encountered in the chronic recurring form of Langerhans cell histiocytosis.

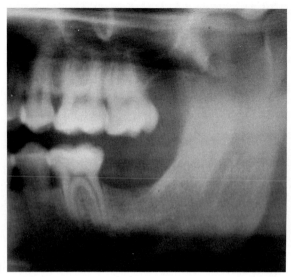

B

Question 102

Concerning osteosclerotic odontogenic lesions of the jaw,

    (A) condensing osteitis occurs in response to dental infection
    (B) about 10% of odontomas have an amorphous appearance
    (C) cemental dysplasia progresses from osteosclerotic to osteolytic
    (D) hypercementosis is excessive formation of cementum on the surface of the tooth root
    (E) ossifying fibroma causes tooth migration

Condensing osteitis, also termed chronic focal sclerosing osteomyelitis, is a sclerotic reaction of alveolar bone to adjacent infection **(Option (A) is true).** Bacteria entering bone from an adjacent carious tooth induce a proliferative tissue response rather than causing tissue destruction. This is thought to occur when the bacteria are of low virulence or the host tissue response is unusually vigorous. Radiography demonstrates a nearly pathognomonic well-circumscribed radiopaque zone of sclerotic bone surrounding and extending beyond the apex of one or more tooth roots (Figure 23-10). It occurs outside the periodontal ligament and is continuous with the lamina dura. Treatment is focused on the infected tooth, since the osteosclerosis is a secondary reaction.

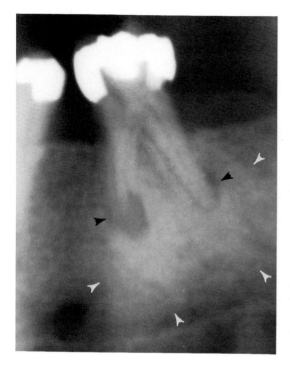

Figure 23-10. Condensing osteitis. The periapical lucencies (black arrowheads) adjacent to the roots of this mandibular molar are periapical abscesses or granulomas. The sclerotic alveolar bone (white arrowheads) surrounding this infected tooth is the region of condensing osteitis.

Odontomas occur in one of two patterns: either as a compound odontoma, characterized by a cluster of toothlike structures, or as a complex odontoma, manifested as an amorphous radiopaque mass. The two types occur with nearly equal frequency, although the compound type has a slight predominance **(Option (B) is false).**

The compound odontoma is a hamartoma of the jaw. It consists of enamel produced by ameloblasts of epithelial origin and dentin produced by odontoblasts of mesenchymal origin. Morphologically, it has a central area containing toothlike structures (ranging in number from a few to several dozen) surrounded by a radiolucent dental sac. Compound odontomas occur more frequently in the maxilla than in the mandible and favor the anterior portions of both. They are often associated with impacted or unerupted teeth and may displace teeth. The unerupted teeth are most often structurally normal but may be malformed.

If the odontoma consists of an irregular mass of calcified dental tissues that is not differentiated into toothlike elements, it is a complex odontoma (Figure 23-11). In this case a specific radiographic diagnosis may not be possible because cementoblastomas, osteomas, and fibromas may have a similar appearance. Both types of odontoma are treated by simple excision, and recurrence is rare. These hamartomas have no malignant potential.

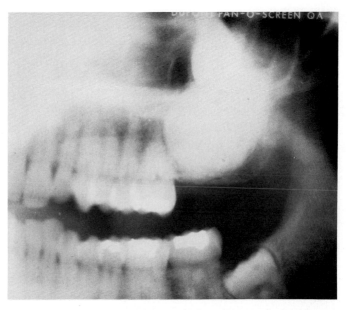

Figure 23-11. Complex odontoma. A large, amorphous, radiodense mass fills the maxillary tuberosity and extends into the maxillary sinus.

Disorders of cementum, the hard substance that lines the outer surface of tooth roots, occur principally at the periapical region of teeth. In general, cemental lesions evolve through three stages, from osteolytic to cementoblastic to osteosclerotic **(Option (C) is false).** The first (osteolytic) stage is characterized by areas of bone rarefaction adjacent to the tooth roots. The second (cementoblastic) stage begins with the appearance of a radiopaque cemental mass in the center of the lucent lesion. The third (osteosclerotic or mature) stage is identified when several cemental masses coalesce to form a solid radiopaque core. A radiolucent rim separates the radiopaque mass from the adjacent bone. No cemental lesions are malignant.

Periapical cemental dysplasia is a benign condition in which cementum is laid down adjacent to the roots of teeth, usually the mandibular incisors. Radiographically, mature cemental dysplasia is characteristically crescentic and surrounded by a radiolucent rim (Figure 23-12). The appearance is similar to that of condensing osteitis, but in periapical cemental dysplasia the adjacent tooth is not infected and remains vital. (A tooth is vital when the nerve in the pulp space is alive so that the tooth is sensitive to pressure and temperature.) When cemental dysplasia develops in edentulous areas, the outline is circular or ovoid rather than crescentic. In the osteolytic stage, the radiographic appearance of

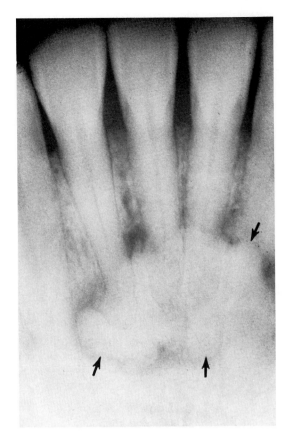

Figure 23-12. Periapical cemental dysplasia (sclerotic form). Masses of cementum (arrows) form sclerotic crescents around the apices of the roots of the mandibular incisors. A radiolucent rim surrounds this mature cemental lesion. (Courtesy of Charles W. Pemble III, D.M.D., Armed Forces Institute of Pathology, Washington, D.C.)

cemental dysplasia is similar to that of a periapical granuloma or cyst (Figure 23-13). It is important to recognize cemental dysplasia because it requires no treatment and is not associated with infection.

Cementoblastoma is a benign neoplasm of functioning cementoblasts. These cells deposit a large, round mass of cementum on a tooth root. Cementoblastomas occur more frequently in the mandible than in the maxilla and are more common posteriorly, with the first molar region being the most common location. Like cemental dysplasia, the cementoblastoma evolves from a radiolucent to a radiopaque lesion. In all stages, it is well circumscribed and well demarcated with respect to the adjacent bone. In the mature stage, the mass may be sufficiently dense to obscure adjacent tooth roots (Figure 23-14). Displacement of adjacent teeth is common and does not indicate malignant behavior. Cementoblastomas are treated by simple excision.

Hypercementosis is defined as deposition of excessive amounts of cementum on the roots of teeth **(Option (D) is true).** This deposition

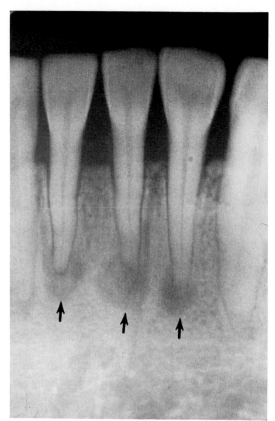

Figure 23-13. Periapical cemental dysplasia (osteolytic form). Small radiolucencies (arrows) surround the apices of the roots of the mandibular incisors in this immature cemental lesion. (Courtesy of Charles W. Pemble III, D.M.D.)

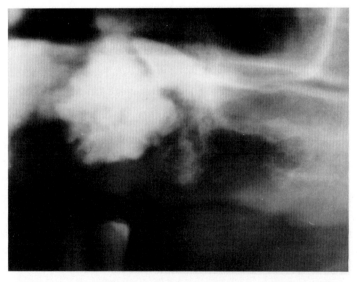

Figure 23-14. Cementoblastoma. This sclerotic mass of the maxillary alveolus completely obscures adjacent teeth. Such extreme density is seen only with cementoblastoma. Note the sharp margin and thin lucent zone separating this lesion from the normal bone.

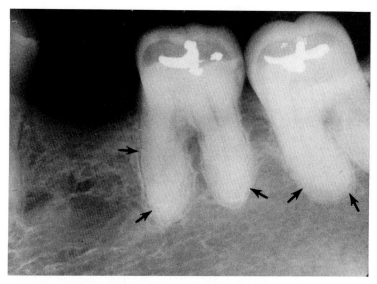

Figure 23-15. Hypercementosis. Sclerotic cementum is deposited along the tooth roots (arrows) within the periodontal ligament. (Courtesy of Suleyman Gulmen, D.M.D., St. Louis, Mo.)

occurs as a reparative response to inflammation or injury in the affected tooth. Alternatively, a generalized hypercementosis of all teeth may occur; it is of unknown etiology. The radiographic appearance is that of thickening and blunting of the tooth roots within the periodontal ligament (Figure 23-15). The condition has no associated symptoms and requires no treatment. If localized hypercementosis is the result of an adjacent infection, therapy is directed at the infected tooth.

Ossifying fibroma, cementifying fibroma, and cemento-ossifying fibroma are closely related benign neoplasms that cannot be differentiated on the basis of their clinical or radiographic features. They occur with a strong female predominance and may be found in either the maxilla or the mandible. They are slow-growing masses that may become quite large, up to 7 cm, although most remain less than 4 cm in diameter. They are initially asymptomatic but present later with swelling. They tend to grow in a spherical fashion and usually enlarge the bone without perforating the cortex. Displacement of teeth occurs early in the course (Figure 23-16) **(Option (E) is true).** Like most other cemental lesions, these evolve from radiolucent to radiopaque. In all cases, the fibromas are well demarcated. In the intermediate stages, the fibromas may resemble fibrous dysplasia in terms of the pattern of matrix mineralization, but the sharply marginated fibromas (Figure 23-17) do not blend in with the ad-

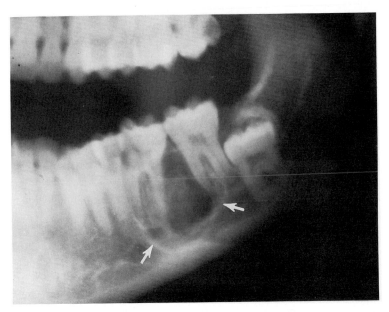

Figure 23-16. Cemento-ossifying fibroma. This small, primarily radiolucent lesion (arrows) displaces the roots of the first and second mandibular molars.

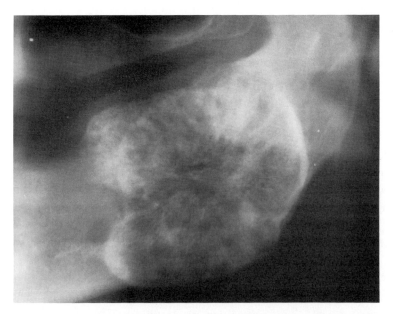

Figure 23-17. Cemento-ossifying fibroma. This mature 4-cm spherical mass in the posterior body of the mandible is sharply demarcated from the surrounding bone and causes considerable bone expansion and cortical thinning.

jacent bone as does fibrous dysplasia. Simple excision of the neoplasm is the preferred treatment.

Question 103

Concerning osteolytic odontogenic lesions of the jaw,

(A) at least 60% of jaw cysts occur at the apex of a tooth root
(B) radicular cysts arise most often in association with the roots of vital teeth
(C) dentigerous cysts develop in association with unerupted teeth
(D) odontogenic keratocysts should be surgically excised rather than curetted
(E) ameloblastomas metastasize in about 20% of cases

Cysts of the jaw constitute a heterogeneous group of radiolucent lesions. A cyst is defined as an epithelium-lined cavity usually containing fluid or semisolid material. Odontogenic cysts are derived from the epithelium associated with development of the teeth. Important odontogenic cysts include the radicular cyst, the dentigerous cyst, the residual cyst, the odontogenic keratocyst, the gingival cyst, and the calcifying odontogenic cyst. Of these, the most common is the radicular cyst, a lesion that occurs at the apex of a tooth root and represents more than 60% of all jaw cysts **(Option (A) is true).**

Radicular cysts (also called apical periodontal cysts) develop toward the end stage of long-standing tooth infection. The sequence begins with a caries. If the infection spreads into the tooth pulp, the condition is called acute pulpitis. At this stage, the infection kills the tooth's nerve by interrupting pulp blood supply. As a result, the tooth is nonvital (i.e., it is unable to sense temperature or pressure). As the infection spreads beyond the tooth, a granulomatous response (periapical granuloma) develops at the root apex. Later, epithelial proliferation creates an apical radicular cyst at the site of the preexisting granuloma. The tooth adjacent to the radicular cyst is always nonvital **(Option (B) is false).**

The radiographic appearance of a radicular cyst is that of a well-circumscribed radiolucent lesion with a sclerotic margin, intimately associated with the apex of a diseased tooth root (Figure 23-18). The radicular cyst cannot be distinguished from the related periapical granuloma on the basis of radiologic features, and both conditions occur in the same clinical setting. The cyst often remains the same size for months, but it may enlarge. Treatment is tooth extraction or root canal therapy with removal of the lucent lesion. If the cyst is not removed, it will not resolve spontaneously and is called a residual cyst. There is no tendency for either the radicular cyst or the residual cyst to transform into an ameloblastoma.

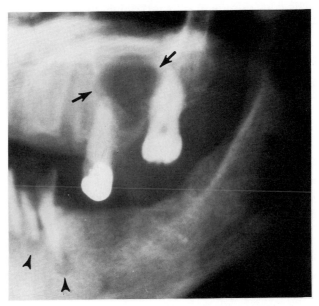

Figure 23-18. Radicular and residual cysts. The small periapical radiolucencies adjacent to the carious mandibular incisor and canine teeth (arrowheads) are due to periapical abscess, granuloma, or cyst. These related entities cannot be differentiated on radiographs. Between the maxillary premolar and the second molar is a larger lucent lesion, a residual cyst, at the site of a previously extracted tooth (arrows). Such a cyst occurs if a radicular cyst is left behind when the tooth is extracted.

A dentigerous or follicular cyst develops from the normal follicular sac that surrounds a developing tooth. If the space between the tooth and the sac wall is more than 3 mm wide, the sac has undergone cystic transformation. Dentigerous cysts arise in a pericoronal location around the crown of an unerupted, impacted, or embedded tooth **(Option (C) is true).** Although these cysts occur most often around unerupted third molars or maxillary canines, they may originate with any unerupted tooth (Figure 23-19). The cyst commonly enlarges to surround the entire tooth or may become large enough to occupy an entire mandibular segment or fill the entire maxillary antrum (Figure 23-20). Involved or adjacent teeth may be displaced, sometimes greatly. Bone expansion and cortical thinning also occur when dentigerous cysts become large. An infrequent but widely recognized complication of an untreated dentigerous cyst is transformation into an ameloblastoma, a squamous cell carcinoma, or a mucoepidermoid carcinoma. Therefore, it is recommended that every dentigerous cyst be treated by complete excision if small or by surgical drainage if large.

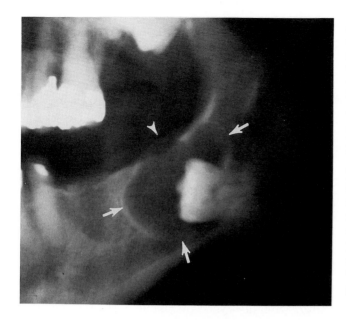

Figure 23-19 (left). Dentigerous cyst. This is the classic appearance of a dentigerous cyst. An unerupted mandibular third molar is surrounded by an enlarged pericoronal dental sac (arrows) with a very well defined border. The cyst causes expansion and cortical thinning along the alveolar margin (arrowhead).

Figure 23-20 (right). Dentigerous cyst. This dentigerous cyst of the maxillary tuberosity (arrows) has expanded into the maxillary sinus. The associated unerupted molar tooth (arrowhead) is markedly displaced.

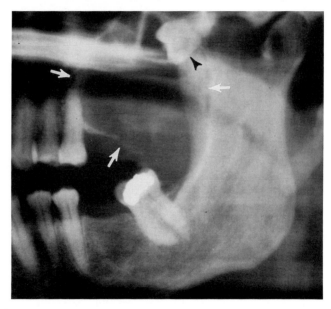

The odontogenic keratocyst is distinguishable from other odontogenic cysts by its characteristic histologic appearance and its high risk of recurrence. In general, it does not occur periapically but may appear in a pericoronal location or laterally along a tooth root. The radiographic appearance of the keratocyst may mimic other odontogenic cysts. The

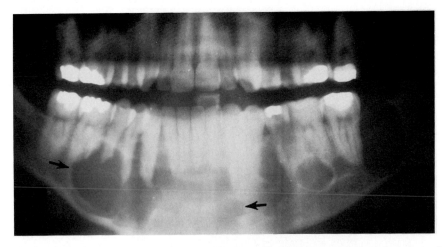

Figure 23-21. Odontogenic keratocysts. This 29-year-old man has basal cell nevus syndrome. Note the numerous cysts in the mandible. The largest extends from the right first molar to the left canine tooth (arrows) and has a scalloped margin. Smaller cysts are visible in the left mandibular body. All cysts have sharp, dense borders.

keratocyst is characteristically radiolucent with a well-defined, commonly scalloped border and a resultant multilocular appearance. These cysts often grow more rapidly than other odontogenic cysts, expand bone, perforate the cortex, and displace and resorb teeth.

When they are multiple, odontogenic keratocysts may be associated with basal cell nevus syndrome (Figure 23-21). This syndrome includes a spectrum of cutaneous abnormalities such as basal cell carcinoma, benign dermal cysts and tumors, palmar pitting, palmar and plantar keratoses, and dermal calcinosis. Dental and osseous anomalies in addition to odontogenic keratocysts include mandibular prognathism, rib and vertebral anomalies, and brachymetacarpalism. Ophthalmologic, neurologic, and gonadal abnormalities are also encountered.

The most important clinical aspect of the odontogenic keratocyst is its high rate of recurrence. The cyst must be completely eradicated to achieve a cure. Thus, surgical excision is recommended instead of curettage **(Option (D) is true).** On average, 25% of treated cysts will recur within 5 years of definitive surgery. Regular radiologic follow-up is recommended to ensure early detection of recurrence.

Ameloblastoma is a benign neoplasm that arises from ectodermal odontogenic cells that have not differentiated sufficiently to form enamel. The classic radiographic appearance is that of a multilocular, expansile radiolucency of the mandible (80%), especially in the region of molar

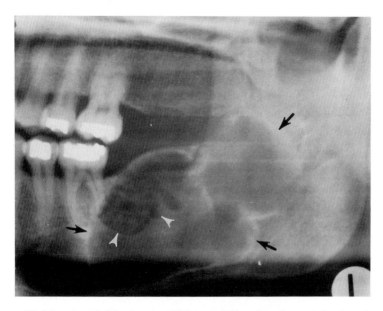

Figure 23-22. Ameloblastoma. This multilocular lucent lesion (arrows) fills the posterior body and angle of the mandible. The margin is well defined and dense, and the bone is expanded along the alveolar margin. Note the small locules anteriorly giving a "honeycomb" appearance (arrowheads), whereas the rest of the lesion consists of large locules with a "soap bubble" appearance.

teeth and the ramus. Early lesions tend to be unilocular with well-corticated rounded margins, and they therefore resemble odontogenic cysts. With growth, several locules may form, each locule maintaining an individual cortical outline. If the locules are small and numerous, a "honeycomb" appearance is evident. Larger and less numerous locules produce a "soap-bubble" appearance. Bone expansion with cortical thinning is typical, and the tumor may perforate the cortex and extend to involve adjacent soft tissues. Associated tooth migration and root resorption are common (Figure 23-22).

Ameloblastoma occurs in young adults, and the average age at diagnosis is approximately 33 years. The stimulus to ameloblastoma formation is unknown. However, up to 20% occur in association with an impacted tooth or a dentigerous cyst. Complete removal of an ameloblastoma is required to attain a cure. Otherwise, the lesion may have a locally invasive behavior pattern. A small fraction of ameloblastomas (<2%) are aggressive enough to develop pulmonary metastases **(Option (E) is false).**

Question 104

Concerning mandibular trauma,

    (A) a panoramic radiograph is an adequate examination
    (B) a widened periodontal ligament space indicates a loosened tooth
    (C) single mandibular fractures are twice as common as multiple fractures
    (D) malocclusion resulting from fracture requires fracture reduction and stabilization
    (E) clinical and radiologic evidence of fracture healing occur simultaneously

The mandible is difficult to image because of its complex U shape. Panoramic radiography is a tomographic technique employing a parabolic plane of focus and a collimated slit beam to image the entire jaw. Under ideal circumstances, the panoramic radiograph shows the jaw from one temporomandibular joint to the other, including the symphysis, with all parts in focus and with no important artifacts. The resultant image provides an excellent global view of the jaw with both osseous and dental anatomy fairly well displayed. Central portions of the maxilla and mandible may be difficult to depict because the plane of focus is narrowest at the apex of the parabolic zone, at times permitting this anatomic region to rest outside the focal plane. In addition, a radiopaque scanning artifact is often present in the symphyseal region. Metal in the mouth may also contribute important artifacts. On occasion, the mandible is too large for the film size and one or both temporomandibular joints are omitted from the image. Finally, fractures of the mandibular body and angle are difficult to detect when there is no fracture fragment displacement perpendicular to the plane of scanning (Figure 23-23). Thus, the panoramic radiograph is an excellent method for evaluating jaw trauma but should not be considered an adequate single examination when fracture is suspected **(Option (A) is false).** It should be part of a mandibular trauma series.

    A standard mandibular trauma series usually consists of frontal, lateral, Towne, and bilateral oblique projections in addition to the panoramic radiograph. Each projection optimizes assessment of a different part of the mandible. The frontal projection gives a global impression of the mandible and the tooth-bearing portions of the maxilla. The condyles are often obscured by the overlying skull. This view is particularly useful for assessing the symphysis and mediolateral fracture displacement. The lateral projection shows the subcondylar, ramus, angle, and body regions. The airway is also assessed on this view. The Towne projection demonstrates the mandibular condyles, subcondylar regions, and coronoid processes. The oblique projections depict the condyle, ramus, angle, and posterior body. On oblique projections, the side closest to the film

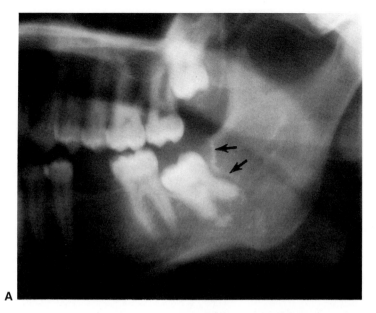

A

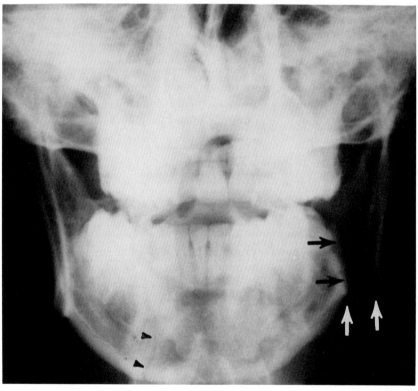

B

Figure 23-23. Mandibular angle fracture. (A) The panoramic radiograph shows a subtle widening of the periodontal ligament space posterior to the second mandibular molar (arrows). No fracture line or fragment displacement is evident. With this panoramic radiograph as the only image, a fracture would not be diagnosed. (B) The frontal radiograph shows a 1-cm displacement at the fracture site in the left mandibular angle (arrows). A hairline fracture is present in the right parasymphyseal region (arrowheads).

609

should be evaluated most carefully, because the opposite side tends to be distorted and partially obscured. If the standard series and panoramic radiograph do not depict the symphysis and incisors adequately, an intraoral dental radiograph may be helpful. For patients with complex mandibular injury, CT with or without multiplanar or three-dimensional reconstruction may be useful in detailed analysis and surgical planning.

Tooth injury is best assessed by a combination of physical examination and radiographs. The panoramic radiograph is a good screening examination of the teeth, but intraoral dental radiographs frequently are needed for better detail. An important radiographic finding is widening of the periodontal ligament space. Since the periodontal ligament attaches the tooth to the alveolar bone, widening of its space indicates damage to the ligament and correlates with loosening of the tooth on physical examination **(Option (B) is true)** (Figure 23-24). The Bennett classification of tooth fractures is as follows:

I.   Traumatized tooth without crown or root fracture
     A. Tooth firm in alveolus
     B. Tooth subluxated in alveolus
II.   Crown fracture
     A. Involving enamel
     B. Involving enamel and dentin
III. Crown fracture with pulpal exposure
IV. Root fracture
     A. Without crown fracture
     B. With crown fracture
V.   Avulsion of tooth

When external forces are applied to it, the mandible fractures at sites of tensile strain (Figure 23-25). The ramus is thick and is protected by the overlying masseter muscle, whereas the coronoid process is protected by the zygomatic arch and muscles of mastication. Neither of these areas is prone to fracture. Inherently weak areas that are prone to fracture include the subcondylar region, angle, and parasymphyseal region. Multiple fractures occur twice as often as single fractures **(Option (C) is false)**. Therefore, a second fracture should be suspected if one fracture of the mandible is found. Single fractures are most common at the mandibular angle.

Of all mandibular fractures, condylar-subcondylar fractures are the most frequent (25 to 40%, depending on the series reported). Fractures of the mandibular angle (11 to 30%), body (16 to 36%), and symphysis (12 to 24%) are also common. Coronoid process and ramus fractures are rare, each representing 1 to 2% of mandibular fractures. Isolated alveolar pro-

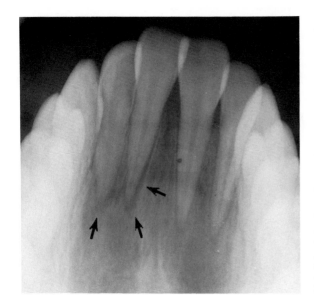

Figure 23-24. Loosened teeth. This intraoral occlusal view of the central maxillary teeth demonstrates widening of the periodontal ligament space of the right maxillary central and lateral incisors (arrows). Compare this with the normal periodontal ligament space on the contralateral side. No associated fracture of the crown or roots is present. These are Bennett class IB injuries.

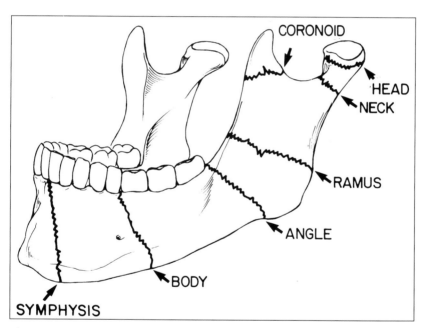

Figure 23-25. Mandibular fractures. Fractures of the condyle (head or neck), angle, body, and symphysis are frequently encountered, either alone or in combination. The coronoid process and ramus are protected by overlying structures and are not often fractured. (Reprinted with permission from Murphy WA. The temporomandibular joint. In: Resnick D, Niwayama G (eds), Diagnosis of bone and joint disorders, 2nd ed. Philadelphia: WB Saunders; 1988:1816–1863.)

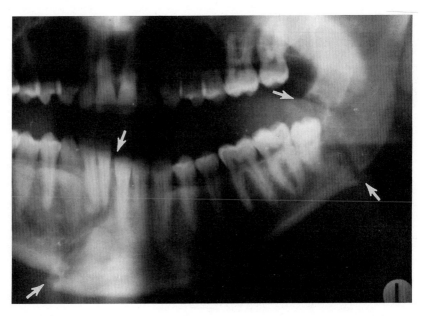

Figure 23-26. Mandibular angle and parasymphyseal fractures. Fractures of the left angle and right parasymphyseal regions (arrows) result in a free segment, which is displaced inferiorly. Such fractures usually require operative reduction and fixation to correct malocclusion. Since the fracture lines pass through periodontal ligament spaces, the fractures are potentially contaminated with oral bacteria and are considered open.

cess fractures (3 to 4%) are also uncommon and usually require intraoral radiographs for diagnosis.

Mandibular angle fractures occur most often along the posterior aspect at the last molar and extend downward and posteriorly to the anatomic angle of the mandible. Angle fractures are the result of a blow to the chin from the contralateral side or a blow to the ipsilateral mandibular body. A second fracture is often present, particularly in the contralateral mandibular body, parasymphyseal region, or subcondylar region (Figure 23-26).

Condylar neck or subcondylar fractures are the result of a direct blow and may occur in isolation or in combination with fractures in the anterior portion of the mandible (Figure 23-27). The subsequent relationships of the condylar head to the temporomandibular joint and to the remainder of the mandible is important in determining treatment. Condylar head fractures that occur within the capsule at the temporomandibular joint usually result from a blow to the chin. Deformity of the condylar head is frequently complicated by internal derangement, osteoarthritis, or even ankylosis of the joint.

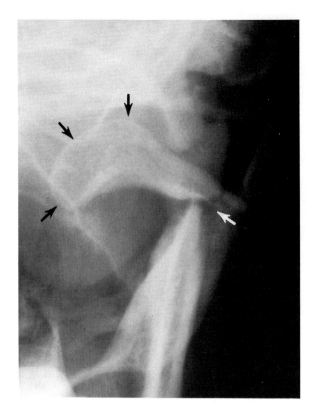

Figure 23-27. Isolated fracture of the condyle. The condylar head (black arrows) is angulated medially and dislocated from the mandibular fossa of the temporal bone. The white arrow indicates the site of fracture.

Mandibular body fractures more commonly result from motor vehicle accidents than from falls or altercations. They are often associated with a second fracture. Fractures of the mandibular symphysis usually run an oblique course and may be difficult to detect on panoramic radiographs as a result of midline unsharpness or artifacts. On occasion, an intraoral radiograph is the only view that demonstrates a nondisplaced fracture in this area.

Fractures that pass through the alveolar ridge involve the periodontal ligament space and allow contamination of the fracture by the oral flora. These fractures are considered open or compound and require antibiotic therapy in all cases.

The neurovascular bundle within the mandibular canal may be injured by a mandibular fracture. Less frequently, the facial or lingual nerves may be damaged by sharp fracture fragments.

Airway obstruction may occur when the support for the tongue and other soft tissues provided by the mandibular symphysis is lost, thereby permitting the musculature of the floor of the mouth to fall back into the

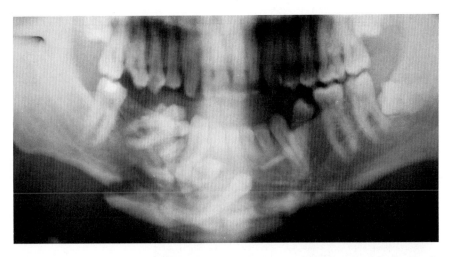

Figure 23-28. Flail mandible. The symphysis and both mandibular bodies are crushed in this victim of a high-speed motor vehicle accident. Such fractures allow the suprahyoid muscles to pull posteriorly, which may result in airway compromise as the floor-of-the-mouth musculature fills the oropharynx.

airway. This occasionally occurs with bilateral mandibular body fractures in edentulous patients. Patients with bilateral subcondylar, ramus, or body fractures in conjunction with a complete or comminuted symphysis fracture are considered to have a flail mandible and may develop airway compromise (Figure 23-28).

Malocclusion is a clinical finding that results from displacement of a tooth-bearing segment of the jaw. Such fractures require operative reduction and fixation to restore normal jaw mechanics and mastication **(Option (D) is true).** Segmental displacement identified on radiographs indicates malocclusion and usually requires open reduction and stabilization.

Compared with fractures of long bones, fractures of the mandible and facial bones usually show less callus formation during normal bone healing. Typically, fracture lines are visible for months to years after there is clinical evidence of solid union **(Option (E) is false).** Radiographic features of fracture union eventually become evident. In the meantime, clinical decisions rely heavily on knowledge of the biology of fracture healing and assessment of physical findings.

Question 105

Concerning periodontal disease,

    (A) it is the principal cause of tooth loss prior to age 30
    (B) it is typically painful
    (C) it is caused by loosening of the teeth
    (D) dentists rely on oral radiographs for early diagnosis
    (E) resorption of the alveolar crest is a typical radiologic feature
    (F) control of bacterial plaque is the most important preventive measure

Periodontal disease is an increasingly important cause of tooth loss, but dental caries remain the most common cause of tooth loss in children and young adults **(Option (A) is false)**. Periodontal disease is the most common cause of tooth loss in adults over the age of 40. In large population studies, some degree of periodontal disease is present in about 80% of adult men and over 70% of adult women.

Periodontal disease represents a spectrum of inflammatory conditions of the gingiva and underlying alveolar bone. Early disease is termed gingivitis and is characterized by redness and swelling of the gums. There is some migration of the gingival margin toward the tooth apex. The gums bleed easily when the teeth are brushed or when they are probed with a dental instrument. When inflammation extends into and destroys the periodontal ligament and alveolar bone, the condition is termed periodontitis. When sufficient bone and ligament are destroyed, the periodontal attachment of the tooth is lost and the tooth becomes loosened and is finally shed. The clinical hallmark of periodontitis is a deep periodontal pocket, which forms as the gingival epithelium migrates toward the apex of the tooth, filling in the space caused by bone destruction. Even with severe bone loss, periodontal disease is usually not painful **(Option (B) is false)**. Periodontal disease is a progressive condition characterized by episodes of worsening followed by periods of remission.

Periodontal disease is caused by the accumulation of bacterial plaque on the surface of the tooth under the gingiva. There is a change in the oral flora in the gingival recess, from primarily facultative gram-positive organisms to anaerobic microaerophilic gram-negative organisms. Bacterial toxins in the periodontal pocket mediate tissue destruction. In addition, as with other chronic inflammatory diseases, some of the tissue destruction is immunologically mediated as part of the host response. Tooth loosening is a late consequence of the underlying alveolar inflammatory condition of the gingiva and alveolar bone and is not a cause of periodontal disease **(Option (C) is false)**.

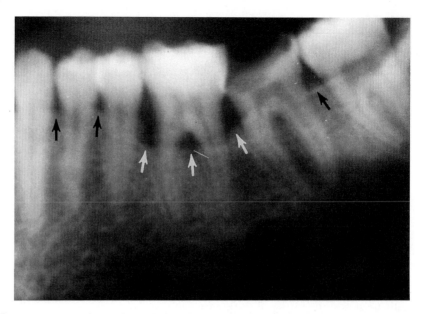

Figure 23-29. Periodontal disease with horizontal bone loss. The alveolar ridge around the first mandibular molar is resorbed (white arrows). The normal relationship between the cemento-enamel junction and the alveolar crest is seen between the other teeth (black arrows). Note the normal width of the periodontal ligament space around the roots of all teeth, including the diseased ones. The second molar has extensive caries of its crown.

Gingivitis can be detected only by oral physical examination; there are no radiographic findings **(Option (D) is false).** Thus, radiographs do not have a role in the early diagnosis of periodontal disease. The earliest detectable radiographic finding is the loss of height of the alveolar crest **(Option (E) is true).** Normally, the alveolar crest extends to within 1 or 2 mm of the line formed by connecting the cemento-enamel junctions of adjacent teeth. In patients with periodontal disease, the dense horizontal cortical plate of alveolar bone is destroyed but the vertically oriented lamina dura adjacent to the tooth root initially remains intact. This first stage of bone destruction is termed horizontal bone loss (Figure 23-29). As the disease progresses, vertical bone loss develops and the alveolar crest becomes V-shaped (Figure 23-30). As vertical bone loss progresses with widening of the periodontal space beyond its normal 0.3 to 0.4 mm, the tooth is shed. In advanced disease, the bone loss may extend beyond the tooth apex, causing a periapical lucency very similar to the periapical abscess seen with tooth pulp infection (Figure 23-31).

The first line of defense against periodontal disease is prevention of bacterial plaque accumulation by daily tooth brushing and dental floss-

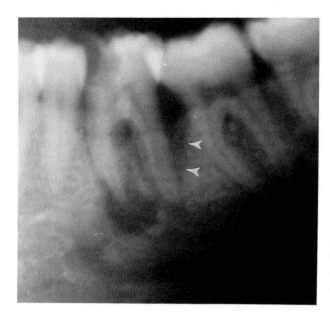

Figure 23-30. Periodontal disease with vertical bone loss. The carious first mandibular molar has a widened periodontal ligament space along its posterior roots (arrowheads). The process extends beyond the apex of these roots. Also note the periapical lucency adjacent to the anterior roots. The hypereruption of this molar is evidence of loosening.

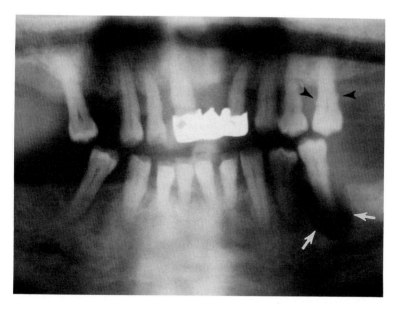

Figure 23-31. Advanced periodontal disease. The maxillary and mandibular alveolar ridges are markedly resorbed. The left second mandibular premolar (arrows) could be shed at any moment. Note the calculus deposited near the cemento-enamel junction of the left second maxillary premolar (arrowheads).

ing. This personal oral hygiene should be combined with periodic removal of accumulated plaque, particularly in the subgingival region, by scaling and tooth polishing performed by a dentist or dental hygienist **(Option (F) is true).** Once periodontal disease is present, treatment depends on the severity of the disease. The single most important factor is mechanical removal of bacteria. Scaling alone is sufficient in cases of gingivitis and mild periodontitis. Root planing is used to remove infected cementum in more severe cases. Periodontal surgery involves incising the gingiva near its attachment to the crown of the tooth to expose the tooth roots and alveolar bone. This allows scaling and planing of the root and allows bone reshaping and bone grafting. Healing of the incision reduces the depth of the periodontal pocket. Antibiotics also play a role in the eradication of pathogenic bacteria. These techniques usually halt the progression of the disease.

O. Clark West, M.D.
William A. Murphy, Jr., M.D.

SUGGESTED READINGS

GENERAL

1. Gibilisco JA. Stafne's oral radiographic diagnosis, 5th ed. Philadelphia: WB Saunders; 1985
2. Hallikainen D, Paukku P. Panoramic zonography. In: Delbalso AM (ed), Maxillofacial imaging. Philadelphia: WB Saunders; 1990:1–33
3. Halstead CL, Hoard BC. Dental radiology and oral pathology. Curr Probl Diagn Radiol 1991; 20:187–235
4. Langlais RP. Radiology of the jaws. In: Delbalso AM (ed), Maxillofacial imaging. Philadelphia: WB Saunders; 1990:313–373
5. Osborn AG, Hanafee WH, Mancuso AA. Normal and pathologic CT anatomy of the mandible. AJR 1982; 139:555–559
6. Seldin EB. Radiology of the mandible. In: Taveras JM, Ferrucci JT (eds), Radiology. Diagnosis—imaging—intervention. Philadelphia: JB Lippincott; 1991; 3; 14:1–21
7. Shafer WG, Hine MK, Levy BM, Tomich CE. A textbook of oral pathology, 4th ed. Philadelphia: WB Saunders; 1983

OSSEOUS LESIONS

8. Clark JL, Unni KK, Dahlin DC, Devine KD. Osteosarcoma of the jaw. Cancer 1983; 51:2311–2316
9. Garrington GE, Scofield HH, Cornyn J, Hooker SP. Osteosarcoma of the jaws. Analysis of 56 cases. Cancer 1967; 20:377–391
10. Hartman KS. Histiocytosis X: a review of 114 cases with oral involvement. Oral Surg Oral Med Oral Pathol 1980; 49:38–54
11. Horner K. Central giant cell granuloma of the jaws: a clinico-radiological study. Clin Radiol 1989; 40:622–626

12. Obisesan AA, Lagundoye SB, Daramola JO, Ajagbe HA, Oluwasanmi JO. The radiologic features of fibrous dysplasia of the craniofacial bones. Oral Surg Oral Med Oral Pathol 1977; 44:949–959

13. Ratner V, Dorfman HD. Giant-cell reparative granuloma of the hand and foot bones. Clin Orthop 1990; 260:251–258

14. Stull MA, Kransdorf MJ, Devaney KO. Langerhans cell histiocytosis of bone. RadioGraphics 1992; 12:801–823

OSTEOSCLEROTIC ODONTOGENIC LESIONS

15. Budnick SD. Compound and complex odontomas. Oral Surg 1976; 42:501–506

16. Cherrick HM, King OH Jr, Lucatorto FM, Suggs DM. Benign cementoblastoma: a clinicopathologic evaluation. Oral Surg 1974; 37:54–63

17. Eversole LR, Merrell PW, Strub D. Radiographic characteristics of central ossifying fibroma. Oral Surg Oral Med Oral Pathol 1985; 59:522–527

18. Hamner JE III, Scofield HH, Cornyn J. Benign fibro-osseous jaw lesions of periodontal membrane origin. An analysis of 249 cases. Cancer 1968; 22:861–878

19. Zegarelli EV, Kutscher AH, Budowsky J, Hoffman PJ. The progressive calcification of the cementoma: a roentgenographic study. Oral Surg 1964; 18:180–183

OSTEOLYTIC ODONTOGENIC LESIONS

20. Eversole LR, Leider AS, Strub D. Radiographic characteristics of cystogenic ameloblastoma. Oral Surg Oral Med Oral Pathol 1984; 57:572–577

21. Hertzanu Y, Mendelsohn DB, Cohen M. Computed tomography of mandibular ameloblastoma. J Comput Assist Tomogr 1984; 8:220–223

22. Hodgkinson DJ, Woods JE, Dahlin DC, Tolman DE. Keratocysts of the jaw. Clincopathologic study of 79 patients. Cancer 1978; 41:803–813

23. Shear M. Cysts of the oral regions. Bristol: John Wright & Sons; 1976

24. Stockdale CR, Chandler NP. The nature of the periapical lesion—a review of 1108 cases. J Dent 1988; 16:123–129

25. Ueda M, Kaneda T, Imaizumi M, Abe T. Mandibular ameloblastoma with metastasis to the lungs and lymph nodes: a case report and review of the literature. J Oral Maxillofac Surg 1989; 47:623–628

FRACTURES

26. Delbalso AM, Hall RE, Margarone JE. Radiographic evaluation of maxillofacial trauma. In: Delbalso AM (ed), Maxillofacial imaging. Philadelphia: WB Saunders; 1990:35–128

27. Ellis E III, Moos KF, el-Attar A. Ten years of mandibular fractures: an analysis of 2,137 cases. Oral Surg Oral Med Oral Pathol 1985; 59:120–129

28. Haug RH, Prather J, Indresano AT. An epidemiologic survey of facial fractures and concomitant injuries. J Oral Maxillofac Surg 1990; 48:926–932

29. Olson RA, Fonseca RJ, Zeitler DL, Osbon DB. Fractures of the mandible: a review of 580 cases. J Oral Maxillofac Surg 1982; 40:23–28

PERIODONTAL DISEASE

30. Williams RC. Periodontal disease. N Engl J Med 1990; 322:373–382

Notes

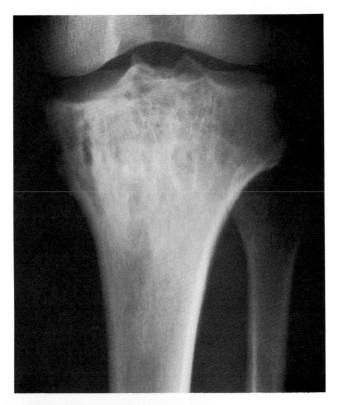

Figure 24-1

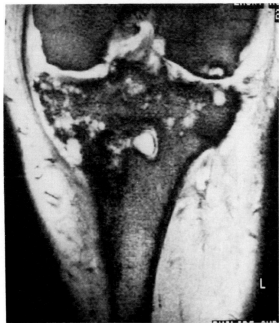

GRE 509/20/40°

Figure 24-2

Figures 24-1 and 24-2. This 33-year-old man has had pain and swelling of the knee for approximately 1 year. You are shown an anteroposterior radiograph obtained at initial evaluation (Figure 24-1) and a T2-weighted gradient-echo MR image obtained 9 months later (Figure 24-2).

Case 24: Fungal Infection

Question 106

Which *one* of the following is the MOST likely diagnosis?

(A) Fungal infection
(B) Bone infarction
(C) Langerhans cell histiocytosis
(D) Pigmented villonodular synovitis
(E) Subchondral cysts

The anteroposterior radiograph and coronal MR image of the knee (Figures 24-1 and 24-2) show numerous fluid-filled lytic areas of different sizes within the cancellous bone of the proximal tibia. These cavities are surrounded by thick, poorly defined zones of reactive bone sclerosis and by a more generalized sclerosis of the adjacent cancellous bone. There is also erosion of the subarticular cortex of the medial and lateral tibial plateaus and the lateral femoral condyle, as well as narrowing of both joint compartments (Figure 24-3). The presence of such multiple, interconnecting lytic areas accompanied by marginal and diffuse sclerosis strongly suggests osteomyelitis. The lytic pattern reflects multiple intraosseous abscesses and interconnecting sinus tracts. The osteomyelitis has invaded the adjacent joint, eroded the subarticular cortical and cancellous bone, and partially destroyed the articular cartilage. This radiographic appearance could be produced by a slowly progressive pyogenic infection, but this option was not offered. Therefore, fungal infection is the most likely diagnosis **(Option (A) is correct).**

The test patient sustained a deep laceration over the left knee when he fell against a pipe in a shallow canal of water in Thailand. Five years later he noticed swelling of the left knee followed by severe pain. The initial radiograph (Figure 24-1) was obtained at that time. Aspirated joint fluid revealed no infection, and arthroscopy with biopsy of bone and synovial tissue was not definitive, but the diagnosis of chronic osteomyelitis was considered. The patient continued to have pain until reevaluation 9 months later, when the MR image (Figure 24-2) was obtained, showing

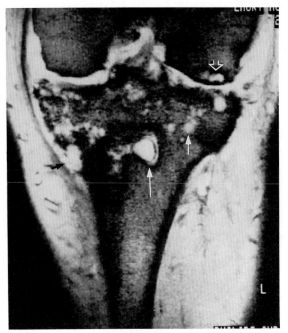

GRE 509/20/40°

Figure 24-3 (Same as Figure 24-2). Fungal osteomyelitis. A coronal T2-weighted gradient-echo MR image shows joint space narrowing, multiple fluid-filled cavities in the tibia (solid white arrows), destruction of the medial tibial cortex (black arrow), destruction of subarticular bone along both tibial plateaus, and involvement of the lateral femoral condyle (open white arrow).

progression of disease with destruction of subarticular bone and joint space. A radiograph taken at the same time also showed progressive destruction (Figure 24-4A).

At the time of reevaluation, culture of biopsy tissue obtained from the proximal tibia and the synovium grew *Pseudoallescheria boydii*. This soil fungus is not one of the more common fungal pathogens in general, but it is the most common cause of fungal mycetoma in the United States.

CT and MR images are helpful in diagnosing fungal osteomyelitis because they show the multiplicity and various sizes of abscess cavities and sinus tracts more clearly than radiographs do. CT (Figure 24-4B) and MR (Figure 24-2) images of the test patient showed the multiple abscess cavities and sinus tracts, sclerotic margins, sequestra, diffuse cancellous sclerosis, cortical destruction, narrowing of the joint spaces, and invasion of the femoral condyle. Sectional imaging studies are also useful to the surgeon in planning local debridement of the infected tissues, in conjunction with systemic antifungal drug treatment. The test patient underwent above-knee amputation because of the advanced bone, joint, and soft tissue involvement.

Bone infarcts (medullary osteonecrosis) (Option (B)) appear as elongated, metadiaphyseal sclerotic areas with irregular, serpentine mar-

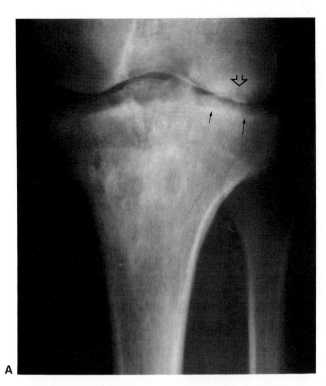

A

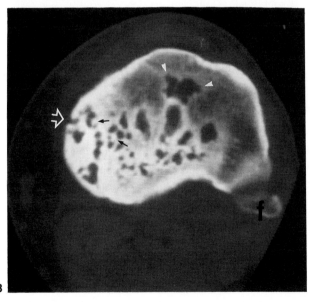

B

Figure 24-4. Same patient as in Figures 24-1 through 24-3. Fungal osteomyelitis. (A) A radiograph obtained at 9-month follow-up (at same time as Figure 24-2) shows progressive erosion of the subarticular cortex of both tibial plateaus but especially in the lateral compartment (solid arrows). The infection has narrowed the lateral joint space and crossed the joint to invade the lateral femoral condyle, where it has eroded subarticular bone and produced a subarticular lucency with surrounding sclerosis (open arrow). (B) A CT image through the proximal tibia obtained at 9-month follow-up clearly shows the multiple abscess cavities, sinus tracts, and surrounding sclerotic reaction within cancellous bone. The largest lytic area demonstrates the typical shape of a bone abscess, with a lobulated outline and fingerlike extensions into the surrounding bone (arrowheads). There are several sequestra (black arrows). Medially, the infection has eroded through the cortex (open arrow). The proximal tip of the fibula is visible laterally (f).

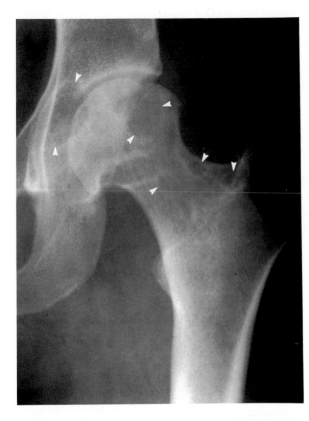

Figure 24-5. Pigmented villonodular synovitis in the hip. An anteroposterior radiograph shows multiple, well-marginated erosions of the femoral head and neck and the acetabulum (arrowheads) in a 22-year-old woman. There is also early degenerative disease indicated by slight narrowing of the articular cartilage, minimal subarticular sclerosis, and small marginal osteophytes around the the femoral head.

gins. They may contain irregular lucent areas, but they do not appear as multiple, small lytic areas and sinus tracts. Moreover, uncomplicated infarcts do not destroy the cortex, as occurred in the test patient.

Langerhans cell histiocytosis (LCH) (Option (C)) does destroy bone, but it typically produces a fairly large oval or rounded lytic lesion, not a series of tiny ones. It rarely, if ever, affects subarticular bone. LCH can cause periosteal reaction, but it does not typically produce diffuse cancellous sclerosis.

Pigmented villonodular synovitis (Option (D)) can cause juxta-articular bony erosions. Such osseous invasion occurs early in its course in small, tight joints such as the hip or ankle (Figure 24-5), whereas in the knee it usually causes marked intra-articular swelling but erodes bone only in its very advanced stages (Figure 24-6). Furthermore, the erosions of pigmented villonodular synovitis tend to be larger, located along the joint margins at capsular insertions, and associated with a soft tissue mass.

Subchondral cysts (Option (E)) can be multiple, but they are usually centered along the subarticular cortex, are larger than the lytic lesions

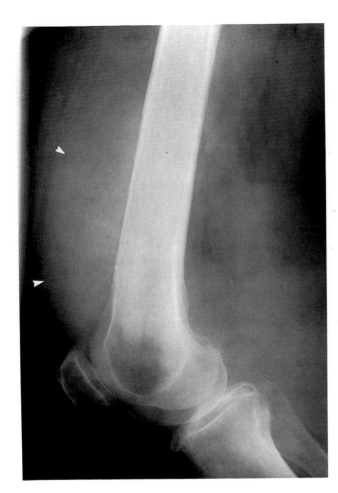

Figure 24-6. Pigmented villonodular synovitis in the knee of an 89-year-old woman. In spite of a 10-year history of increasing pain and swelling, the lateral radiograph shows only massive swelling within the knee (arrowheads) but no bony erosions or joint destruction.

seen in the test patient, and do not penetrate as deeply into bone as does the process in the test patient (Figure 24-7). They also do not cause the bone destruction manifested in the test images.

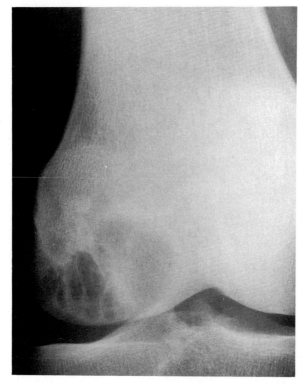

Figure 24-7. Subchondral cyst, or intraosseous ganglion. An anteroposterior radiograph shows a large, multiloculated-appearing radiolucency in the subarticular region of the lateral femoral condyle of a 19-year-old man. It was treated by curretage, and the pathologic diagnosis was "intra-osseous ganglion." However, other pathologists might have used the term "subchondral cyst."

Question 107

Concerning fungal osteomyelitis,

(A) sporotrichosis of bone occurs primarily in immunocompromised patients
(B) the incidence in the United States is decreasing
(C) mycetoma most commonly affects the jaws
(D) most opportunistic fungal infections are acquired from the hospital environment
(E) coccidioidal osteomyelitis usually follows a primary pulmonary infection

Fungi that cause infection in humans can be divided into two broad categories: true (or primary) pathogens, which affect normal individuals, and opportunistic pathogens, which affect immunocompromised individuals. Sporotrichosis is caused by a true pathogenic fungus, *Sporothrix schenckii*, not an opportunistic one **(Option (A) is false).**

Accurate figures are not available, but there is no reason to believe that the incidence of fungal bone infections (already rare) is decreasing in the United States. First, pulmonary and other infections due to the primary pathogenic fungi, such as *Histoplasma*, *Blastomyces*, and *Coccidioides* species, remain prevalent in the areas where they are endemic. In contrast to viral and bacterial infections, fungal diseases have not been substantially reduced by public sanitation measures and immunizations are not available. Furthermore, opportunistic fungal infections in general have increased in frequency because of the wider use of immunosuppressive drugs in conjunction with organ transplantation and the treatment of malignancies. Also, deep-seated mycotic infections have become more common in recent years as a result of the increased use of broad-spectrum antibiotics, more invasive surgical procedures, the widespread use of indwelling catheters, and the substantial increase in the number of immunocompromised patients. Nosocomial fungal infections (usually due to *Candida* species) are now fairly frequent, usually in the urinary tract or the blood. Because of the general increase in the incidence of serious, deep-seated fungal infections, at least some of which will spread to the bones, it is reasonable to conclude that there will also be an increase in the incidence of fungal osteomyelitis **(Option (B) is false).**

Although actinomycotic infections most commonly affect the jaws, this form of infection is not called "mycetoma." The term mycetoma refers to a chronic granulomatous infection caused by a puncture wound, in which there is localized subcutaneous swelling with sinus draining to the skin surface. The diagnostic triad consists of (1) tumefaction, (2) draining sinuses, and (3) the presence of "grains" (or "granules") within the granulomatous abscesses and in the draining exudate. It can be caused by either true fungi or by *Actinomycetes* species. Mycetoma syndrome affects the foot 70% of the time **(Option (C) is false).** Mycetoma begins in the subcutaneous tissue and may extend to involve deep soft tissues and even bone. Craniofacial actinomycotic infections, on the other hand, begin deep in the jaws and form sinus tracts, which burrow outward to drain through the skin.

Opportunistic fungal infections can be caused by two categories of fungi: those that normally live on the human body (commensal, or endogenous) and those that are present in the surrounding environment (exogenous). Accurate statistics regarding the relative incidence of various opportunistic fungi that cause osteomyelitis are not readily available. However, probably the most common organisms that cause opportunistic fungal infections are the *Candida* species, which are normally present on the human body **(Option (D) is false).**

The true (primary) pathogenic fungi usually enter the human body by inhalation. This may cause no clinical infection at all, or a primary pulmonary infection may be established. Occasionally, the fungus disseminates via the bloodstream to infect various organs, including bone. *Coccidioides immitis* is one of the true fungal pathogens that behave in this way **(Option (E) is true).**

Fungi. The fungi make up their own kingdom, separate from animals, plants, and other organisms. Fungi grow on organic material in water or soil. They are ubiquitous and very hardy, thriving in a wide range of environments throughout the world. Fungal spores form a substantial part of the normal suspended particulate matter found in the air. In nature, fungi help recycle organic debris by breaking it down. Fungi also normally inhabit the human body as harmless commensals; these include *Candida* species in the mouth and gastrointestinal tract and *Pityrosporum* species on the skin.

The metabolic pathways and enzyme contents of fungi differ substantially from those of bacteria and other organisms. Unlike bacteria, fungi contain nuclei. Most fungi grow in the form of hyphae, i.e., elongated tubular structures that group together to form a mycelium, which is the fuzzy growth known more commonly as a mold. Other fungi grow in the form of single-cell yeasts. Fungi are often classified as either "perfect" or "imperfect" forms, the perfect forms exhibiting sexual reproduction and the imperfect forms undergoing asexual reproduction. One confusing aspect of fungal classification is that the perfect and imperfect forms of the same organism have different species names.

Fungi can harm humans who ingest food contaminated with mycotoxins or who accidentally ingest toxic mushrooms. Also, many people suffer allergic reactions through skin contact with or inhalation of fungi. Finally, fungi can directly infect the human body. Infections in humans can be divided into four main clinical types: (1) superficial infections affecting the keratin layer of the skin, such as pityriasis versicolor; (2) cutaneous infections affecting the skin or mucous membranes, including such common diseases as ringworm and candidiasis; (3) subcutaneous infections such as sporotrichosis and mycetoma; and (4) systemic infections. A fifth category includes miscellaneous and rare mycoses. The systemic infections are of greatest relevance to the musculoskeletal radiologist.

Systemic mycoses. The fungi that cause systemic infections can be divided into two broad categories. (1) The true (primary) pathogenic fungi can infect normal humans who are exposed to a sufficient quantity of the fungi by the appropriate route to overcome normal defense mechanisms. These infections most commonly involve the lungs and are caused by organisms such as *Histoplasma, Blastomyces,* and *Coccidioides* species. (2) The opportunistic fungi infect individuals with severe systemic illness or immune deficiency. These fungi are not virulent enough to cause infection in normal individuals; they include *Aspergillus* and *Can-*

dida species. Of course, true pathogenic fungi can also infect immuno-compromised persons. The diagnosis of infections caused by primary pathogens is based on the fairly predictable extraskeletal clinical manifestations characteristic of the fungus. On the other hand, the diagnosis of opportunistic fungal infections depends more on the nature of the underlying disease, the associated clinical presentations, and the sites of fungal infections.

There are more than 100,000 species of fungi, but only about 275 species cause infections in humans. Furthermore, only about 200 species have been implicated in systemic infections. About 20 species of fungi account for most systemic infections, about 20 cause most skin infections, and only about 12 commonly cause subcutaneous infections; however, a very large number of fungi can cause opportunistic infections.

True (primary) pathogenic fungi. These fungi are widely distributed soil saprophytes; they often grow best in bird or bat droppings. They can cause infections (for example, blastomycosis, coccidioidomycosis, cryptococcosis, and histoplasmosis) in normal individuals, usually after being inhaled into the lungs. Although humans have a high natural resistance to fungi, infection occurs if a sufficient number of fungal conidia are inhaled. In 90% of infected patients, there is either an asymptomatic or very mild pulmonary infection, but the fungi occasionally disseminate throughout the body to infect visceral organs or, infrequently, bones or joints. The initial infection confers specific resistance on the infected person, since fungi contain abundant antigens, which stimulate a strong cellular immunity. Human-to-human transmission of deep fungal infections is unknown or extremely rare. These organisms can, of course, also infect debilitated persons, in which case the clinical course is more severe.

These fungi are generally encountered outdoors; therefore, the infected individuals are often active and healthy persons in the prime of life, engaging in outdoor occupations or recreation. These infections are more common at certain times of the year and vary in incidence with age, sex, and race. They have strong geographic associations. Histoplasmosis in the United States is confined largely to the Mississippi and Ohio River Valleys. Blastomycosis has a less well-defined distribution but generally occurs in the same area. Coccidioidomycosis is typically found in the desert southwest.

Some fungal infections occur by direct inoculation into the tissues rather than by inhalation. For example, sporotrichosis typically results from a puncture wound by a thorn. *Aspergillus* species live in compost and therefore often infect gardeners or farmers through a puncture wound. Various wounds can also directly inoculate *Eumycetes* species into the subcutaneous tissue, and these can then invade deep soft tissues and bone, causing a mycetoma.

Opportunistic pathogenic fungi. These fungi rarely cause infection in normal hosts; instead, they infect patients who are severely ill or immunodeficient. The outcome of the infection depends more on the course of the predisposing, underlying disease than on the specific fungal infection itself. Opportunistic fungi, like the primary pathogens, are commonly exogenous fungi that enter the body by inhalation. Unlike infections by true pathogens, the occurrence of opportunistic fungal infections does not seem to be related to the age, sex, or race of the patient, and they do not confer specific immune resistance following the primary infection.

By far the most common opportunistic pathogenic infections are those due to *Candida* species, normal inhabitants of the human gut and mucous membranes, and *Aspergillus* species, which are ubiquitous in the environment. *Cryptococcus* species can act as either primary or opportunistic pathogens. In recent years, there has been a striking increase in the number of fungal species identified as causes of opportunistic infections. This will most probably continue, and it is possible that all fungi are potentially pathogenic under the right circumstances.

A number of local or systemic anatomic or physiologic abnormalities predispose to opportunistic fungal infection. These include the surgical implantation of prosthetic devices with their accompanying physiologic and immunologic consequences, total parenteral alimentation, and focal structural abnormalities such as the presence of a foreign body or an abnormal cavity. Intravenous drug abuse can lead to fungal infection, such as candidal infection of the spine. Candidiasis has also been known to complicate peritoneal dialysis, prosthetic implants, and vascular grafts. Endocrine diseases can predispose to fungal infections, but this is rare except for candidal urinary tract infections in diabetic patients. Systemic antibiotic administration can also lead to superinfection by fungi, usually when there is also immune deficiency or an anatomic abnormality. Immunodeficiency commonly predisposes to fungal infection. Cell-mediated immunity, primarily through T cells, provides human immune defense against fungal infections. Humeral antibodies play little or no role. The deficiency may be due to a systemic disease that causes diminished immune response or to the administration of steroids or other immunosuppressive drugs, often for the treatment of malignancies.

Musculoskeletal infections. Musculoskeletal fungal infections are rare, but when they occur they tend to be chronic, indolent, and quite destructive and can cause a great deal of disability. They may occur secondary to a disseminated fungal infection or to superinfection in an immunocompromised host, following trauma or surgery, or by deep extension from a primary skin infection.

Although this discussion focuses on fungal osteomyelitis, fungal arthritis is at least as common as fungal osteomyelitis. Fungal arthritis causes a chronic erosive synovitis that commonly affects weight-bearing joints, especially the knee, which accounts for 70% of infections. Culture of synovial fluid is often negative, and the fluid should be examined directly with appropriate stains. *Candida* species are a frequent cause, and *Blastomyces dermatiditis* is an uncommon cause. Joint infections due to *Coccidioides* species are less common than osteomyelitis, but hematogenous arthritis can occur and sometimes a primary bone infection can spread into the adjacent joint.

Actinomycetes ("false fungi"). *Actinomyces* and *Nocardia* species cause chronic granulomatous infections, which are clinically and pathologically similar to fungal infections. These are bacteria of the order *Actinomycetales*, and they have characteristics of both fungi and bacteria.

Actinomyces species are anaerobic gram-positive bacilli found in the soil, like pathogenic fungi. Also like some fungi, they are normal commensal inhabitants of the human body, residing in and around the teeth and tonsilar crypts, gastrointestinal tract, and pelvic organs. Aspiration of organisms can cause lung infection, but active infection is more commonly triggered by dental disease or tooth extraction. The organism then invades the mucosal surface of the mouth and extends into the deeper structures, especially the mandible and sometimes the maxilla. This is the craniofacial form of infection, which is the most common clinical presentation and accounts for more than half of all actinomycotic infections. The infection leads to chronic suppurative granulomas and fibrosis in the deep soft tissues and to the formation of sinus tracts, which drain to the skin surface. Fistulae can drain to the skin surface or dissect through the soft tissues to invade the chest cavity or even extend below the diaphragm to the abdomen, where ileocecal infection is probably the most common manifestation. Fistulae can also lead to invasion of the skull, vertebrae, or ribs. Actinomycosis can also cause mycetoma as a result of direct inoculation through laceration or a puncture wound.

The diagnosis can be made by culture. Although *Actinomyces* is a bacterium, it grows in the form of hyphae, like fungi, producing a mycelial appearance on the culture plate. Typically, small, soft, yellow, rounded "sulfur granules" are found within the sinus tract drainage. These are like the "grains" associated with fungal mycetoma.

Nocardia species are gram-positive, partly acid-fast anaerobic bacteria that usually infect the lungs after being inhaled. They often act as opportunists, affecting immunosuppressed patients more seriously. From the lungs, the infection can spread hematogenously to the brain, meninges, peritoneum, subcutaneous tissue, or other deep structures. *Nocardia* can also cause mycetoma by direct puncture or open wound. Like infections by true fungi and by *Actinomyces* species, the infection pro-

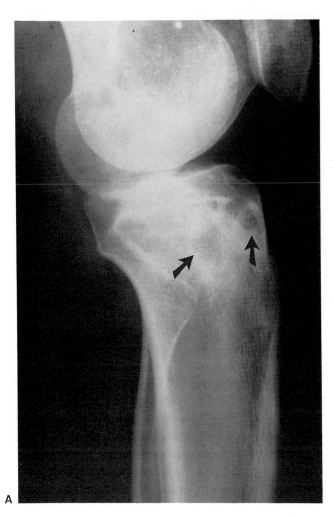

Figure 24-8. Multifocal blastomycotic osteomyelitis. Lateral radiographs of the knee (A) and hind foot (B) show several lytic areas (arrows) surrounded by marginal and diffuse sclerotic bone reaction. There is no evidence of joint involvement.

A

duces suppurative, granulomatous abscesses surrounded by fibrosis and granulation tissue.

Radiologic findings. The radiologic appearance of fungal and actinomycotic osteomyelitis is generally nonspecific, and the diagnosis can rarely be made by radiographic criteria. Although actinomycoses are caused by filamentous bacteria rather than by true fungi, they are usually discussed with fungal infections because they have many clinical and radiologic similarities. In general, however, both these types of infection present a less aggressive appearance and elicit less bony reaction than pyogenic infections do. Their appearance suggests a more indolent, slowly progressive, and less reactive process, much like tuberculosis or LCH. Thus, fungal or actinomycotic infections of bone do not usually

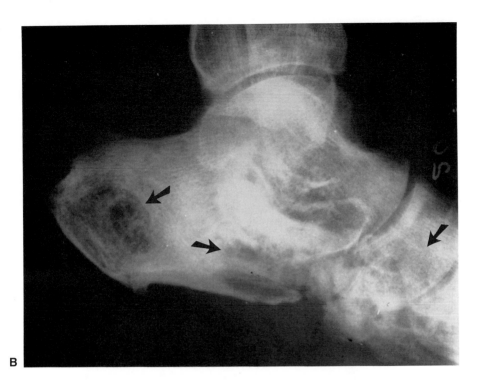

B

cause bone destruction with a moth-eaten or permeated border, nor are they usually associated with mottled cancellous sclerosis or with prominent or extensive sequestrum formation (Figure 24-8). Likewise, they do not tend to stimulate an extensive periosteal reaction, and the periosteal reaction tends to be thick and solid, not thin or lamellated (Figure 24-9). Fungal and actinomycotic osteomyelitis appear as a focal lytic area centered in cancellous bone, usually with geographic margins and a variable amount of marginal sclerotic reaction and sometimes with complete cortical destruction. The appearance may suggest an aggressive tumor, a benign tumor, or a Brodie's abscess. More chronic lesions often produce cortical thickening and "widening" of the bone. However, even chronic fungal infections usually produce less bony sclerosis and cortical thickening than is expected with chronic pyogenic osteomyelitis. The presence of multiple small abscesses and sinus tracts with well-defined sclerotic margins suggests actinomycotic or fungal osteomyelitis. Pyogenic infections typically cause single large abscess cavities, which are often lobulated in outline; multiple sinus tracts can occur, but these are generally not nearly as numerous as those seen in patients with fungal and actinomycotic infections. Fungal and actinomycotic infections of the spine resemble pyogenic, tuberculous, or brucellar infections (Figure 24-10).

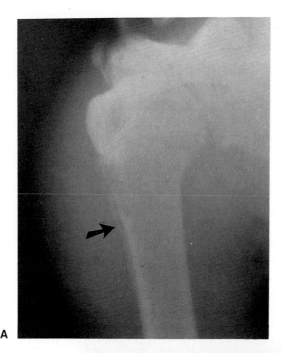

Figure 24-9. Aspergillus osteomyelitis. (A) A shoulder radiograph with the humerus in external rotation shows an ill-defined lytic area within the proximal metaphysis and a single layer of periosteal reaction along the lateral cortex (arrow). (B) A transaxial T2-weighted MR image shows cortical destruction, periosteal reaction (arrowhead), bright T2 signal within the marrow cavity as a result of inflammation and edema (black arrow), and a large area of soft tissue inflammation surrounding the humerus (white arrows).

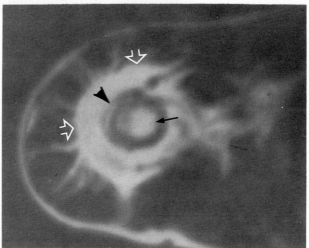

SE 3,000/120

Clinical information may suggest the possibility of fungal or actinomycotic infection. Predisposing factors include serious systemic illness and treatment with steroids or other immunosuppressive drugs. The presence of multiple small sinus tracts draining to the surface of the skin also suggests this type of infection, since pyogenic infections usually produce one or only a few such sinus tracts. There are also some specific fea-

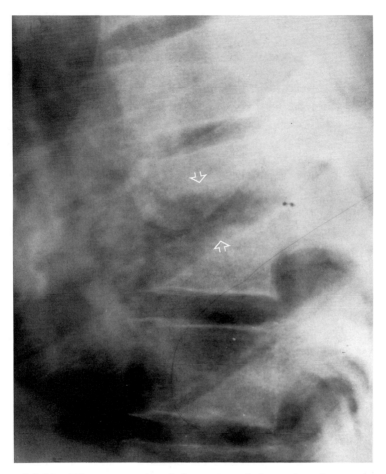

Figure 24-10. Blastomycosis of the spine. A lateral radiograph of the thoracic spine shows destruction of end plates and portions of the vertebral bodies adjacent to a disk space (arrows). The appearance is typical of a disk space infection with vertebral osteomyelitis. However, this infection could be pyogenic or tuberculous rather than fungal.

tures that may be diagnostically helpful. Actinomycotic infections affect the craniofacial region 50% of the time and also commonly affect ribs; therefore, lytic lesions in the jaw, calvarium, facial bones, or ribs suggest this diagnosis. Coccidioidomycosis seems to have a predilection for bony prominences or sites of tendon or ligament attachment, such as the olecranon process, malleoli of the ankle, calcaneus, or tibial tuberosity. Some authors have suggested that cryptococcosis also exhibits such a predilection for bony prominences, but this is not as well documented. When blastomycosis affects the spine, it often erodes the vertebral bodies, causing anterior concavity; it can also spread up and down the spine via a subligamentous route and thus can produce skip lesions at several levels. Sporotrichosis rarely produces bone lesions, but a puncture wound in the hand or foot (especially by a thorn in a gardener) can lead to a chronic infection of the skin and subcutaneous tissues that can eventually spread to the underlying bone.

Radiographically, actinomycotic infection of bones such as the mandible causes cortical erosion or areas of lytic destruction. In the early stages, there is little bone reaction, especially in the jaw. Later, there is more sclerosis as a result of periosteal and endosteal reactive bone formation. When the spine is infected, the appearance is much like that of tuberculosis. There is erosion of the vertebral body and sometimes a "soap bubble" appearance. There may be a paravertebral abscess, and the infection occasionally spreads to the posterior elements and adjacent ribs. Reactive bone formation in the spine sometimes causes large, coarse syndesmophytes. Early in infection the disk is usually spared, but later it may be moderately narrowed.

Of course, there is a higher index of suspicion for fungal diseases in areas where these infections are strongly endemic. However, even in areas where pulmonary infections are likely, such as histoplasmosis in the Mississippi and Ohio River Valleys and coccidioidomycosis in the southwestern deserts and San Joaquin Valley, bone infections secondary to these organisms are still so uncommon that a fungal etiology may not be immediately considered when a patient presents with a bone lesion.

Mycetoma. This clinical syndrome is caused by a puncture wound that introduces the organism, leading to formation of a hard, painless, subcutaneous nodule or plaque, which is followed by swelling and, rarely, pain. After months (for *Actinomyces* infection) or years (for fungal infection), multiple sinuses emerge through the skin, draining pus and blood (Figure 24-11). Some sinuses heal, and new ones appear. The process then slowly extends more deeply to involve the deep soft tissues and bone. The diagnostic triad consists of (1) tumefaction, (2) draining sinuses, and (3) the presence of "grains" (or "granules") within the granulomatous abscesses and in the draining exudate. These grains are aggregates of the causative organisms. Mycetoma can be caused by either true fungi, in which case it may be called eumycetoma, or bacteria of the actinomycetes group ("false fungi"), in which case it is sometimes called actinomycetoma. Mycetoma affects the foot 70% of the time, the hand 12% of the time, and occasionally the knee, leg, trunk, buttock, or scalp. When the disease is due to fungal infection, the causative organisms are soil saprophytes such as *P. boydii* and *Madurella* species. The infection shown in the test patient was not a typical mycetoma, because it did not follow the clinical course for that diagnosis and did not manifest multiple draining sinuses to the skin surface.

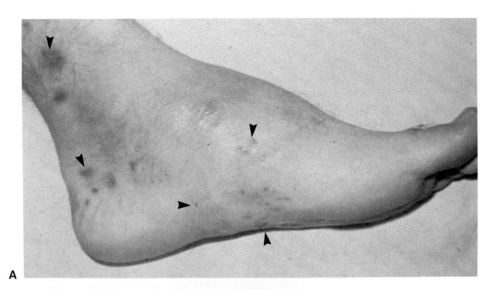

A

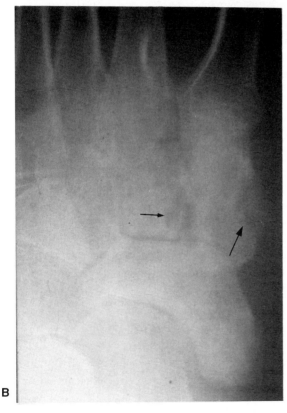

B

Figure 24-11. Mycetoma of the foot caused by *Pseudallescheria boydii.* Gradual swelling of the foot followed a puncture wound in a pig pen, and chronic purulent drainage began 2 years later. (A) A photograph of the foot shows multiple draining sinus tracts (arrowheads). (B) An anteroposterior radiograph shows multiple lytic lesions due to abscesses in the tarsal bones (arrows), with adjacent bone sclerosis. (Panels A, C, D, and F are reprinted with permission from Hudson TM. Radiologic-pathologic correlation of musculoskeletal lesions. Baltimore: Williams & Wilkins; 1987.)

Mycetoma is endemic in tropical and subtropical zones, especially in the Sahara region of Africa and in parts of the Middle East, India, and

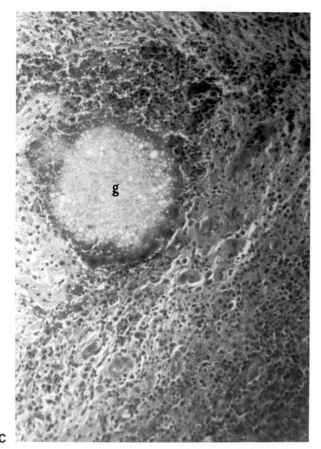

Figure 24-11 (Continued). Mycetoma of the foot caused by *Pseudallescheria boydii.* (C) A photomicrograph (x70) of involved soft tissue shows chronic granulomatous reaction surrounding a fungal grain (g).

c

Central and South America. It is rare in temperate climates. The disease typically occurs in rural areas, especially among people who customarily go barefoot. The foot is the most common anatomic site of mycetoma (named Madura foot after the region in India); this disease is found primarily in boys and men between the ages of 10 and 40 years, probably because of their outdoor occupations and lack of shoes.

Identification of the causative organism of mycetoma is often difficult. The appearance of the grains in the draining exudate can be helpful. Typically, infections caused by true fungi are associated with grains that are more than 0.3 or 0.4 mm in diameter and are black or white. Infections due to the *Actinomycetes* organisms are usually associated with grains that are less than 0.1 mm in diameter and are white, yellow, red, or brown. Worldwide, the most common causative fungus is *Madurella mycetomatis* and the most common actinomycotic organism is *Actinomadura madurae*. In the United States the fungus *P. boydii* is the

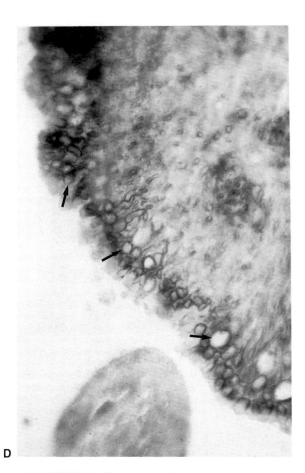

D

Figure 24-11 (Continued). Mycetoma of the foot caused by *Pseudallescheria boydii.* (D) A higher-power view (x280) shows rounded fungal structures (arrows) along the outer edge of the grain. (E) A photomicrograph (x28) of the mycelial culture shows numerous stringlike fungal hyphae.

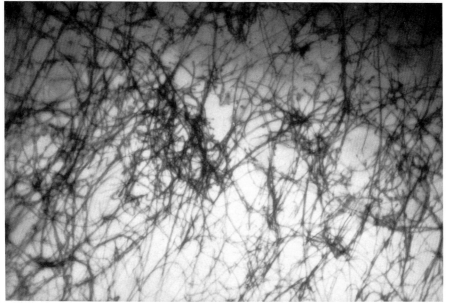

E

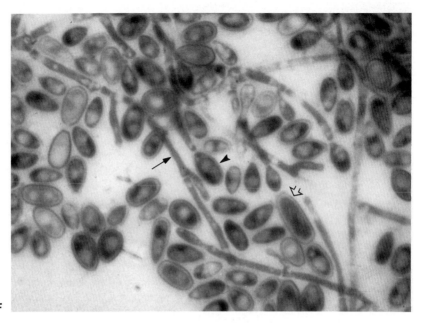

F

Figure 24-11 (Continued). Mycetoma of the foot caused by *Pseudalle-scheria boydii.* (F) A special stain of the cultured fungus shows the typical fungal hyphae (solid arrow), conidia (arrowhead), and ascospores (open arrow) of *P. boydii* (x280).

most common cause of mycetoma, and in Mexico the bacterium *Nocardia brasiliensis* is the most common.

The grains or granules are aggregates of fungal or actinomycotic organisms "cemented" together. To identify the organism, the grains can be examined microscopically after treatment with potassium hydroxide, and other stains of the exudate may be helpful. A biopsy specimen stained with hematoxylin and eosin may reveal the causative organism. Culture is necessary for definitive diagnosis, but culture of the exudate is often negative because the grains are not viable in about 30% of cases.

When the infection spreads into bone, radiographs may reveal lytic bone lesions, bone expansion, and periosteal reaction. The typical radiographic appearance is that of extensive soft tissue swelling, multiple small lytic lesions in the bone as a result of multiple abscesses, variable amounts of sclerosis around the abscesses, expansion of the bones, and periosteal reaction.

It is rare for mycetoma to progress to a systemic infection, and death is also very rare. When death does occur, it is usually caused by an infection of the scalp that extends into the brain. Infections clinically similar to mycetoma but caused by various bacteria are called "botryomycosis" and affect the skin, deep soft tissues, and even viscera.

Laboratory diagnosis. As with other infections, the diagnosis of fungal osteomyelitis requires identification of the causative organism, which may be difficult. It is important to obtain the diagnostic specimen carefully, so that it is representative of the infection itself and is not contaminated by clinically insignificant organisms from the skin. Material for culture and microscopic examination should be obtained from fluid or pus draining from deep within the infection or from curettage or biopsy of infected tissue. A swab of exudate from the crusted edge at the opening of a sinus tract will be contaminated by normal skin organisms, which are abundant in such sites.

Microscopic examination of the specimen is the most rapid means of diagnosis. However, organisms may be scarce, especially in patients with chronic fungal infections. Furthermore, it can be difficult to distinguish fungi (especially yeasts) from other cells. Smears of pus or serous exudate can be treated with 10% KOH, which dissolves and clears most organic material, in order to demonstrate the fungi clearly.

Histologic slides can be prepared from deep tissue specimens obtained by curettage or biopsy. Some fungi stain with routine hematoxylin-and-eosin preparation or with special stains, such as methionine silver or periodic-acid Schiff. However, it can still be very difficult to identify a specific species of fungus on morphologic grounds. Furthermore, the microscopic features must still be correlated with the clinical situation to ascertain the significance of any fungi observed.

Specimens should be submitted for culture as well as microscopic examination. Primary pathogenic fungi are usually recoverable on culture, although it can take so long for the organisms to grow that the identification is retrospective, with treatment already well under way. It is fairly easy to grow these organisms but much harder to make a specific identification of the species and determine the clinical significance. Opportunistic fungi may grow very slowly or not at all in culture, and incubation for 4 to 6 weeks is required to exclude their presence. Even then, growth of some of these organisms, especially *Candida* species, is of questionable relevance unless it correlates well with the clinical situation, because *Candida* species are normal commensal residents of the human body and are common laboratory contaminants. The presence of opportunistic pathogenic fungi on culture is very significant if the specimen was obtained from a normally sterile site or fluid and was not contaminated during collection. Multiple cultures can be useful, and results, of course, are more significant if the same organism grows from multiple sites in the same patient or from the same site multiple times and if organisms are also identified on direct microscopic examination of fluid or tissue specimens.

Serologic tests are usually not very useful for clinical diagnosis. Fungi are weakly antigenic, and serial determinations must be made to determine whether there is a rising antifungal titer. This is a complicated procedure and often takes too long to be useful for treatment of the patient. Fluorescent antibodies are available and can be useful, but the tests are difficult to perform and are not reliably available in many medical centers.

Treatment. The treatment of fungal or actinomycotic osteomyelitis, like that of bacterial osteomyelitis, often requires surgery supplemented by antimicrobial drugs. Cure may involve debridement of dead and diseased bone, excision of infected synovial tissue, and drainage of pus and exudate from abscess cavities. Successful treatment of opportunistic fungal infections in patients who are immunosuppressed or have serious disease depends heavily on control of the primary abnormality and not just the secondary fungal infection.

Despite their side effects, antifungal drugs are essential for the effective treatment of systemic or deep fungal infections. There are three main types of antifungal drugs (as well as several miscellaneous drugs).

(1) Polyenes. The polyene antifungal drugs include the most common and useful one, amphotericin B. This broad-spectrum drug remains the mainstay of treatment of serious, deep fungal infections. However, it must be given intravenously. In addition, up to 40% of patients experience side effects ranging from minor ones, such as fever, chills, and myalgia, to serious ones, such as renal toxicity, edema, and (rarely) anaphylaxis.

(2) Pyrimidine analogs. Flucytosine (5-fluorocytosine) is the most widely used pyrimidine analog. It can be administered orally or intravenously and is used to treat candidal, cryptococcal, and some other infections, almost always in combination with amphotericin B. If peak levels in blood are too high, serious bone marrow suppression can occur.

(3) Azoles. These are synthetic, broad-spectrum drugs, which can be very useful. Ketoconazole, which can be given orally, can be used for certain infections such as histoplasmosis, coccidioidomycosis, and some mycetomas. Very serious infections, however, usually require the addition of amphotericin B. Miconazole must be given intravenously but is currently the drug of choice for treatment of infections due to *P. boydii*, the cause of infection in the test patient. Itraconazole, recently introduced, is especially useful because it is active against aspergillosis. Several other agents in this group have been used, but there is limited experience with them. A third generation of azoles has been developed, and these drugs may prove to be more specific and exhibit fewer side effects.

Actinomyces and *Nocardia* species are, of course, bacteria. Nocardiosis is treated with sulfonamides, tetracycline, streptomycin, and some other drugs, and actinomycosis is treated with penicillin and some other drugs. Like other infections, osteomyelitis due to either of these organisms can also require extensive surgical drainage and debridement.

Individual fungal infections. Blastomycosis most commonly affects the lungs, skin, and skeleton. Musculoskeletal infections with *Blastomyces dermatidis* occur in up to 20% of patients with disseminated blastomycosis and are the presenting problem in about 10% of patients. As in most fungal infections, a primary lung infection spreads hematogenously to the bones and, less commonly, to the joints. Rarely, musculoskeletal infections occur by direct innoculation.

The radiographic appearance of blastomycosis is not pathognomonic. The ribs are most commonly involved, followed by the vertebrae and tibia. A focal or diffuse lytic lesion tends to occur in the subarticular or epiphyseal-metaphyseal region of long bones. The infection sometimes extends into the contiguous soft tissues. In about one-third of patients, there are two or more bone lesions (Figure 24-8). In up to three-quarters of patients with a bone lesion, a pulmonary infection is visible radiographically. Vertebral infections appear much like tuberculosis (Figure 24-10). They tend to affect the anterior part of the vertebral body but may affect the body, pedicle, or spinous processes. A paraspinal mass and spread beneath the anterior longitudinal ligament can occur, producing skip lesions in the adjacent spine. Unlike tuberculosis, blastomycosis can spread to an adjacent rib.

C. immitis produces a wide spectrum of musculoskeletal disease. As with other fungi, infection usually involves the lungs through inhalation. Up to 70% of persons living in some areas of endemicity have positive skin tests, and about 60% of patients with a primary pulmonary infection remain asymptomatic. A small percentage of patients develop a hypersensitivity arthritis ("desert rheumatism"), which is usually self-limited, resolves in 2 to 4 weeks, and exhibits no radiographic abnormalities. Disseminated coccidioidomycosis, which occurs in less than 1% of patients with primary pulmonary infection, leads to an acute febrile illness. It can involve the meninges, skin, bone, liver, spleen, or genital organs. Bone or joint involvement occurs in 20% of patients with the disseminated form. Septic arthritis or tenosynovitis is rare (less common than osteomyelitis) and occurs by hematogenous spread or invasion from adjacent osteomyelitis.

However, coccidioidal skeletal infections occur more commonly in the nondisseminated form of the disease, in which patients are less acutely ill. Usually there is a single focus of osteomyelitis, but in about 10% of patients as many as four to eight bones are involved. The spine is affected most commonly, followed by the tibia, skull, metatarsals, femur, and ribs. Radiographically, coccidioidal osteomyelitis appears as a rounded, well-demarcated lytic lesion in the diaphysis or metaphysis of a long bone. In the skull, the lesion can be well circumscribed or have irregular margins, and it involves either the outer table or both tables. Coccidioidal osteomyelitis seems to have a predilection for bony prominences, especially points of tendinous or ligamentous attachment such as the greater trochanters of the proximal femurs and the olecranon process of the ulna. Older, resolving bone lesions become more sclerotic as a result of reactive bone formation. When the process involves the spine, it tends to spare the disk.

Paracoccidioidomycosis ("South American blastomycosis") is a rare cause of musculoskeletal infections. Occasionally, focal lytic osteomyelitis occurs. Acute juvenile paracoccidioidomycosis refers to a fulminant disease in which the organism is present widely throughout the body, often with several lytic bone lesions.

Aspergillus species occasionally infect the lungs and can spread to contiguous vertebrae, especially as a postoperative complication of laminectomy or in patients taking steroids or antibiotics. Occasionally, lung infections spread contiguously to the ribs or sternum or hematogenously to other bones, such as the tibia and metatarsals (Figure 24-9).

Candida species are now the most frequent cause of deep mycotic infection in immunocompromised patients. Candidiasis is not an unusual infection in patients who have a serious systemic illness or who have undergone a complex surgical procedure. Other predisposing factors include immunosuppression (especially granulocytopenia), steroid treatment, administration of broad-spectrum antibiotics, and total parenteral alimentation. There are many different clinical manifestations depending on the site of infection. The fungus usually invades via the gastrointestinal tract or an intravenous catheter and can cause infection of the skin, muscles, retinas, prosthetic heart valves, brain, kidneys, or esophagus, as well as other areas. Intravenous drug abuse can also lead to *Candida* infections, especially vertebral or costochondral.

Septic arthritis due to candida is rare but is more common than osteomyelitis. It most commonly affects the hips, knees, shoulders, or elbows by hematogenous seeding. In contrast to other fungal infections, candidal osteomyelitis usually occurs secondary to septic arthritis by direct invasion into the adjacent bones. Therefore, the osteomyelitis is usually found in a long bone adjacent to a joint. Osteomyelitis that is not preceded by septic arthritis is rare. The radiographic appearance of candidal osteomyelitis is not characteristic; it shows nonspecific bone destruction. Typical locations include the ribs, humerus, and ilium.

When the infection involves the vertebral column, it destroys both the disk and adjacent vertebrae.

Histoplasma capsulatum is a common cause of a mild and self-limited pulmonary infection in areas where it is endemic. This infection leads to calcified granulomata in the lungs and spleen, which are common incidental observations on radiographs. A self-limited reactive polyarthritis is fairly common, but actual septic arthritis is extremely rare. Disseminated histoplasmosis, usually occurring in immunosuppressed patients, can affect the reticuloendothelial cells of the bone marrow diffusely, but it rarely causes osteomyelitis. Osteomyelitis occurs in less than 0.01% of patients with histoplasmosis. When osteomyelitis does occur in a child, there are usually multiple patchy lytic areas in various bones. In adults, the lesions tend to appear as sharply marginated lytic areas in the long bones.

Histoplasma dubosii infection is rarely seen in the United States, except in recent immigrants from central and west Africa. It affects primarily the skin, lymph nodes, and skeleton (which is involved in 40 to 60% of patients). In contrast to other fungi, pulmonary infections are rare. When the skeleton is involved, lytic areas may be seen in the metaphyses of long bones, the small bones of the hands, flat bones, ribs, vertebrae, and skull.

Cryptococcus neoformans can behave as either a true or an opportunistic pathogen. In Europe, most patients with active cryptococcosis do have a predisposing disease, so the fungus behaves as an opportunistic pathogen; however, in the United States, only about half of the patients have some predisposing disease. Bone is involved in 5 to 10% of patients with extrapulmonary spread of the disease. Cryptococcal arthritis is rare, but it has been reported in patients who are being given high doses of steroids or in patients with AIDS.

Radiographically, cryptococcal osteomyelitis causes well-defined lytic lesions without significant periosteal reaction. It affects the long bones, scapula, pelvis, skull, and vertebrae and, like histoplasmosis, can occur at bony prominences. The lesions are usually multiple and widely disseminated, and they change slowly. They resemble the "cold abscesses" of tuberculosis.

Sporotrichosis is usually acquired by direct inoculation of *Sporothrix schenckii* rather than by inhalation. Thorn punctures are a common source of infection. The typical clinical syndrome consists of a lymphocutaneous complex with nodular ulcerating skin lesions extending into the draining lymph nodes. Infection can then secondarily invade deep tissues, including muscle, bone, joints, and bursae. Infection of the knee joint by a direct puncture wound is fairly common. Sometimes there is no history of penetrating trauma, and it is possible that bone and joint infections are acquired through hematogenous spread from a primary pulmonary focus.

Radiographically, bone infection produces lytic lesions with periosteal reaction but with little sclerotic reaction within the bone. It can affect both long bones and the smaller bones of the hands and feet, especially the metacarpals, phalanges, tibia, and ribs. Multiple-joint involvement often occurs in patients who are immunocompromised or who have serious systemic illness. If there is no obvious skin or lung disease, diagnosis of bone or joint involvement can be delayed by as much as 2 years.

Question 108

Concerning diametaphyseal bone marrow infarction,

   (A) its radiologic appearance is easily confused with that of fibrous dysplasia
   (B) a lytic area nearly always represents cyst formation
   (C) pathologic fracture is a frequent complication
   (D) most patients also develop subarticular epiphyseal infarcts
   (E) it is usually associated with systemic corticosteroid therapy

A mature diametaphyseal bone infarct is typically located centrally within the medullary cavity and is characterized by a dense serpentine rim of sclerosis surrounding irregular lucent areas of variable size, which may contain scattered flecks of dense calcification (Figure 24-12). The peripheral sclerosis corresponds pathologically to a rim of dense fibrous connective tissue, which condensed around the infarct and in which calcium salts were deposited. Reactive bone formation around the lesion also contributes to the peripheral density, and calcification within the infarct contributes to the central density. This matrix calcification is due to formation of an insoluble "soap" by combination of calcium with free fatty acids released from the dead marrow lipocytes. Diametaphyseal infarcts may be solitary but are often bilateral and sometimes symmetric (Figure 24-13).

Fibrous dysplasia can exhibit many different radiographic appearances, but it seldom resembles a bone marrow infarct **(Option (A) is false).** Fibrous dysplasia is sometimes surrounded by a zone of sclerotic reaction, but this zone is generally smooth. The overall shape of a fibrous dysplasia lesion is typically ovoid or rounded (Figure 24-14), and the margin does not resemble the very irregular, dense, serpentine border of a bone infarct. Furthermore, fibrous dysplasia is often eccentric, whereas an infarct is usually central within the medullary cavity. When fibrous dysplasia comes in contact with the cortex, it can produce either cortical thinning or thickening (Figure 24-15). Sometimes it produces a very characteristic appearance, obliterating the cortical-medullary junction

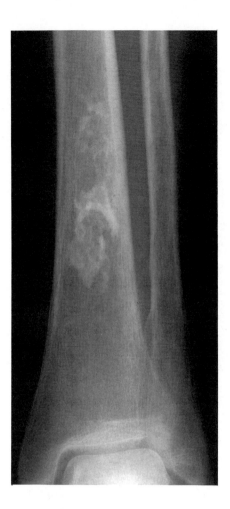

Figure 24-12 (left). Diametaphyseal bone marrow infarct. An anteroposterior radiograph shows typical mature medullary infarct within the distal tibial shaft. The densely mineralized lesion has an irregular margin and contains multiple lucent areas.

Figure 24-13 (below). Bilateral bone marrow infarcts. An anteroposterior radiograph of the knees shows multiple, radiographically typical infarcts in both distal femurs and both proximal tibias.

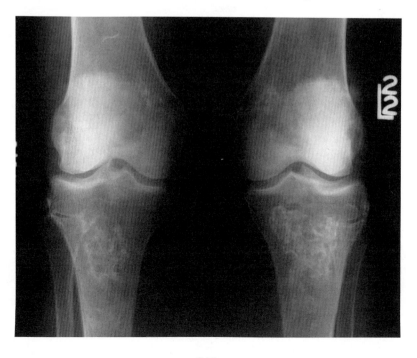

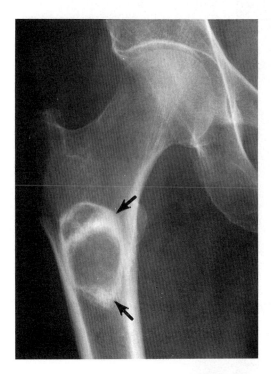

Figure 24-14 (left). Fibrous dysplasia. An anteroposterior radiograph of the proximal femur shows an ovoid sclerotic rind at the periphery of a focus of fibrous dysplasia (arrows).

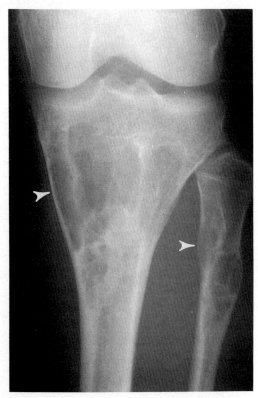

Figure 24-15 (right). Fibrous dysplasia. An anteroposterior radiograph of the proximal tibia and fibula shows foci of fibrous dysplasia characterized by eccentric lucent areas with cortical thinning (arrowheads).

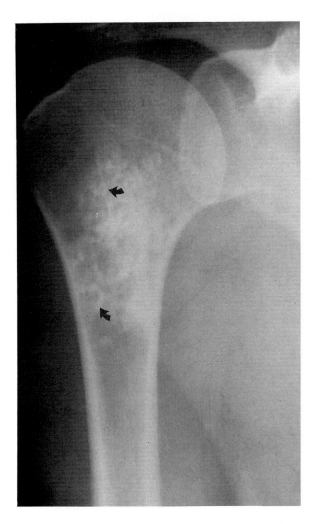

Figure 24-16. Typical enchondroma. An anteroposterior radiograph of the shoulder shows ring and arc mineralization (arrows) characteristic of cartilage tissue.

by replacing both cortical and cancellous bone with abnormal homogeneous tissue. Fibrous dysplasia often exhibits a characteristic homogeneous "ground-glass" appearance, which is not seen in bone infarcts. Focal calcific densities rarely appear within areas of solitary fibrous dysplasia but may appear in areas of polyostotic fibrous dysplasia. Such matrix densities are foci of calcified cartilage tissue. However, these densities are not as extensive or prominent as the focal densities found in and around a bone infarct.

The appearance of a medullary bone infarct may closely resemble that of an enchondroma (Figure 24-16). These two conditions can be differentiated because the thick serpentine sclerotic rim typical of an infarct does not usually occur around an enchondroma. Moreover, an

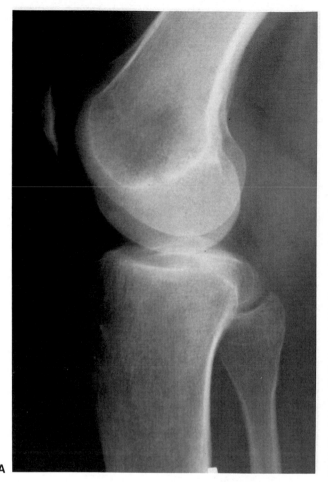

Figure 24-17. Diametaphyseal infarcts. (A) A lateral radiograph of the left knee shows no abnormalities. (B) A sagittal T1-weighted MR image of the same knee shows classic features of medullary bone infarcts. The infarcts are delineated by moderately thick, very irregular, serpentine, low-intensity margins (arrows).

A

enchondroma tends to have typical ring- and/or arc-pattern cartilage calcifications. However, despite these different features, some lesions are diagnostically indeterminate on radiographs alone.

Immediately after infarction, the radiographic appearance of the bone remains normal, since altered, dead bone appears the same as living bone. During repair, vascular connective tissue grows into the periphery of the infarct, resorption of dead trabeculae occurs, new bone is laid down, and calcification within the necrotic marrow fat takes place. Radiographically, the mineral pattern of the bone can then develop a mottled appearance, with small lucencies intermingled among ill-defined areas of increased density. Pathologically, in the early stages of a bone marrow infarct there is an elongated, pale, well-demarcated abnormal area in the marrow surrounded by a hyperemic border. The necrotic fat cells break down, and hemorrhage occurs, especially around the periph-

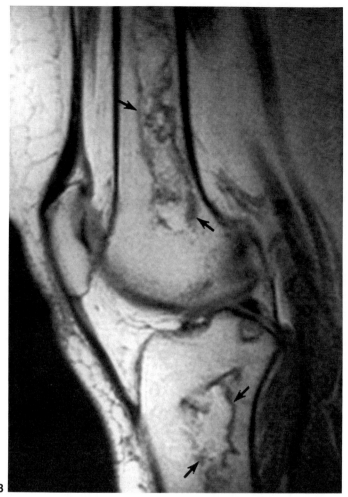

ery of the infarct. MRI can detect infarcts in their early stages, when the radiograph is still normal (Figure 24-17). Presumably, in the early stages of the infarct the MR examination displays some combination of the reactive hyperemic rim and the fibrous wall at the periphery of the infarct.

Liquefaction of bone marrow necrosis can occur in the center of an infarct and can lead eventually to formation of an intraosseous cyst. Such postinfarction cysts can appear radiographically as small lucent areas within the infarct. They can also be larger, with erosion and expansion of the cortex and with sharply outlined thin shells of reactive bone. Occasionally, very dense, peculiar, corkscrew-like calcification is present within the cyst (Figure 24-18). Ordinarily, such cysts do not require any special management.

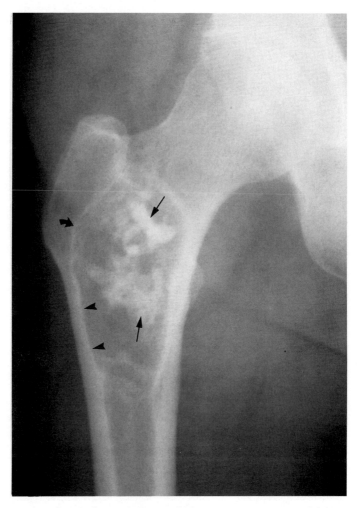

Figure 24-18. Cystic bone infarct. An anteroposterior radiograph of the hip shows a proximal femoral lesion characterized by endosteal cortical erosion (arrowheads), a nearly complete sclerotic rim (curved arrow), and peculiar, branching, dense matrix calcifications (straight arrows). (Reprinted with permission from Hudson TM. Radiologic-pathologic correlation of musculoskeletal lesions.)

It is important to realize that not all lytic areas within bone infarcts are cysts. Malignant transformation can occur within bone infarcts (Figure 24-19). When a lytic area associated with an infarct has an irregular margin, when it enlarges on serial radiographs, or when there is cortical destruction or an extra-osseous mass, it is likely that a malignant tumor is superimposed on the infarct. If a secondary sarcoma is suspected, it is important to obtain additional imaging studies, such as CT or MRI, and to initiate appropriate treatment. Malignant fibrous histiocytoma, fibro-

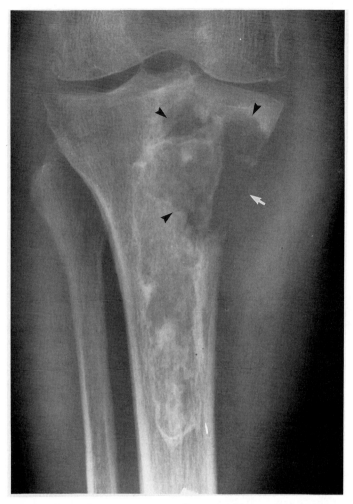

Figure 24-19. Transformation to malignant fibrous histiocytoma within a bone infarct. An anteroposterior radiograph of the proximal tibia shows an irregular, aggressive-appearing lytic area (arrowheads) that has destroyed cortex (arrow) adjacent to a typical medullary infarct. (Reprinted with permission from Hudson TM. Radiologic-pathologic correlation of musculoskeletal lesions.)

sarcoma, and, more rarely, osteosarcoma have been reported to arise in association with a bone infarct. Encystification and malignant transformation of bone infarcts are uncommon but of similar frequency **(Option (B) is false).** When a lucent region is discovered in what otherwise appears to be an infarct, the features must be studied carefully and a biopsy performed if indicated.

The results of devascularization of bone can be divided into two broad categories based on the location of the event within the involved bone. "Osteonecrosis" is now the preferred term to encompass both types of bone devascularization. The first type, diametaphyseal osteonecrosis, affects the cancellous bone in the shaft or metaphysis of long bones or within flat bones, and such lesions are usually termed bone infarcts. The second type, epiphyseal-metaphyseal osteonecrosis, affects the subarticular bone. This type has been termed avascular necrosis, aseptic necrosis, or ischemic necrosis.

Medullary infarcts are commonly asymptomatic but occasionally cause pain. No predisposing cause can be found in many patients, but many different etiologies have been identified in the remainder. These causes include barotrauma, sickle-cell anemia, marrow storage diseases, and vascular occlusive diseases of various types. Systemic steroid therapy is also associated with medullary bone marrow infarction.

Diametaphyseal osteonecrosis typically does not affect cortical bone; therefore, it does not weaken the structural integrity of the bone and does not lead to long-term mechanical complications such as fractures **(Option (C) is false).**

Epiphyseal-metaphyseal osteonecrosis is clinically more important than diametaphyseal osteonecrosis because it affects subarticular bone. As the healing response takes place, resorption of dead bone trabeculae, "creeping substitution," weakens the bone and can lead to pathologic fracture (Figure 24-20). The most familiar form of this type of osteonecrosis is avascular necrosis of the femoral head, leading to collapse and deformity of the articular surface and hence to severe secondary degenerative arthritis.

Small, button-shaped areas of epiphyseal osteonecrosis occur in children and young adults and are termed osteochondritis dissecans. Idiopathic osteonecrosis of the femoral condyle is well recognized in older individuals. These types of osteonecrosis also affect subarticular bone and can therefore lead to degenerative arthritis or formation of loose bodies in the joint. Epiphyseal osteonecrosis is often idiopathic, but it can follow trauma such as femoral neck fracture and can accompany systemic diseases such as sickle-cell disease, marrow-packing disorders, barotrauma, various forms of vascular occlusive disease, and heavy alcohol use. Patients commonly have multiple diametaphyseal infarcts without subarticular osteonecrosis **(Option (D) is false).** A major cause of epiphyseal-metaphyseal osteonecrosis is systemic steroid administration. Patients undergoing systemic corticosteroid therapy usually develop epiphyseal-metaphyseal osteonecrosis rather than diametaphyseal bone infarcts **(Option (E) is false).** The pathogenesis of steroid-induced osteonecrosis has not been unequivocally established, but explanations have been offered. One theory holds that microscopic fat emboli arise from the fatty liver induced by steroids and lodge in marrow vessels to cause infarcts. Another hypothesis holds that steroids cause enlargement of marrow fat

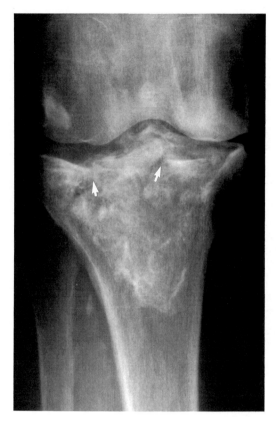

Figure 24-20. Subarticular osteonecrosis. An anteroposterior radiograph of the proximal tibia shows a typical medullary infarct in the metaphysis. The infarct involved the subarticular cortex, and this led to fracture and collapse of the tibial plateaus (arrows). The result was severe knee joint disability.

cells, which then impinge on marrow sinusoids in the closed space of medullary bone. The resulting increased pressure leads to venous stasis, reduced blood flow, and infarction.

Question 109

Concerning Langerhans cell histiocytosis of bone,

(A) a solitary bone lesion requires treatment by curettage or intralesional steroid injection
(B) disseminated bone disease is usually treated with systemic chemotherapy
(C) the spine is the most common site of bone involvement
(D) the development of marginal sclerosis on serial radiographs suggests healing of a lesion
(E) the lesions exhibit low signal intensity on T2-weighted MR images

LCH is currently the preferred name for the condition formerly known as histiocytosis X. It is a granulomatous disease characterized by

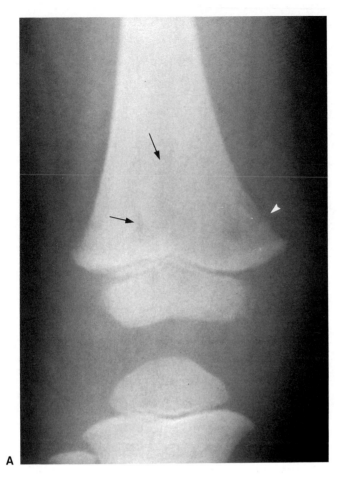

A

Figure 24-21. Polyostotic LCH. Radiographs of the knee (A) and hip (B) show subtle and ill-defined lytic lesions (arrows) with probable cortical penetration of the distal femoral metaphysis (arrowhead). (C) In the skull, the lytic lesions (arrows) are more clearly defined than those encountered in the long bones.

the presence of specific Langerhans cells, along with other inflammatory cells. It may affect only bones, only nonskeletal organs, or both.

Bones are involved at some time in 80 to 90% of patients with LCH. The disease affects only bone in 60 to 80% of patients with this condition. Bone involvement is usually solitary but is sometimes multifocal (Figure 24-21). Solitary bone lesions carry an excellent prognosis and tend to heal within 3 to 12 months regardless of the treatment used or even with no treatment at all (Figure 24-22) **(Option (A) is false).**

As lesions heal, laminated periosteal reaction develops and then tends to condense into a solid layer. Sclerotic margins form around lytic areas, and lytic areas gradually fill in with trabecular bone **(Option (D) is true).** Over months to years, the involved area may return to normal, or minimal cortical thickening and a coarsened trabecular pattern may persist (Figure 24-23).

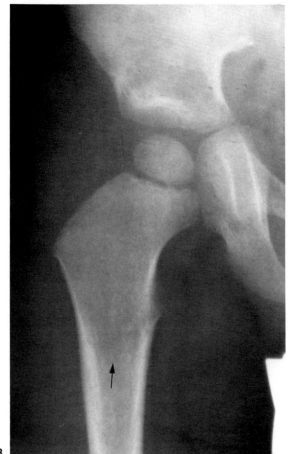

B

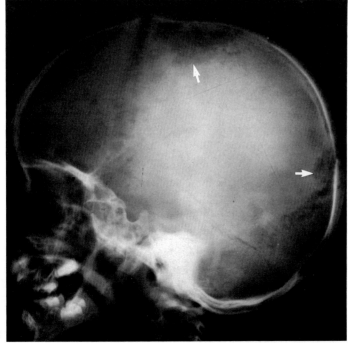

C

659

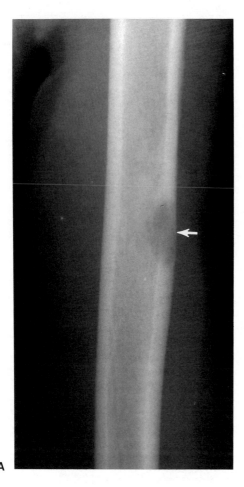

Figure 24-22. Natural history of LCH. (A) An anteroposterior radiograph of the humerus of a 29-year-old man shows an eccentric, well-defined, ovoid lytic area (arrow) at the time of diagnosis. (B) One year later, the lesion has enlarged. (C) Two years after obtaining the original radiograph, the lesion has healed, leaving some residual, faint medullary lucency and a thickened lateral cortex.

A

Patients with several bone lesions but without any other organ involvement also have an excellent prognosis and do not generally require systemic treatment **(Option (B) is false).** Some bone lesions can penetrate the cortex to invade the adjacent soft tissues, but this does not indicate general dissemination of disease and does not significantly affect the prognosis.

LCH primarily affects individuals in the first three decades of life, with a peak incidence between 5 and 10 years of age. There is a slight male predominance. Up to 85% of patients with LCH present initially with a solitary bone lesion. Of these, about 10 to 20% develop multiple bone lesions and about 1% develop disseminated visceral disease.

Symptoms of bone lesions include pain, limp, a palpable mass, and occasionally neurologic problems. About half of all bone lesions are asymptomatic. In the skull, the disease commonly affects the temporal

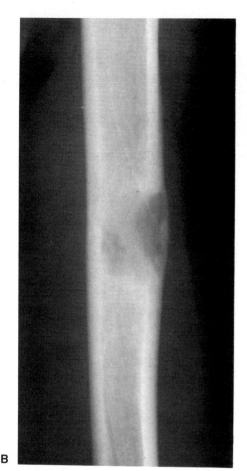
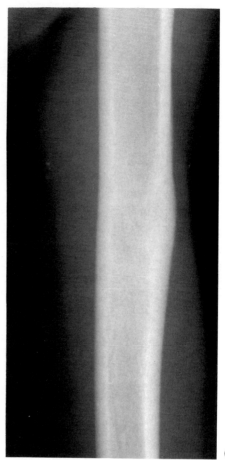

B

C

bone and can simulate otitis media, presenting with chronic drainage from the external ear. Lesions of the jaw can present as focal bone destruction or can simulate periodontal disease. A few patients have peripheral eosinophilia.

The skull is the most commonly affected bone (Figure 24-24), followed by the femur, ribs, pelvis, scapula, jaw, vertebra, and other long bones **(Option (C) is false).** Half of all bone lesions of LCH affect the skull, spine, pelvis, ribs, or mandible. The femur, tibia, and humerus are the most commonly affected long bones. In the spine, the thoracic area is the most commonly involved, followed by the lumbar region and finally the cervical region.

CT scans can show the extent of bone destruction more clearly than radiographs in areas of complex anatomy such as the scapula and pelvis

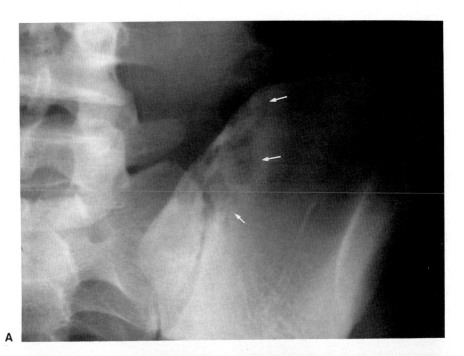

A

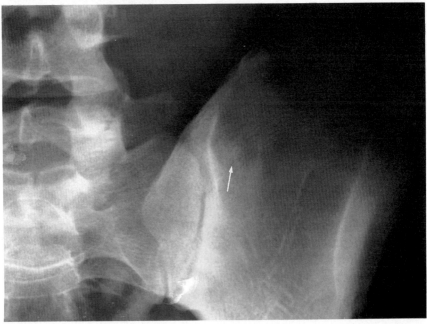

B

Figure 24-23. Spontaneous healing of LCH. An anteroposterior radiographs of the left ilium of a 23-year-old man show a large lytic lesion surrounded by some bony sclerosis (arrows) at the time of diagnosis (A) and a healed lesion with only faint residual sclerosis (arrow) 7 years later (B). The patient received no treatment.

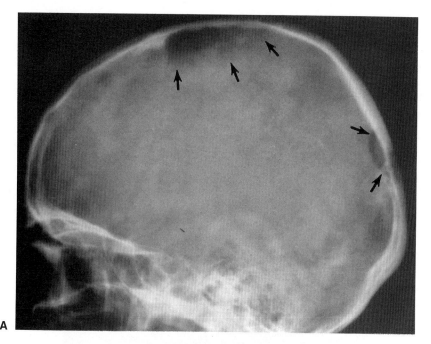

A

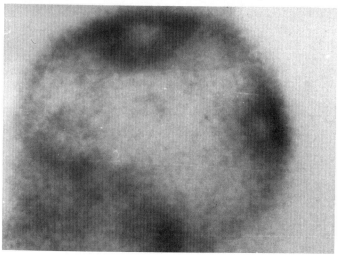

B

Figure 24-24. LCH of the skull. (A) A lateral radiograph shows well-defined, rounded, lytic lesions with broad irregular margins (arrows). (B) A lateral scintigram shows a "doughnut" pattern of focal uptake around the periphery of the lesions. Transaxial CT images windowed for bone (C) and soft tissue (D) show the occipital lesion. It is characterized by a very wide area of destruction of the outer table of the skull (white arrows) compared with a much smaller area of destruction of the inner table (black arrows). This creates a "beveled-edge" appearance that is also evident on the radiograph. The occipital lesion has completely destroyed the outer table, but it seems to be contained by periosteum (white arrowheads). A small piece of bone, a so-called sequestrum, is visible in the center of the lytic area (open white arrow).

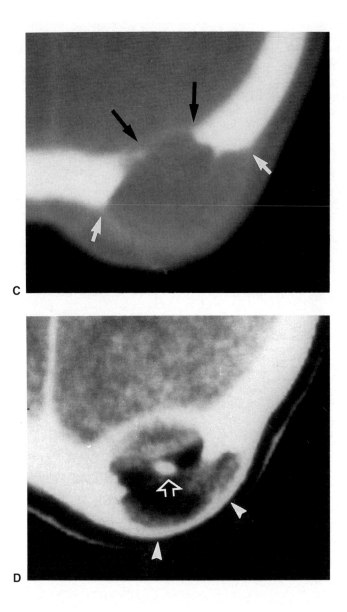

C

D

(Figure 24-25). MRI demonstrates the intraosseous extent, cortical penetration, and soft tissue spread of the condition. As with most active bone lesions, the cellular tissue typically exhibits high signal intensity on T2-weighted images **(Option (E) is false).**

Beltran et al. and De Schepper et al. have recently described the MR characteristics of eosinophilic granuloma of bone. On T1-weighted images, the abnormal tissue usually exhibits signal intensity near or slightly greater than that of skeletal muscle (Figure 24-26), though it is

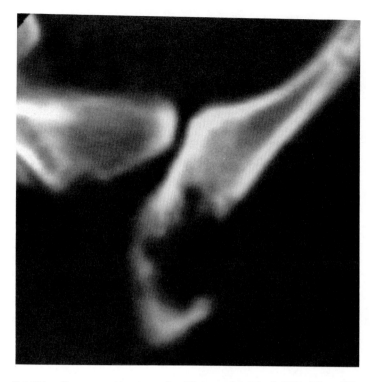

Figure 24-25. Same patient as in Figure 24-23. LCH. The CT section shows the extent of destruction of the posterior ilium particularly well.

occasionally slightly lower. The tissue typically enhances markedly with gadolinium. On T2-weighted images, the tissue exhibits a very high signal intensity. In most lesions, there is also diffuse abnormal signal in the adjacent marrow, and in nearly half the lesions there is abnormal signal in the surrounding soft tissues. This surrounding abnormal signal is low in intensity on T1-weighted images and high on T2-weighted images and is thought to be due to edema in the adjacent marrow and soft tissues. On T2-weighted images, the tissue of the lesion itself usually exhibits a higher signal intensity than that within the surrounding reactive tissue. About half of the lesions exhibit a rim of low signal intensity. Because of the common occurrence of this surrounding reactive or "flare" phenomenon, eosinophilic granuloma of bone may be confused with diseases that also tend to elicit such a reaction, including more-aggressive processes such as osteomyelitis or Ewing's tumor, or with benign tumors such as osteoid osetoma and chondroblastoma.

Nomenclature. Traditionally, three general forms of the disease that is now called LCH have been recognized: Letterer-Siwe disease, Hand-

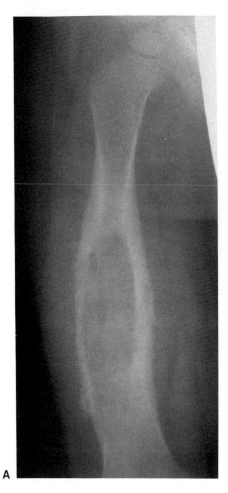

A

Figure 24-26. LCH of the femur in a 2-year-old boy with a limp and a palpable mass. (A) An anteroposterior radiograph shows a large, expansile, lytic lesion with cortical thickening and irregular periosteal reaction. (B) A transaxial T1-weighted MR image shows periosteal reaction, cortical erosion, and cortical penetration (arrow). (C) A coronal T2-weighted MR image shows high-intensity cellular tissue within the lesion (curved arrow). High signal in adjacent muscle (straight arrows) is presumed to be due to edema.

Schüller-Christian disease, and eosinophilic granuloma of bone. These were originally thought to be three different diseases, but they were later considered different clinical manifestations of the same basic disease, which was termed histiocytosis X. These three forms have recently been labeled the fulminant form, the chronic recurring form, and the localized form of LCH, respectively. The fulminant form, which makes up only 10% of all cases, occurs in children up to 3 years of age; involves the liver, spleen, and lymph nodes; and often rapidly results in death from hemorrhage or infection. The chronic recurring form makes up 15 to 45% of cases, typically occurs between the ages of 5 and 10 years, and affects the bones (especially the skull), liver, spleen, lymph nodes, marrow, skin, and, less commonly, lungs, heart, brain, kidneys, and other organs. The mortality rate is high, and the prognosis worsens as more organ systems

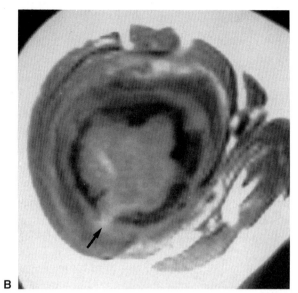

B

SE 750/17

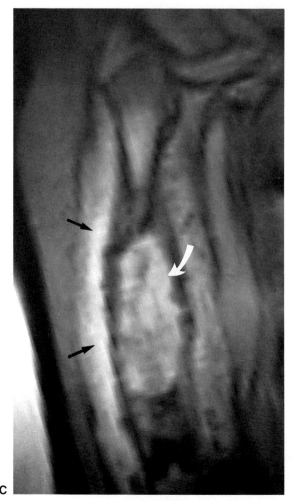

C

SE 2,000/80

667

are involved and with younger patients. A classic triad of diabetes insipidus, exophthalmos, and skull lesions was described, but this combination is unusual and actually occurs in only 10% of patients with the chronic recurring form of the disease. Localized LCH of bone makes up 60 to 80% of cases, has a peak incidence at 5 to 10 years of age, and most often affects the skull and axial skeleton. Most lesions are solitary, though some are multiple, but all carry an excellent prognosis if there is no evidence of visceral involvement.

Etiology. The etiology of LCH remains unknown. In recent years, the disease was staged and treated much like a generalized malignancy of lymphoid or bone marrow tissue. However, it is not malignant in the classic pathologic sense. (It does not involve an uncontrolled proliferation of a unified population of cells, and there is no reliable correlation between the degree of differentiation of the abnormal cells and the clinical course of the disease.) It is probably best considered a nonmalignant disorder of immune regulation, perhaps affecting cell migration.

Prognosis and clinical course. Patients with LCH present with skin lesions, eye abnormalities, respiratory symptoms, fever, or other signs of systemic illness. About one-half of patients have skin lesions, about one-third have lymph node involvement, and about one-fourth have hepatosplenomegaly.

A variety of staging or scoring systems have been used to try to determine the prognosis and select the appropriate treatment. It seems clear that the prognosis is related to the patient's age and to functional impairment of organs (especially the liver and bone marrow). Bone marrow dysfunction involves manifestations such as anemia, leukemia, and thrombocytopenia. Impaired liver function causes hypoproteinemia, edema, ascites, or hyperbilirubinemia. Pulmonary dysfunction can cause tachypnea or dyspnea, cyanosis, cough, pleural effusion, pneumothorax, or subclinical impairment of pulmonary function tests, with decreased compliance and decreased lung volume.

Patients older than 2 years with no organ dysfunction have about a 90% 5-year survival, whereas those with organ dysfunction have a 45 to 50% 5-year survival. Patients with the fulminant clinical syndrome (organ dysfunction, patient younger than 2 years) do poorly. About 30% survival is expected without treatment, but this can be increased to about 65% with systemic chemotherapy. Half of the survivors will have residual disability, such as diabetes insipidus, short stature, deafness, or pulmonary or orthopedic complications.

Patients with disease limited to bones have an excellent prognosis. They rarely develop disseminated disease, and their disease takes a generally benign course except in some patients younger than 3 years.

Treatment of systemic illness. There has been a recent trend toward less-aggressive treatment of systemic disease when there is no organ dysfunction. Such patients generally do well, and aggressive treatment may be worse than the disease. However, when there is generalized visceral disease with organ dysfunction, especially involving the lungs, liver, or bone marrow, the prognosis is quite grim and aggressive treatment with systemic chemotherapy is indicated. The least toxic drug is usually selected, most commonly one of the vinca alkaloids or antimetabolites and sometimes steroids. Newer drugs such as etoposide are also being evaluated. In patients with particularly bad prognostic signs, very aggressive treatments such as cyclosporine and bone marrow transplantation have been tried.

Disease limited to the bones is much less serious than visceral disease and generally does not require intensive treatment. Furthermore, even when multiple bone lesions are present, systemic treatment is not required. Attention to any bone lesions is directed toward maintaining musculoskeletal function, controlling symptoms, and preventing pathologic fractures. Radiographic survey of the skeleton is useful because of the relatively high false-negative rate of bone scintigraphy. On the other hand, scintigraphy sometimes detects a few bone lesions that are not clearly visible on radiographs because of their location in complex anatomic areas, such as the pelvis or spine. It is not clear which imaging studies should be used for following up these patients or how frequently they should be done. Generally, repeated radiographic skeletal surveys are used.

Radiology. The bone lesions of LCH are typically lytic, round to oval, and generally smoothly marginated and well defined, although they sometimes have irregular margins. A few even have ill-defined, permeated margins, especially in the ribs and clavicle. About one-quarter appear initially as mixed lytic and blastic lesions. Periosteal reaction occurs in about 10% of all lesions, more commonly in the long bones. Cortical expansion is present in 60% of long-bone lesions.

The skull is most commonly involved, but 20% of all skeletal lesions appear in the long bones. Long-bone lesions are usually centered in the diaphysis, less commonly in the metaphysis, and only rarely in the epiphysis. The open physeal plate acts as a relative barrier to the spread of the disease. The lesion generally arises centrally in the medullary cavity and quite commonly produces endosteal erosion, frequently completely penetrates the cortex, and can invade the adjacent soft tissues. Occasionally, lesions arise in cortical bone.

The periosteal reaction can form a single layer, or it may be laminated, onion-skinned, or thick and undulating. When it is mature and well consolidated, the result is cortical thickening. In early stages, only

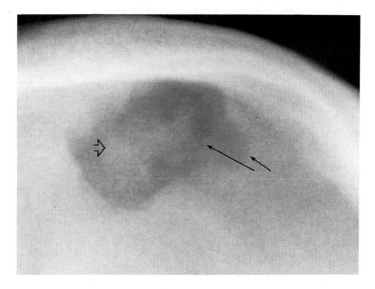

Figure 24-27. Typical skull lesion in a 21-year-old woman with LCH. A close-up view of a region from a lateral skull radiograph shows a beveled edge (solid arrows) where the inner and outer tables form two edges as a result of an unequal extent of destruction of the two tables. There also is a sequestrum (open arrow) of engulfed, undestroyed bone within the lytic area.

periosteal reaction may be visible on radiographs, but visible bone destruction appears later. In flat bones, there is less periosteal reaction and sometimes a multiloculated appearance as a result of thick ridges in the bony walls around the lesions.

In the skull, the margin of the lytic area may have a beveled appearance as a result of a different extent of cortical destruction at the inner and outer tables. In the pelvis, the same appearance may result from differential destruction of the inner and outer cortices. Skull lesions are typically 1 to 4 cm in diameter, but multiple separate bone lesions can coalesce into a large area of irregular lytic destruction. A segment of preserved bone can appear as a "sequestrum" within a lytic skull lesion (Figure 24-27). Skull lesions can destroy portions of the mastoid process, the petrous bone, and the sphenoid bone. Pituitary dysfunction occurs in about one-third of patients with sphenoid destruction.

In the mandible, the lesions tend to arise around the roots of the teeth, typically destroying the lamina dura to simulate periodontal disease. As destruction coalesces to a large lytic area surrounding several roots, it can produce the appearance of "floating teeth." Lesions in the

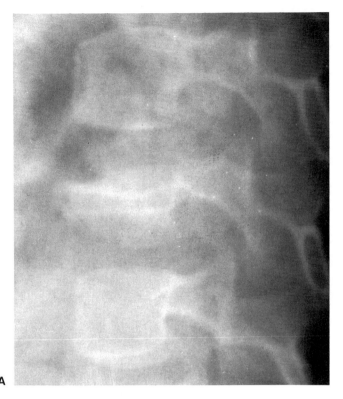

A

Figure 24-28. Typical vertebral lesion in a 7-year-old boy with LCH who had multiple bone lesions and lymphadenopathy. (A) A lateral radiograph of the lumbar spine shows the typical "vertebra plana" configuration. Following chemotherapy the patient was clinically well. (B) After 4 years of skeletal growth, the affected vertebral body (arrow) had returned to nearly normal height. (Reprinted with permission from Hudson TM. Radiologic-pathologic correlation of musculoskeletal lesions.)

ribs and clavicle are commonly expansile and exhibit permeated margins. In the pelvis, lesions typically arise in the iliac neck region.

In the spine, the vertebral body is most commonly affected and usually collapses to produce the "vertebra plana" appearance (Figure 24-28). Occasionally, lesions affect the posterior elements with or without extension into the vertebral body. Despite the frequent severe vertebral-body collapse, neurologic complications are unusual.

Most bone lesions exhibit increased tracer uptake on bone scintigraphy, and up to 11% of lesions have been reported to cause abnormal "cold" areas of decreased uptake. However, unlike most active bone diseases, 30 to 35% of bone lesions of LCH have a normal scintigraphic appearance. Therefore, radiographic skeletal surveys remain useful for

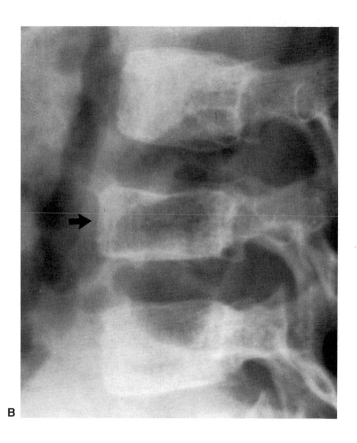

B

detecting and monitoring bone lesions, even though, in a few instances, scintigraphy discloses lesions not readily apparent on radiographs.

The radiographic differential diagnosis of a typical skull lesion includes venous lake, parietal foramen, epidermoid cyst, and hemangioma. The differential diagnosis of poorly marginated permeative lesions (such as those commonly seen in the clavicle, ribs, and long-bone metaphyses) includes osteomyelitis, Ewing's sarcoma, leukemia, lymphoma, and metastatic neuroblastoma. The differential diagnosis of vertebra plana includes trauma, Gaucher's disease, Hodgkin's disease, leukemia, osteoporosis, and hemangioma. The differential diagnosis of cortical long-bone lesions includes osteoid osteoma and Ewing's sarcoma. The differential diagnosis of multiple bone lesions includes osteomyelitis, metastases, leukemia, lymphoma, Gaucher's disease, and brown tumors of hyperparathyroidism. Clues to the correct diagnosis of LCH include well-defined margins, endosteal scalloping, beveled edges, thick periostitis, periosteal buttressing, and location in the pelvis or skull.

Treatment of bone lesions. Bone lesions generally heal spontaneously. No difference in the rate of healing has been demonstrated for untreated

672 / *Musculoskeletal Disease*

lesions and those treated by chemotherapy, chemotherapy combined with radiation therapy, or radiation therapy alone. A variety of other treatments have been used as well. Bone lesions are commonly curetted. More recently, percutaneous intralesional steroid injection has been used, allegedly with rapid resolution of symptoms and perhaps an increased rate of healing, although the evidence for the latter is questionable. Radiation therapy, in low doses of 500 to 800 rads, has been reported to provide local control of up to 88% of lesions limited to bone but only 69% of bone lesions that have invaded adjacent soft tissues. Some of the treated bone lesions recur within the radiation field for unknown reasons. Radiation of the sphenoid bone does not reverse the syndrome of diabetes insipidus, even when local control of the bone lesion is achieved. Potential complications of surgery, radiation, or local injection, and the fact that most lesions heal spontaneously, should be considered carefully before undertaking treatment.

Treatment seems clearly indicated when bone lesions cause significant pain or when there is a risk of anatomic instability or pathologic fracture of large-bone lesions in critical areas, such as the proximal femur. In such instances, curettage or steroid injection may be indicated in an attempt to prevent complications and preserve function. As an alternative, radiation therapy can be used when the site of bone involvement is inaccessible to injection, especially when there is a threat to the function of the spinal cord, optic nerve, or other vital structure. Symptomatic bone lesions in expendable areas such as the fibula or clavicle have been resected, but since the lesions heal spontaneously, there seems to be little reason to do this. Practically speaking, solitary bone lesions are often treated at the time of diagnosis in the form of open biopsy and curettage or needle biopsy and steroid injection. Patients with bone lesions but without structural risk factors should be monitored closely with sequential radiographs to detect enlargement or extension of bone lesions so that complications such as pathologic fracture can be anticipated and prevented.

Pathologic and laboratory features. Histologically, the presence of the typical Langerhans cell is required to make the diagnosis. This cell resembles other histiocytes. It is large and ovoid, and it contains abundant pale cytoplasm and a grooved, oval, or reniform nucleus, with a low nuclear/cytoplasmic ratio. Mitotic figures are rare. The Langerhans cell can be specifically identified by electron microscopy and immunocytochemical staining.

Other cells scattered throughout the abnormal tissue include occasional multinucleated giant cells and a variable number of inflammatory cells, including eosinophils, lymphocytes, plasma cells, and neutrophils. Despite the name "eosinophilic granuloma," in some lesions eosinophils are sparse, whereas in others they are abundant. The large number of inflammatory and histiocyte-appearing cells may make it difficult to distinguish LCH from infection or lymphoma by light microscopy.

Terry M. Hudson, M.D.

SUGGESTED READINGS

FUNGAL OSTEOMYELITIS

1. Cockshott WP, Lucas AO. Radiographic findings in *Histoplasma dubosii* infections. Br J Radiol 1964; 37:653–660.
2. Dalinka MK, Dinnenberg S, Greendyke WH, Hopkins R. Roentgenographic features of osseous coccidioidomycosis and differential diagnosis. J Bone Joint Surg (Am) 1971; 53:1157–1164
3. Dalinka MK, Lally JF, Koniver G, Coren GS. The radiology of osseous and articular infection. CRC Crit Rev Clin Radiol Nucl Med 1975; 7:1–64
4. Gruninger RP. Fungal injections in bones and joints. In: Gustilo RB, Gruninger RP, Tsukayama DT (eds), Orthopedic infections: diagnosis and treatment. Philadelphia: WB Saunders; 1989:211–223
5. Harwood-Nash DC, Kirks DR, Howard BA, et al. Image interpretation session: 1991. RadioGraphics 1992; 12:171–198
6. Johnson PC, Sarosi GA. Fungal synovitis and osteomyelitis. In: D'Ambrosia RD, Marier RL (eds), Orthopedic infections. Thorofare, NJ: Slack; 1989:283–302
7. Lewall DB, Ofole S, Bendl B. Mycetoma. Skeletal Radiol 1985; 14:257–262
8. MacDonald PB, Black GB, MacKenzie R. Orthopaedic manifestations of blastomycosis. J Bone Joint Surg (Am) 1990; 72:860–864
9. McGinnis MR, Fader RC. Mycetoma: a contemporary concept. Infect Dis Clin North Am 1988; 2:933–954
10. Oyston JK. Madura foot. J Bone Joint Surg (Br) 1961; 43:259–267
11. Rippon JW. Medical mycology, 3rd ed. Philadelphia: WB Saunders; 1988:1–11
12. Roberts SOB, Hay RJ, Mackenzie DWR. Systemic mycoses. In: A clinician's guide to fungal disease. New York: Marcel Dekker; 1984:133–187
13. Rosen RS, Jacobson G. Fungus disease of bone. Semin Roentgenol 1966; 1:370–391
14. Sharif HS, Clark DC, Aabed MY, et al. Mycetoma: comparison of MR imaging with CT. Radiology 1991; 178:865–870
15. Travis LB, Roberts GD, Wilson WR. Clinical significance of *Pseudoallescheria boydii*: a review of 10 years' experience. Mayo Clinic Proc 1985; 60:531–537

BONE INFARCTION

16. Bullough PG, Kambolis CP, Marcove RC, Jaffe HL. Bone infarctions not associated with caisson disease. J Bone Joint Surg (Am) 1965; 47:477–491

17. Edeiken J, Hodes PJ, Libschitz HI, Weller MH. Bone ischemia. Radiol Clin North Am 1967; 5:515–529

18. Furey JG, Ferrer-Torells M, Reagan JW. Fibrosarcoma arising at the site of bone infarcts. A report of two cases. J Bone Joint Surg (Am) 1960; 42:802–810

19. Mankin HJ. Nontraumatic necrosis of bone (osteonecrosis). N Engl J Med 1992; 326:1473–1479

20. Mirra JM, Bullough PG, Marcove RC, Jacobs B, Huvos AG. Malignant fibrous histiocytoma and osteosarcoma in asssociation with bone infarcts: report of four cases, two in caisson workers. J Bone Joint Surg (Am) 1974; 56:932–940

21. Munk PL, Helms CA, Holt RG. Immature bone infarcts: findings on plain radiographs and MR scans. AJR 1989; 152:547–549

22. Norman A, Steiner GC. Radiographic and morphological features of cyst formation in idiopathic bone infarction. Radiology 1983; 146:335–338

LANGERHANS CELL HISTIOCYTOSIS

23. Beltran J, Aparisi F, Bonmati LM, Rosenberg ZS, Present D, Steiner GC. Eosinophilic granuloma: MRI manifestations. Skeletal Radiol 1993; 22:157–161

24. Bollini, G, Jouve JL, Gentet JC, Jacquemier M, Bouyala JM. Bone lesions in histiocytosis X. J Pediatr Orthop 1991; 11:469–477

25. Crone-Münzebrock W, Brassow F. A comparison of radiographic and bone scan findings in histiocytosis X. Skeletal Radiol 1983; 9:170–173

26. David R, Oria RA, Kumar R, et al. Radiologic features of eosinophilic granuloma of bone. AJR 1989; 153:1021–1026

27. De Schepper MA, Ramon F, Van Marck E. MR imaging of eosinophilic granuloma: report of 11 cases. Skeletal Radiol 1993; 22:163–166

28. Dimentberg RA, Brown KL. Diagnostic evaluation of patients with histiocytosis X. J Pediatr Orthop 1990; 10:733–741

29. Ennis JT, Whitehouse G, Ross FG, Middlemiss JH. The radiology of the bone changes in histiocytosis X. Clin Radiol 1973; 24:212–220

30. Komp DM. Concepts in staging and clinical studies for treatment of Langerhans' cell histiocytosis. Semin Oncol 1991; 18:18–23

31. McLelland J, Broadbent V, Yeomans E, Malone M, Pritchard J. Langerhans cell histiocytosis: the case for conservative treatment. Arch Dis Child 1990; 65:301–303

32. Parker BR, Pinckney L, Etcubanas E. Relative efficacy of radiographic and radionuclide bone surveys in the detection of the skeletal lesions of histiocytosis X. Radiology 1980; 134:377–380

33. Sartoris DJ, Parker BR. Histiocytosis X: rate and pattern of resolution of osseous lesions. Radiology 1984; 152:679–684

34. Siddiqui AR, Tashjian JH, Lazarus K, Wellman HN, Baehner RL. Nuclear medicine studies in evaluation of skeletal lesions in children with histiocytosis X. Radiology 1981; 140:787–789

35. Stull MA, Kransdorf MJ, Devaney KO. Langerhans cell histiocytosis of bone. RadioGraphics 1992; 12:801–823

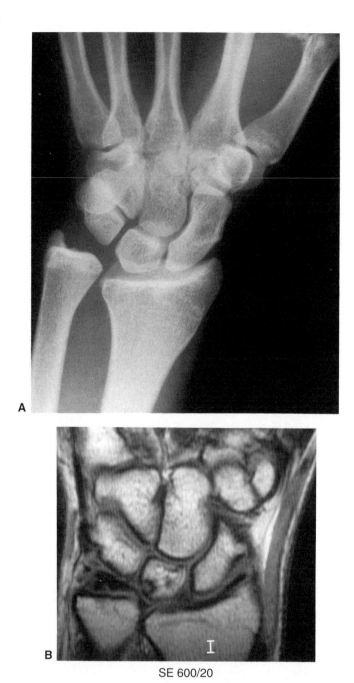

SE 600/20

Figure 25-1. This 17-year-old baseball player presented with wrist pain. You are shown a conventional posteroanterior radiograph (A) and coronal T1-weighted (B) and gradient-echo (C) MR images of the wrist.

Case 25: Ulnolunate Impaction
Syndrome

Question 110

Which *one* of the following is the MOST likely diagnosis?

(A) Kienböck's disease
(B) Ulnar-minus variance
(C) Ulnolunate impaction syndrome
(D) Subluxation of the distal radioulnar joint
(E) Scapholunate ligament tear

The conventional posteroanterior radiograph of the wrist (Figure 25-1A) demonstrates the distal articular surfaces of the radius and ulna to be at different levels, with the ulna projecting distal to the radius. This is referred to as ulnar-positive or ulnar-plus variance. Therefore, ulnar-minus variance (Option (B)) is an incorrect diagnosis. There is also a flattened contour of the medial or ulnar aspect of the proximal surface of the lunate where it apposes the ulna (Figure 25-2A). This appearance is caused by bone remodeling in response to chronic stress on this portion of the lunate from the adjacent ulna. The T1-weighted spin-echo (Figure 25-1B) and gradient-echo (Figure 25-1C) MR images demonstrate the incongruity of the distal ulnar and radial articular surfaces secondary to the unequal lengths of the bones. The triangular fibrocartilage is draped over the distal articular surface of the head of the ulna. Also, there is a small partial-thickness tear of the proximal surface of the triangular fibrocartilage on its ulnar aspect (Figure 25-2B), and the fibrocartilage is abnormally thinned centrally. There is a small subchondral degenerative cyst in the lunate, caused by chronic mechanical impingement of the ulna on the lunate (Figure 25-2C). These findings make ulnolunate impaction syndrome the most likely diagnosis **(Option (C) is correct).**

Kienböck's disease (Option (A)), or osteonecrosis of the lunate, initially appears as diminished bone marrow signal intensity on T1-

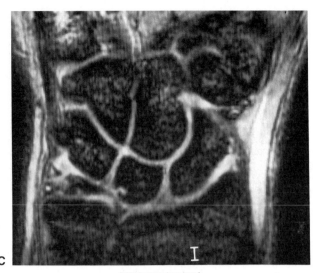

GRE 350/20/30°

Figure 25-1 (Continued)

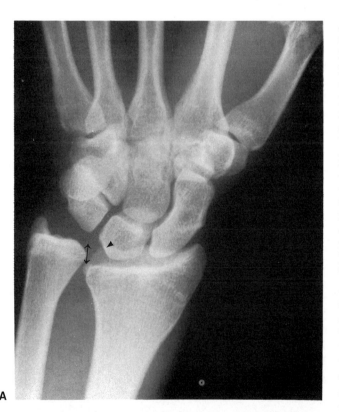

Figure 25-2 (Same as Figure 25-1). Ulnolunate impaction syndrome. (A) A posteroanterior radiograph shows the ulna to be longer than the radius (double-headed arrow) and the surface of the lunate to be flattened adjacent to the prominent ulna (arrowhead). Coronal T1-weighted (B) and gradient-echo (C) MR images confirm the ulnar-positive variance. The triangular fibrocartilage is stretched over the distal ulna and has a partial-thickness tear of its proximal surface (curved arrow). The triangular fibrocartilage is thinned where it is interposed between the lunate and ulna (solid arrow). A small subchondral cyst is present in the lunate (open arrow) at the point of the apposition between the ulna and the lunate.

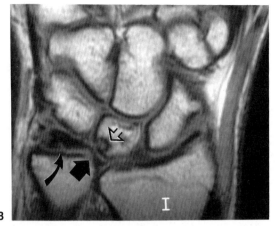

B

SE 600/20

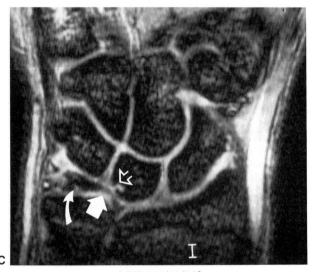

C

GRE 350/20/30°

weighted MR images in combination with increased signal intensity on T2-weighted images. All or only a portion of the lunate bone marrow may be affected. In later stages of Kienböck's disease, the lunate undergoes repair, which is manifested as new bone formation, partial collapse of the bone, and a variable amount of bone fragmentation. These alterations appear as low-intensity regions on both T1- and T2-weighted images. Except for the small cyst, the marrow signal within the lunate is nearly normal in the test patient. Therefore, Kienböck's disease is not a likely diagnosis.

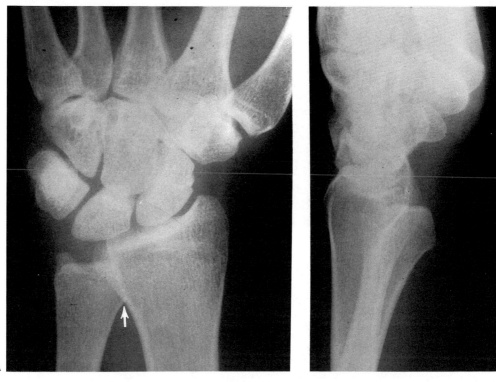

A

Figure 25-3. Distal radioulnar joint dislocation. (A) A posteroanterior radiograph of the wrist demonstrates malalignment of the distal radioulnar joint manifested by overlap of the radius and ulna (arrow) associated with a relatively short ulna. (B) A lateral radiograph shows volar displacement of the distal ulna.

Subluxation of the distal radioulnar joint (Option (D)) refers to abnormal volar or, more commonly, dorsal displacement of the distal ulna relative to the distal radius. This malalignment indicates ligamentous laxity or disruption of the distal radioulnar joint. Isolated subluxation or dislocation at the distal radioulnar joint is unusual (Figures 25-3 and 25-4). It is usually associated with trauma, fractures (Figure 25-5) of the distal radius (e.g., Colles, Smith, or Galeazzi fracture), or comminuted impacted fractures of the proximal radius (e.g., Essex-Lopresti fracture).

Dislocations of the distal radioulnar joint result from severe rotational forces, either supination or pronation, causing anterior or posterior displacements of the ulna. On a true lateral view of the normal wrist, the distal ulna is superimposed over the radius and the ulnar dorsal cortex projects about 2 mm dorsal to the radial dorsal cortex. As a general rule, the dorsal cortex of the ulna should be in the same plane as

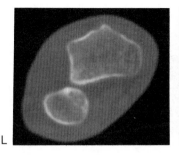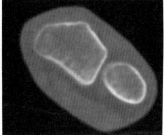

L   R

Figure 25-4. Same patient as in Figure 25-3. Volar dislocation of the ulna. A transaxial CT scan shows volar dislocation of the left ulna at the distal radiolunate joint. The contralateral (right) distal radioulnar joint is normal. (Courtesy of Camelia G. Whitten, M.D., University of Iowa, Iowa City.)

the dorsal cortex of the triquetrum on the lateral projection. Small degrees of pronation or supination of the wrist subtly alter this alignment, often making the diagnosis of minor distal radioulnar joint malalignment difficult. Posteroanterior radiographs of the wrist can be useful in suggesting a diagnosis of distal radioulnar joint malalignment by showing abnormal overlapping (Figure 25-3A), widening (Figure 25-5A), or angulation of the joint space between the distal ulna and radius, which are normally parallel. Also, the ulna may appear too short or too long relative to the radius.

Transaxial CT or MR images can also be used to assess the alignment at the distal radioulnar joint (Figure 25-4) and are often more accurate than radiographs, particularly for subtle subluxation of the ulna. The subluxation may not be evident without comparison images with the hand in neutral, pronated, and supinated positions. The range of wrist motion must be tested to discover malalignments that are transient and position dependent. Other than ulnar-positive variance, the relationship of the distal ulna and radius at the joint appears normal in the test images. Thus, subluxation of this joint is not a likely diagnosis.

On coronal MR images of the wrist, the normal scapholunate interosseous ligament is a low-intensity band that connects the proximal aspects of the lunate and scaphoid bones (Figure 25-6). The MR signs of a scapholunate ligament abnormality are discontinuity of the ligament; distorted ligament morphology with fraying, thinning, and irregularity; complete absence of the ligament; elongation of the ligament; and a wide scapholunate joint space (Figure 25-7). The scapholunate ligament may become stretched to 200% of its normal length without losing continuity (Figure 25-8). Clinically, this has the same importance as a disrupted lig-

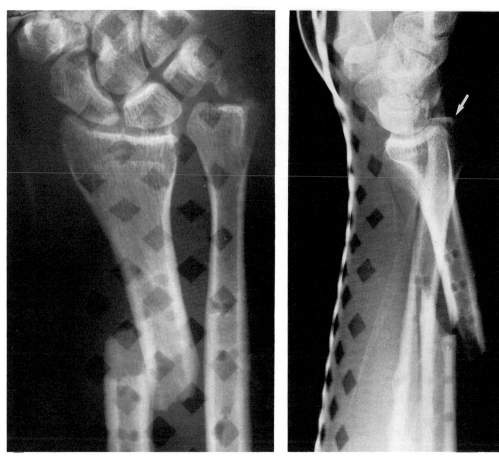

A

Figure 25-5. Distal radioulnar joint dislocation associated with radial fracture. (A) An anteroposterior radiograph of the wrist shows an abnormally long ulna relative to the radius with widening of the distal radioulnar joint. Both features are associated with a fracture of the distal radial shaft. (B) A lateral radiograph shows the dorsal position of the ulna (arrow) as a result of the disruption of the distal radioulnar joint, which occurred in conjunction with the radial fracture (Galeazzi fracture).

ament. With arthroscopy as the standard of reference, Zlatkin et al. reported that MRI was 86% sensitive and 100% specific in the detection of scapholunate ligament tears. When compared with wrist arthrography, MRI had a sensitivity of 93% and specificity of 89% in evaluation of these tears. The MR images of the wrist in the test patient demonstrate an intact scapholunate interosseous ligament. Thus, a tear of this ligament (Option (E)) is unlikely.

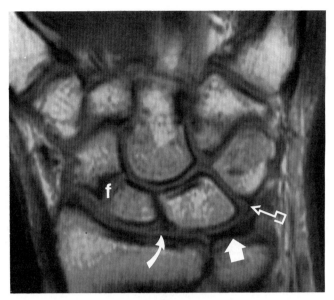

SE 600/20

Figure 25-6. Normal intercarpal ligaments of the wrist. A coronal T1-weighted image in a patient with an ununited scaphoid fracture (f) shows the scapholunate ligament as a low-intensity band bridging the proximal aspects of the scaphoid and lunate bones (curved arrow). There is a similar-appearing low-intensity structure representing the lunotriquetral ligament (open arrow). The biconcave low-intensity triangular fibrocartilage (solid arrow) is interposed between the ulna and the carpal bones and attaches to the articular cartilage on the ulnar aspect of the radius and to the ulnar styloid process.

The ulnolunate impaction or abutment syndrome is the result of chronic mechanical impingement of the ulna upon the lunate. This condition occurs in association with ulnar-positive variance. The juxtaposed lunate articular cartilage is affected by the chronic stress and becomes softened and fibrillated and hence degenerates prematurely. Additionally, the abnormal alignment results in increased stress on the triangular fibrocartilage, causing thinning and ultimately tears within the substance of the fibrocartilage (Figure 25-9).

Radiographs show the ulnar-positive variance and may also reveal sclerosis and subchondral cyst formation in the adjacent ulna and lunate. MRI simultaneously shows the osseous and soft tissue abnormalities associated with this condition and does so earlier than other imaging techniques do. All these soft tissue and osseous abnormalities lead to ulnar-sided wrist pain. Patients with symptoms that do not respond to

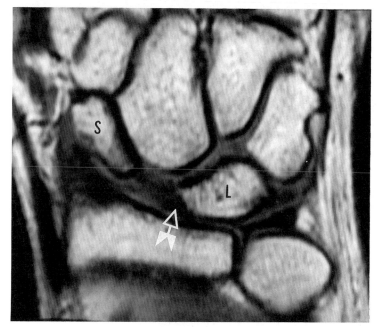

SE 600/20

Figure 25-7. Scapholunate ligament tear. A coronal T1-weighted MR image shows disruption of the scapholunate ligament with a portion of the ligament still attached to the lunate (arrow). There is a wide gap between the two bones. Note the normal triangular fibrocartilage interposed between lunate and ulna. S = scaphoid; L = lunate.

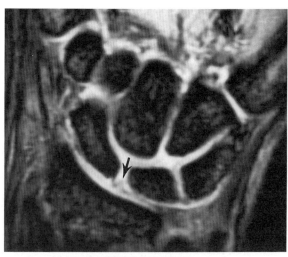

GRE 385/20/30°

Figure 25-8. Stretched scapholunate ligament. A coronal gradient-echo MR image shows a wavy, redundant scapholunate ligament (arrow), which is stretched but not torn. The scapholunate joint space is widened.

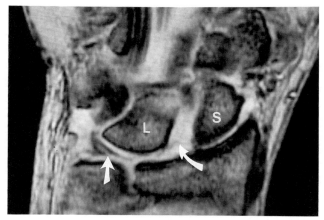

GRE 350/20/30°

Figure 25-9. Large scapholunate ligament tear with partial triangular fibrocartilage tear. A coronal gradient-echo MR image of the wrist shows a ruptured scapholunate ligament with a thin, frayed, and indistinct fragment attached to the lunate (curved arrow). The scapholunate space is abnormally wide. The oblique high-intensity line in the medial aspect of the triangular fibrocartilage extending to its proximal surface (straight arrow) represents a partial tear. L = lunate; S = scaphoid.

conservative management may require a surgical ulnar shortening procedure for relief of their symptoms.

Question 111

MRI of the wrist is a sensitive method for detecting:

    (A) Kienböck's disease
    (B) radiographically occult fractures
    (C) triangular fibrocartilage tears
    (D) deQuervain's tenosynovitis
    (E) chondrocalcinosis

    MRI of the wrist has significantly altered the diagnostic workup of wrist pain of undetermined cause in many institutions. Many physicians have accepted wrist MRI as the imaging technique of choice following conventional radiographs if a diagnosis remains in doubt or if a patient does not respond to conservative therapy. One basis for this approach is that MRI provides a global evaluation of all structures of the wrist, both osseous and soft tissue, in a single noninvasive examination. Another basis is that MRI may solve diagnostic dilemmas that previously would have required several different imaging studies (arthrography, bone scintigraphy, CT, etc.) that cumulatively cost considerably more than an MR examination.

Kienböck's disease (osteonecrosis of the lunate) is an uncommon entity of uncertain etiology. Patients are typically men between 20 and 40 years of age who experience pain over the dorsal surface of the wrist. Patients with advanced disease may have decreased wrist motion and grip strength.

Potential explanations for lunate osteonecrosis include traumatic interruption of blood supply, commonly from unnoticed or chronic repetitive minor trauma or an increase in the axial-loading forces transmitted across the lunate. With a normal relationship between the radius and ulna, 80% of axial-loading forces across the wrist are transmitted to the radius by way of the capitate and lunate and 20% of forces are transmitted to the ulna. When the distal ulna is located proximal to the distal radius (ulnar-minus variance), nearly all the axial-loading force across the wrist is borne by the radial side. In addition, the radial side of the wrist is less compliant than the ulnar side because the ulna is covered by the triangular fibrocartilage, which acts as a cushion or shock absorber. These alterations in force distribution and rigidity may explain the association of Kienböck's disease with ulnar-minus variance. Indeed, 80% of patients with Kienböck's disease also have an ulnar-minus variance. However, the percentage of individuals with ulnar-minus variance who also have Kienböck's disease of the lunate is much smaller.

The appearance of osteonecrosis of the lunate on the various imaging studies depends on the point in the course of the condition when the particular imaging study is obtained. Early in the disease process, conventional radiographs are normal. Scintigraphy may show increased radiotracer uptake. MRI is also highly sensitive in the diagnosis of early osteonecrosis of the lunate. Additionally, it can delineate the extent of bone involvement **(Option (A) is true).** Decreased bone marrow signal intensity on T1-weighted images and high signal intensity on T2-weighted images in all or a portion of the lunate bone marrow are the earliest changes detected by MRI (Figure 25-10).

Later in the course of osteonecrosis, conventional radiography shows increased bone density of the lunate and eventually loss of volume secondary to fracture and collapse of the bone (Figure 25-11). Collapse of the lunate results in premature degenerative changes involving the surrounding carpal joints. It is important to diagnose lunate osteonecrosis early so that treatment can be instituted in an effort to prevent structural changes.

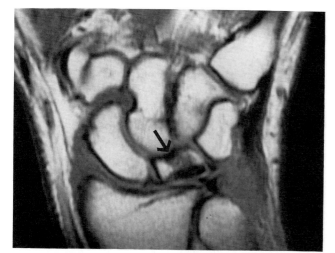

SE 600/20

Figure 25-10 (left). Kienböck's disease. A coronal T1-weighted MR image of the wrist shows abnormally low intensity bone marrow in a portion of the lunate (arrow). The ulna is short relative to the radius.

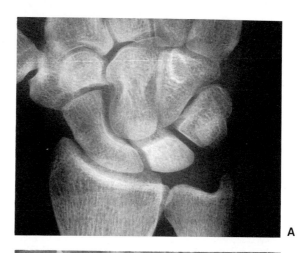

A

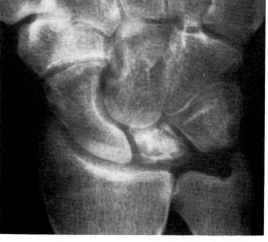

B

Figure 25-11 (right). Kienböck's disease. (A) A posteroanterior radiograph shows slightly increased bone density of the entire lunate. (B) One year later there are fractures and partial collapse of the lunate. Disuse osteoporosis is present, with the exception of the persistently dense lunate.

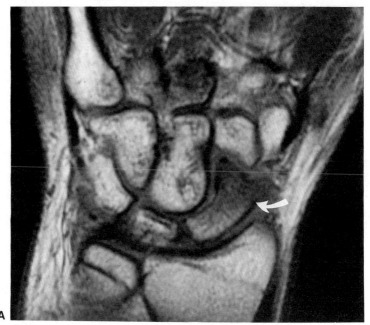

SE 600/20

Figure 25-12. Scaphoid bone marrow contusion. This patient had persistent wrist pain following trauma. Coventional radiographs were normal. (A) A coronal T1-weighted MR image shows focal low-intensity bone marrow (arrow) in the distal half of the scaphoid bone. (B) The corresponding gradient-echo image shows a corresponding high-intensity area (arrow). This focal bone marrow abnormality is considered a contusion (presumably a combination of subtle trabecular fractures, local hemorrhage, and reactive bone marrow edema).

Carpal fractures are usually detected by conventional radiography. However, stress and insufficiency fractures, nondisplaced fractures, and contusions may be very subtle or completely occult on a radiograph. MRI is an excellent imaging tool for detection of nondisplaced or occult carpal fractures because of its ability to image bone marrow directly in a tomographic fashion and its great sensitivity to physical and chemical changes in tissues that are displayed as contrast differences **(Option (B) is true).** Carpal fractures not detected on conventional radiographs but revealed by MRI may be bone marrow contusions, stress fractures, or occult linear fractures.

Bone marrow contusions manifest as focal areas of abnormal signal intensity within the bone marrow, presumably reflecting a combination of edema and trabecular microfractures associated with bone marrow

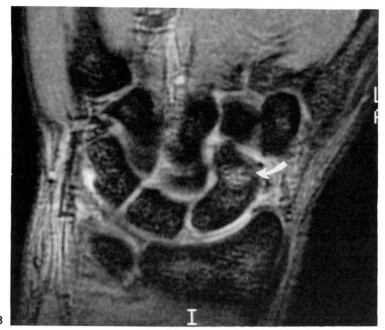

B

GRE 350/20/30°

hemorrhage (Figure 25-12). Stress fractures and linear occult fractures are manifested as lines of abnormal signal intensity that traverse the bone marrow (Figure 25-13). Typically, contusions, stress, and linear fractures exhibit low signal intensity on T1-weighted images and high signal intensity on T2-weighted images. The degree of signal intensity abnormality depends on the severity of the injury and the interval since the injury occurred. Signal intensity alterations peak during the healing process, and the marrow pattern eventually returns to normal.

CT cannot diagnose bone marrow contusions. It is an excellent method of diagnosing linear occult fractures, but if the fracture is oriented within the same plane as the CT section, it may be impossible to detect. Bone scintigraphy can detect radiographically occult fractures with a sensitivity comparable to that of MRI. However, bone scintigraphy has relative disadvantages. Scintigrams are occasionally falsely negative during the first 72 hours after the fracture, and the anatomic definition may be insufficient for a specific diagnosis. Both bone scintigraphy and CT are much less effective at demonstration of nonosseous (tendon, ligament, cartilage) abnormalities than is MRI. These associated injuries may account for some of the patient's symptoms after trauma.

The triangular fibrocartilage complex is a composite structure consisting of the triangular fibrocartilage, the dorsal and volar radioulnar

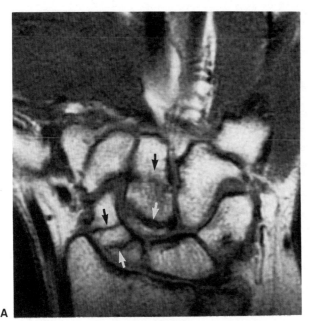

SE 600/20

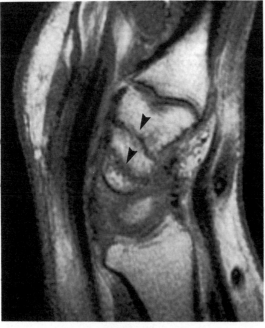

SE 600/20

Figure 25-13. Occult linear fractures of the capitate and scaphoid. This patient had wrist pain following significant trauma. Conventional radiographs were normal. (A) A coronal T1-weighted MR image of the wrist shows two nondisplaced linear fractures of the scaphoid and another two fractures of the capitate (arrows). (B) A sagittal T1-weighted MR image provides additional definition of the two capitate fractures (arrowheads).

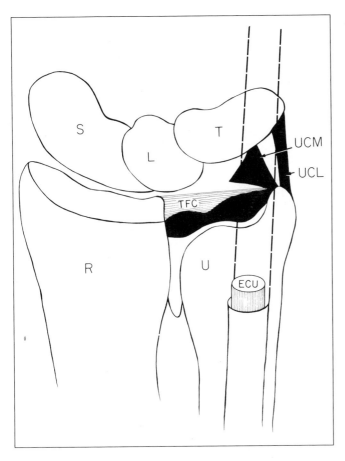

Figure 25-14. Triangular fibrocartilage complex. The stability of the distal radioulnar joint and the ulnar side of the wrist is maintained by the triangular fibrocartilage complex, which is composed of the following: triangular fibrocartilage (TFC), dorsal and palmar radioulnar ligaments (not shown), the ulnar collateral ligament (UCL), ulnocarpal meniscus (UCM), and the fibrous sheath of the extensor carpi ulnaris tendon (dashed lines). S = scaphoid; L = lunate; T = triquetrum; R = radius; U = ulna; ECU = extensor carpi ulnaris tendon.

ligaments, the ulnar collateral ligament, the ulnocarpal meniscus, and the sheath for the extensor carpi ulnaris tendon (Figure 25-14). The complex is the primary stabilizer of the distal radioulnar joint and the ulnar side of the wrist. The triangular fibrocartilage has a relatively thin central zone surrounded by thicker peripheral margins, which are referred to as the dorsal and volar radioulnar ligaments. These ligaments in turn blend with the volar and dorsal capsule of the distal radioulnar joint. The triangular fibrocartilage is attached laterally to the ulnar aspect of the distal radius and medially to the ulnar styloid process.

MRI depicts the triangular fibrocartilage as a biconcave, triangular structure very similar in appearance to the disk of the temporomandibular joint. It has homogeneously low signal intensity on all MR pulse sequences. A thin margin of articular hyaline cartilage is present at the attachment of the triangular fibrocartilage to the medial aspect of the radius, and this hyaline cartilage appears as a linear area of higher sig-

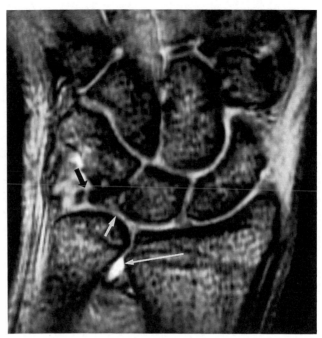

GRE 350/20/30°

Figure 25-15. Peripheral and central triangular fibrocartilage tears. A gradient-echo coronal MR image of the wrist shows a vertical complete tear at the periphery of the triangular fibrocartilage manifested as a high-intensity line (black arrow). A degenerative-type central perforation is also present (short white arrow). Fluid in the distal radioulnar joint (long white arrow) is a secondary sign of a triangular fibrocartilage tear.

nal intensity precisely where the fibrocartilage attaches to the radius. This feature should not be mistaken for a tear or detachment of the fibrocartilage.

Most triangular fibrocartilage tears or perforations occur in the central region of the fibrocartilage and are degenerative. The prevalence of triangular fibrocartilage tears or perforations increases with age, being almost universal after age 50. Degenerative tears are often asymptomatic. Conversely, acute traumatic tears of the fibrocartilage are typically peripheral and are associated with pain. MR criteria for triangular fibrocartilage tears are similar to those used to evaluate menisci in the knee. Linear areas of higher signal intensity within the low-intensity triangular fibrocartilage that extend to a surface, abnormal morphology, and focal areas of discontinuity are all MR features of triangular fibrocartilage tears (Figures 25-15 and 25-16). A common secondary sign of a triangular fibrocartilage tear is the presence of fluid in the distal radioul-

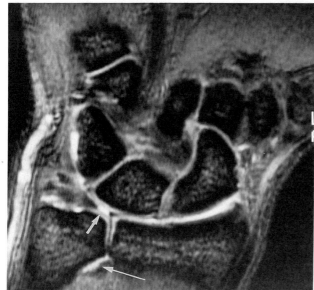

Figure 25-16.
Central triangular fibrocartilage tear. A gradient-echo coronal MR image of the wrist shows a tear through the central thin portion of triangular fibrocartilage. Note that high-intensity fluid fills the hole (short arrow). Fluid is also present in the distal radioulnar joint (long arrow).

GRE 350/20/30°

nar joint. In the series by Zlatkin et al., MRI was shown to be 100% sensitive and 89% specific for detection of tears when compared with arthrography as the standard of reference. MRI also compared favorably with surgery as the standard method of documenting tears, with sensitivities and specificities over 90% **(Option (C) is true).**

MRI can demonstrate abnormalities involving the flexor and extensor tendons as they pass along the volar and dorsal surfaces of the wrist. Tendons are normally low-intensity structures on all pulse sequences. Inflammation or trauma can alter the morphology of the tendon or cause abnormally increased signal intensity within the substance of a tendon or in the fat surrounding tendons. Tenosynovitis refers to inflammation of the tendon sheath and manifests as fluid surrounding the tendon on MRI. Tendinitis or partial tendon tears cause enlargement, thinning, or irregularity of the involved tendon with or without associated abnormal signal intensity within the tendon.

Tendinitis or tenosynovitis affecting the abductor pollicis longus and extensor pollicis brevis tendons is known as deQuervain's stenosing tenosynovitis or deQuervain's syndrome and is easily detected by MRI **(Option (D) is true).** These tendons occupy the first extensor compartment and pass through a restrictive fibro-osseous tunnel at the level of the radial styloid. The tendons may become inflamed. Any small amount of swelling of the tendons or their sheaths causes the restrictive tunnel

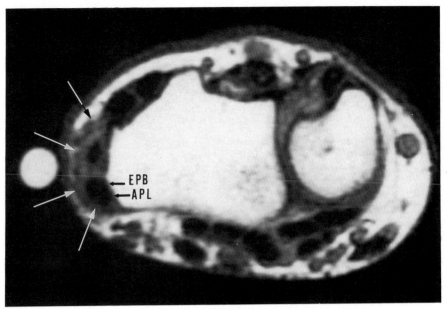

SE 600/20

Figure 25-17. deQuervain's stenosing tenosynovitis. A recently post-partum woman had a small mass and severe pain over the radial styloid process. A T1-weighted transaxial MR image shows tendons traversing the wrist as low-intensity oval structures imaged in cross section. Normal high-intensity subcutaneous fat has been replaced by intermediate-intensity inflammatory swelling (arrows) over the radial styloid and surrounding the underlying extensor pollicis brevis (EPB) and abductor pollicis longus (APL) tendons. The circular high-intensity structure extrinsic to the wrist is a marker to localize the region of the patient's symptoms.

to become constrictive, resulting in pain. The pain that occurs with thumb movement and over the radial aspect of the wrist may be difficult to distinguish clinically from degenerative joint disease in the wrist.

deQuervain's syndrome occurs most commonly in young women during their third trimester of pregnancy or during lactation, but it usually regresses spontaneously with cessation of lactation. Repetitive occupational trauma is another common cause. MRI may show abnormal size or signal intensity of the affected tendons, fluid surrounding the tendons, or no abnormality. Often the only MR finding is obliteration of the high-intensity fat surrounding the tendons (Figure 25-17).

Chondrocalcinosis results from deposition of calcium pyrophosphate dihydrate or calcium hydroxyapatite crystals in hyaline and fibrous cartilage. It is most commonly due to calcium pyrophosphate dihydrate crystal deposition, which is usually idiopathic or associated with hyperparathyroidism or hemochromatosis, adult hypophosphatasia, or other rarer conditions. In the wrist, chondrocalcinosis most commonly occurs in the triangular fibrocartilage and is recognized on conventional radiographs as linear calcification running horizontally in the space between the ulna and the carpus. If MRI can detect chondrocalcinosis at all, the crystal will appear as tiny foci of very low signal intensity similar to cortical bone. The triangular fibrocartilage is normally a low-intensity structure, and so it is not surprising that MRI is very insensitive for the detection of superimposed low-intensity calcification **(Option (E) is false).**

Question 112

Concerning ulnar variance,

(A) positive variance is associated with triangular fibrocartilage tears
(B) negative variance is associated with Kienböck's disease
(C) its assessment is not influenced by wrist positioning during radiography
(D) both proximal and distal radial fractures are associated with positive variance
(E) with a normal relationship between the distal ulna and radius, 50% of the axial-loading forces pass through the radial side of the wrist

Ulnar variance refers to the position of the distal ulna relative to the distal radius (Figure 25-18). Neutral-ulnar variance is the normal situation, in which the distal articular surfaces of the radius and ulna are perfectly aligned. A small amount of variation is permitted, but the ulna should be no more than 2 mm proximal to the radius. Positive and negative variances indicate more distal or more proximal positions, respectively, of the ulna.

The relationship of the distal ulna and radius, and thus the determination of ulnar variance, is influenced by the position of the forearm during radiography **(Option (C) is false).** Relative to the radius, the ulna moves distally with pronation and proximally with supination. Variance is determined by using the standard posteroanterior wrist radiograph with full pronation. Neutral variance refers to the normal orientation of these two bones on a pronated posteroanterior radiograph in which the distalmost cortex of the head of the ulna lies 0 to 2 mm proximal to the distal surface of the radius at the radioulnar joint. Ulnar-positive or ulnar-plus variance is present when the distal ulna projects beyond the distal radius; ulnar-negative or ulnar-minus variance is noted when the ulna is more than 2 mm shorter than the adjacent radius. The determi-

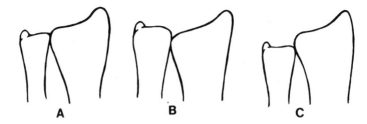

Figure 25-18. Ulnar variance. (A) Neutral-ulnar variance refers to the normal orientation of the distal radius and ulna. The distal ulna is aligned with the distal radial articular surface or is no more than 2 mm proximal to it. Positive variance (B) and negative variance (C) correspond to situations in which the ulna is relatively long or short, respectively, relative to the distal radius.

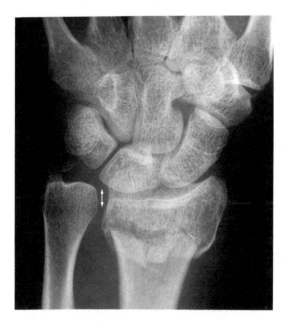

Figure 25-19. Posttraumatic ulnar-positive variance. A posteroanterior wrist radiograph demonstrates Colles-type distal radial and ulnar styloid fractures. Positive-ulnar variance has resulted from impaction at the radial fracture site, with relative shortening of the radius compared with the ulna (double-headed arrow).

nation of variance is important because the relative position of the distal ulna has been implicated in certain disorders of the wrist.

Normally there is an asymmetric distribution of the axial-loading force across the wrist, with the radius and ulna receiving 80 and 20% of the force, respectively **(Option (E) is false).** A relatively short ulna, ulnar-negative variance, alters the distribution of this force, which may explain its association with Kienböck's disease **(Option (B) is true).** A relatively long ulna, ulnar-positive variance, is frequently associated with triangular fibrocartilage tears and the ulnolunate impaction syndrome **(Option (A) is true).** Fractures of the radius or ulna may also disrupt the normal neutral variance of the distal articular surfaces.

Fractures involving the distal or proximal radius associated with some component of impaction or fragment overlap may heal in such a fashion that the radius is shortened and the ulna is relatively long. This posttraumatic ulnar-positive variance may exhibit all the sequelae of idiopathic ulnar-positive variance **(Option (D) is true).** The degree of ulnar variance is an important feature to note during assessment and follow-up of the common distal radial fracture (Figure 25-19).

Craig W. Walker, M.D.
Phoebe A. Kaplan, M.D.

SUGGESTED READINGS

ULNOLUNATE IMPACTION SYNDROME

1. Bowers WH. The distal radioulnar joint. In: Green DP (ed), Operative hand surgery, 2nd ed. New York: Churchill Livingstone; 1988:939–989
2. Taleisnik J. Pain on the ulnar side of the wrist. Hand Clin 1987:51–69

KIENBÖCK'S DISEASE

3. Koenig H, Lucas D, Meissner R. The wrist: a preliminary report on high-resolution MR imaging. Radiology 1986; 160:463–467
4. Reinus WR, Conway WF, Totty WG, et al. Carpal avascular necrosis: MR imaging. Radiology 1986; 160:689–693

ULNAR VARIANCE

5. Epner RA, Bowers WH, Guilford WB. Ulnar variance—the effect of wrist positioning and roentgen filming techniques. J Hand Surg (Am) 1982; 7:298–305
6. Palmer AK, Glisson RR, Werner FW. Ulnar variance determination. J Hand Surg (Am) 1982; 7:376–379

DISTAL RADIOULNAR SUBLUXATION/DISLOCATION

7. Space TC, Louis DS, Francis I, Braunstein EM. CT findings in distal radioulnar dislocation. J Comput Assist Tomogr 1986; 10:689–690
8. Wechsler RJ, Wehbe MA, Ritkin MD, Edeiken J, Branch HM. Computed tomography diagnosis of distal radioulnar subluxation. Skeletal Radiol 1987; 16:1–5

FIBROCARTILAGE AND LIGAMENT TEARS

9. Golimbu CN, Firooznia H, Melone CP Jr, Rafii M, Weinreb J, Leber C. Tears of the triangular fibrocartilage of the wrist: MR imaging. Radiology 1989; 173:731–733
10. Kang HS, Kindynis P, Brahme SK, et al. Triangular fibrocartilage and intercarpal ligaments of the wrist: MR imaging. Cadaveric study with gross pathologic and histologic correlation. Radiology 1991; 181:401–404
11. Zlatkin MB, Chao PC, Osterman AL, Schnall MD, Dalinka MK, Kressel HY. Chronic wrist pain: evaluation with high-resolution MR imaging. Radiology 1989; 173:723–729

GENERAL

12. Reicher MA, Kellerhouse LE (eds). MRI of the wrist and hand. New York: Raven Press; 1990:107–127

Notes

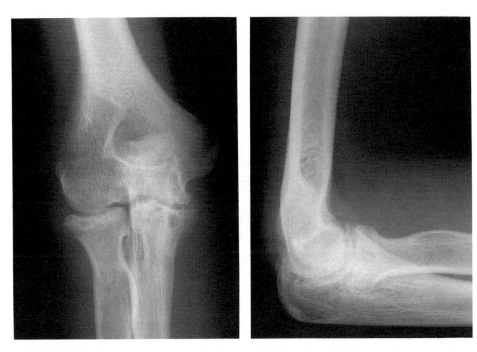

Figure 26-1. This 24-year-old man with human immunodeficiency virus infection has elbow pain. You are shown anteroposterior and lateral radiographs.

Case 26: Hemophilia

Question 113

Which *one* of the following is the MOST likely diagnosis?

(A) Rheumatoid arthritis
(B) Gout
(C) Pigmented villonodular synovitis
(D) Hemophilia
(E) HIV arthropathy

The anteroposterior and lateral radiographs of the elbow joint show evidence of arthritis (Figure 26-1). The specific radiographic findings include displacement of the anterior and posterior elbow fat pads by radiodense synovitis and perhaps an associated joint effusion; nonuniform joint space narrowing; irregular subchondral surfaces; and subchondral cysts and erosions (Figure 26-2). There is slight periarticular osteopenia on the humeral side, and the radial head is mildly enlarged. These radiographic features indicate a chronic arthropathy secondary to recurrent or unresolved hemarthrosis. In a 24-year-old man, the most likely diagnosis is hemophilia **(Option (D) is correct).** The patient's infection with human immunodeficiency virus (HIV) can be surmised to represent a complication of treatment for hemophilia.

Rheumatoid arthritis (Option (A)) and chronic juvenile arthritis are important considerations in the differential diagnosis, but the elbow joint is an infrequent site of involvement, joint space narrowing typically would be diffuse and uniform, and radiodense synovium would not be a feature. Joint space narrowing is usually uniform in patients with rheumatoid arthritis because the diffuse pannus formation and the presence of proteolytic enzymes act globally throughout an involved joint.

Idiopathic gout (Option (B)) is a disease of adult men (20:1 male preponderance). The specific radiographic changes, which include eccentric focal soft tissue density nodules or masses (tophi) (Figure 26-3), usually become apparent 6 to 10 years after symptoms begin. The characteristic bony lesions seen in patients with chronic gout are well-defined para-

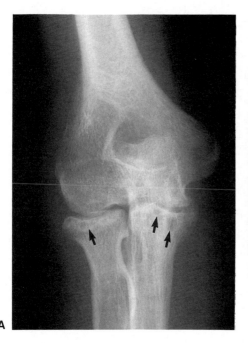
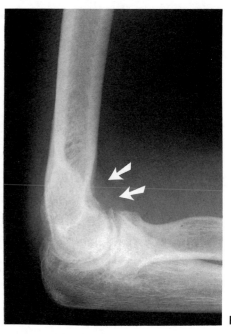

A

B

Figure 26-2 (Same as Figure 26-1).   Hemophilia. An anteroposterior radiograph of the elbow (A) shows mild osteopenia of humeral condyles, nonuniform cartilage loss, and small subchondral lucencies (arrows). A lateral radiograph (B) shows radiolucent elbow fat pad displacement and underlying dense synovium (arrows).

articular erosions with sclerotic margins and overhanging edges. The joint involvement is asymmetric and polyarticular. The joint space thickness is often preserved until secondary degenerative arthritis occurs. The clinical history and age of the test patient, the absence of soft tissue mass, and the articular surface erosive pattern do not favor gout as the most likely diagnosis.

Pigmented villonodular synovitis (PVNS) (Option (C)) occurs most frequently in the third and fourth decades of life. Most cases involve the knee. The most frequent radiographic manifestation is soft tissue swelling as a result of a combination of joint effusion and hypertrophic synovial mass. Other radiographic features include multiple subchondral osseous pressure erosions and, in later stages, nonuniform joint space narrowing. Osseous pressure erosions are present in about 85% of joints, other than the knee, affected by PVNS. Because the joint is capacious and decompresses into the suprapatellar bursa, pressure erosions occur in only about 25% of knees with PVNS. The site of involvement and the absence of pressure erosions do not favor the diagnosis of PVNS.

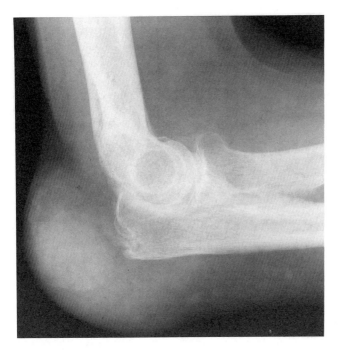

Figure 26-3. Gout. A lateral radiograph of the elbow shows a partially calcified nodular soft tissue mass of the olecranon bursa. Small spurs are present at the triceps tendon insertion on the olecranon.

Although the test patient is HIV positive, HIV arthropathy (Option (E)) is an unlikely diagnosis. Arthritic abnormalities in HIV-positive patients have radiologic features of a seronegative arthropathy, predominantly affect the lower extremity joints, and are often associated with extensive periostitis. These characteristics are absent in the test patient.

Question 114

Concerning pigmented villonodular synovitis,

    (A) the affected synovium has low signal intensity on MR images
    (B) the combination of bone erosions and intact joint space is a characteristic radiographic appearance
    (C) polyarticular involvement is the rule
    (D) bone erosions are found in about 50% of affected elbow joints
    (E) the elbow is the most commonly involved joint

PVNS is a disease of unknown origin that arises in synovium-lined joints, tendon sheaths, and bursae. It has both diffuse and localized forms. Histologically, the villous or nodular changes of the thickened synovium are highly vascular and are characterized by a fibrous stroma containing variable numbers of histiocytic epithelioid cells, giant cells, xanthoma cells, and focal areas of hemosiderin deposition. The histologic variability has resulted in many terms for this entity, particularly in its localized form, including giant cell tumor, xanthoma, and fibroxanthoma. The diffuse form of PVNS is most commonly found in joints. The focal nodular form occurs only occasionally in joints; however, it is the most common pattern encountered in extra-articular locations such as tendon sheaths (Figure 26-4).

PVNS of a joint is almost invariably monoarticular **(Option (C) is false)**. It most frequently involves the knee joint (60 to 80% of cases), followed by the hip, ankle, and shoulder joints. The elbow is an unusual site for diffuse PVNS **(Option (E) is false)**.

The characteristic radiographic features of PVNS are soft tissue swelling, bone erosions, preservation of joint space thickness, and absence of focal osteopenia **(Option (B) is true)** (Figure 26-5A). More than half of all involved joints have multiple subchondral lytic lesions and pressure erosions of intracapsular cortices, yet they maintain an intact joint space thickness. Later, as the disease progresses, nonuniform joint space narrowing may develop. In small-capacity joints such as the elbow joint, osseous lytic lesions and cortical erosions are an early and more common feature than they are in the knee joint and are seen in about 85% of cases **(Option (D) is false)**.

Aspirated joint fluid classically appears "rusty" or brown tinged. The fluid is typically serosanguinous, and clinical chemistry reveals elevated cholesterol levels. Opacification of the joint for arthrography demonstrates distension of the joint capsule by multiple lobulated soft tissue masses of variable shape and size (Figure 26-5B).

The tendency of PVNS to cause recurrent bleeding results in deposition of hemosiderin in the synovial masses; this is a characteristic histo-

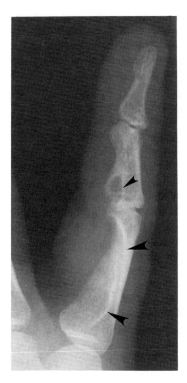

Figure 26-4. Focal nodular pigmented villonodular synovitis (giant cell tumor of tendon sheath). An oblique radiograph of the index finger shows a soft tissue mass causing cortical erosion (arrowheads) of the proximal and middle phalanges.

pathologic feature. The hemosiderin deposits are detected as areas of decreased signal intensity on both T1- and T2-weighted MR images **(Option (A) is true)** (Figure 26-6). However, any intra-articular tumor may contain hemosiderin deposits as a result of intralesional hemorrhage; therefore, synovial biopsy is required for a definitive diagnosis of a joint mass.

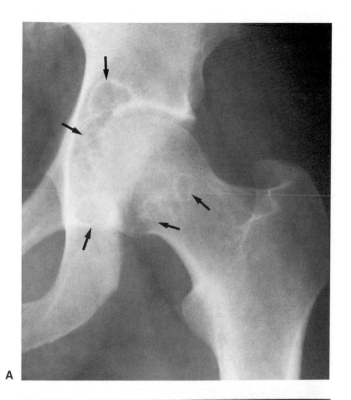

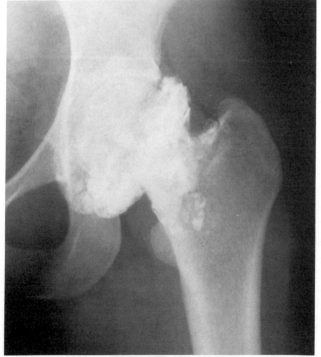

Figure 26-5. Pigmental villonodular synovitis. (A) An anteroposterior radiograph of the left hip shows erosions of the acetabulum and femoral head-neck junction (arrows) with preservation of a normal joint space. (B) A hip arthrogram shows nodular intra-articular masses in the contrast-filled joint.

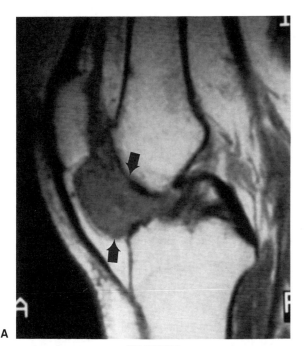

A

SE 600/20

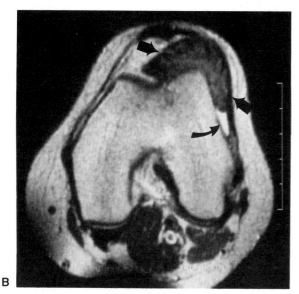

B

SE 2,000/80

Figure 26-6. Pigmented villonodular synovitis. (A) A sagittal T1-weighted MR image shows a low-intensity intra-articular soft tissue mass inferior to the patella (arrows). (B) An axial T2-weighted MR image also shows the mass (arrows) to be of low intensity and demonstrates high-intensity joint effusion (arrowhead).

Question 115

Concerning the elbow,

    (A) hemophilia affects the elbow more commonly than does juvenile chronic arthritis

    (B) degenerative joint disease of the elbow is usually idiopathic

    (C) degenerative arthritic abnormalities of the elbow joint in a young man suggest the possibility of AIDS

    (D) golfer's elbow, tennis elbow, and Little Leaguer's elbow are all the same entity

    (E) the distal tendon of the brachialis muscle is the most commonly ruptured tendon about the elbow

The elbow joint actually consists of three different articulations. The ulnohumeral and radiohumeral articulations form hinge joints for flexion and extension of the elbow; the proximal radioulnar joint allows supination and pronation of the forearm. Being a hinge articulation, without weight-bearing stresses, the elbow is not commonly involved with idiopathic degenerative joint disease **(Option (B) is false).**

Degenerative joint disease of the elbow is commonly caused by previous trauma. Old trauma is often obvious because deformities are evident where fractures have healed. Traumatic osteochondral or chondral fracture may lead to degenerative joint disease with intra-articular loose bodies (Figure 26-7); the latter is particularly common in those who pitch or throw. Less likely etiologies to be considered in elbows with a general appearance of degenerative joint disease are neuropathic joint disease or calcium pyrophosphate dihydrate (CPPD) crystal deposition disease. Chronic, repetitive, unnoticed trauma from loss of proprioception and sensation can lead to a neuropathic joint with destruction, fragmentation, subluxation, and disorganization of the joint. A neuropathic joint anywhere in the upper extremity is most likely to be secondary to syringomyelia. CPPD arthropathy generally manifests with chondrocalcinosis superimposed on the degenerative process.

Inflammatory arthritides, gout, septic arthritis, and hemophilia are the most likely causes of elbow arthropathy other than degenerative joint disease. Inflammatory arthritis and septic arthritis have radiographic features similar to one another and are easily distinguishable from degenerative arthritis. Degenerative joint disease causes cartilage destruction, osteophytes, loose bodies, subchondral sclerosis, and cysts, whereas inflammatory arthritides cause osteoporosis, diffuse uniform joint space narrowing, marginal erosions that lead to diffuse erosions, subluxations, and joint effusion (Figure 26-8). Elbow joint involvement is more common in hemophilia than in juvenile chronic arthritis **(Option (A) is true).** The most common sites of involvement in hemophilia are

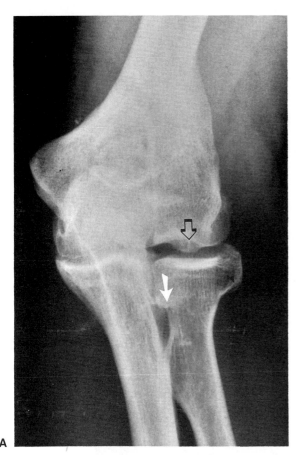

A

Figure 26-7. Degenerative joint disease with osteocartilaginous bodies in a 35-year-old male baseball enthusiast. Anteroposterior (A) and lateral (B) radiographs show osteophytes at the radial head-neck junction (arrowheads in panel B), irregularity of the articular surface of the capitellum (open arrow in panel A), and osteocartilaginous bodies (arrows in panels A and B). (C) A coronal T1-weighted MR image shows irregular capitellum (open arrows) from previous trauma, osteochondral fracture, and degenerative change. (D) A sagittal gradient-echo MR image through the humero-ulnar joint demonstrates many osteocartilaginous bodies (arrows) surrounded by joint effusion.

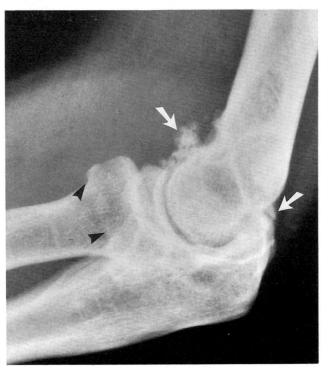

B

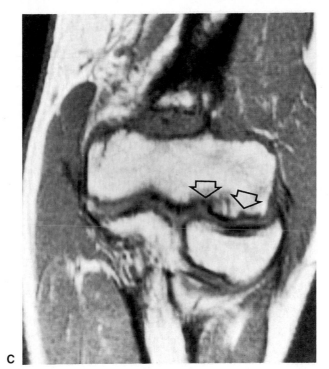

C

SE 600/20

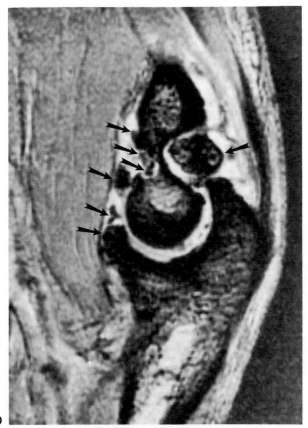

D

GRE 700/20/30°

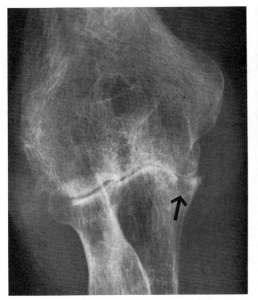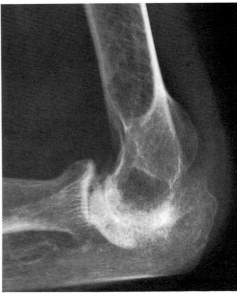

B

Figure 26-8. Rheumatoid arthritis. Anteroposterior (A) and lateral (B) radiographs show diffuse, uniform cartilage loss throughout the elbow joint with generalized osteopenia and marginal erosion (arrow in panel A), typical of inflammatory arthritis.

the knee, elbow, and ankle. In juvenile chronic arthritis, the hands, wrists, knees, and ankles are frequently involved. Both juvenile chronic arthritis and hemophilia may share similar radiographic features such as bulbous overgrowth of the epiphyses, osteoporosis, joint effusion, and cartilage loss.

Seronegative spondyloarthropathies infrequently affect the elbow. AIDS-related arthritis most commonly has features of a seronegative arthritis but usually affects the lower extremities rather than the elbow **(Option (C) is false).**

The elbow is often affected in patients with gout. Indeed, the most common cause of an olecranon bursitis is gout (Figure 26-9). Articular manifestations of gout in the elbow are similar to those in any other joint and consist of erosions of bone with overhanging edges, intact joint space, and soft tissue masses from tophi (urate crystal deposits); a swollen olecranon bursa is frequently noted.

The elbow joint is a frequent site of sport-related injury, often as a result of chronic, repetitive trauma. Golfer's elbow and tennis elbow both represent inflammation at the site of insertion of the common extensor tendon on the lateral epicondyle of the humerus. Radiographic features are usually absent; however, soft tissue swelling, calcification in the

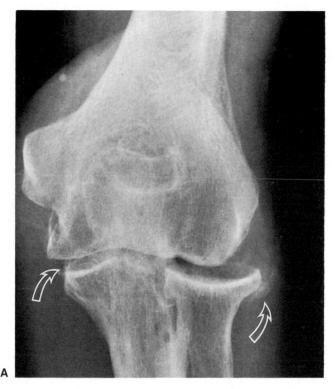

A

Figure 26-9. Calcium pyrophosphate dihydrate crystal deposition disease superimposed on gout. Anteroposterior (A) and lateral (B) radiographs of a 62-year-old man with elbow pain and swelling show calcification (open arrows) of synovium, cartilage, and triceps tendon. The marked soft tissue swelling over the dorsum of the elbow (solid arrow in panel B) is a manifestation of olecranon bursitis. The head of the radius is smoothly eroded and ventrally subluxed. Coronal T1-weighted (C) and gradient-echo (D) MR images show a large erosion of the trochlea secondary to a mass (straight arrow) with an overhanging edge (curved arrow) typical of gout. Other tophi with bone erosions were evident on other images. (E) An axial gradient-echo MR image shows both distension of the olecranon bursa by fluid (arrow) and the presence of a joint effusion (arrowheads). O = olecranon.

extensor tendon at its insertion on the lateral epicondyle, fragmentation of the lateral epicondyle, or bone marrow edema may be seen (Figures 26-10 and 26-11).

Unlike golfer's elbow and tennis elbow, Little Leaguer's elbow is secondary to valgus stress on the elbow during pitching, especially the pitching of curve balls **(Option (D) is false).** This throwing action places traction on the medial epicondyle by the common flexor tendon

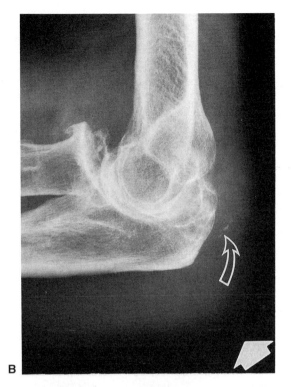

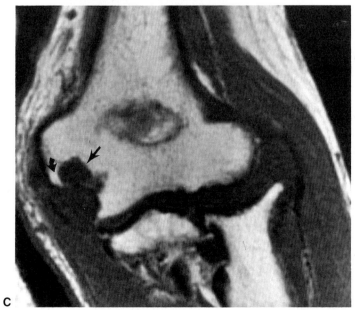

SE 600/20

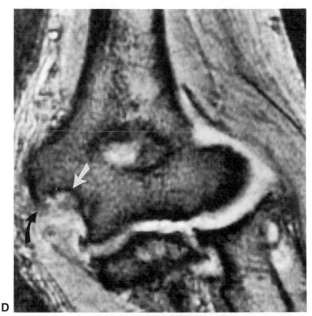

GRE 450/20/30°

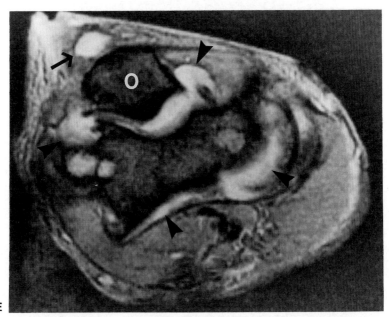

GRE 450/20/30°

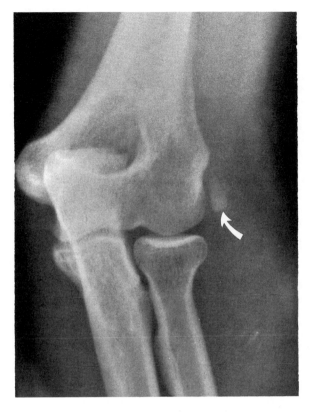

Figure 26-10. Tennis elbow. An anteroposterior radiograph shows calcification (arrow) at the site of insertion of the common extensor tendon on the lateral epicondyle.

and the ulnar collateral ligament, and this force can cause avulsion of the epicondyle. The avulsed medial epicondyle may be displaced by various amounts or may be trapped within the elbow joint between the trochlea and the ulna. Valgus forces on the elbow also cause compression of the lateral structures of the joint, which may lead to the other manifestations of Little Leaguer's elbow, especially osteochondral fractures and avascular necrosis of the capitellum (Figure 26-12). In the adult, traction spurs on the medial epicondyle may occur as a result of repetitive throwing.

The brachialis muscle is the major flexor of the forearm. It originates from the anterior aspect of the middle third of the humerus, crosses the elbow joint, and inserts onto a tuberosity of the ulna, distal to the coronoid process. The muscle belly of the brachialis extends all the way to its insertion, with its central tendon embedded within the muscle. In contrast, the two bellies of the biceps brachii muscle converge distally into a

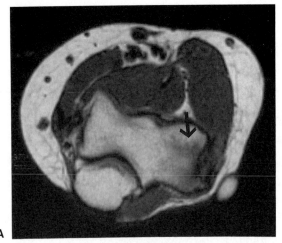

SE 600/20

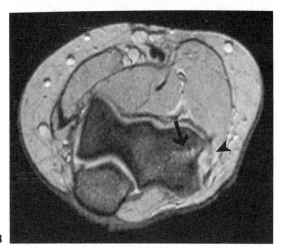

GRE 430/20/30°

Figure 26-11. Tennis elbow. (A) A transaxial T1-weighted MR image demonstrates low-intensity lateral epicondyle bone marrow (arrow) with adjacent soft tissue edema. (B) A transaxial gradient-echo (T2*) MR image confirms the presence of high-intensity bone marrow (arrow) and soft tissue edema (arrowhead).

flattended tendon that has no surrounding muscle in the region of the elbow (Figure 26-13). The distal biceps tendon is superficial to the brachialis muscle and inserts onto the radial tuberosity. The biceps tendon is more subject to rupture than is the brachialis tendon **(Option (E) is false)** (Figure 26-14). A biceps tendon rupture is associated with pain and tenderness at the radial tuberosity and loss of ability to contract the biceps muscle. If the rupture is not repaired, other muscles, particularly the brachialis, will assume most of the function of the biceps.

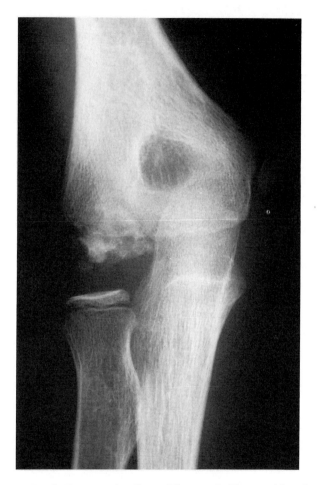

Figure 26-12. Little Leaguer's elbow. The capitellar ossification center is heterogeneously mineralized and shows evidence of fragmentation, features of osteochondral injury, and avascular necrosis.

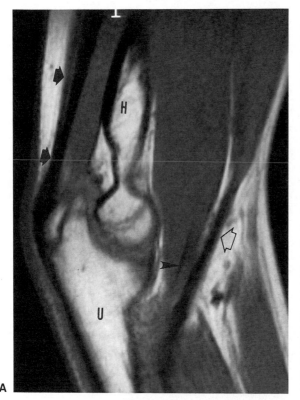

SE 600/20

Figure 26-13. Normal elbow anatomy. (A) T1-weighted sagittal MR image of the elbow in a child. The low-intensity central tendon of the brachialis (arrowhead) is embedded within the muscle belly. The distal biceps brachii tendon (open arrow) is located superficial to the brachialis muscle. The dorsal triceps tendon (solid arrows) inserts on the olecranon. (B) A T1-weighted transaxial MR image of the elbow depicts the low-intensity tendon of the brachialis (white arrow) and the more anterior biceps brachii tendon (curved black arrow). H = humerus; O = olecranon; U = ulna.

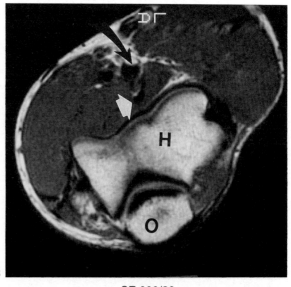

SE 600/20

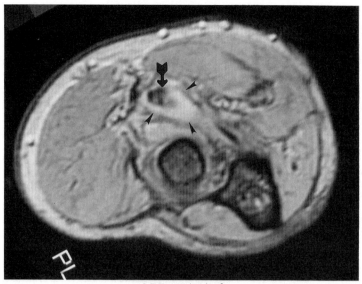

GRE 430/20/30°

Figure 26-14. Ruptured distal biceps tendon. A transaxial gradient-echo (T2*) MR image of the elbow shows an increase in the signal intensity of the biceps brachii tendon (arrow), indicative of a partial tendon tear at this level. On a more distal image, the tendon was completely absent; i.e., it was ruptured. High-intensity fluid (arrowheads) surrounds the abnormal tendon.

Question 116

Populations of patients with human immunodeficiency virus infection show an increased prevalence of:

(A) ankylosing spondylitis
(B) Reiter's syndrome
(C) psoriasis
(D) rheumatoid arthritis
(E) septic arthritis

HIV infection has been associated with various forms of arthritis. Reiter's syndrome, psoriatic arthritis, undifferentiated articular syndromes, polymyositis, vasculitis, or the sicca syndrome may herald the clinical onset of HIV infection or may develop in patients who already have a full-blown illness. Several studies have shown an increased prevalence of psoriasis, psoriatic arthropathy, and Reiter's syndrome in these

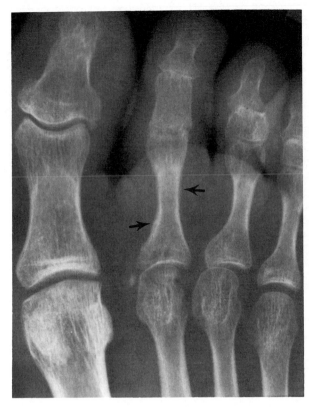

Figure 26-15. AIDS-related arthropathy. Cartilage destruction of the metatarsophalangeal and interphalangeal joints of the second toe, in association with fusiform soft tissue swelling, indicates an inflammatory arthritis in this 47-year-old man with AIDS. There is also subtle periosteal reaction along the shaft of the proximal phalanx (arrows) that is similar to that found in reactive arthropathies such as Reiter's syndrome and psoriatic arthropathy.

patients **(Options (B) and (C) are true).** Systemic opportunistic infections are highly prevalent during the course of HIV infection. However, septic joint involvement seldom occurs, despite the profound immunodeficiency **(Option (E) is false).**

HIV-associated arthritis is a relatively new diagnostic consideration for radiologists. Its radiographic presentation is that of an inflammatory arthropathy that may mimic either a seronegative arthritis or rheumatoid arthritis with proliferative periostitis (Figure 26-15). The seronegative-type arthritis has an asymmetric distribution and predominantly affects the lower extremities. Sites of involvement include the feet, ankles, knees, wrists, and hands. The axial skeleton is generally spared, but asymmetric sacroiliitis is occasionally found. There is no increased prevalence of ankylosing spondylitis in patients with HIV infection **(Option (A) is false).** Joint involvement consists of joint effusions, enthesopathy, periostitis, and bone erosions. Erosions usually occur at tendon insertion sites rather than at the margins of joints or in subchondral bone as would be expected of the typical inflammatory arthritides. Joint space narrowing is rare, but osteopenia is common and severe.

The other type of HIV-associated arthritis is an acute symmetric polyarthritis that resembles rheumatoid arthritis. In this form of HIV-associated arthritis, the upper extremities are more commonly and severely involved. The radiographic findings include soft tissue swelling, joint effusions, osteopenia, marginal erosions, joint space narrowing, and joint malalignment. Characteristic findings are the presence of proliferative bone formation and periostitis, which are not features of typical rheumatoid arthritis. Conventional rheumatoid arthritis shows no increased prevalence in patients with HIV infection **(Option (D) is false).** Of potential importance, rheumatoid arthritis is believed to require the interaction of helper-inducer T lymphocytes and B cells, whereas HIV infection is associated with loss of helper T-cell activity. These observations suggest that rheumatoid arthritis and HIV-associated inflammatory arthritis are two separate conditions.

Discussion

Hemophilia A (classic hemophilia) and hemophilia B (Christmas disease) are X-linked recessive disorders of blood coagulation. In classic hemophilia there is a plasma clotting-factor deficiency of factor VIII (antihemophiliac factor), and in Christmas disease (named after the first patient with the entity who was studied) there is a deficiency of factor IX (plasma thromboplastin component). Hemophilia manifests itself clinically almost exclusively in men and is genetically carried by women.

Recurrent bleeding is characteristic of hemophilia. Hemarthrosis is a very frequent feature of the disease and often occurs in the first decade of life. The most commonly affected joints are the knee, elbow, and ankle, in that order, but any joint can be involved. Acute hemarthrosis is manifested radiographically by distension of the joint capsule, as shown by displacement of periarticular fat planes. Radiographic features of chronic hemophilic arthropathy result from repeated hemarthroses. The synovial membrane becomes hypertrophic, hyperplastic, and hypervascular with absorption of hemosiderin and phagocytosed erythrocytes. This inflammatory synovitis or pannus lines the joint capsule and extends over the margins of the articular cartilage. The hemosiderin-laden hypertrophied synovium may be identified as a somewhat radiodense capsular distension on plain radiographs (Figure 26-2) or CT scans.

Increased intra-articular pressure from hemarthrosis may cause occlusion of epiphyseal blood vessels and hence avascular necrosis. Hyperemia secondary to synovial inflammation leads to periarticular osteopenia, often manifested by a coarsening of the local trabecular pattern. In

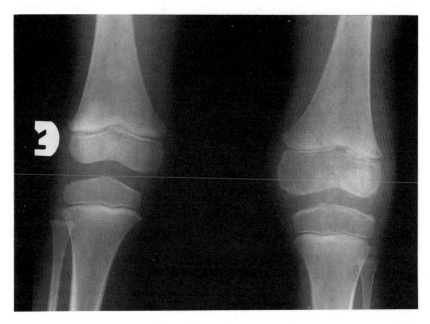

Figure 26-16. Hemophilia. An anteroposterior radiograph of both knees shows the effects of hyperemia on the left knee, including periarticular soft tissue swelling and epiphyseal overgrowth (femoral overgrowth is most obvious, but tibial and patellar overgrowths are also present). There are also irregular subchondral surfaces of the left femoral and tibial epiphyses.

the growing skeleton, the hyperemia may induce premature ossification of epiphyses, epiphyseal overgrowth (Figure 26-16), or premature fusion of growth plates with resultant limb shortening and joint deformity. Pannus invades bone directly and causes marginal erosions, subchondral "cystlike" lytic lesions, and, eventually, joint space narrowing. Intraosseous hemorrhage in the load-bearing central areas of a joint results in subchondral lucencies and destruction of subchondral bone. Secondary osteoarthritis occurs early and presents with nonuniform joint space narrowing, subarticular "cysts," bone sclerosis, and irregular subchondral surfaces.

MRI displays synovial hypertrophy as areas of low signal intensity on T1- and T2-weighted images because of the hemosiderin deposited in the synovium (Figure 26-17). There occasionally are focal areas of increased signal intensity within the soft tissues on T2-weighted images; these areas probably represent fluid collections or inflammation. Erosions and subchondral cysts exhibit low signal intensity on T1-weighted images but high signal intensity on T2-weighted images (Figure 26-18). MRI can also show focal or diffuse thinning of articular cartilage.

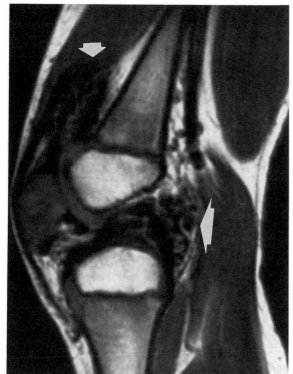

A

SE 600/20

Figure 26-17. Hemophilia. (A) A sagittal T1-weighted MR image of the knee shows massive synovial hypertrophy, which has low signal intensity because of hemosiderin deposition (arrows). (B) A corresponding sagittal T2-weighted MR image shows persistent low signal intensity of the hypertrophic synovium.

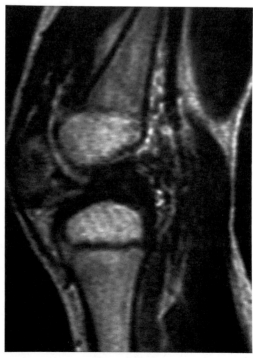

B

SE 2,000/80

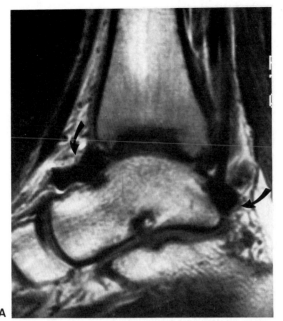

A

SE 600/20

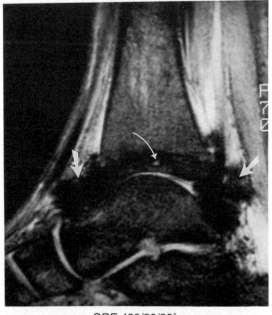

B

GRE 430/20/30°

Figure 26-18. Hemophilia. (A) A sagittal T1-weighted MR image shows the extraordinarily low signal intensity of the joint capsule (arrows) in the anterior and posterior recesses of the ankle joint as a result of hemosiderin deposition in the synovium. (B) The corresponding sagittal gradient-echo (T2*) MR image shows persistent low signal intensity of the joint capsule (straight arrows). Degenerative subchondral sclerosis and loss of articular cartilage are seen. There is also a small tibial subchondral cyst (curved arrow).

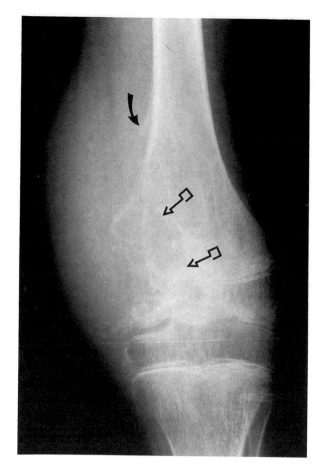

Figure 26-19. Hemophilic pseudotumor. An anteroposterior radiograph of the knee shows a geographic osteolytic lesion of the medial distal femoral metaphysis and epiphysis, with cortical destruction (open arrows), a Codman's triangle (curved arrow) superiorly, and a large soft tissue mass. Associated osteopenia, nonuniform joint space narrowing, and irregularity of the subchondral surface of the distal femur are present.

Hemorrhage into large muscles is relatively common in patients with hemophilia and most frequently involves the iliopsoas, quadriceps, and gastrocnemius muscles. Bleeding into the iliacus muscle sheath is often complicated by femoral nerve palsy. The developing mass consists of a slowly expanding, encapsulated coagulum of acute, subacute, and chronic hemorrhage. This pseudotumor formation in soft tissue and bone occurs in fewer than 2% of patients. The bones involved, in decreasing order of frequency, are the femur, pelvis, and tibia (Figure 26-19).

The soft tissue hemophilic pseudotumor can be evaluated well by ultrasonography, CT, or MRI. An osseous hemophilic pseudotumor is shown well by radiographs, CT, or MRI. In the acute and subacute stages of pseudotumor, sonography shows a well-delineated hypoechoic mass with posterior enhancement. On a contrast-enhanced CT scan, a pseudotumor is hypodense with a thick wall and may appear similar to an abscess.

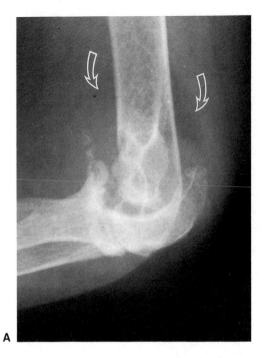

Figure 26-20. Rheumatoid arthritis. (A) A lateral radiograph of the elbow shows a large joint effusion manifested by displaced fat pads (arrows). Diffuse osteopenia, extensive bone erosions, and a few small bone fragments are also present. (B) An anteroposterior radiograph confirms diffuse osteopenia and shows uniform joint space narrowing with global articular erosions.

The MR signal characteristics of soft tissue hemorrhage depend on the age of the blood. In the acute stage (1 to 6 days), hematomas have intermediate signal intensity (similar to that of muscle) on T1-weighted images and high signal intensity on T2-weighted images. After about 7 days, the peripheral portion of the hemorrhagic mass becomes hyperintense on T1- and T2-weighted images and the center gradually becomes hyperintense but in a patchy distribution. Much later, the peripheral and central portions of the mass exhibit low signal intensity on all pulse sequences because of progressive fibrosis and hemosiderin deposition.

The main condition in the differential diagnosis of hemophilic arthropathy is juvenile chronic arthropathy, in particular juvenile rheumatoid arthritis. Both hemophilic and juvenile rheumatoid arthropathies may present with soft tissue swelling, periarticular osteopenia, subchondral "cysts" and bone erosions, joint space narrowing (Figure 26-20), and epiphyseal overgrowth. Clinical history and the distribution of joint involvement are the most useful distinguishing features. Juvenile rheumatoid arthritis usually affects the hands, wrists, knees, ankles, and spine, whereas hemophilic arthropathy usually affects the knees, ankles, and elbows. An HIV-associated arthropathy should be considered in patients with hemophilia presenting with an acute arthropathy, since a large fraction of hemophiliacs, up to 90% of those with hemophilia A

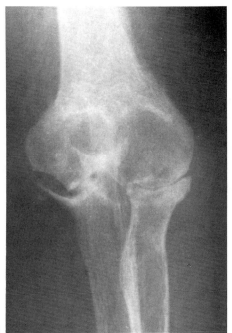

B

and 50% of those with hemophilia B, have been shown to have antibodies to HIV.

Robert G. Dussault, M.D.
Phoebe A. Kaplan, M.D.

SUGGESTED READINGS

HEMOPHILIA

1. Arnold WD, Hilgartner MW. Hemophilic arthropathy. Current concepts of pathogenesis and management. J Bone Joint Surg (Am) 1977; 59:287–305
2. Hermann G, Gilbert MS, Abdelwahab IF. Hemophilia: evaluation of musculoskeletal involvement with CT, sonography, and MR imaging. AJR 1992; 158:119–123
3. Pettersson H, Ahlberg A, Nilsson IM. A radiologic classification of hemophilic arthropathy. Clin Orthop 1980; 149:153–159
4. Stehr-Green JK, Holman RC, Jason JM, Evatt BL. Hemophilia-associated AIDS in the United States, 1981 to September 1987. Am J Public Health 1988; 78:439–442

4m.

Case 26 / 727

5. Stoker DJ, Murray RO. Skeletal changes in hemophilia and other bleeding disorders. Semin Roentgenol 1974; 9:185–193
6. Yulish BS, Lieberman JM, Strandjord SE, Bryan PJ, Mulopulos GP, Modic MT. Hemophilic arthropathy: assessment with MR imaging. Radiology 1987; 164:759–762

RHEUMATOID ARTHRITIS

7. Ansell BM, Kent PA. Radiological changes in juvenile chronic polyarthritis. Skeletal Radiol 1977; 1:129–144
8. Cassidy JT, Levinson JE, Bass JC, et al. A study of classification criteria for a diagnosis of juvenile rheumatoid arthritis. Arthritis Rheum 1986; 29:274–281
9. el-Khoury GY, Larson RK, Kathol MH, Berbaum KS, Furst DE. Seronegative and seropositive rheumatoid arthritis: radiographic differences. Radiology 1988; 168:517–520
10. Martel W, Holt JF, Cassidy JT. Roentgenologic manifestations of juvenile rheumatoid arthritis. AJR 1962; 88:400–423
11. Wilkinson RH, Weissman BN. Arthritis in children. Radiol Clin North Am 1988; 26:1247–1265

GOUT

12. Bloch C, Hermann G, Yu TF. A radiologic reevaluation of gout: a study of 2,000 patients. AJR 1980; 134:781–787
13. Cornelius R, Schneider HJ. Gouty arthritis in the adult. Radiol Clin North Am 1988; 26:1267–1276
14. Rubenstein J, Pritzker KP. Crystal-associated arthropathies. AJR 1989; 152:685–695
15. Watt I, Middlemiss H. The radiology of gout. Review article. Clin Radiol 1975; 26:27–36

PIGMENTED VILLONODULAR SYNOVITIS

16. Dorwart RH, Genant HK, Johnston WH, Morris JM. Pigmented villonodular synovitis of synovial joints: clinical, pathologic, and radiologic features. AJR 1984; 143:877–885
17. Goldman AB, DiCarlo EF. Pigmented villonodular synovitis. Diagnosis and differential diagnosis. Radiol Clin North Am 1988; 26:1327–1347
18. Jelinek JS, Kransdorf MJ, Utz JA, et al. Imaging of pigmented villonodular synovitis with emphasis on MR imaging. AJR 1989; 152:337–342

HIV ARTHROPATHY

19. Espinoza LR, Aguilar JL, Berman A, Gutierrez F, Vasey FB, Germain BF. Rheumatic manifestations associated with human immunodeficiency virus infection. Arthritis Rheum 1989; 32:1615–1622
20. Kaye BR. Rheumatologic manifestations of infection with human immunodeficiency virus (HIV). Ann Intern Med 1989; 111:158–167

21. Rosenberg ZS, Norman A, Solomon G. Arthritis associated with HIV infection: radiographic manifestations. Radiology 1989; 173:171–176

ELBOW

22. Bunnell DH, Fisher DA, Bassett LW, Gold RH, Ellman H. Elbow joint: normal anatomy on MR images. Radiology 1987; 165:527–531
23. Middleton WD, Macrander S, Kneeland JB, Froncisz W, Jesmanowicz A, Hyde JS. MR imaging of the normal elbow: anatomic correlation. AJR 1987; 149:543–547

SPORT-RELATED ELBOW INJURY

24. Gore RM, Rogers LF, Bowerman J, Suker J, Compere CL. Osseous manifestations of elbow stress associated with sports activities. AJR 1980; 134:971–977
25. Keats TE. Radiology of musculoskeletal stress injury. Chicago: Year Book Medical Publishers; 1990:16–22

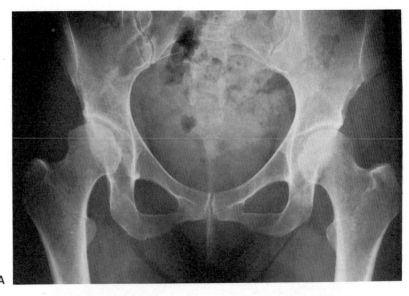

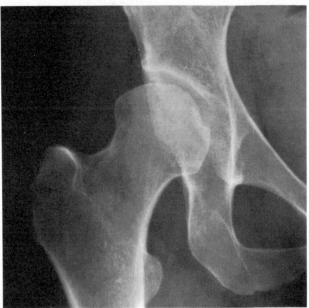

Figure 27-1. This 35-year-old woman complained of right hip pain. You are shown an anteroposterior radiograph of the pelvis (A) and a close-up view of the right hip (B).

Case 27: Developmental Dysplasia of the Hip

Question 117

Which *one* of the following is the MOST likely diagnosis?

(A) Synovial chondromatosis
(B) Healed Legg-Calvé-Perthes disease
(C) Transient osteoporosis
(D) Infection
(E) Developmental dysplasia of the hip

Anteroposterior radiographic views of the pelvis and right hip (Figure 27-1) in a 35-year-old woman with right hip pain show a normal left acetabulum and femoral head. On the right, the acetabulum is shallow, and there is incomplete coverage of the lateral femoral head by the bony acetabulum (Figure 27-2). Minimal joint space narrowing and mild superior acetabular sclerosis are consistent with early degenerative disease. The center-edge angle of Wiberg (CE angle) is decreased (Figures 27-3 and 27-4). These findings are most consistent with developmental dysplasia of the hip **(Option (E) is correct).**

Synovial chondromatosis (Option (A)) is an idiopathic disorder resulting from cartilage formation by metaplastic synovial membrane. Radiographically, joints affected by synovial chondromatosis can appear normal or the bones can be osteopenic. Later, when the cartilaginous bodies begin to mineralize, synovial chondromatosis is seen as multiple juxta-articular radiodense shadows ranging from a few millimeters to several centimeters in size. At this stage, the condition is termed synovial osteochondromatosis. There will be various degrees of mineralization (either chondrification or ossification) within the hyperplastic cartilaginous nodules, which then can appear as either small specks of calcification or large calcified bodies. The larger calcified bodies can show peripheral linear dense areas with radiolucent bodies. In the most mature ossified lesions, internal trabeculations can be seen. Uncalcified

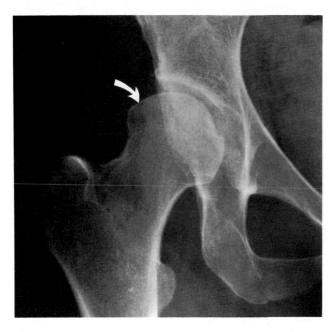

Figure 27-2
(Same as Figure
27-1B). Develop-
mental dysplasia
of the right hip.
The acetabulum
is shallow, and
the lateral aspect
of the femoral
head (arrow) is
not covered by the
acetabulum.

synovial chondromatosis has soft tissue or water density on radiographs and is best detected by MRI or by conventional arthrography, where displacement of contrast material will show multiple filling defects. Synovial chondromatosis does not cause acetabular dysplasia; acetabular morphology is normal. Therefore, synovial chondromatosis is not a likely consideration in the test patient. In the later stages of synovial chondromatosis or osteochondromatosis, secondary osteoarthritis can occur as a result of irritation from loose bodies. Joint space narrowing, ebernation, and osteophyte formation are characteristic of secondary osteoarthritis.

Legg-Calvé-Perthes disease (Option (B)) develops in boys five times as frequently as in girls and is most common in children between the ages of 3 and 12 years (peak incidence at 6 to 8 years). It is characterized by osteonecrosis of the femoral head, the pathogenesis of which is not fully understood. Initial radiographic features include slight to mild lateral displacement of the femoral head. This lateral displacement is thought to be secondary to synovial thickening. The superoanterior portion of the femoral head becomes vulnerable to pressure by the margin of the acetabular roof. A fracture develops, resulting in a curvilinear fissure in the subchondral region of the femoral head.

The Catterall classification is used to stage Legg-Calvé-Perthes disease and is based on radiographic findings. Group I, the mildest form of the disease, shows mineralization abnormalities in the anterolateral seg-

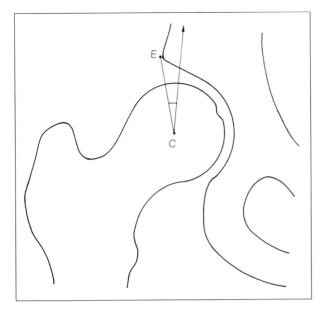

Figure 27-3 (left). Center-edge angle of Wiberg. The CE angle is used to evaluate the degree of lateral coverage of the femoral head. A large CE angle correlates with a deep acetabulum (normal range 20° to 46°), whereas a small CE angle correlates with a steeper and shallower acetabulum. With progressive subluxation, the angle may decrease to 0° or even a negative value. (Reprinted with permission from Tonnis [9].)

Figure 27-4 (right). (Same as Figure 27-1B). The center-edge angle of Wiberg measured in the test image yields a value of 15°, which confirms the diagnosis of developmental dysplasia of the hip.

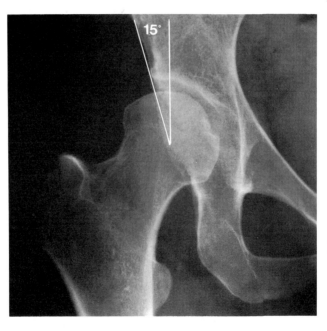

ment of the femoral head in the frog-leg projection. Group II is characterized by partial involvement, collapse, and femoral-head sequestration. Later, absorption and healing can result in mild deformity, but the prog-

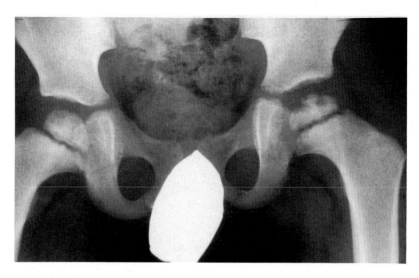

Figure 27-5. Legg-Calvé-Perthes disease. An anteroposterior radiograph of the pelvis in a 4-year-old boy shows irregular contour and early fragmentation of the left femoral head. These features are categorized as Catterall Group II.

nosis is good (Figure 27-5). At Catterall Group III, the disease shows almost complete involvement of the epiphysis, advanced deformity of the femoral head and neck, and collapse of the femoral head. The femoral neck is shortened and widened, and metaphyseal changes are prominent. Group IV disease shows widening of the entire physis, total collapse and loss of height of the femoral head, and extensive metaphyseal change. The prognosis for Groups III and IV is poor, with a high frequency of ultimate deformity of the femoral head (Figure 27-6).

The appearance of the hip in healed Legg-Calvé-Perthes disease is variable; in some cases, the involved head is indistinguishable from that of the uninvolved femoral head, whereas in others, coxa plana, shortening and widening of the femoral head and neck, osteochondroma-like lesions of the femoral neck, degenerative joint disease, and intra-articular osseous bodies are seen. Metaphyseal cysts and sclerosis can also be seen; cysts are thought to be indicative of either necrosis or a disturbance of enchondral bone formation in the metaphysis adjacent to the weakened growth plate. These metaphyseal lucencies will heal, and some residual sclerosis may be present.

A short, wide femoral neck is frequently seen in healed Legg-Calvé-Perthes disease. Some researchers have attributed these changes to overall increased apposition of bone throughout the length of the bone,

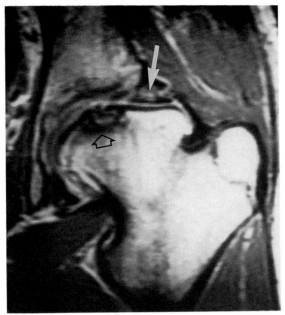

SE 2,500/23

Figure 27-6. Healed Legg-Calvé-Perthes disease. A proton-density coronal MR image of the left hip in a 14-year-old boy shows that the femoral head is flattened, widened, and distorted, with a focal region of low signal intensity in the middle portion of the femoral epiphysis (open arrow). On radiographs, this region was fragmented, representing a persistent area of osteonecrosis. Note the synovial thickening in the region of the labrum (solid arrow). The acetabulum only partially covers the femoral head, and the osteonecrosis is in the region of maximum femoral-head stress.

whereas others have attributed these changes to focal widening of the metaphyseal neck and overall increased appositional growth. A diminished femoral-head blood supply might cause not only epiphyseal necrosis but also a decrease in cartilage-cell production in the germinal layer of the growth plate. This should result in diminution of longitudinal bone growth but continued metaphyseal appositional bone growth, since the metaphyseal vascular supply is intact. Measurement of the length and width of the femoral neck and comparison of these measurements with the degree of disease seen on radiographs show a correlation between disease severity and metaphyseal abnormality. Although Legg-Calvé-Perthes disease can lead to joint space narrowing and degenerative joint disease, there is no evidence of femoral-head deformity or femoral-neck widening to suggest Legg-Calvé-Perthes disease in the test images. Therefore, Legg-Calvé-Perthes disease is an unlikely diagnostic option.

A prospective study by Henderson et al. comparing MRI with conventional radiographs in the evaluation of Legg-Calvé-Perthes disease suggested that MRI is more sensitive than radiography in detecting early disease. MR technique for the evaluation of Legg-Calvé-Perthes disease should include coronal T1- and T2-weighted images of the femoral head. Surface-coil images of the femoral head may provide better anatomic detail of the hips than would images obtained with a body coil; however, this necessitates two separate acquisitions if both femoral heads are to be evaluated, and this is not always feasible when imaging young children. The abnormalities are most striking on the T1-weighted images, where the normally bright-signal fatty marrow within the femoral epiphysis is replaced by a much lower signal intensity tissue.

MRI may be best for evaluating early healing in Legg-Calvé-Perthes disease, where the correlation of radiographic and MR findings in patients scanned during the active phase and early in the healing process showed a return to normal marrow signal intensity on T1-weighted images that corresponds to healing and reossification on radiographs. Increased epiphyseal signal on T2-weighted images corresponds to regions of femoral healing and typically precedes a return to normal marrow signal intensity on T1-weighted images. This increased signal intensity may correspond to granulation tissue, as is seen with avascular necrosis, and does not represent transient marrow edema. T2-weighted MR images are therefore useful to evaluate for healing or progression of disease. MRI is also useful for evaluating the unossified femoral and acetabular structures.

Transient osteoporosis of the hip (Option (C)) is characterized by hip pain without antecedent trauma or infection. The pain can be severe enough to result in a limp or restricted joint function. Radiographically, regional osteopenia is present, but there should be no additional abnormalities. CT and MRI can reveal evidence of joint fluid. Bone scintigraphy shows increased regional tracer uptake. Decreased marrow signal intensity is prominent on T1-weighted MR images and is accompanied by morphologically similar increased signal intensity on T2-weighted images. These MR findings are typical of bone marrow edema. Initial symptoms can mimic those of avascular necrosis, infection, and neoplasm. However, the clinical and radiographic findings regress spontaneously in 6 to 12 months without sequelae. Therefore, transient osteoporosis is frequently a diagnosis of exclusion. Transient osteoporosis is not a likely diagnosis for the dysplastic features shown in the test images.

In the adult, osseous infection (Option (D)) is most frequently seen in the spine, pelvis, and small bones. This differs from hematogenous osteomyelitis found in children, where most cases occur in the metaphyses of the long bones. When infection does occur in a long bone of an adult, the

Table 27-1: Developmental dysplasia of the hip[a]

Developmental dislocation	Other developmental or congenital dysplasias
Developmental subluxation	Acetabular dysplasia
Unstable hip	Coxa vara
Dislocatable	Coxa valga
Subluxatable	Femoral anteversion
Clicking hip	Other

[a] New terminology accepted by Pediatric Orthopedic Society of North America to describe various hip conditions previously known as congenital dislocation of the hip (CDH). The term developmental dysplasia of the hip (DDH) is now used to describe these disorders.

free communication of the metaphyseal and epiphyseal vessels through the closed growth plate results in an infection that localizes in the subchondral region of the bone. Septic arthritis is frequently a sequela of this subchondral infection.

In children, increased intraosseous pressure generated by the infection can drive the infection through the Haversian canals of the cortex and into the subperiosteal space. The periosteum is lifted off the cortex, forming subperiosteal abscesses. The firm attachment of the periosteum to the cortex in adult patients resists this displacement, and the formation of subperiosteal abscess is infrequent. Extensive periostitis, involucrum formation, and sequestration are therefore not common features of adult osteomyelitis. Instead, there is cortical destruction, atrophy, and osseous weakening, often resulting in pathologic fracture. Epiphyseal, metaphyseal, and diaphyseal destruction results in radiolucent regions of various size within the bone. Endosteal scalloping, cortical tunneling, and a poorly defined subperiosteal region are all signs of acute osteomyelitis. Eventually, the infection will spread into the joint, where secondary septic arthritis is accompanied by joint space narrowing and bone lysis on both sides of the joint. In the test patient, subtle joint space narrowing is present but there is no evidence of bone destruction. Infection is thus an unlikely diagnosis.

Developmental dysplasia of the hip (DDH) was previously referred to by a number of terms, including congenital dislocation of the hip (CDH), teratogenic hip, and acetabular dysplasia. The Pediatric Orthopedic Society of North America recently accepted a change in the terminology used to describe various hip conditions that had been known as CDH. The term DDH was chosen to describe the condition as a whole (Table 27-1). This change in nomenclature is intended to include all forms of hip dysplasia that are thought to be congenital, neonatal, infantile, or developmental in etiology. It does not include pathologic displacement of the hip caused by neuromuscular disease.

DDH is an often overlooked cause of osteoarthritis in the adult. The development and anatomy of the human hip joint represents an imperfect evolutionary solution to the bipedal gait. In quadripeds, the plane of the acetabular inlet is almost perpendicular to the femoral neck axis, and the massive posteroinferior lip of the acetabulum provides support for the weight of a vertical load. In contrast, the primary bony abutment for the femoral head in humans is posterosuperior and anterosuperior, and complete joint closure anteriorly must rely on the cartilaginous labrum or capsular and ligamentous elements. This, and the need to support all weight on two instead of four limbs, creates a biomechanically more complex pattern of stress transfer across the human hip joint. A balance must be maintained between the stresses acting on the joint and the ability of the joint to withstand those stresses. If this balance is disrupted, osteoarthritis develops. The factors that allow the development of osteoarthritis in the human hip can be either intrinsic or extrinsic to the joint. Intrinsic factors relate primarily to the biologic quality of the articular structures or to developmental defects and anomalies, most notably hip dysplasia. Hip dysplasia is considered a predisposing factor for osteoarthritis since the load borne by the hip is concentrated in a smaller, more localized area, and this gradually erodes the articular surface of the hip and leads to osteoarthritis (Figure 27-7).

The acetabulum forms during the early embryonic period, from precursors of the ilium, ischium, and pubis. The ossification centers for these three bones appear early in the second trimester of intrauterine life, and all three are joined by the triradiate cartilage. The triradiate cartilage fuses between 13 and 16 years of age in girls and between 15 and 18 years of age in boys. Centralized pressure from the femoral head is essential for normal acetabular growth, which occurs as appositional bone growth along the acetabular roof and triradiate cartilage. The appositional bone growth occurring along the triradiate cartilage is a result of columns of actively growing cartilaginous cells that form on both sides of the triradiate cartilage. Growth along the lower border of the ilium is both transverse and longitudinal, accounting for the lateral and caudal growth pattern of the superior acetabular rim. Another aspect of superior acetabular rim growth that becomes clinically important is the fact that enchondral and periosteal bone formation merge at the superior acetabular rim and must proceed concurrently. Any disruption of this superior acetabular rim growth results in deficient marginal ossification of the acetabulum and consequent acetabular dysplasia.

The depth of the acetabulum and its spherical contour depends largely on the response of the acetabulum to the presence of a spherical

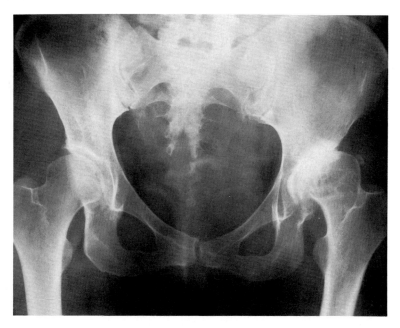

Figure 27-7. Developmental dysplasia with secondary osteoarthritis. An anteroposterior radiograph of the pelvis in a 32-year-old woman shows abnormalities of both hips. On the right side, the acetabulum is shallow and the lateral aspect of the femoral head is not covered by acetabulum. On the left side, secondary osteoarthritis is manifested as destruction of articular cartilage, remodeling of the apposing bone surfaces, sclerosis, and craniolateral subluxation of the femoral head.

femoral head. If that spherical femoral head is not present within the joint or is not in the optimum position within the joint, the acetabulum does not develop properly in depth and surface area; the triradiate cartilage does continue to grow and thus maintains the overall length of the iliac wing. All of the actively growing parts of the hip must exist in an environment of physiologic joint function and loading for normal development to occur.

Several radiographic techniques can be used to evaluate the acetabulum in the adult. Two views are commonly used; the standard anteroposterior pelvic view and the antetorsion view of Rippstein (AT view). The anteroposterior pelvic radiograph is taken with the legs in neutral position. The CE angle gives a numerical value useful in assessing acetabular coverage of the femoral head in the adult. The CE angle is the angle between a line parallel to the longitudinal body axis through the femoral-head center and a line from the femoral-head center to the superior acetabular rim (Figure 27-3). In adults, the CE angle varies from 20° to

46°. Values below 20°, as in the test patient, are considered diagnostic of hip dysplasia (Figure 27-4). When using the CE angle to diagnose dysplasia of the hip, the size of the femoral head should be taken into consideration. In the normal hip, intermediate femoral-head radii correlate with intermediate CE angles, whereas large CE angles are associated with smaller femoral-head radii and small CE angles are associated with larger femoral-head radii. The combination of a small femoral-head radius and a small CE angle amplifies the joint stress, and thus smaller CE angles (20° to 25°) that are associated with smaller femoral-head radii would result in a greater frequency of osteoarthritis than would smaller CE angles associated with larger femoral-head radii.

Another indicator of joint stress is the subchondral bony condensation that occurs as a response to increased joint stress in the acetabular roof. This is sometimes referred to as a "sourcil." When the distribution of joint pressure is normal, the sourcil appears thin and even, but as the joint pressure becomes more concentrated (corresponding to a lack of femoral-head coverage), this area of dense bone thickens toward the acetabular margin and assumes a more triangular shape (Figure 27-8). In advanced stages, localized sclerosis of the femoral head is also present due to impaired blood flow to the femoral head. As blood flow becomes increasingly impaired, osteonecrosis and bone loss occur, and cystic changes of the femoral head develop.

When femoral-head coverage is horizontal, the weight-bearing area is greatest and the compressive stresses are widely and evenly distributed. With increasing steepness of the acetabulum or with deficient anterior coverage, the stresses increase and the weight-bearing area shifts laterally toward the acetabular margin. This ultimately results in osteoarthritis (Figure 27-7).

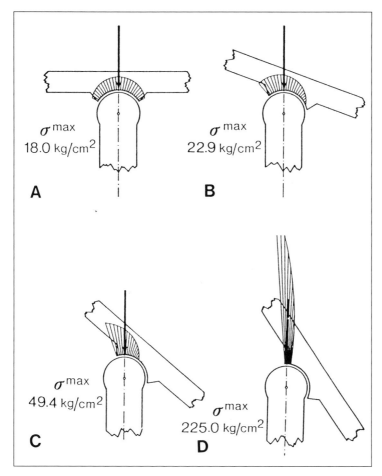

Figure 27-8. Evolution of bony condensation in the acetabular roof ("sourcil") as shown by schematic drawings with the magnitude and distribution of joint pressure as a function of head coverage, or the weight-bearing area of the joint. (A) Horizontally covered joint with a large weight-bearing area. The compressive stresses are small and evenly distributed; the sourcil is narrow and even. (B and C) As acclivity increases and the weight-bearing area dwindles, compressive stress is built toward the superior acetabular rim and the sourcil tips toward the acetabular margin. (D) The weight-bearing area is minimal in this subluxated hip, where all compressive stresses are concentrated at the acetabular margin. (Reprinted with permission from Tonnis [9].)

Question 118

Concerning synovial chondromatosis,

- (A) it is almost invariably a monoarticular disorder
- (B) the synovium is hypoplastic
- (C) conventional radiographs are frequently diagnostic
- (D) ossified intra-articular loose bodies are common
- (E) malignant transformation is rare

Synovial chondromatosis is essentially a monoarticular disorder **(Option (A) is true).** The knee, hip, elbow, and shoulder are most frequently involved. This disorder is a result of synovial metaplasia that generates foci of cartilage within the synovial membrane. The synovium is not hypoplastic **(Option (B) is false);** rather, it is hyperplastic, with multiple foci of cartilage and metaplasia. These cartilaginous nodules project into the joint on delicate pedicles, which may break as a result of trauma, permitting the cartilaginous nodules to become loose bodies. Since the cartilage is nourished by the synovial fluid, these loose bodies will enlarge within the joint capsule.

Enchondral bone formation typically occurs within the cartilage nodules, giving the distinctive radiographic pattern of multiple calcified or ossified densities within the joint capsule. The pattern of mineralization can range from small specks of calcification to large calcified bodies. These larger calcified bodies can have peripheral linear dense areas and radiolucent centers. Trabeculation can be seen within the more mature ossified nodules. This mineralization, called synovial osteochondromatosis, is readily recognized on radiographs.

Since cartilage cannot be differentiated from surrounding soft tissue by conventional radiography, synovial chondromatosis cannot be diagnosed on conventional radiographs **(Option (C) is false).** In patients who have chronic hip pain, no evidence of a radiculopathy, a physical examination consistent with an intrinsic hip abnormality, and normal hip radiographs (except for osteopenia), synovial chondromatosis should be prominent in the differential diagnosis. Additional imaging is necessary to confirm or exclude this condition. CT, MRI, and conventional arthrography are all options. CT may fail to demonstrate the cartilage particles because of insufficient contrast difference with surrounding tissues. MRI is more likely to detect the cartilage abnormality, but if a body coil is utilized, MRI might not have sufficient spatial resolution to detect the cartilage nodules. Therefore, conventional arthrography remains an important diagnostic method for this condition. The cartilage nodules are demonstrated in bold relief by the intra-articular contrast agent (Figure 27-9). For synovial chondromatosis to be evident on conventional radio-

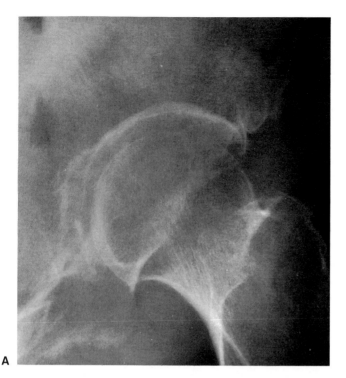

A

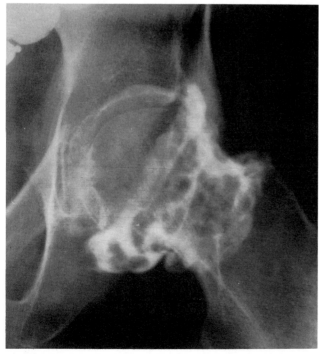

B

Figure 27-9.
Synovial chon-
dromatosis.
This 61-year-old
woman had
chronic left hip
pain and no evi-
dence of radicul-
opathy and was
otherwise
healthy. (A) A
frog-leg lateral
radiograph of
the left hip is
normal except
for the presence
of osteopenia.
(B) A similarly
positioned ar-
throgram shows
multiple filling
defects, a finding
diagnostic of
cartilaginous
nodules. A CT
examination did
not detect these
nodules, and
MRI was not
performed.

graphs, the cartilage nodules must begin to mineralize; once that happens, the condition is no longer synovial chondromatosis, but synovial osteochondromatosis.

While mineralization of the nodule chondroid matrix is common, actual bone formation or ossification develops much less frequently **(Option (D) is false)**. When ossification does occur, the ossified nodules frequently develop fatty marrow.

Synovial chondromatosis occurs twice as frequently in men as in women and is usually diagnosed in the third to fifth decades of life. Clinical symptoms are frequently insidious,, and patients often present with a several-year history of joint pain and limitation of motion. Joint effusion, when present, may be bloody, and secondary osteoarthritis occurs as a result of mechanical destruction of the articular cartilage by the loose bodies. Focal recurrence of synovial chondromatosis after surgery is common. Malignant transformation to chondrosarcoma, although extremely rare, can occur **(Option (E) is true)**. Histologically, the benign cartilaginous nodules tend to be hyaline cartilage, although some reports confirm a myxoid type of cartilage. Cellular proliferation with atypical nuclei is common in the subcapsular region and can be misinterpreted by the pathologist as a sign of aggressiveness.

Question 119

Concerning transient osteoporosis of the hip,

(A) it is most common in young women
(B) conventional radiographs are usually normal
(C) it predisposes to fracture of the femoral neck
(D) MRI shows marrow edema

Transient osteoporosis of the hip is characterized radiographically by osteopenia of the femoral head and sometimes of the acetabulum and femoral neck. The condition was originally described as a condition in pregnant women, but young or middle-aged men are most frequently affected **(Option (A) is false)**. Hip pain is the predominant clinical symptom; the pain presents without an antecedent history of infection or trauma and can be severe enough to produce a limp or restricted joint function. Conventional radiographs can appear normal, but close inspection of the films almost invariably reveals osteopenia of the femoral head and acetabulum **(Option (B) is false)**.

While the etiology of transient osteoporosis is unknown, bone biopsy in cases of transient osteoporosis can show necrosis, increased bone turnover, and inflammatory change. Histologic evaluation of the synovium can show a normal synovium or thickened synovial tissue with chronic inflammatory cellular reaction.

In young women, the left side is almost exclusively involved, although the etiology of this asymmetric involvement is not known. In other groups of patients, either hip may be involved. The cause of transient osteoporosis is uncertain, but the clinical course is characterized by debilitating pain. The pain is self-limited and resolves without treatment unless complicated by femoral neck fracture, to which patients with this disorder are predisposed **(Option (C) is true)**. The clinical and radiographic findings typically regress within 6 to 12 months. Scintigraphic examination with Tc-99m diphosphonates shows increased uptake in the femoral head, often extending into the acetabulum. On CT, the osteopenia of the femoral head and acetabulum can be seen, especially in comparison with the unaffected side. An accompanying joint effusion is also frequently seen.

MR examination of the hip in transient osteoporosis shows a characteristic pattern typical of marrow edema **(Option (D) is true)**. In general, decreased signal intensity of marrow is seen on T1-weighted images with an accompanying increased signal intensity on T2-weighted images. A joint effusion is typically identified on the T2-weighted images as increased-intensity intra-articular fluid. Several patterns of marrow abnormality have been described, including focal regions of abnormal marrow signal intensity along the primary trabeculae (Figure 27-10), regional marrow abnormality, and diffuse abnormality of the entire femoral head. This can frequently be accompanied by similar marrow signal abnormalities in the juxta-articular acetabulum and in the femoral neck (Figure 27-11).

The marrow signal abnormalities on MR examination most likely represent nonspecific marrow edema and are frequently indistinguishable from those due to other causes of marrow edema. The extent and degree of signal intensity abnormality depend upon the severity of marrow hypervascularity and hyperperfusion and consequent increased extracellular water. Increased marrow signal is also seen on fat-saturated T2-weighted images, as well as short-tau inversion-recovery (STIR) images. In addition to the transient osteoporosis seen in adults, "transient" marrow abnormalities have been reported to occur in children with hip pain. Abnormal low-signal-intensity femoral-head marrow detected on T1-weighted images eventually resolves and reverts to a normal marrow signal intensity. This resolution of marrow signal abnormality coincides with improvement in the child's clinical condition. Other disorders that can present as "edema" on MR images include early avascular necrosis, early Legg-Calvé-Perthes disease, reflex sympathetic dystrophy, and stress fracture or trabecular microfracture. To distinguish these entities,

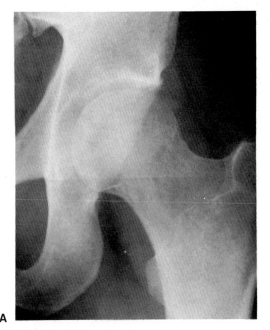

A

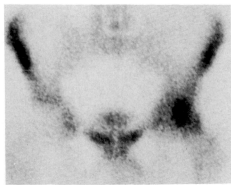

B

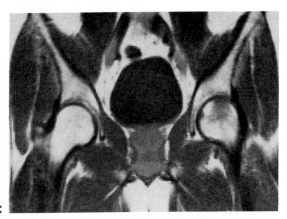

C

SE 500/35

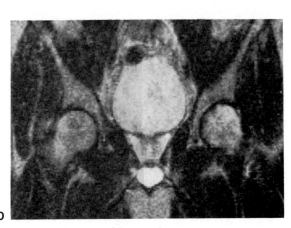

D

SE 1,500/120

Figure 27-10. Transient osteo-porosis of the hip in a 38-year-old man with severe left hip pain and no other relevant history. (A) An anteroposterior radiograph shows subtle osteopenia with unsharp trabeculae. (B) An anterior scinti-gram shows focally increased tracer accumulation in the weight-bearing portion of the hip joint, greatest in the femoral head. (C) A T1-weighted coronal MR image shows a focal zone of low signal intensity at the apex of the left femoral head. (D) A T2-weighted image shows the corre-sponding zone of high signal in-tensity.

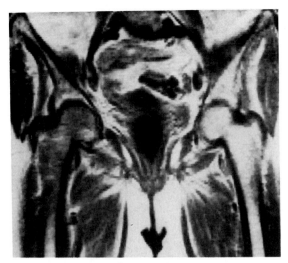

SE 1,500/35

Figure 27-11. Transient osteporosis of the hip. A proton-density coronal MR image of a 77-year-old woman with right hip pain shows a regional pattern of marrow edema with low-intensity marrow throughout the right ilium and proximal right femur. This patient's condition resolved spontaneously.

the presence of specific symptoms suggestive of infection, trauma, or tumor is helpful.

Question 120

Concerning developmental dysplastic hip disease in adults,

    (A) it usually develops during late adolescence
    (B) osteoarthritis is a common sequela
    (C) there is diminished weight-bearing area in the acetabulum
    (D) conservative management will diminish symptoms
    (E) the center-edge angle of Wiberg is increased

DDH encompasses a spectrum of hip abnormalities that range from mild acetabular dysplasia to irreducible dislocation of the femoral head. DDH affects 1 to 2% of the Caucasian population in the United States; it is less frequently seen in African Americans and other ethnic groups. Although girls are affected five times more frequently than boys overall, the female-to-male ratio is only 2:1 following breech delivery. Detection and treatment of DDH at birth is desirable; however, the diagnosis is frequently missed and many children subsequently present for evaluation and therapy months to years later. The acetabular dysplasia, subluxation, and dislocation of the developing hip are all part of the spectrum of dynamic morphologic alterations that occur in the growing hip; abnormalities in this development can be insidious in onset and subtle in clinical and radiographic presentation and can result in both short- and long-term disability even if diagnosed and treated during the earliest stages of development.

The etiology and pathogenesis of DDH are not completely understood, but in most cases DDH results from abnormalities in the alignment of the femoral head within the acetabulum. Abnormal laxity of the hip joint rather than structural abnormality is most likely responsible for DDH, and this abnormal laxity can be exacerbated during the third trimester of pregnancy when the hormonal effects of maternal estrogen increase tissue laxity. Extreme flexion of the fetal hip and knee *in utero*, with sudden extension of the hip joint during birth, tends to promote femoral-head subluxation and dislocation. The hyperflexion of the hip joint during breech presentation, with subsequent shortening and contracture of the iliopsoas muscle, exacerbates these changes. A suboptimal placement of the developing femoral head within the acetabulum affects not only the contour and size of the femoral head, but also the subsequent growth and remodeling of the acetabulum. This frequently leads to an acetabulum that is more shallow and less well formed, with incomplete femoral-head coverage.

Typically, DDH is classified into one of three major groups. Type 1 DDH, the most common group, is characterized by a dislocatable and unstable hip. There is increased femoral anteversion and mild acetabular cartilaginous abnormalities with early labral eversion. In type 2 DDH, the femoral head is partially dislocated or subluxated and there is a loss of femoral-head sphericity, an increase in femoral anteversion, and an early labral inversion and hypertrophy. The acetabulum is typically shallow. Type 3 DDH is characterized by flattening of the femoral head and the acetabular contour, with inward growth and hypertrophy of the labrum to yield the "inverted limbus." While these changes usually occur in the prenatal or antenatal period, DDH can occasionally develop during the pubertal growth spurt, when a disturbance in the development of the superior acetabular rim can result from deformities of the hip such as coxa valga or deformities secondary to osteochondrosis or osteonecrosis. In these instances, deficiency of femoral-head coverage by acetabulum can arise in a previously normal hip. Abnormalities do not develop during late adolescence **(Option (A) is false).**

Osteoarthritis is a common sequela of DDH in both treated and untreated patients **(Option (B) is true),** depending on the severity of the initial dysplasia. In children with moderate-to-severe subluxation or dislocation, even appropriate treatment may not prevent long-term disability and the need for subsequent total hip arthroplasty in the fifth or sixth decade. Patients with mild and undiagnosed dysplasia may experience the onset of osteoarthritis at an earlier age than in the general population. Earlier onset of osteoarthritis also is expected in patients with more severe DDH, in whom the diagnosis is delayed or in whom treatment is not adequate.

The primary factor that leads to the osteoarthritis seen in patients with DDH is the diminished weight-bearing area in the acetabulum **(Option (C) is true).** With deficient anterior coverage or increasing steepness of the acetabulum, the stresses on the acetabulum and consequently on the femoral head increase. There is a progressive lateral shifting of the stress forces toward the acetabular margin, and, as the weight-bearing area decreases, the joint pressure increases dramatically. The bone responds with increasing bone formation and sclerosis in the region of the stress overload, usually the superior and lateral aspects of the acetabulum. The "sourcil" or bony condensation identified in the acetabular roof on conventional radiographs can pinpoint the region of the acetabulum under excessive compressive force. As these compressive stresses are distributed over a smaller area of the acetabulum, the underlying articular cartilage becomes progressively affected, with eventual erosion of this cartilage as the degenerative process progresses.

Early treatment is necessary to ameliorate or prevent the sequelae of DDH. Neonatal diagnosis and reduction are necessary to reestablish normal chondro-osseous development in the hip. In the neonate, conservative treatment such as closed reduction can frequently result in satisfactory development of the hip; however, once DDH is identified in an adult patient, conservative management is much less likely to be effective in diminishing the symptoms and improving the outcome **(Option (D) is false).**

The sequelae of DDH become most apparent after the cessation of bone growth. Time since onset of pain, limitation in motion, and the development of osteoarthritis are all important factors in determining patient prognosis. The clinical symptoms, radiographic features, and ultimate outcome are not always concordant. Some patients with mild dysplasia and relatively normal appearing joints on radiographs experience pain at an early age, whereas others with comparable pathology do not experience pain until middle-age or later. However, when there is significant pathology in the hip, most patients become symptomatic by about age 40.

In the adult, pain in the hip is often the most compelling reason to consider surgical intervention. Mild and moderate degrees of hip dysplasia can present with pain very early in some cases and much later in others. Because it is presently impossible to distinguish patients who will present with early pain from those who will present with late pain, operative treatment is best deferred until the hip does become painful. In patients with severe grades of dysplasia, pain and other complaints are generally manifested by 35 years of age. In these cases of severe dysplasia, treatment before or near the end of the growth period is desirable to delay further deterioration of the articular cartilage. Surgical treatment for DDH in the adult includes acetabular rotation procedures, other osteotomy procedures, and hip arthroplasty.

Several radiographic measurements are useful in the evaluation of DDH in the adult. In particular, the CE angle is used as a screening procedure on an anteroposterior pelvis radiograph. The normal CE angle is positive and should be greater than 20°. A CE angle that is decreased or negative in value is indicative of DDH **(Option (E) is false).** The greater the degree of subluxation of the hip, the smaller the CE angle, until negative values are reached with more-advanced cases of subluxation.

Question 121

Concerning developmental dysplasia of the hip in the neonate,

(A) the cartilaginous femoral head should normally be completely covered by the bony acetabular roof on coronal sonographic images
(B) dynamic ultrasonography is best performed by the application of posterior force to assess posterior-to-anterior movement of the femoral head
(C) MR diagnosis of "hourglass capsule" is made by identification of the iliopsoas muscle anterior to the femoral head
(D) loss of the characteristic "rose thorn" appearance of the labrum on hip arthrography is seen in inverted limbus
(E) ischemic necrosis occasionally occurs in the contralateral normal hip when both hips are immobilized

In the past, the radiologist and the orthopedic surgeon were forced to rely on clinical evaluation and analysis of conventional radiographs to diagnose DDH. This was particularly difficult in the neonatal period, when the lack of ossification of the femoral head, lateral acetabulum, and greater trochanter meant that only indirect evidence of DDH was obtained. The radiographic evaluation of DDH in the neonate frequently relies on the recognition of lateral migration of the femoral head as measured using the horizontal line of Hilgenreiner (a horizontal line drawn through the triradiate cartilage) and its intersection with the Ombrédanne-Perkins line (a vertical line drawn from the lateral rim of the acetabulum inferiorly to intersect with the line of Hilgenreiner) (Figure 27-12). The intersection of these two lines divides the hip joint into quadrants. The femoral ossific nucleus or the medial aspect of the femoral metaphysis should lie within the lower-inner quadrant. If it lies within the upper-outer quadrant, the hip is likely to be dislocated. Alternatively,

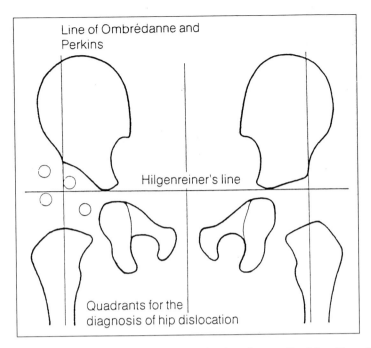

Line of Ombrédanne and Perkins

Hilgenreiner's line

Quadrants for the diagnosis of hip dislocation

Figure 27-12. Hilgenreiner's line and Ombrédanne-Perkins line. Imaginary capital ossification centers are shown in the different quadrants of the hip. Location in the lower-inner quadrant is normal; other locations are abnormal. (Reprinted with permission from Tonnis [9].)

Shenton's line, a line drawn between the medial border of the femoral neck and the superior border of the obturator foramen, should present a continuous arc. In the dislocated hip with proximal displacement of the femoral head, this arc is interrupted (Figure 27-13).

Since first reported in the 1980s by Graf, sonography has been increasingly used in the evaluation of neonatal hip dysplasia. With its dynamic assessment of the hip and lack of ionizing radiation, sonography has become the screening method of choice for DDH in most clinical settings. Infants from birth until 8 to 10 months of age can be easily examined by sonography; beyond 8 to 10 months the ossified femoral-head nucleus will frequently obscure the underlying anatomy. Since normal neonates show an increased degree of mobility of the femoral head, sonography of the neonatal hip during the first few days of life can result in a false-positive study. It is therefore preferable to delay performance of the sonographic examination of the hips until the baby is 1 to 2 weeks of age.

The examination is performed with the infant lying in the decubitus position. A high-frequency linear-array transducer gives optimal image

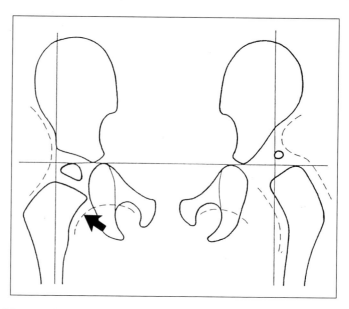

Figure 27-13. Auxiliary line of Shenton. On the right, Shenton's line (arrow) is smooth and forms a continuous arc. On the left, where the femoral head is dislocated, the line is broken. Lateral rotation of the femoral neck will alter the course of the arc. The lines of Hilgenreiner and of Ombrédanne-Perkins have been added for reference. (Reprinted with permission from Tonnis [9].)

quality, and the examination of the hip should be performed with the hip in the neutral (extended) and flexed positions. When the infant's hip is in the flexed position, coronal images of the hip are obtained in both the abducted and adducted positions. In addition, a modified Barlow maneuver is performed to elicit any instability in the hip. To perform this maneuver, the examiner adducts the infant's flexed hip and applies gentle pressure directed posteriorly while maintaining the transducer in a fixed position. Once the coronal scans are completed, the transducer is turned 90° and the hip is examined in the transverse plane. Both hips should be examined to look for clinically silent abnormalities in the contralateral hip. When evaluating the hip, one should examine the coverage of the femoral head by the acetabular roof, the symmetry between the left and right hips, the stability of the joint, the shape of the acetabulum, and the appearance of the labrum.

The lateral aspect of the iliac bone should be a straight echogenic structure, or iliac "line," that is seen in its entirety on the coronal image. Only when the iliac line is straight can the examiner be assured that the position and coverage of the femoral head is evaluated accurately. The

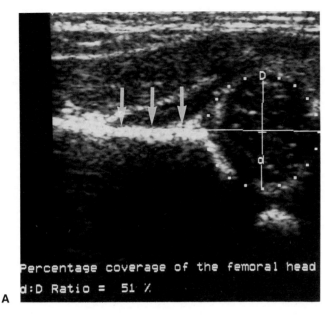

Figure 27-14. Subluxatable femoral head in coronal sonographic images of the right hip in a newborn with a hip click. (A) A coronal image with the hip in neutral position shows the echogenic iliac crest (arrows) defining the lateral aspect of the bony acetabulum. The cartilaginous femoral head (defined by dots) is identified, and quantitative evaluation of the acetabular coverage of the cartilaginous femoral head is 51%. (B) The same patient, with the leg in adduction, shows only 36% coverage of the femoral head. This finding is consistent with a subluxatable right femoral head. At least 50% of the femoral head should be covered by the bony acetabulum. (C) With the hip reduced, in abduction, the coverage is again 50%.

normal acetabulum on the coronal image is gently curved, and at least 50% of the femoral head should lie medial to a line drawn along the iliac bone and extending inferiorly through the femoral head **(Option (A) is false)** (Figure 27-14). These measurements are repeated with the hip in the abducted and adducted positions. In the normal hip, coverage during abduction and adduction remains at 50% or greater. In hips that are subluxatable (Figure 27-14), coverage may be normal in the neutral or abducted view but will decrease in the adducted view to less than 50%. In the subluxated or dislocated hip, coverage will be less than 50% on the neutral and adducted coronal views and may be less than 50% in the abducted view (Figure 27-15). Dynamic scanning using gentle pressure directed posteriorly with the infant's flexed hip in the abducted position

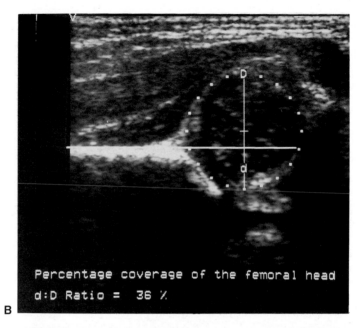

Percentage coverage of the femoral head
d:D Ratio = 36 %

B

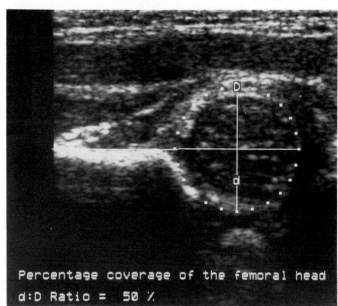

Percentage coverage of the femoral head
d:D Ratio = 50 %

C

will identify posterior and lateral subluxation of the femoral head **(Option (B) is false).**

After examination of the hip in the coronal plane, the transducer is turned 90° and the hip is scanned in the transverse plane. With the hip

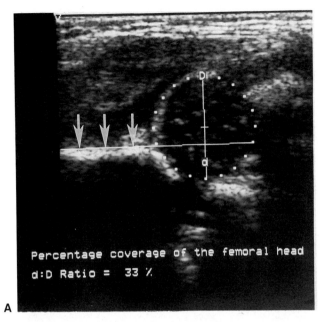

A

Percentage coverage of the femoral head

d:D Ratio = 33 %

Figure 27-15. Subluxated femoral head in coronal sonographic images of the left hip in a newborn infant. (A) The echogenic bony ilium (arrows) and the cartilaginous femoral head (enclosed dots) are identified. Calculation of the percent coverage of the femoral head with the leg in a neutral position shows only 33% coverage. This is consistent with a subluxated left femoral head. (B) Abduction of the leg results in a near relocation of the femoral head within the acetabulum, with 48% coverage of the femoral head.

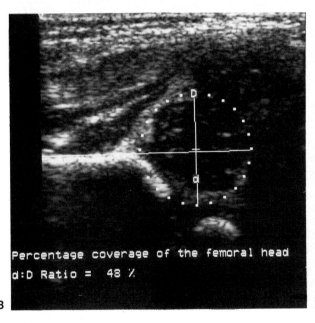

B

Percentage coverage of the femoral head

d:D Ratio = 48 %

extended and in neutral position, the femoral head is identified between the pubis and ischium, well seated within the acetabulum and abutting the triradiate cartilage (Figure 27-16). The modified Barlow maneuver is then performed with the hip flexed, and posterior motion of the femoral

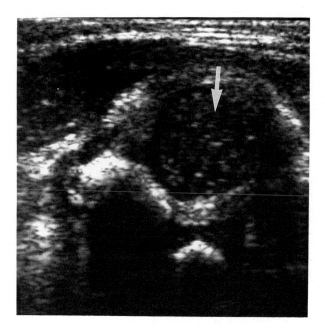

Figure 27-16. Normal hip. A transverse image of the hip in a neonate shows normal sonographic anatomy. The cartilaginous femoral head can be identified (arrow) and is well seated within the bony acetabulum.

head is assessed. A few millimeters of posterior motion of the femoral head can be normal in the first few days of life; 1 to 6 mm of posterior displacement is not uncommon when the hip is stressed. After 2 to 4 weeks of age, the femoral head should not move posteriorly when stress maneuvers are performed.

An additional indicator of hip dysplasia on sonographic examination is an irregular and only slightly curved acetabulum, which differs from the smooth and cup-shaped acetabulum of the normal hip. The femoral head may have an abnormal position or may be subluxatable or dislocatable with the modified Barlow maneuver. Increased amounts of fibrofatty pulvinar (fibrofatty tissue within the acetabulum) and an abnormally formed or inverted labrum are also associated with chronic dislocation. Delayed ossification, if recognized on sonography, also suggests the presence of DDH. The transverse view of the subluxatable or dislocatable hip shows lateral and posterior movement of the femoral head with respect to the triradiate cartilage when the hip is stressed.

MR evaluation of DDH can be especially useful in the neonate or young infant, because cartilaginous structures are readily identified on MRI. The advantage of MRI over sonography is the relative ease with which the examination can be performed on a patient in a full spica cast, without the presence of artifacts or the need to cut an acoustic window in the cast. MR provides additional information when compared with sonography and is not operator dependent. Even dynamic assessment of the hip is possible with newer MR techniques, but it is more cumbersome than the dynamic assessment of the hip with sonography. The greater cost of MRI versus sonography means that sonography remains the screening method of choice for DDH in the neonate and young infant.

Probably the greatest potential for MRI is as a replacement for arthrography in the diagnosis of failed hip reduction. MRI can detect features that prevent acceptable reduction, including an hourglass capsule (indentation of the capsule by the iliopsoas muscle), inverted limbus, infolding of the capsule, and hypertrophy of both the fatty pulvinar and the ligamentum capitis femoris. The ligamentum capitis femoris (ligamentum teres) is a normally flat, ribbonlike structure that extends from the acetabulum to the femoral head and serves as a source of vascular supply to the femoral head. It generally follows the contour of the femoral head, but in DDH it can become pathologically elongated and hypertrophied, resulting in an impediment to closed reduction. In addition to defining the anatomy of the cartilaginous femoral head, MRI is useful in defining both the bony and cartilaginous acetabulum and in further delineating acetabular dysplasia.

The anatomy of the infant hip can be clearly defined on MR images (Figure 27-17). Routine MR evaluation of the pediatric hip can be performed with both coronal and transverse T1-weighted images. The field-of-view should be approximately 10% larger than the diameter of the pelvis. Interleaved sections of 5 mm and a 256×128 image matrix usually give satisfactory images. When attempting to diagnose causes of failed closed reduction, such as inverted limbus or hourglass capsule, a 5" or 3.5" circular surface coil may be required to achieve adequate spatial resolution for imaging of the symptomatic hip. Both T1- and T2-weighted images are obtained using a field-of-view of 12 to 16 cm; noninterleaved, 5-mm-thick sections with two excitations; and an imaging matrix of 256×128.

The normal iliopsoas tendon can be difficult to see on MR images in the infant hip because the normal tendon lies close to the capsule and the anterior portion of the labrum may obscure the tendon. The abnormal iliopsoas tendon, such as is seen with the hourglass capsule, is more readily identified, since the tendon often becomes shortened, rounded, and more vertically oriented when it invaginates the capsule. On transaxial images, the iliopsoas tendon is seen as a rounded structure with an intermediate signal intensity (equal to that of muscle) in the medial and anterior aspect of the joint, interposed between the acetabulum and the femoral head **(Option (C) is true)** (Figure 27-18). Both inverted limbus and enfolded capsule are seen as structures with low (limbus) or intermediate (capsule) signal intensity invaginating the superior aspect

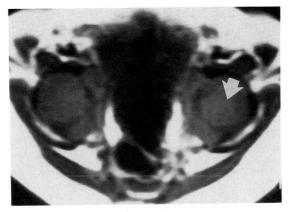

Figure 27-17 (left).
Normal hips. A T1-
weighted transaxial MR
image through the hips
in a 2-month-old infant
with suspected congeni-
tal dislocation of the left
hip shows a normal ana-
tomic position of both
femoral heads within
the acetabula. The ar-
row identifies the left
femoral head.

SE 300/20

Figure 27-18 (right). Hip dislocation. A proton-density transaxial MR image through the left
hip of an infant with a dislocated femoral head demon-
strates the intermediate-signal-
intensity iliopsoas tendon (arrow) within the joint. (Reprinted
with permission from Johnson
et al. [4].)

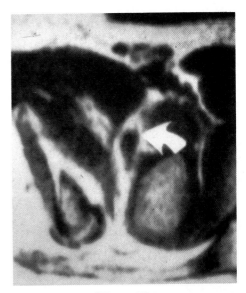

SE 1,500/25

of the hip joint. Both structures become interposed between the acetabulum and the femoral head. When joint fluid is present, the inverted limbus or enfolded capsule is more easily seen on T2-weighted images, since
the labrum or capsule will be surrounded by high-signal-intensity fluid.
The presence of hypertrophied fatty pulvinar can be identified on both
T1- and T2-weighted images as increased-signal-intensity fat in the
medial aspect of the joint.

Arthrography of the hip is still useful in DDH, particularly in the
operating room when closed reduction of the hip has failed and a sus-

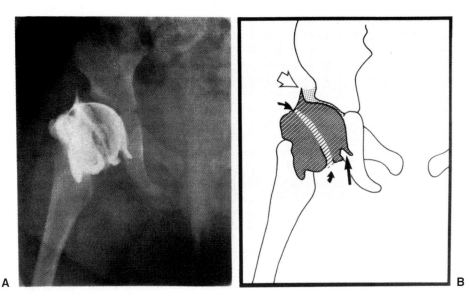

Figure 27-19. Normal arthrogram. (A) Arthrogram in a 7-month-old infant. (B) Schematic drawing of the arthrogram. The straight black arrow points to the "groove" of the ligamentum transversum. The open arrow indicates the "rose thorn" projection of the contrast agent. The curved arrows show the "zona orbicularis." (Reprinted with permission from Grech [2].)

pected mechanical impediment to reduction requires evaluation. With use of sterile technique, a contrast agent is injected into the synovial cavity, where it renders the joint space radiopaque and outlines the bony, fibrous, and cartilaginous structures within the joint. There are several structures that should be recognized in the normal hip arthrogram (Figure 27-19). These include the cartilaginous, partially ossified, or ossified femoral head; the labrum; the joint capsule; and the synovial membrane. The labrum is a ring of fibrocartilage that is attached to the brim of the acetabulum and enhances joint stability. It is particularly prominent on the posterosuperior aspect of the acetabulum, where it is lined by synovial membrane. This free margin of fibrocartilage is termed the limbus and is recognized on the arthrogram as a projection into the contrast agent in the superolateral aspect of the joint. The contrast agent trapped between the limbus and the adjacent joint capsule resembles a rose thorn. In cases of inverted limbus, where the labrum has hypertrophied, turned inward into the joint, and prevented closed reduction of the hip, the typical "rose thorn" appearance is not seen **(Option (D) is true)** (Figure 27-20).

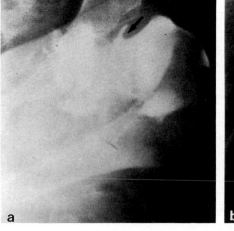
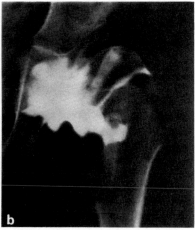
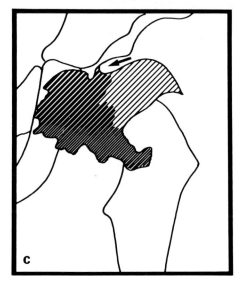

Figure 27-20. Dislocated left femoral head. A left hip arthrogram in a 10-month-old girl shows an inverted limbus (arrow) obstructing reduction of the head of the femur: adduction and flexion (a), neutral position (b), and a line drawing of the image in panel b (c). In panel c, the arrow indicates the inverted limbus, the light shading represents the femoral epiphysis, and the dark shading represents the contrast agent within the joint. (Reprinted with permission from Grech [2].)

The capsule should also be evaluated on the hip arthrogram. The capsule is a closely fitting fibrous sleeve that attaches to the brim of the acetabulum, to the labrum, and to the transverse ligament. It covers the head and neck of the femur and attaches inferiorly to the intertrochanteric region of the femur at the junction of the middle and distal thirds of the femoral neck. It is constricted around the narrowest part of the femoral neck by the zona orbicularis. These circular fibers help to strengthen and stabilize the hip joint and will be seen as an indentation in the contrast material at the level of the femoral neck. A third impression in the contrast material can be seen in the medial aspect of the joint on arthrography. This impression on the synovial membrane is caused by the transverse ligament as it crosses the synovium.

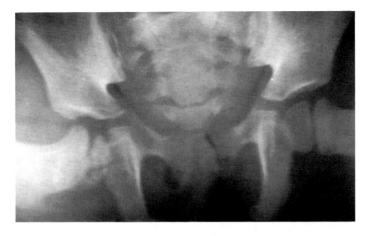

Figure 27-21. Ischemic necrosis in an 11-month-old infant after treatment for developmental dysplasia of the hip. An anteroposterior radiograph of the pelvis with femora in frog-leg lateral position shows a dense, fragmented right femoral capital epiphysis.

Of the many complications that can occur as a result of treatment for DDH, ischemic (avascular) necrosis is one of the most devastating (Figure 27-21). When the femoral head becomes ischemic, normal growth is impaired and the head becomes flattened and irregular in contour. This results in a secondary deformation of the acetabulum and in the development of acetabular slope as a result of deficient growth of the superior acetabular rim. Early degenerative disease with its lifelong morbidity is the result. Ischemia can affect any portion of the femoral head following treatment, causing either generalized or localized growth retardation. Both coxa vara and coxa valga deformities can develop, as can growth retardation of the entire femoral head coupled with overgrowth of the greater trochanter (Figure 27-22). There appears to be a relationship between the position of the femur during treatment for DDH and the subsequent development of ischemic necrosis. Medial rotation of the leg with concomitant abduction can compromise blood flow to the femoral head. In addition, pressure from an inverted limbus or the acetabular margin in cases of subluxation or dislocation can result in mechanical trauma to the femoral head and neck in certain positions. Vessels particularly affected by these factors include the medial circumflex, lateral circumflex, and superior and inferior ascending arteries. The posterolateral retinacular vessels can also be affected.

In healthy individuals, contralateral femoral-head ischemic necrosis can occasionally complicate treatment for DDH. This may be secondary to excessive medial rotation and abduction of the unaffected immobilized femur. Contralateral necrosis probably occurs when treatment is delayed

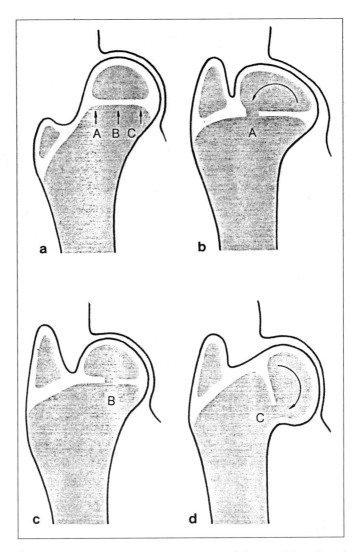

Figure 27-22. Morphologic complications of femoral-head ischemia in developmental dysplasia of the hip. (a) This diagram shows the normal proportion and growth of the proximal femur. Lettered arrows point to foci that may lead to specific growth disturbances. (b) Tilting of the head into the valgus ("head in neck" position) and shortening of the femoral neck and coxa plana result from necrosis involving the lateral segment of the physis (A). (c) Central necrosis or total necrosis of the physis further retards growth of the femoral neck (B), which remains short. Note the marked relative overgrowth of the greater trochanter. (d) Necrosis involving the medial segment of the physis (C) arrests neck growth medially while allowing it to proceed laterally and superiorly. The result is coxa vara with a short femoral neck and greater trochanteric overgrowth. (Reprinted with permission from Tonnis [9].)

in children with unstable dislocations, and these children consequently put most of their weight on the undislocated side prior to treatment. This increased weight and pressure on the unaffected femoral head could result in femoral-head necrosis or in an increased susceptibility to ischemia when this unaffected hip is immobilized **(Option (E) is true).**

Sheila G. Moore, M.D.

SUGGESTED READINGS

DEVELOPMENTAL DYSPLASIA OF THE HIP

1. Beim GM, Sartoris DJ, Resnick D. Interventional radiology: congenital dysplasia of the hip. Appl Radiol 1991; 20(1):10–21
2. Grech P. Hip arthrography. Philadelphia: JB Lippincott; 1977:1–106
3. Harcke HT, Grissom LE. Performing dynamic sonography of the infant hip. AJR 1990; 155:837–844
4. Johnson ND, Wood BP, Jackman KV. Complex infantile and congenital hip dislocation: assessment with MR imaging. Radiology 1988; 168:151–156
5. Johnson ND, Wood BP, Noh KS, Jackman KV, Westesson PL, Katzberg RW. MR imaging anatomy of the infant hip. AJR 1989; 153:127–133
6. Moore SG. Pediatric musculoskeletal imaging. In: Stark DD, Bradley WG Jr (eds), Magnetic resonance imaging. St. Louis: Mosby-Year Book; 1992:2223–2330
7. Ogden JA. Congenital dysplasia of the hip. In: Resnick D, Niwayama G (eds), Diagnosis of bone and joint disorders, 2nd ed. Philadelphia: WB Saunders; 1988:3336–3373
8. Share JC, Teele RL. Ultrasonography of the infant hip: a practical approach. Appl Radiol 1992; 21(6):27–34
9. Tonnis D. Congenital dysplasia and dislocation of the hip. Berlin: Springer-Verlag; 1987:1–288

SYNOVIAL CHONDROMATOSIS

10. Madewell JE, Sweet DE. Tumors and tumor-like lesions in or about joints. In: Resnick D, Niwayama G (eds), Diagnosis of bone and joint disorders, 2nd ed. Philadelphia: WB Saunders; 1988:3889–3943
11. Tuckman G, Wirth CZ. Synovial osteochondromatosis of the shoulder: MR findings. J Comput Assist Tomogr 1989; 13:360–361

LEGG-CALVÉ-PERTHES DISEASE

12. Catterall A, Pringle J, Byers PD, et al. A review of the morphology of Perthes' disease. J Bone Joint Surg (Br) 1982; 64:269–275
13. Henderson RC, Renner JB, Sturdivant MC, Greene WB. Evaluation of magnetic resonance imaging in Legg-Perthes disease: a prospective, blinded study. J Pediatr Orthop 1990; 10:289–297

14. Silverman FN. The limbs. Legg-Perthes disease. In: Silverman FN, Kuhn JP (eds), Caffey's pediatric x-ray diagnosis: an integrated imaging approach, 9th ed. St. Louis: Mosby-Year Book: 1993:1821–1824

TRANSIENT OSTEOPOROSIS

15. Bloem JL. Transient osteoporosis of the hip: MR imaging. Radiology 1988; 167:753–755
16. Pay NT, Singer WS, Bartal E. Hip pain in three children accompanied by transient abnormal findings on MR images. Radiology 1989; 171:147–149
17. Wilson AJ, Murphy WA, Hardy DC, Totty WG. Transient osteoporosis: transient bone marrow edema? Radiology 1988; 167:757–760

Notes

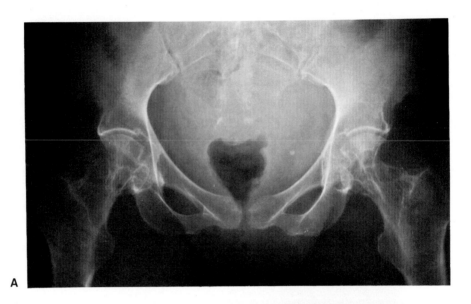

A

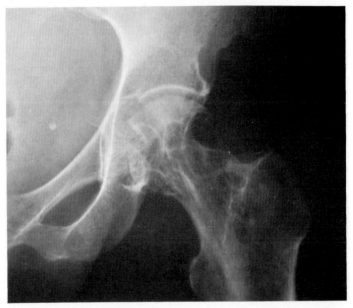

B

Figure 28-1. This 57-year-old woman with plasma cell (multiple) myeloma complained of bilateral hip pain. You are shown an anteroposterior
radiograph of the pelvis (A) and a detail image of the left hip (B).

Case 28: Amyloidosis

Question 122

Which *one* of the following is the MOST likely explanation for the radiographic changes in the hips?

(A) Tuberculosis
(B) Amyloidosis
(C) Plasma cell myeloma
(D) Hemochromatosis
(E) Gout

The test images show nearly symmetric involvement of the hip joints, characterized by osteopenia, preservation of the joint spaces, and well-circumscribed large marginal erosions or lytic lesions (Figure 28-1). Bilateral bulky soft tissue masses are also present but are more difficult to appreciate (Figure 28-2). These features are characteristic of amyloidosis, which is a known complication of plasma cell myeloma **(Option (B) is correct).**

Tuberculous arthritis (Option (A)) does affect large joints such as the hip, but it is usually monoarticular. Plasma cell myeloma (Option (C)) has many skeletal manifestations; however, bilateral articular involvement is distinctly unusual in uncomplicated cases.

Hemochromatosis (Option (D)) is often associated with joint abnormalities; however, its arthropathy typically includes joint space narrowing, subchondral bony sclerosis, and formation of small marginal osteophytes (Figure 28-3). Therefore, hemochromatosis is an unlikely cause of the radiographic changes in the test patient. Loss of the articular cartilage in patients with hemochromatosis does not predominate in stress-bearing areas, as it does in patients with osteoarthritis, but tends to be more uniform throughout the involved joint. Another important, although variable, feature of hemochromatosis, and one that is absent in the test patient, is articular cartilage calcification (Figure 28-4).

Gouty arthritis (Option (E)) (Figure 28-5), like amyloid joint disease, tends to produce well-circumscribed marginal or para-articular erosions

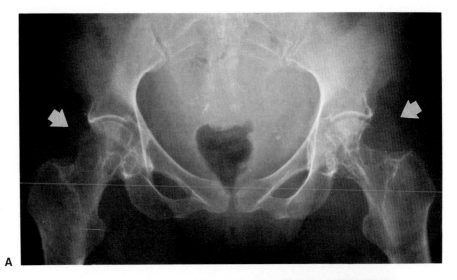

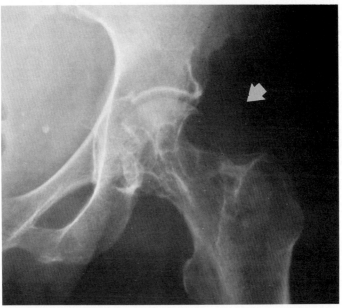

Figure 28-2 (Same as Figure 28-1). Amyloidosis. (A) Well-circumscribed lytic lesions or erosions are present in both femoral heads, but joint spaces are preserved. Periarticular soft tissue masses (arrows) surround both hips. (B) A close-up view of the left hip emphasizes the soft tissue mass (arrow).

and may spare the joint space. However, because gout is only intermittently inflammatory, it is usually not associated with periarticular osteoporosis. Gout also tends to be bilaterally asymmetric. It commonly

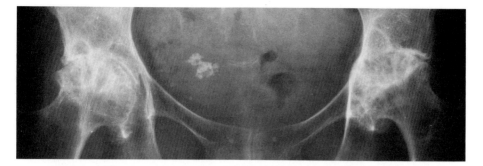

Figure 28-3. Hemochromatosis in a 64-year-old woman. The radiographic features include moderate-sized subarticular lucent lesions, mild sclerosis, uniform loss of articular cartilage, and little bony proliferation.

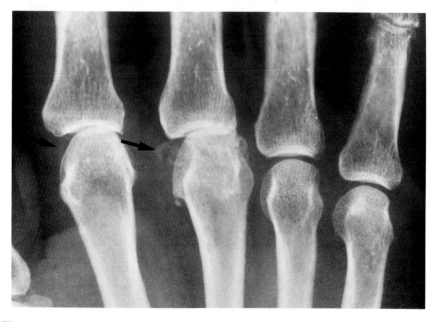

Figure 28-4. Hemochromatosis in a 76-year-old man. In the hands, radiographic changes characteristically involve the metacarpophalangeal joints, particularly of the index and long fingers. Features include cartilage loss, flattening of the metacarpal heads, and development of tiny bone fragments. These features may be associated with chondrocalcinosis and related periarticular calcifications (arrows).

involves the hands, wrists, feet, ankles, knees, and elbows, but it rarely involves the hips. Therefore, gout is unlikely in the test case.

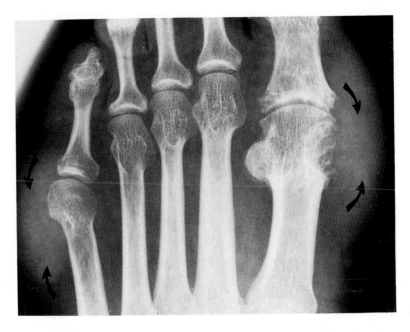

Figure 28-5. Chronic tophaceous gout. Subtle, hazy calcification is present in tophi adjacent to the first and fifth metatarsal heads (arrows). Despite partial destruction of the medial eminence of the head of the first metatarsal, the joint space is only moderately thinned and there is no osteoporosis.

Question 123

Concerning joint tuberculosis,

   (A) radiographically apparent pulmonary tuberculosis is also present in most patients
   (B) it is associated with severe periarticular osteopenia
   (C) destruction of articular cartilage precedes marginal erosion
   (D) the hip is the most commonly affected appendicular joint
   (E) it is common in patients with AIDS

Most cases of musculoskeletal tuberculosis are the result of hematogenous spread of the mycobacteria from a primary pulmonary focus of infection. However, in approximately half of the patients with musculoskeletal infection by *M. tuberculosis hominis,* concomitant pulmonary tuberculosis cannot be demonstrated in radiographs **(Option (A) is false).** Therefore, a negative chest radiograph does not exclude the possi-

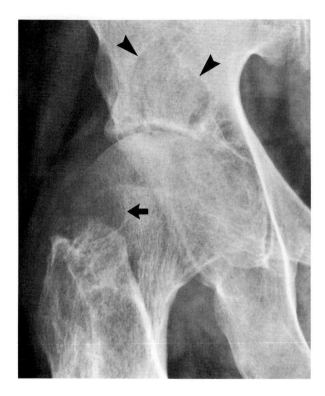

Figure 28-6. Tuberculosis of the hip in a 53-year-old man. A marginal erosion (arrow) is present along the lateral surface of the femoral neck. Lucent lesions (arrowheads) in the acetabulum reflect invasion of the supra-acetabular ilium by the tuberculous pannus.

bility of tuberculous osteomyelitis or arthritis. The infection has a predilection for bones in young children and for joints in adults.

Joint tuberculosis, unlike pyogenic infection of joints, progresses slowly. Tuberculous arthropathy commonly exhibits the diagnostic triad of Phemister: profound osteopenia, marginal erosions, and preservation of contacting articular cartilage despite the presence of large osseous erosions (Figures 28-6 and 28-7) **(Option (B) is true; Option (C) is false).** Although radiographs often show that the joint width is preserved, osteolytic lesions in the subchondral bone are common and reflect undermining of the articular cartilage and subarticular bone plate by tuberculous pannus. Articular cartilage is preserved because contact between opposing articular surfaces, in combination with the normal motion of the joint, tends to minimize the spread of the granulomatous pannus along the surface of the cartilage. Instead, the pannus attacks the cartilage and adjacent para-articular bone primarily at its periphery, at the joint margins. The pannus, having destroyed the joint margin, progressively undermines the articular cartilage and destroys the subchondral cancellous bone (Figures 28-6 and 28-7). The articular cartilage may then undergo separation from the adjacent bone followed by fragmentation and resorption.

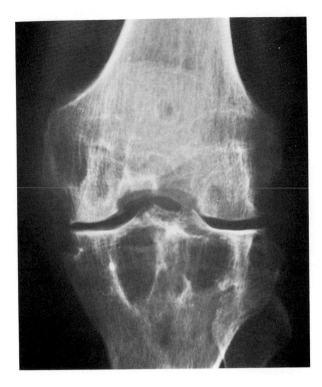

Figure 28-7. Tuberculosis of the knee in a 46-year-old man. The changes consist of osteoporosis, marginal erosions, and relative preservation of contacting articular cartilage (Phemister's triad). Note the osteolytic lesions in the subchondral bone of the tibia, similar to those in Figure 28-6.

The hip is the most common appendicular joint infected by *M. tuberculosis* **(Option (D) is true)** (Figure 28-6). An early radiographic manifestation may be lateral displacement of the femoral head, the result of joint distension by increasing amounts of intra-articular fluid or exudate. In a child, enlargement and accelerated maturation of the femoral head may occur in association with long-standing inflammation.

If the lesion originates in a juxta-articular location such as within the acetabulum or the intracapsular portion of the femur, bone destruction about the hip may be detected relatively early. A tendency to greater destruction of the acetabulum than of the femoral head and neck contrasts with the reverse order of destruction found in association with infections by other organisms. Resorption of the acetabulum results in protrusio acetabuli and ultimately acetabular perforation, which allows exudate to enter the pelvis.

The soft tissue abscess may extend distal to the hip joint into the region of the femoral triangle. Sharply demarcated shadows in the soft tissues of the thigh or leg may represent loculated collections of exudate. Many years after the onset of infection, calcified caseous debris may develop in the joint and in the dependent part of the abscess. The sharp demarcation of a tuberculous "cold" abscess signifies a lack of inflamma-

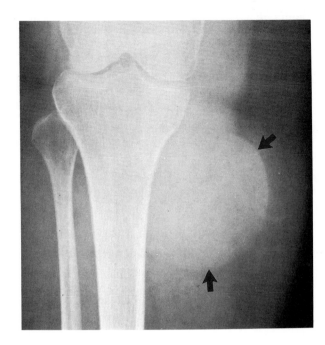

Figure 28-8. Tuberculous cold abscess of the leg of a 58-year-old woman. The abscess (arrows) had dissected from a long-standing tuberculous infection of the hip.

tory edema (Figure 28-8). This characteristic sharp demarcation is not a feature of abscesses caused by other organisms, which tend to be associated with considerable edema in the adjacent soft tissues. Other common sites of tuberculous arthropathy are the knee, elbow, and wrist.

Despite a decline in the incidence of infections caused by *M. tuberculosis* in the past several decades, tuberculosis remains a serious health problem in the United States. Groups at special risk for tuberculosis include the homeless, intravenous-drug abusers, certain immigrants and refugees, and residents of prisons and nursing homes. A recent resurgence of pulmonary tuberculosis appears to be related to the epidemic of acquired immunodeficiency syndrome (AIDS), resulting from infection with the human immunodeficiency virus (HIV). In a report from New York State in 1986, tuberculosis was found to have developed in 8.6% of 280 patients with AIDS. AIDS is a defect in cell-mediated immunity, and pulmonary tuberculosis is relatively common in patients with AIDS; therefore, tuberculous osteomyelitis would also be expected to occur in these patients. However, whereas individual cases of muscle, bone, and joint tuberculosis in patients with AIDS have been reported, musculoskeletal involvement with tuberculosis is not common in these patients. A review of 560 patients with AIDS revealed that only 2% had proven osteomyelitis, usually caused by *Staphylococcus* or *Salmonella* species; tuberculous osteomyelitis was not reported among these cases **(Option (E) is false).**

Question 124

Concerning musculoskeletal amyloidosis,

(A) it occurs in about 15% of patients with plasma cell myeloma
(B) intra-articular amyloidosis is characterized by preservation of the joint space
(C) joint involvement is associated with periarticular soft tissue masses
(D) it is associated with carpal tunnel syndrome
(E) joint involvement is usually monoarticular

In 1854, Virchow published the first histologic description of amyloid infiltration. Amyloid is a proteinaceous material, which, as shown by electron microscopy, is composed of aggregated fibrils arranged in sheets. Amyloid consists primarily of fibril proteins (90%), with the remainder composed of glycoproteins. Two classes of amyloid fibril proteins have been identified: amyloid light chain (AL), derived from plasma cells; and amyloid associated (AA), a nonimmunoglobulin synthesized by the liver. The AL type is associated with plasma cell myeloma and is derived from the circulating light chains (Bence Jones protein). Although amyloidosis has been classified in several ways, the most important distinction is between the primary and secondary forms. One popular system of classification is as follows: (1) primary amyloidosis occurs without antecedent or coexistent diseases and predominates in the heart, muscle, tongue, synovium, and perivascular connective tissues. It is associated with plasma cell myeloma, as the two disorders tend to have a simultaneous onset; (2) secondary amyloidosis, the type most commonly associated with musculoskeletal involvement, tends to occur late in the course of chronic diseases, including rheumatoid arthritis and other inflammatory arthritides, tuberculous and nontuberculous osteomyelitis, neoplasms (excluding plasma cell myeloma, which has a simultaneous onset, as noted above), long-term hemodialysis, and familial Mediterranean fever, and predominates in the liver, spleen, kidneys, and adrenals; (3) heredofamilial amyloidosis is associated with neuropathies, nephropathies, or cardiomyopathies; and (4) localized amyloid tumors (amyloidomas) usually affect the larynx or tracheobronchial tree.

The radiographic changes of musculoskeletal amyloidosis reflect amyloid deposition in bone, synovium, and soft tissue and may be superimposed upon the changes of the inciting disease process. Primary musculoskeletal amyloidosis occurs concomitantly in approximately 15% of patients with plasma cell myeloma **(Option (A) is true).** Secondary

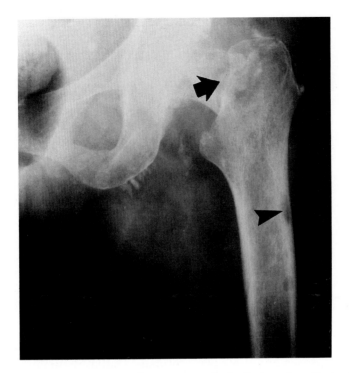

Figure 28-9. Amyloidosis producing osteolytic foci and pathologic fracture. This 58-year-old woman had been diagnosed with plasma cell myeloma on the basis of Bence Jones proteinuria and osteolytic bone lesions. An anteroposterior view of the left hip and proximal femur several months later shows a coxa vara deformity due to a fracture at the site of a large lytic lesion (arrow) in the femoral neck and additional lytic lesions (arrowhead) in the femoral shaft. The woman died during surgery. An autopsy revealed amyloidosis as the sole cause of the bone lesions; there was no evidence of plasma cell myeloma. Disturbances in serum electrophoresis and Bence Jones proteinuria can occur in primary amyloidosis, the final diagnosis in this case. (Reprinted with permission from Goldman et al. [1].)

amyloidosis is also seen in patients with long-standing rheumatoid arthritis, ankylosing spondylitis, and other spondyloarthropathies. It has been found in approximately 25% of children with familial Mediterranean fever, a rare disorder characterized by recurrent fever and serositis leading to pleural, peritoneal, and joint pain.

Deposits of amyloid may produce osteolytic foci, which predominate in the humeral and femoral heads and necks. When these deposits result in endosteal scalloping of the cortex, they may simulate changes of plasma cell myeloma (Figure 28-9). Perivascular deposits of amyloid in

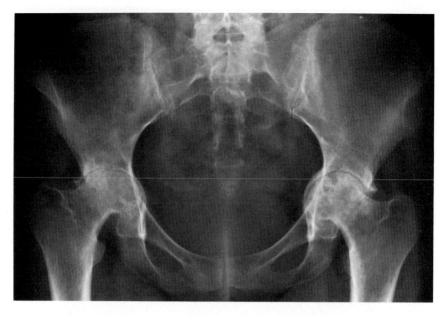

Figure 28-10. Rheumatoid arthritis in a 36-year-old woman. An antero-posterior view of the pelvis shows bilateral hip disease, with uniform loss of the joint space and protrusio acetabuli. Unlike rheumatoid arthritis, amyloidosis tends to spare the joint space (see Figure 28-1).

the subchondral bone may obstruct the vascular supply to the epiphysis, resulting in osteonecrosis. In the hip this may result in ischemic necrosis of the femoral head. Deposits in the vertebrae may lead to their collapse. Localized deposits of amyloid may calcify. Diffuse skeletal amyloidosis leads to pathologic fractures.

Although the clinical and radiographic findings of amyloid joint disease may resemble those of rheumatoid arthritis (and, indeed, the two disorders may coexist), the two conditions can usually be distinguished because amyloidosis tends to preserve the joint space **(Option (B) is true)** whereas rheumatoid arthritis tends to cause an early and uniform loss of the joint space (Figure 28-10).

The most common sites of periarticular amyloid involvement are the shoulders, olecranon regions, and wrists. Bulky soft tissue masses of amyloid are a hallmark of articular and periarticular amyloidosis **(Option (C) is true)**. In the shoulders these large soft tissue masses, which can be hard and rubbery, resemble the shoulder pads worn by football players. Amyloid accumulation in synovial, peritendinous, and other periarticular tissues of the wrist may lead to the carpal tunnel syn-

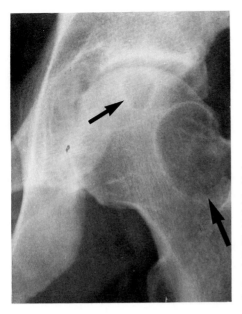

Figure 28-11. Pigmented villonodular synovitis of the left hip of a 32-year-old man. The osteolytic lesions (arrows) have sclerotic margins. Features that distinguish pigmented villonodular synovitis from amyloidosis are the younger age, unilaterality, and absence of periarticular osteopenia.

drome. Up to 8% of patients with the carpal tunnel syndrome have primary amyloidosis as the underlying cause **(Option (D) is true).**

The arthropathy of amyloidosis may also have similarities to that of pigmented villonodular synovitis. However, whereas involvement in amyloidosis is usually bilateral **(Option (E) is false),** pigmented villonodular synovitis is almost always a monoarticular process. In addition, pigmented villonodular synovitis occurs in a younger age group than does amyloidosis and is not associated with periarticular osteopenia or calcification (Figure 28-11). The presence of hemosiderin in the lesion may produce a slight and diffuse increase in X-ray density.

Question 125

Concerning plasma cell myeloma,

    (A) the mandible is involved in about 30% of patients
    (B) skull lesions are more uniform in size than are metastases
    (C) destruction of pedicles is a characteristic feature
    (D) diffuse osteosclerosis is a rare manifestation

Plasma cell (multiple) myeloma is the most common of the plasma cell dyscrasias—disorders that feature uncontrolled proliferation of immunoglobulin-secreting plasma cells in the absence of an identifiable stimulus. Other plasma cell dyscrasias are Waldenström's macroglobulinemia, primary amyloidosis, and heavy-chain disease. These dyscrasias behave as malignant diseases, producing excessive levels of complete or incomplete immunoglobulins in the plasma and/or urine. Plasma cell myeloma is a common malignant disorder that usually originates in the bone marrow, and it is the most common primary cancer of bone. The disorder predominates in men (about 70%); although 98% of patients are over the age of 40 years, the disease is occasionally found in persons as young as 25 years. Most patients are symptomatic when diagnosed. Symptoms and signs include bone pain, loss of height, and kyphosis. Patients may also have constitutional symptoms, such as weakness, fatigue, anorexia, and weight loss. Pathologic fractures occur frequently.

Most patients with plasma cell myeloma undergo an increase in their total protein level in serum as a result of an increase in the globulin fraction. Indeed, the accumulation of immunoglobulin G (IgG) and IgM leads to increased viscosity of the blood serum. Bence Jones proteinuria (the excretion of free light chains) is present in over 50% of the cases. The presence of these proteins in the blood and urine is a key feature of the disease, but the ultimate diagnostic feature is identification of the abnormal aggregates of plasma cells. The major causes of death in patients with plasma cell myeloma are infection and renal failure (myeloma or nephrosis). Metastatic calcifications in the kidneys reflect the bone destruction and resultant hypercalcemia. If untreated, patients with multiple bony lesions rarely survive more than 1 year. Even with chemotherapy in the form of alkylating agents, the median survival is only 2 to 3 years.

Pathologically, focal intraosseous collections of neoplastic plasma cells secrete a substance, lymphotoxin, that stimulates osteoclastic activity, thus causing the characteristic osteolytic changes. Plasma cell infiltration occurs first in bones in which red marrow persists into adulthood, i.e., the bones of the axial skeleton. With gradually advancing erythroid hyperplasia in the appendicular skeleton compensating for the increasing anemia, those bones also become involved.

As might be expected, radiologic features predominate in the axial skeleton; the vertebrae, ribs, skull, pelvis, and femora are involved in decreasing order of frequency. Mandibular involvement, rare in metastatic disease, occurs in about 30% of patients with plasma cell myeloma **(Option (A) is true)**. In the skull, compared with osteolytic metastases, the lesions of plasma cell myeloma tend to appear more discrete and more uniform in size (Figure 28-12) **(Option (B) is true)**. In the spine, myelomatous involvement usually spares the pedicles despite extensive destruction of the vertebral bodies (Figure 28-13) **(Option (C) is false)**; by comparison, early destruction of the pedicles is characteristic in meta-

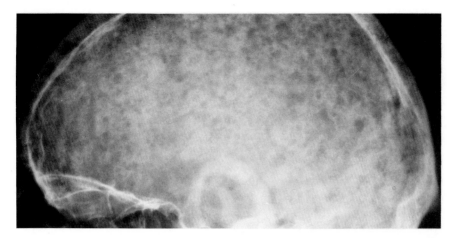

Figure 28-12. Plasma cell myeloma involving the skull of a 60-year-old man. The numerous osteolytic foci are discrete and tend to be uniform in size.

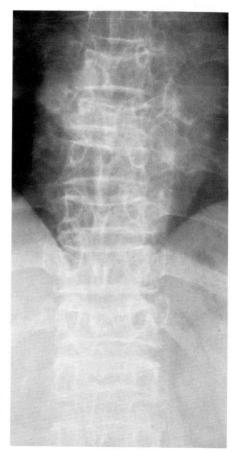

Figure 28-13. Plasma cell myeloma involving the spine of a 71-year-old woman. Despite profound osteopenia with extensive collapse of the vertebral bodies, the pedicles are spared.

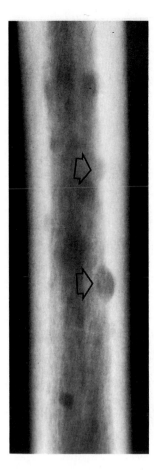

Figure 28-14. Plasma cell myeloma involving the proximal shaft of the femur of a 64-year-old woman. Sharply defined elliptical foci of endosteal cortical destruction (arrows) are characteristic findings in long bones in which the normal marrow has been replaced by tumor cells.

static disease. In long bones, elliptical subcortical foci of destruction associated with endosteal cortical scalloping are a characteristic finding (Figure 28-14).

Another common radiographic presentation of plasma cell myeloma is diffuse skeletal osteopenia in the absence of discrete lesions, often with multiple vertebral compression fractures (Figure 28-15) and rib fractures. This form simulates osteoporosis, except that it has a strikingly more profound and rapidly progressive course.

Focal or diffuse osteolytic lesions are the usual radiographic findings in patients with plasma cell myeloma; however, osteosclerotic lesions or even diffuse osteosclerosis is occasionally encountered (Figure 28-16) **(Option (D) is true).** Interestingly, osteoslerotic myeloma is frequently associated with sensorimotor polyneuropathy. The POEMS syndrome, characterized by single or multiple osteosclerotic lesions, is an unusual multisystem disorder that includes polyneuropathy, organomegaly, endo-

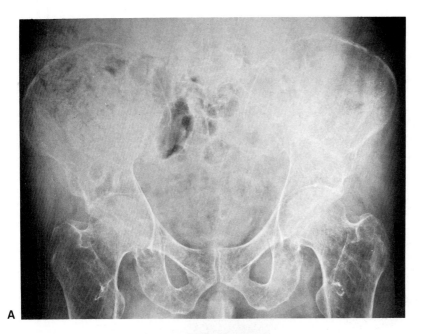

A

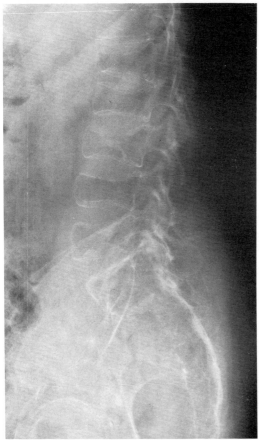

B

Figure 28-15. Plasma cell myeloma producing profound generalized osteopenia in a 33-year-old man. An anteroposterior radiograph of the pelvis (A) and a lateral radiograph of the lumbosacral spine (B) are shown. Although this is one of the characteristic radiographic presentations of plasma cell myeloma, the disorder is uncommon in individuals younger than 40 years of age.

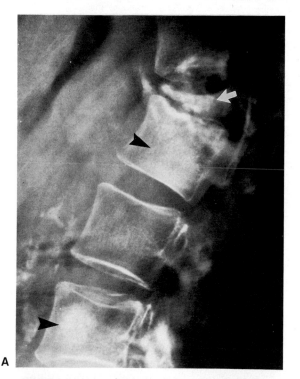

A

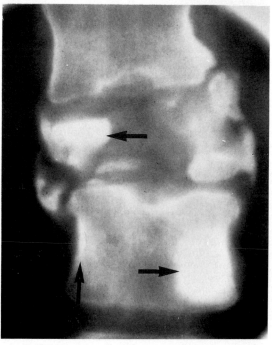

B

Figure 28-16. Osteo-
sclerotic myeloma in a
50-year-old woman with
severe back pain. (A) A
lateral view of the lum-
bar spine shows a com-
pression fracture of L1
(arrow). Sclerotic lesions
(arrowheads) are pres-
ent in the L2 and L4
vertebral bodies. (B) An
anteroposterior tomo-
gram of the L1 fracture
reveals sclerotic lesions
(arrows) in L1 and L2.
(C) A frog-leg lateral
view of the right hip re-
veals a sclerotic lesion in
the proximal femur.
(Courtesy of Harold G.
Jacobson, M.D., Monte-
fiore Medical Center,
Bronx, N.Y.)

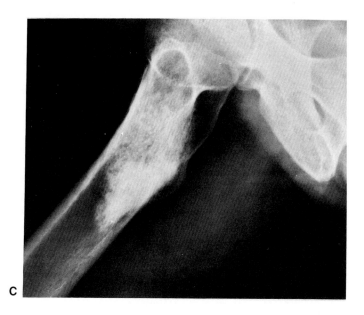

c

crine dysfunction, M-protein abnormalities, and skin changes. The exact relationship of the POEMS syndrome to plasma cell myeloma is uncertain. Bone sclerosis in cases of plasma cell myeloma may also follow chemotherapy or irradiation.

Solitary myeloma (plasmacytoma) is characterized by a single, lytic focus, usually with an expansile, bubbly radiographic appearance. About 25% of patients present with this form of plasma cell myeloma. Almost all cases of solitary plasmacytoma evolve into the disseminated form of plasma cell myeloma, but many years may pass before this occurs.

False-negative bone scintigrams in association with plasma cell myeloma are common. Even in patients with positive findings, scintigraphy usually does not reveal as many lesions as do plain radiographs. This is presumed to reflect the fact that most myelomatous lesions are nearly purely osteolytic and lack significant reactive new bone formation, which is the histopathologic feature most closely associated with increased accumulation of Tc-99m diphosphonate compounds. In many instances, foci of increased activity are due to associated pathologic fractures (e.g., vertebral compression) rather than to the primary effect of the myelomatous lesions.

Richard H. Gold, M.D.
Lawrence W. Bassett, M.D.

SUGGESTED READINGS

AMYLOIDOSIS

1. Goldman AB, Pavlov H, Bullough P. Case report 137. Primary amyloidosis involving the skeletal system. Skeletal Radiol 1981; 6:69–74
2. Kyle RA, Bayrd ED. Amyloidosis: review of 236 cases. Medicine 1975; 54:271–299
3. Mohr W. Amyloid deposits in the periarticular tissue. Z Rheumatol 1976; 35:412–417
4. Ross LV, Ross GJ, Mesgarzadeh M, Edmonds PR, Bonakdarpour A. Hemodialysis-related amyloidomas of bone. Radiology 1991; 78:263–265
5. Subbarao K, Jacobson HG. Amyloidosis and plasma cell dyscrasias of the musculoskeletal system. Semin Roentgenol 1986; 21:139–149
6. Weinfeld A, Stern MH, Marx LH. Amyloid lesions of bone. AJR 1970; 108:799–805
7. Wiernik PH. Amyloid joint disease. Medicine 1972; 51:465–479

TUBERCULOSIS

8. Buckner CB, Leithiser RE, Walker CW, Allison JW. The changing epidemiology of tuberculosis and other mycobacterial infections in the United States: implications for the radiologist. AJR 1991; 156:255–264
9. Chapman M, Murray RO, Stoker DJ. Tuberculosis of the bones and joints. Semin Roentgenol 1979; 14:262–282
10. Fleckenstein JL, Burns DK, Murphy FK, Jayson HT, Bonte FJ. Differential diagnosis of bacterial myositis in AIDS: evaluation with MR imaging. Radiology 1991; 179:653–658
11. Louie E, Rice LB, Holzman RS. Tuberculosis in non-Haitian patients with acquired immunodeficiency syndrome. Chest 1986; 90:542–545
12. Spencer GM, Burgener FA, Hampton BA. Osteomyelitis in AIDS patients. Radiology 1991; 181P:155–156
13. Wolfgang GL. Tuberculosis joint infection. Clin Orthop 1978; 136:257–263

PLASMA CELL MYELOMA

14. Bataille R, Chevalier J, Rossi M, Sany J. Bone scintigraphy in plasma-cell myeloma. A prospective study of 70 patients. Radiology 1982; 145:801–804
15. Hall FM, Gore SM. Osteosclerotic myeloma variants. Skeletal Radiol 1988; 17:101–105
16. Meszaros WT. The many facets of multiple myeloma. Semin Roentgenol 1974; 9:219–228
17. Mirra JM, Picci P, Gold RH. Bone tumors: clinical, radiologic, and pathologic correlations. Philadelphia: Lea & Febiger; 1989:1121–1144
18. Oken MM. Multiple myeloma. Med Clin North Am 1984; 68:757–787
19. Pankovich AM, Griem ML. Plasma-cell myeloma. A thirty-year follow-up. Radiology 1972; 104:521–522

20. Resnick D. Plasma cell dyscrasias and dysgammaglobulonemias. In: Resnick D, Niwayama G (eds), Diagnosis of bone and joint disorders. Philadelphia: WB Saunders; 1988:2358–2403

21. Resnick D, Greenway GD, Bardwick PA, Zvaifler NJ, Gill GN, Newman DR. Plasma-cell dyscrasia with polyneuropathy, organomegaly, endocrinopathy, M-protein, and skin changes: the POEMS syndrome. Distinctive radiographic abnormalities. Radiology 1981; 140:17–22

Index

Where there are multiple page references, **boldface** indicates the main discussion of a topic.

A

Abutment syndrome. *See* Ulnolunate impaction syndrome
Acetabular dysplasia. *See* Hip, developmental dysplasia
Achilles tendon, 503, 510, 514–15, 521
Ackerman biopsy needles, 236
Acquired immunodeficiency syndrome
  AIDS-related arthritis, 711
  cryptococcal arthritis and, 647
  osteomyelitis and, 773
  pulmonary tuberculosis and, 773
Actinomadura madurae, 640
Actinomyces, 633, 638
Actinomycetes, 629
Actinomycotic osteomyelitis
  radiologic findings, 634–38
Acute myelogenous leukemia
  stem cell proliferation as cause, 44
Acute symmetric polyarthritis. *See* HIV-associated arthritis
Adolescent pattern of bone marrow conversion, 19, 40
Adult hypophosphatasia, 335, 337, 339, 341
Adult pattern of bone marrow conversion, 19, 21–22, 40
Age factors
  Achilles tendon ruptures, 521
  ameloblastoma, 607
  aneurysmal bone cysts, 172
  anterior tibial tendon, 529
  bipartite patella, 371–72
  bone marrow conversion, 14, 16–17, 38–40
  calcium pyrophosphate dihydrate crystal deposition disease, 539
  chondroblastomas, 191
  chondromalacia patellae, 382
  chondrosarcomas, 176
  compression type-fractures, 402
  congenital multiple fibromatosis, 243, 260
  cystic angiomatosis, 250

Age factors *(cont'd)*
  epiphyseal osteonecrosis, 656
  fibromatosis, 264
  fibrous dysplasia, 245, 256, 257, 589, 591
  fibroxanthomas, 188–89
  giant cell reparative granuloma, 589
  gout, 702
  hemangiomas, 251, 366
  histoplasmosis, 647
  humeral pseudocysts, 57
  hypophosphatasia, 331, 334–35
  Klippel-Trenaunay-Weber syndrome, 365
  Langerhans cell histiocytosis, 660, 666, 668
  Legg-Calvé-Perthes disease, 732
  mycetoma, 640
  neuropathic arthropathy, 535
  osteitis condensans of the clavicle, 158
  osteoblastomas, 184
  osteochondritis dissecans, 376, 656
  osteogenesis imperfecta tarda, 314
  osteoid osteomas, 195
  osteomyelitis, 736–37
  osteoporosis, 313
  osteosarcomas, 153, 199
  osteosarcomatosis, 200
  Paget's disease, 151, 153
  periodontal disease, 615–16, 618
  pigmented villonodular synovitis, 702, 777
  plasma cell myeloma, 778
  posterior tibial tendon injuries, 522
  regenerate bone, 479
  Reiter's syndrome, 543
  rhabdomyosarcoma, 429, 440
  split-type fractures, 400–402
  sternocostoclavicular hyperostosis, 155
  synovial chondromatosis, 744
  tuberculous osteomyelitis, 771
  X-linked hypophosphatemia, 322
Aggressive fibromatosis. *See* Juvenile fibromatosis

AIDS. *See* Acquired immunodeficiency syndrome
Airway obstruction, 613–14
Alcohol use
    epiphyseal osteonecrosis and, 656
Allogeneic bone marrow transplants, 138
Aluminum intoxication
    osteomalacia and, 147
Alveolar crest
    gingivitis and, 616
Ameloblastomas, 604, 606–7
AML. *See* Acute myelogenous leukemia
Amphotericin B, 644
Amyloidomas, 774
Amyloidosis, 767, 778. *See also* Musculoskeletal amyloidosis
Amyotrophic lateral sclerosis, 445, 446
Anatomic compartments, 228
Anemia. *See* Aplastic anemia; Sickle-cell anemia
Aneurysmal bone cysts, **199**
    differential diagnosis
        well-differentiated osteosarcomas, 172–75, 184
    patellar, 390
Angiography
    angiovenous dysplasias, 360
Angiosarcomas
    patellar, 390
Angiovenous dysplasias of the extremities, **359–60, 363–66**
Angle of Gissane, 418
Angle of Wiberg, 731
Animal studies, 485–86, 487
Ankle
    anatomy, 514–17, 519
    anterior, 519
    lateral, 519
    medial, 516–17, 519
    neuropathic arthropathy, 533–35, 558–59
    posterior, 514–15
    Reiter's syndrome, 544–46
    tendons, **503–5, 519–22, 524, 528–30**
        abnormalities, **505–10, 512–14**
        sheaths, 508–9
Ankylosing spondylitis, and
    HIV infection, 720
    secondary amyloidosis, 775
    sternocostoclavicular hyperostosis, 155
Ankylosis, 546, 613
Antacids
    osteomalacia and, 147
Anterior interbody fixation system, 460
    stable short-segment fixation, 464–66
Anterior tibial tendon, 529
Antibiotics
    fungal infections and, 632, 646
    osteopetrosis skeletal pattern change and, 137

Antifungal drugs, 644
Antihistamines
    systemic mastocytosis, 322
Anti-inflammatory drugs
    osteitis condensans of the clavicle, 159
    plica syndrome, 389
Apical periodontal cysts, 603
Aplastic anemia, 11
    bone marrow changes, 7, 8–9, 43–44
    differential diagnosis
        chronic medullary bone infarct, 3
    leukemia and, 26–27
    treatment, 43
Arachnodactyly, 81–82
Arterial abnormalities
    neurofibromatosis type 1 and, 249
Arteriovenous malformations
    differential diagnosis
        hemangiomas of the extremities, 360, 363
Arthritis. *See also* Osteoarthritis; Pseudogout; Reiter's syndrome
    AIDS-related, 711
    cryptococcal, 647
    fungal, 632–33
    hallux rigidus deformities, 563–64
    hypersensitivity, 645
    inflammatory, 708
    juvenile, 701
    rheumatoid
        anterior femoral pressure erosions, 541
        differential diagnosis
            hemophilia, 701
        hallux valgus deformities and, 577
        HIV infection and, 721
        juvenile, 726
        secondary amyloidosis and, 774–76
        sternoclavicular joint involvement, 163
        tendon injuries and, 520, 522
    secondary degenerative, 702
    septic, 534
        differential diagnosis
            osteomyelitis, 166
        elbow arthropathy, 708
        fungal infections and, 646, 647
        HIV infection and, 720
        intravenous-drug use and, 163, 165–66
        osseous infection and, 736–37
    seronegative-type, 720
    sesamoid bone involvement, 578
    sternoclavicular joint involvement, 159, 163, 166
    sternocostoclavicular hyperostosis and, 155
    tibial plateau fractures and, 402
    tuberculous, 767

Congenital metatarsus primus varus, 570
Congenital multiple fibromatosis, **243–44**,
    260–61, 265–66
  differential diagnosis
    congenital generalized fibromatosis,
        261
    cystic angiomatosis, 250–51
    fibrosarcomas, 260
    fibrous dysplasia, 244–45
    lipomatosis, 243–44
    lymphangiomatosis, 243
    metastatic neuroblastoma, 244
    multiple hemangioma of bone, 251–53
    neurofibromatosis type 1, 245–50
Congenital rubella syndrome
  cardiac anomalies combined with, 79
  patent ductus arteriosus and, 69
Conjunctivitis, 543
Conventional radiography
  acetabulum, 739–40
  aneurysmal bone cysts, 173
  angiovenous dysplasias, 359–60
  chondromalacia patellae, 382–83
  chondrosarcomas, 177–78, 180
  congenital multiple fibromatosis, 243–44,
      260
  hallux valgus deformity, 563, 568–70
  muscles, 445
  osteochondritis dissecans, 378–79
    of the patella, 371
  osteoid osteomas, 195
  sesamoid bones of the great toe, 579
  synovial chondromatosis, **742, 744**
  systemic mastocytosis, 318
  tibial plateau fracture, 397
  tumor staging, 209
Corticotomy
  Ilizarov procedure, 479, 484, 485–86, 488,
      491, 493
  osteotomy comparison, 487
Cosmetic procedures
  fibrous dysplasia, 591
Cotrel-Dubousset fixation system, 460, 465,
    466–67
Coxa valga deformities, 761
Coxa vara deformities, 761
CPPD. *See* Calcium pyrophosphate dihy-
    drate
CPPD crystal deposition disease. *See* Calci-
    um pyrophosphate dihydrate crystal
    deposition disease
Craig biopsy needles, 236
Cryptococcosis, 637
Cryptococcus, 631
Cryptococcus neoformans, 647
CT. *See* Computed tomography
CT arthrography
  shoulder instability, 117, 119–20

Cuboid bone
  crush of, 549, 551
Cuboid dislocation, 549
Cuneiform fractures, 552
Curettage. *See also* Excision; Surgery
  Langerhans cell histiocytosis, 595, 673
Cutaneous abnormalities
  odontogenic keratocysts and, 606
Cutaneous mastocytosis, 317
Cystic angiomatosis
  differential diagnosis
    congenital multiple fibromatosis, 250–
        51
    Rendu-Osler-Weber disease, 250
Cysts. *See also* Aneurysmal bone cysts; Bak-
    er's cysts; Ganglion cysts; Pseudo-
    cysts; Solitary bone cysts
  apical periodontal, 603
  benign dermal, 606
  dentigerous, 604
  follicular, 604
  of the jaw, 603–7
  meniscal, 356–57
  odontogenic keratocyst, 605–6
  radicular, 603
  simple
    differential diagnosis
      calcaneal pseudocysts, 59
  skin, 592
  subchondral, 539, 726
    differential diagnosis
      fungal osteomyelitis, 626–27
  synovial, 355–56

D

DDH. *See* Hip, developmental dysplasia
Degenerative arthritis. *See* Osteoarthritis
Degenerative disk disease
  differential diagnosis
    failed back syndrome, 451
Degenerative joint disease
  elbow, 708
Dentigerous cysts, 604
deQuervain's tenosynovitis, 693–94
Dermal calcinosis, 606
Desert rheumatism, 645
Desmoid tumors
  Gardner's syndrome, 592
Desmoplastic fibromas
  differential diagnosis
    well-differentiated osteosarcomas, 184
Dextrocardia
  radial ray disorders and, 91
Diabetes insipidus
  Langerhans cell histiocytosis and, 668

F

Face
  bone marrow characteristics, 40–41
Facial asymmetry
  fibrous dysplasia and, 589, 591
Failed back syndrome, **458–60**
  differential diagnosis
    degenerative disk disease, 451
    diskogenic pain, 451, 455–57
    postoperative infection, 451
    segmental spine instability, 451, 452,
      455
Failure-to-thrive syndrome, 333
Falls
  tibial plateau fractures and, 398
False fungi, 633, 638
Familial Mediterranean fever
  secondary amyloidosis and, 774–75
Fanconi's anemia
  radial ray disorders and, 92
Femur
  anterior femoral pressure erosion, 541
  bone marrow changes, 42
  Ewing's sarcoma, 205–7, 223
  herniation pits
    differential diagnosis
      pseudocysts, 61
Fibromas
  cementifying, 601, 603
  cemento-ossifying, 601, 603
  composition, 261
  differential diagnosis
    well-differentiated osteosarcomas, 184
  jaw, 601, 603
  ossifying, 601, 603
Fibrosarcomas
  differential diagnosis
    congenital multiple fibromatosis, 260
Fibrous cortical defects. *See* Fibroxantho-
    mas
Fibrous dysplasia, **255–60**, 589, 591
  differential diagnosis
    calcaneal pseudocysts, 59, 61
    congenital multiple fibromatosis, 244–
      45
    diametaphyseal bone marrow infarc-
      tion, 648, 651
    intracortical hemangiomas of bone, 253
    osteitis condensans of the clavicle, 159
    well-differentiated osteosarcomas, 184
  "ground glass" appearance, 244, 255, 651
  malignant transformation, 259–60
  polyostotic
    clinical symptoms, 258–59
    location, 256–57
    soft tissue myxoma and, 255–56
  spine involvement, 257–58

Fibroxanthomas, **188–89**
  differential diagnosis
    well-differentiated osteosarcomas, 175,
      184
    pigmented villonodular synovitis, 704
Flexor digitorum longus tendon, 503, 516,
    522
Flexor hallucis longus tendon, 503, 516, 517,
    528
Flucytosine, 644
Fluoroscopy
  biopsy guidance, 234
Fluorosis, and
  hyperostosis, 145
  osteomalacia, 147
Follicular cyst, 604
Foot. *See also* Calcaneus; Hallux valgus de-
    formities
  anatomy, 514–17, 519
  deformities of the second through fifth
    toes, **580–83**
  mycetoma, 629, 640
  osteoblastomas, 187
  second-digit crossover toe, 582
  sesamoid bones of the great toe, **578–79**
  tendons, **519–22, 524, 528–30**
Footwear, and
  adult forefoot, 583
  bunionettes, 583
  diabetic patients, 559
  hallux rigidus deformities, 565
  hallux valgus deformities, 570
Forefoot. *See also* Foot
  Reiter's syndrome, 546
Fractures. *See also* Looser's zones; Stress
    fractures; Tuberosity fractures
  bicondylar, 400
  bicondylar split, 402
  carpal, 688
  chondral, 708
  condylar neck, 612–13
  condylar-subcondylar, 610, 612
  cortical avulsion, 551
  cuneiform, 552
  distal radius, 680
  distal talus, 533
  fixation rod, 467–68
  Galeazzi, 680
  local compression, 399
  mandibular angle, 610
  mandibular body, 613
  midfoot, **549, 551–52**
  minimally displaced, 398–99, 406
  navicular, 549, 551–52
  nutcracker, 549, 551
  occult complete, 305
  occult linear, 688–89
  open, 408

Giant cell tumors *(cont'd)*
  fibrous dysplasia transformation to, 259
  patellar, 390
  pigmented villonodular synovitis, 704
Gingivitis, 615–16
Glenohumeral joint
  neuropathic arthropathy, 558
  stability of, **117, 119–20, 124–25**
Glenoid labrum
  glenohumeral joint stability and, 117
Golfer's elbow, 711–12
Gout
  differential diagnosis
    hemophilia, 701
  elbow arthropathy, 708, 711
  tendon injuries and, 520
Gouty arthritis, 767–69
Growth arrest lines
  steroid therapy and, 148
Growth plates, 476–77

H

Hallux rigidus deformities
  differential diagnosis
    hallux valgus deformities, 563–64
  sesamoid bones and, 578
Hallux valgus angle, 568
Hallux valgus deformities, **570–72**
  differential diagnosis
    hallux rigidus deformities, 563–65
    hammertoes, 563
    systemic lupus erythematosus, 566
    traumatic dislocations, 566–67
  distal metatarsal articular angle, 569–70,
    572
  incongruent joint and, 572
  second-digit crossover toe and, 582
  sesamoid bones and, 578–79
  surgical correction, 572, **576–78**
Hallux valgus interphalangeal angle, 568
Hamartomas. *See* Compound odontomas
Hammertoes, **580–82**
  differential diagnosis
    hallux valgus deformities, 563
Hands
  osteoblastomas, 187
Hand-Schüller-Christian disease, 594–95,
    665–66
Harrington fixation system, 460, **463–64**,
    465–66
  loss of lumbar lordosis and, 470
Heart disease. *See* Cardiac anomalies; Congenital heart disease
Heavy-chain disease, 778
Heavy metal poisoning
  differential diagnosis
    sclerotic bones, 132

Heel. *See* Calcaneus
Hemangioendotheliomas
  patellar, 390
Hemangiomas
  cavernous
    differential diagnosis
      ganglion cysts, 351–52
  differential diagnosis
    Langerhans cell histiocytosis, 672
    muscle tears, 433–36
Hemangiomas of bone
  capillary type, 253
  cavernous type, 253
  "honeycomb" or "soap bubble" appearance, 251
  intracortical
    differential diagnosis
      Brodie's abscesses, 253
      fibrous dysplasia, 253
      ossifying fibromas, 253
      osteoid osteomas, 253
  multiple
    differential diagnosis
      congenital multiple fibromatosis,
        251–53
  periosteal, 253
Hemangiomas of the extremities, 359
  differential diagnosis
    arteriovenous malformations, 360, 363
    venous malformations, 363
  synovial, 366
Hemangiomas of the patella, 390
Hemarthrosis
  hemophilia and, 721
Hematomas
  hemophilia and, 726
Hemichondrodiatasis, 477
Hemochromatosis, 539, 767
Hemodialysis
  secondary amyloidosis and, 774
Hemophilia, 721–22, 725–26
  associated forms of arthritis, 719–21
  differential diagnosis
    gout, 701–2
    HIV arthropathy, 703
    pigmented villonodular synovitis, 702
    rheumatoid arthritis, 701
  elbow joint involvement, 708
  hemorrhage, 725–26
  radiographic features, 711
Hemophilic arthropathy
  differential diagnosis
    juvenile chronic arthropathy, 726
    neuropathic arthropathy, 536
Hemosiderin deposits
  pigmented villonodular synovitis, 704–5,
    777
Hereditary sensory motor neuropathy, 446

Infections *(cont'd)*
  intravenous drug use and, 166
  osseous
    differential diagnosis
      developmental dysplasia of the hip, 736–37
    osteochondritis dissecans, 375
    pin tract, 485–86, 488
    postoperative
      differential diagnosis
        failed back syndrome, 451
    sesamoid bone involvement, 578
Inflammatory arthritis
  elbow arthropathy, 708
Intermetatarsus angle, 568–69
Internal derangement, 613
Internal disk derangement. *See* Diskogenic pain
Internal disk disruption. *See* Diskogenic pain
Intestinal polyposis
  Gardner's syndrome, 592
Intra-articular calcification, and
  steroid therapy, 148
  tuberculosis, 148
Intraoral dental radiograph, 610, 613, 616
Intraosseous lipomas
  differential diagnosis
    calcaneal pseudocysts, 59, 61
Intravenous drug use
  fungal infections, 632, 646
  septic arthritis, 163, 165–66
Ischemic necrosis
  developmental dysplasia of the hip and, 761, 763
  of the medial end of the clavicle
    differential diagnosis
      osteitis condensans of the clavicle, 159
Isotretinoin
  hyperostosis and, 145
Itraconazole, 644

J

Jamshidi biopsy needles, 236
Jaw. *See also* Mandible
  Langerhans cell histiocytosis
    differential diagnosis
      periodontal disease, 661
  osseous portion lesions, **589, 591–95**
  osteolytic odontogenic lesions, **603–7**
  osteosclerotic odontogenic lesions, **596–99, 601, 603**
Joint involvement
  articular and periarticular amyloidosis, 776

Joint involvement *(cont'd)*
  HIV-associated arthritis, 720–21
Joint malalignment
  Ilizarov procedure complication, 489, 494
Joint space narrowing
  hemophilia, 722
  hemophilic arthropathy, 726
  juvenile rheumatoid arthropathy, 726
  pigmented villonodular synovitis, 702, 704
  Reiter's syndrome, 545
  rheumatoid arthritis, 701
Joint tuberculosis, **770–74**
Jumper's knee, 292
Juvenile arthritis
  chronic, 701, 708, 711
Juvenile chronic arthropathy, 726
Juvenile fibromatosis, **261, 263–64**, 266

K

Keratoderma blennorrhagica
  Reiter's syndrome, 543
Ketoconazole, 644
Kienböck's disease
  differential diagnosis
    ulnolunate impaction syndrome, 677, 679
  magnetic resonance imaging of the wrist, 686
  ulnar variance and, 696
Klebsiella, 166
Klippel-Trenaunay-Weber syndrome, 365
Knee. *See also* Patella
  CPPD arthropathy, 541
  ganglion cysts, 351
  meniscal cysts, 356–57
  pigmented villonodular synovitis, 704
  pyrophosphate arthropathy, 540
  Reiter's syndrome, 544–45
  synovial cysts, 355–56
Knee injuries
  anterior cruciate ligament, 271, 299, 301–2, 304, 308, 403, 407
  bone marrow contusions, 271, 273, **305–8**
    anterior cruciate ligament tears and, 302, 304
  lateral collateral ligament, 276, 278, 296, 401, 403
  ligaments, **296–97, 299, 301–2, 304**
  lipohemarthrosis, 273–74
  medial collateral ligament, 278, 296–97, 400
  meniscus
    bicondylar type fractures, 400
    MR appearance, 274, 276, **279–82, 284, 286–89, 291**

Magnetic resonance imaging
  aneurysmal bone cysts, 174–75
  angiovenous dysplasias, 363–65
  ankle tendons, 503–5
    abnormalities, **505–10, 512–14**
    "magic angle" phenomenon, 507
  biopsy guidance, 235
  bone marrow, 3–5, **28–31, 33–38**
    distribution patterns, **14, 16–19, 21–23**
  carpal fractures, 688
  chemical shift techniques, 26
  chondroblastomas, 192, 194
  chondrocalcinosis, 695
  chondromalacia patellae, 383–85, 387
  cysts of the knee, 357
  deQuervain's tenosynovitis, 693–94
  developmental dysplasia of the hip, 756–58
    hourglass capsule, 757
    inverted limbus, 757–58
  eosinophilic granulomas of bone, 664–65
  Ewing's sarcoma of the femur, 205–7
  fast-acquisition spin-echo imaging, 34–37
  fat-fraction images, 26
  fat suppression, 37–38
  fibromatosis, 261, 263
  fibrous dysplasia, 257
  fibroxanthomas, 189
  gadolinium enhancement of the spine, 41
  ganglion cysts, 351
  glenoid labrum, 120, 124
  gradient-recalled-echo imaging, 29–31
  impingement syndrome of the shoulder, 113–14
  knee injuries, 271, 273–74, 276, 278
    meniscus, **279–82, 284, 286–89, 291**
  Legg-Calvé-Perthes disease, 736
  leukemic bone marrow, **23–27**
  medullary bone infarcts, 3–5, 6
  muscles, **443–45**
  muscle tears, 429, 436–39
  myxomas, 255–56
  neurofibromatosis type 1, 250
  neuromuscular disorders, 446–47
  nonosseous abnormalities, 689
  osseous hemophilic pseudotumors, 725
  osteoblastomas, 187–88
  osteochondritis dissecans, 379–80
  osteochondromas, 198
  osteoid osteomas, 196–98
  osteosarcomas, 200
  rhabdomyosarcomas, 441–43
  scapholunate ligament tears, 680–81
  shoulder, 105, 107
  soft tissue hemangiomas, 434–36
  soft tissue hemophilic pseudotumors, 725

Magnetic resonance imaging *(cont'd)*
  spin-echo technique, 28–38
  STIR imaging, 10–11, 13–14, 33–34
  synovial chondromatosis, 742, 744
  synovial hypertrophy, 722
  transient osteoporosis of the hip, 745, 747
  tumor staging
    cortical bone involvement, 216, 218
    CT comparison, 209, 225–27
    distinguishing marrow edema from tumor infiltration of marrow, 212, 215
    extent of marrow involvement, 211–12
    extent of tumor, 228
    hemorrhage signal intensity, 210–11
    joint involvement, 225–26
    lymph node involvement, 228
    neurovascular involvement, 227–28
    periosteal reaction, 219, 222–25
    physeal and/or epiphyseal involvement, 215–16
    soft tissue mass and edema, 226–27
    typical protocol, 209–10
  water-fraction images, 26
  wrist, 683, **685–86, 688–89, 691–95**
Malocclusion, 614
Mandible. *See also* Jaw
  Langerhans cell histiocytosis, 670–71
  plasma cell myeloma, 778
  radiation therapy-induced osteonecrosis, 142–43
Mandibular trauma, **608, 610, 612–14**
Manubrosternal articulation
  sternocostoclavicular hyperostosis and, 155
Marfan's syndrome
  cardiac anomalies combined with, 79–82
  differential diagnosis
    homocystinuria, 82
Mastocytosis, **317–18, 320–22**
  differential diagnosis
    hypophosphatasia, 314
Maxilla. *See* Jaw
Medullary thyroid carcinoma
  neurofibromatosis type 1 and, 249
Melanomas
  neurofibromatosis type 1 and, 248–49
Membranous bone formation, 487
Meningomyeloceles, 554
Meniscal cysts
  differential diagnosis
    ganglion cysts, 352
Metastases
  ameloblastomas, 607
  differential diagnosis
    osteitis condensans of the clavicle, 159
  skeletal, 440–41

Metatarsus adductus, 570
Methylmethacrylate, 485
Miconazole, 644
Midfoot fractures, **549, 551–52**. *See also* Foot
Mitochondrial myopathy, 432, 446
Mixed hemangiomas, 433
Moore and Hohl's classification of tibial plateau fractures, 398–400
Mortality rates
    Ellis-van Creveld syndrome, 95
    hypophosphatasia, 331–32, 333
    Langerhans cell histiocytosis, 666, 668
    mycetoma, 642
MRI. *See* Magnetic resonance imaging
Mucoepidermoid carcinoma, 604
Multiple myeloma. *See* Plasma cell myeloma
Muscle contracture
    Ilizarov procedure complication, 488
Muscles, **443–45**. *See also* Muscle tears
Muscle tears, **429, 436–39**
    differential diagnosis
        hemangiomas, 433–36
        muscular dystrophy, 431–32
        plexiform neurofibromas, 432–33
        rhabdomyosarcomas, 429, 431
Muscular dystrophy, 445
    differential diagnosis
        muscle tears, 431–32
Musculoskeletal amyloidosis, **774–77**
Musculoskeletal tuberculosis. *See* Joint tuberculosis
Mycetoma, **638–40, 642**
    grain or granule appearance, 638, 642
    treatment, 644
Myonecrosis, 444, 445, 446
Myositis
    "hair-on-end" periosteal reaction, 223
Myxomas
    fibrous dysplasia and, 255–56

N

Navicular bone fractures, 533, 549, 551–52
Neer classification for proximal humeral fractures, 54
Neonates. *See* Infants
Nephropathies
    heredofamilial amyloidosis and, 774
Neuroblastomas, 440
    differential diagnosis
        Langerhans cell histiocytosis, 672
    metastatic
        differential diagnosis
            congenital multiple fibromatosis, 244
    neurofibromatosis type 1 and, 248
Neurofibromas, 246

Neurofibromatosis type 1
    bone lesion pathophysiology, 245–49
    coarctation of the aorta and, 69
    diagnostic criteria, 245
    differential diagnosis
        congenital multiple fibromatosis, 245–50
    imaging characteristics, 249–50
Neurilemmomas, 246–48
Neurologic injury
    Ilizarov procedure complication, 488
Neuropathic arthropathy
    atrophic form, 556
    diabetic, 556
    differential diagnosis
        calcium pyrophosphate arthropathy, 535
        hemophilic arthropathy, 536
        Reiter's arthropathy, 535–36
        septic arthropathy, 534
    etiology, 553
    hypertrophic form, 555–56
    microscopic features, 555
    pathophysiology, 553–54
    related disorders, 554–55
    syphilitic neuropathic arthropathy, 556–57
    syringomyelia and, 558
Neuropathic joint disease, 708
Neuropathies
    heredofamilial amyloidosis and, 774
Neutral-ulnar variance, 695
Nocardia, 633–34
Nocardia brasiliensis, 642
Non-Hodgkin's lymphoma
    bone marrow involvement, 13–14
Nonossifying fibromas. *See* Fibroxanthomas
Nonsteroidal anti-inflammatory drugs
    hallux rigidus deformities, 565
    tendon injuries, 512
Noxious agents
    withdrawal of
        osteopetrosis skeletal pattern change and, 137
Nutcracker fractures, 549, 551

O

Occult complete fractures, 305
Occult linear fractures, 689
Occupational factors
    impingement syndrome of the shoulder, 111
    osteitis condensans of the clavicle, 159
    tendon injuries, 520
OCD. *See also* Osteochondritis dissecans

Ocular manifestations
Reiter's syndrome, 543
O'Donahue's triad of knee injuries, 297
Odontogenic cysts. *See also* Osteolytic odon-
togenic lesions of the jaw
keratocysts, 605–6
Odontomas. *See also* Compound odontomas
complex, 597
Olecranon bursitis, 711
Oncogenous osteomalacia, 343–44
1,25-dihydroxyvitamin D_3, 137, 329
Osgood-Schlatter disease, 292
Osseous anomalies
congenital heart disease and, 83
Osseous infections
differential diagnosis
osteomyelitis, 736–37
Osseous lesions of the jaw, **589, 591–95**
Osseous pressure erosions
pigmented villonodular synovitis, 702
Ossifying fibromas
differential diagnosis
compound odontoma, 587
intracortical hemangiomas of bone, 253
well-differentiated osteosarcomas, 184
Osteitis condensans of the clavicle, **158–59**
differential diagnosis
bone island, 159
fibrous dysplasia, 159
infection, 159
ischemic necrosis of the medial end of
the clavicle, 159
metastasis, 159
osteoarthritis of the sternoclavicular
joint, 159
osteoid osteomas, 159
osteomyelitis, 151
osteosarcomas, 153, 159
Paget's disease, 151, 153
sternocostoclavicular   hyperostosis,
151, 157–58, 159
Osteoarthritis
anterior femoral pressure erosions, 541
condylar head fractures, 612–13
developmental dysplasia of the hip and,
738, 740, 748–49
differential diagnosis
osteitis condensans of the clavicle, 159
pyrophosphate arthropathy and, 539–40
synovial chondromatosis and, 744
Osteoarthropathy
diabetic, 556
Osteoblastomas, **184–88**
differential diagnosis
osteoid osteomas, 184–85
well-differentiated osteosarcomas, 170,
172
patellar, 390

Osteocartilaginous   exosstosis.   *See*   Osteochondromas
Osteochondral fractures, 305
Osteochondritis dissecans, **375–76, 378–80,**
656
Osteochondritis dissecans of the patella. *See*
Patella
Osteochondromas, **198**
patellar, 390
Osteogenesis imperfecta tarda
differential diagnosis
hypophosphatasia, 314
Osteoid osteomas, **195–98**
differential diagnosis
eosinophilic granuloma of bone, 665
intracortical hemangiomas of bone, 253
Langerhans cell histiocytosis, 672
osteitis condensans of the clavicle, 159
osteoblastomas, 185
osteochondritis dissecans of the patella, 374
of the elbow, 196
radiographic appearance, 195
Osteolytic metastases
comparison to plasma cell myeloma, 778
Osteolytic odontogenic lesions of the jaw,
603–7
Osteomalacia, **342–48**
aluminum intoxication and, 147
antacids and, 147
differential diagnosis
osteoporosis, 342
phenytoin and, 145, 147
sodium fluoride and, 147
Thorotrast and, 147
X-linked hypophosphatemia and, 322,
323
Osteomas. *See also* Gardner's syndrome; Osteoid osteomas
endosteal, 592
periosteal, 592
Osteomyelitis. *See also* Fungal osteomyelitis
AIDS and, 773
chronic focal sclerosing, 596
differential diagnosis
eosinophilic granuloma of bone, 665
Langerhans cell histiocytosis, 672
osseous infection, 736–37
osteitis condensans of the clavicle, 151
sternoclavicular joint septic arthritis,
166
Ilizarov procedure complication, 484, 486,
488
osteopetrosis and, 138
sclerotic bone, 484
tuberculous, 771, 773–74

Patella *(cont'd)*
    differential diagnosis
        bipartite patella, 371–72
        chondromalacia patellae, 372
        dorsal defect of the patella, 372, 374
        osteoid osteomas, 374
    primary tumors, 390
Patellar plicae, 387–89
Patent ductus arteriosus
    cerebrohepatorenal syndrome and, 69
    chondrodysplasia punctata and, 69
    congenital rubella syndrome and, 69
    differential diagnosis
        septal defect, 68–69
    Down's syndrome and, 69
    radial ray disorders and, 91
    Rubenstein-Taybi syndrome and, 69
    trisomy 13 and, 69
    trisomy 18 and, 69
PDA. *See* Patent ductus arteriosus
Pedicles. *See also* Transpedicular screw fixation system
    plasma cell myeloma, 778, 780
Periapical cemental dysplasia, 598–99
Perinatal hypophosphatasia, 331–32
Periodontal disease, **615–16, 618**
Periosteal new bone, 479, 484
Periosteal reactions
    complex, 222, 223–24
    continuous, 219, 222
    description, 219
    "hair-on-end," 222, 223
    interrupted, 222, 223
    Langerhans cell histiocytosis, 669–70
    MR features, 224–25
    "onion skin," 205
        chondroblastomas, 192
    single lamellar, 222, 223
    "sunburst," 222, 224
Periosteum
    radiation therapy effect, 139
Periostitis, 703
    prostaglandin E$_1$ and, 147–48
Peripheral arthritis. *See* Reiter's syndrome
Peroneus brevis tendon, 519, 529
Peroneus longus tendon, 529
Phenytoin
    osteomalacia and, 145, 147
Pheochromocytomas
    neurofibromatosis type 1 and, 248
Phleboliths, and
    angiovenous dysplasias, 359
    Maffucci's syndrome, 366
Phosphate
    hypophosphatasia, 331, 339
    osteomalacia and, 342–43, 347–48
    X-linked hypophosphatemia and, 322, 329

Phosphorus poisoning, 132
Physical therapy
    tibial plateau fractures, 407
Pigmented villonodular synovitis, **704–5**
    differential diagnosis
        fungal osteomyelitis, 626
        hemophilia, 702
    similarity to amyloidosis, 777
Pin tract infection
    Ilizarov procedure complication, 485–86, 488
Plantar arch, 533
Plantar keratoses, 606
Plantar stress injury, 551
Plasma cell dyscrasias, 777–78
Plasma cell myeloma, 767, 775, **777–78, 780, 783**
    musculoskeletal amyloidosis and, 774
Plasmacytoma, 783
Plexiform neurofibromas. *See also* Neurofibromatosis type 1
    differential diagnosis
        muscle tears, 432–33
Plica syndrome, 389
POEMS syndrome
    plasma cell myeloma and, 780, 783
Poliomyelitis, 447
"Polka dot" spine, 41–42
Polydactyly, 98
    classification, 86
    Ellis-van Creveld syndrome, 67
Polymyositis, 445
Polysyndactyly, 87
Popliteal cysts. *See* Baker's cysts
Posterior tibial tendon, 503, 516
Posttraumatic clavicular sclerosis. *See* Osteitis condensans of the clavicle
Pregnancy
    deQuervain's tenosynovitis and, 694
    fibrous dysplasia reactivation, 257
Premature consolidation
    Ilizarov procedure complication, 490
Premature epiphyseal closure
    retinoids and, 145
Premature sternal fusion
    congenital heart disease and, 84
Prevalence
    bipartite patella, 371
    dorsal defect of the patella, 372, 374
    patellar plicae, 388
Prostaglandin E$_1$
    periostitis and, 147–48
Pseudarthrosis, 467–68, **470**
Pseudocysts
    calcaneal
        differential diagnosis
            chondroblastomas, 59, 61
            chondromyxoid fibromas, 59, 61
            enchondromas, 59, 61

Sarcomas. *See also* Chondrosarcomas;
    Ewing's sarcoma; Osteosarcomas;
    Rhabdomyosarcomas
  radiation therapy-induced, 143–44
Scapholunate collapse, 540–41
Scapholunate ligament tear
  differential diagnosis
    ulnolunate impaction syndrome, 681–
      82
Schatzker's classification of tibial plateau
      fractures, 400–402
Schwannomas, 246–48
Sclerotic bones. *See* Osteosclerosis
Scoliosis, 466–67, 470, 557
  congenital heart disease and, 84–85
  osteoid osteomas, 195
  radiation therapy-induced, 139–40
Segmental spine instability
  diagnosis, 459–60
  differential diagnosis
    failed back syndrome, 452, 455
Sensorimotor polyneuropathy, 780
Septal defects
  differential diagnosis
    coarctation of the aorta, 69
    patent ductus arteriosus, 68–69
    peripheral pulmonic stenosis, 68
    tetralogy of Fallot, 67–68
  radial ray disorders and, 91
Septic arthropathy
  differential diagnosis
    neuropathic arthropathy, 534
Sequestration, 484
Seronegative arthropathy, 703
Seronegative spondyloarthropathies, 711
Serratia, 166
Sesamoid bones of the great toe, **578–79**
Sexually acquired reactive arthritis. *See* Re-
    iter's syndrome
Shoes. *See* Footwear
Shoulder. *See also* Rotator cuff
  abnormalities, 105, 107–10
  dislocations
    tuberosity fractures and, 54
  glenohumeral joint stability, **117, 119–20,
    124–25**
  impingement syndrome, 105, **111–15**
Sickle-cell anemia, 11
  bone marrow changes, 5, 7–8, 9, 44
  differential diagnosis
    chronic medullary bone infarct, 3
    epiphyseal osteonecrosis and, 656
    medullary infarcts and, 44, 656
Skeletal anomalies
  cardiac anomalies combined with, 67, **70–
    73, 76–82**
Skeletal maturation
  congenital heart disease and, 84

Skin cysts
  Gardner's syndrome, 592
Skull
  bone marrow characteristics, 40–41
  bone marrow conversion, 19
  Langerhans cell histiocytosis, 669–70
    differential diagnosis
      epidermoid cysts, 672
      hemangiomas, 672
      otitis media, 661
      parietal foramen, 672
      venous lake, 672
  osteoblastomas, 186
  parietal foramen
    differential diagnosis
      Langerhans cell histiocytosis, 672
  plasma cell myeloma, 778
  venous lake
    differential diagnosis
      Langerhans cell histiocytosis, 672
Smith fractures, 680
Smoking
  regenerate bone production and, 487
Sodium fluoride
  osteomalacia and, 147
Soft tissue hemangiomas, 433–36
Solitary bone cysts
  patellar, 390
Solitary myeloma, 783
South American blastomycosis, 646
Spherocytosis
  bone marrow changes, 44
Spina bifida
  radial ray disorders and, 91–92
Spinal arthropathy, 557
Spinal fusion
  failed back syndrome, 458–60
  fixation rod fracture, 467–68
  fixation systems, 460, 462–68, 470
  pseudarthrosis, 467–68, **470**
Spine
  bone marrow changes, 9–10, 41–42
  bone marrow conversion, 22–23
  compression injuries
    calcaneal fractures and, 414
  fibrous dysplasia involvement, 257–58
  gadolinium enhancement, 41
  Langerhans cell histiocytosis, 671
  osteoblastomas, 186
  "polka dot" spine, 41–42
  radiation therapy effect, 139
  "soap bubble" appearance of actinomy-
    cotic infection, 638
  syphilitic neuropathic arthropathy, 557
Splay foot, 570
Spondyloarthropathy
  sternocostoclavicular hyperostosis and,
    155

Synovial joints
Reiter's syndrome, 544
Synovitis
inflammatory, 535, 721
Synovium-lined joints
pigmented villonodular synovitis, 704
Syphilis
"hair-on-end" periosteal reaction, 223
Syphilitic neuropathic arthropathy, 554, 556–57
Syringomyelia
neuropathic arthropathy, 554, 558
neuropathic joints, 708
Systemic lupus erythematosus
differential diagnosis
hallux valgus deformities, 566
Systemic mastocytosis
bone changes, 320–21
description, 317–18
differential diagnosis
diffuse osteopenia, 318
mineralization pattern, 321
radiographic appearance, 318
treatment, 322

T

Tailor's bunions, 582–83
Talonavicular joints
CPPD arthropathy, 541
TAR syndrome. *See* Thrombocytopenia-absent radius syndrome
Teeth. *See also* Compound odontomas; Jaw; Mandible; Osseous lesions of the jaw
Bennett classification of tooth fractures, 610
extraction, 603
fungal infections and, 633
hypophosphatasia, 334
mandibular trauma and, 608, 610, 612–14
osteolytic odontogenic lesions of the jaw, 603–7
osteosclerotic odontogenic lesions of the jaw, 596–99, 601, 603
periodontal disease, 615–16, 618
X-linked hypophosphatemia, 328–29
Tendinitis, 503, 510, 512
Tendon degeneration, 512, 513–14
Tendon ruptures, 512
Tendon sheaths
ankle, 508–9
pigmented villonodular synovitis, 704
Tendon tears, 512
Tennis elbow, 711–12
Tenosynovitis, 503, 509–10
Tension-stress concept, 475, 477
Teratogenic hip. *See* Hip, developmental dysplasia

Tetralogy of Fallot
differential diagnosis
septal defect, 67–68
Down's syndrome and, 68
Thalassemia
bone marrow changes, 44
periosteal reaction, 223
Thalidomide embryopathy
radial ray disorders and, 92
Thorotrast
osteomalacia and, 147
Thrombocytopenia-absent radius syndrome
radial ray disorders and, 92
Tibia
bone marrow changes, 42
Tibialis anterior tendon, 519
Tibial plateau fractures
angular deformity of the leg following reduction, 406–7
anterior cruciate ligament tears, 403
distal fibula involvement, 402
early motion treatment, 402, 407
knee instability and, 402, 407
lateral collateral ligament rupture and, 398
malunion, 405
mechanism, 397–98
meniscal tears, 404–5
Moore and Hohl's classification, 398–400
nonunion, 405
open, 408
peroneal nerve palsy, 403
Schatzker's classification, 400–402
treatment, 406–8
Tissue transplantation
osteopetrosis skeletal pattern change and, 137–38
Tophaceous CPPD crystal deposition, 541, 543
Trabeculae
fibrous dysplasia, 591
longitudinally oriented, 479, 487
osteitis condensans of the clavicle, 159
Transpedicular screw fixation system, 460, 462
categories, 465
stable short-segment fixation, 464
Trauma. *See also* Barotrauma
bipartite patella, 372
bone marrow contusions, 305–8
deQuervain's tenosynovitis, 693–94
differential diagnosis
Langerhans cell histiocytosis, 672
elbow, 708
epiphyseal osteonecrosis and, 656
knee injuries, 271
mandibular, **608, 610, 612–14**
muscle tears, 436, 445, 446
second-digit crossover toe and, 582
sesamoid bone involvement, 578

Trauma *(cont'd)*
  subluxation of the distal radioulnar joint, 680–81
  tendon subluxation or dislocation, 514
  tendon tears, 512
  tuberosity fractures, 54–55
Trephine biopsy needles, 236–37
Triangular fibrocartilage tears, 683
  magnetic resonance imaging, 689, 691–93, 695
  ulnar variance and, 696–97
Trisomy 13
  patent ductus arteriosus and, 69
Trisomy 18
  patent ductus arteriosus and, 69
Trisomy 21. *See* Down's syndrome
Tuberculosis. *See also* Joint tuberculosis; *M. tuberculosis hominis*
  groups at risk, 773
  intra-articular calcification and, 148
Tuberculous arthritis, 767
Tuberculous arthropathy, 771
Tuberculous osteomyelitis, 771
Tuberosity fractures
  calcaneal, 421
  differential diagnosis
    calcific peritendinitis of the rotator cuff, 55
    chondroblastomas, 51–52
    giant cell tumors, 51–52
    Hill-Sachs deformity, 52–53
    humeral pseudocysts, 52
  trauma and, 54–55
  treatment, 55–56
Tumor staging, 209–28
Turf toe, 563
Turkel biopsy needles, 236
Turner's syndrome
  cardiac anomalies combined with, 72–73, 76
  coarctation of the aorta and, 69
  Madelung deformity and, 91
  osteopenia and, 83

U

Ulcers
  oral mucosal and tongue, 543
Ulna
  pseudocysts, 62
Ulnar-minus variance, 695–96
  differential diagnosis
    ulnolunate impaction syndrome, 677
Ulnar-plus variance, 677, 695–97
Ulnar variance, **695–97**
Ulnolunate impaction syndrome
  differential diagnosis
    Kienböck's disease, 677–79
    scapholunate ligament tear, 681–82

Ulnolunate impaction syndrome *(cont'd)*
  subluxation of the distal radioulnar joint, 680–81
  ulnar-minus variance, 677
  ulnar variance and, 697
Ultrasonography
  developmental dysplasia of the hip, 751–56
  modified Barlow maneuver, 752, 755–56
  muscles, 444, 445
  new bone formation, 479
  pseudotumors, 725
  soft tissue hemophilic pseudotumors, 725
Upper extremity musculoskeletal anomalies, **86–87, 89, 91–92, 94**
Urethritis, 543

V

Vascular damage
  Ilizarov procedure complication, 489–90
Vascular occlusive disease
  epiphyseal osteonecrosis and, 656
VATER association
  radial ray disorders and, 92, 94
Venous malformations
  differential diagnosis
    hemangiomas of the extremities, 363
Vertebrae. *See* Spine
Vitamin D. *See also* Hypervitaminosis A and D
  osteomalacia, 342–43, 347
  X-linked hypophosphatemia, 322
Vitamin D-resistant rickets. *See* X-linked hypophosphatemia

W

Waldenström's macroglobulinemia, 778
Wilms' tumors
  neurofibromatosis type 1 and, 249
  radiation therapy-induced scoliosis, 139
Wrist. *See also* Ulnolunate impaction syndrome
  magnetic resonance imaging, 683, **685–86, 688–89, 691–95**
  pyrophosphate arthropathy, 540

X–Z

Xanthoma
  pigmented villonodular synovitis, 704
XLH. *See* X-linked hypophosphatemia
X-linked Duchenne muscular dystrophy, 432, 446
X-linked hypophosphatemia, **322–24, 326, 328–29**
X-linked hypophosphatemia *(cont'd)*
  differential diagnosis
    hypophosphatasia, 314–15